Diseases of Bones
and Joints

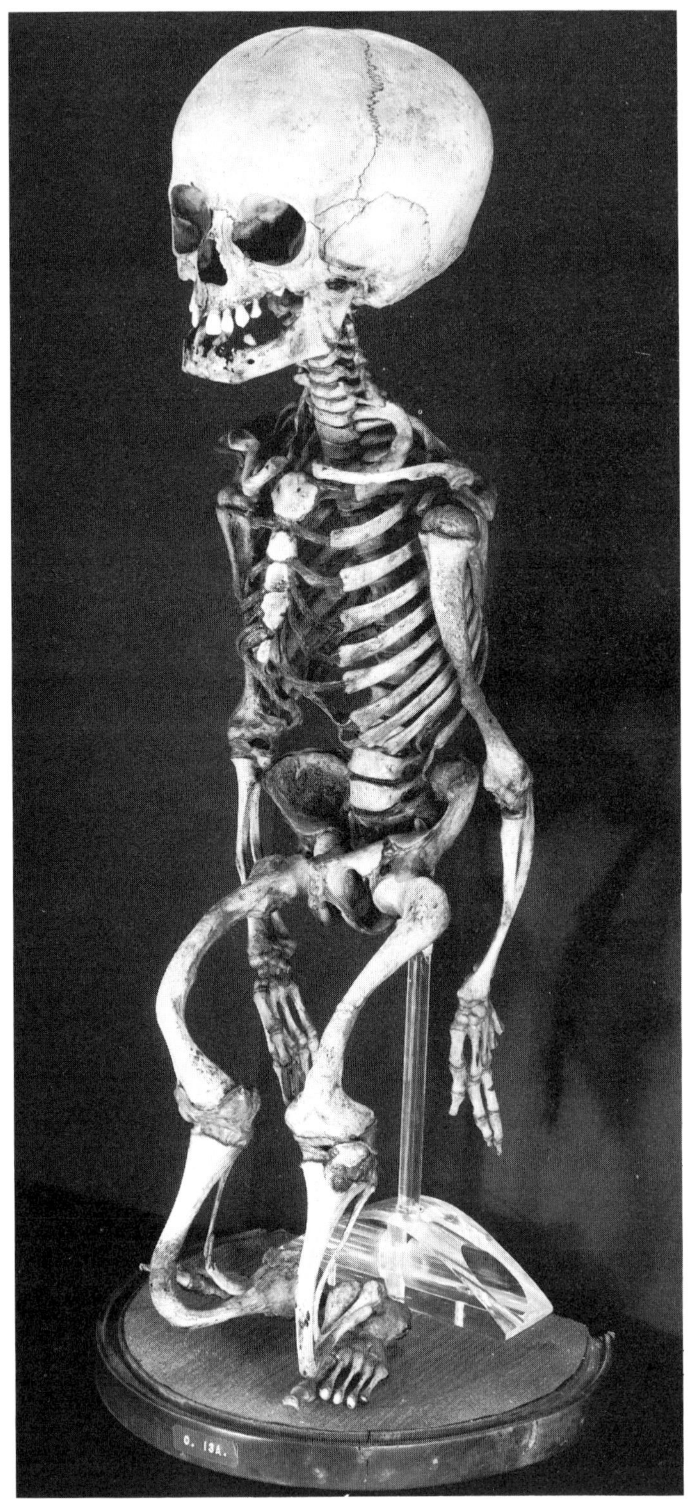

Frontispiece: This skeleton, in spite of the features suggestive of severe rickets, is an example of osteogenesis imperfecta. In this skeleton, bending of the limbs is severe but there are few fractures. The tri-radiate pelvis is also a well recognized feature of osteogenesis imperfecta. The specimen formed part of Lord Lister's collection and came from the old King's College Hospital in Portugal Street.

Diseases of Bones and Joints

Edited by

Jonathan R. Salisbury BSc, MD, MRCPath

Senior Lecturer in Histopathology
King's College School of Medicine and Dentistry
London
UK

Colin G. Woods BSc, MB, ChB, FRCPath

Honorary Consulting Pathologist
Nuffield Orthopaedic Centre
Oxford
UK

and

Paul D. Byers BSc, MD, CM, DCM, FRCPath

Reader Emeritus
Institute of Orthopaedics
University of London
UK

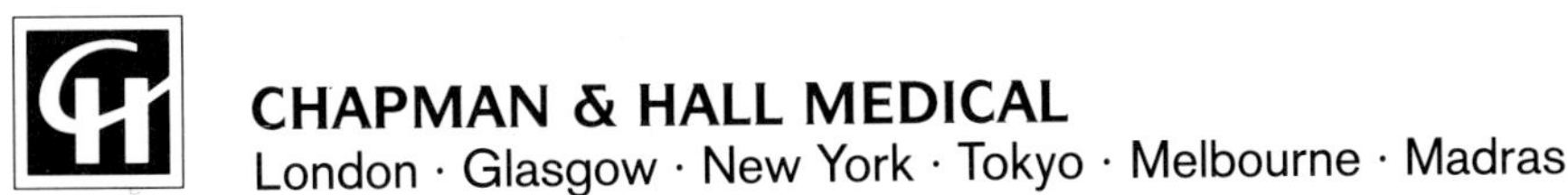

CHAPMAN & HALL MEDICAL
London · Glasgow · New York · Tokyo · Melbourne · Madras

Published by Chapman & Hall, 2–6 Boundary Row, London SE1 8HN

Chapman & Hall, 2–6 Boundary Row, London SE1 8HN, UK

Blackie Academic & Professional, Wester Cleddens Road, Bishopbriggs, Glasgow G64 2NZ, UK

Chapman & Hall Inc., One Penn Plaza, 41st Street, New York, NY10119, USA

Chapman & Hall Japan, Thomson Publishing Japan, Hirakawacho Nemoto Building, 6F, 1-7-11 Hirakawa-cho, Chiyoda-ku, Tokyo 102, Japan

Chapman & Hall Australia, Thomas Nelson Australia, 102 Dodds Street, South Melbourne, Victoria 3205, Australia

Chapman & Hall India, R. Seshadri, 32 Second Main Road, CIT East, Madras 600 035, India

First edition 1994

© 1994 Chapman & Hall

Typeset in 10/12 Palatino by Falcon Graphic Art, Wallington, Surrey

Printed in Great Britain at Cambridge University Press, Cambridge

ISBN 0 412 48010 7

A catalogue record for this book is available from the British Library

Library of Congress Cataloging-in-Publication data available

CONTENTS

CONTRIBUTORS

Paul D. Byers
18 Wimpole Street
London
W1M 7AD

Alan J. Darby
Department of Pathology
Robert Jones & Agnes Hunt
Orthopaedic Hospital
Oswestry
Shropshire
SY10 7AG

Anthony J. Freemont
Department of Pathological Sciences
University of Manchester
Oxford Road
Manchester
M13 9PT

Jonathan R. Salisbury
Department of Histopathology
King's College School of Medicine
Denmark Hill
London
SE5 8RX

Dennis J. Stoker
Department of Radiology
Royal National Orthopaedic Hospital
45–51 Bolsover Street
London
W1P 8AQ

Colin G. Woods
Department of Pathology
Nuffield Orthopaedic Centre
Oxford

FOREWORD

Diseases of Bones and Joints, reflecting the vast experience of the authors, provides a complete discussion of the complex field of pathology of the skeletal system and the joints. Unique in its total coverage, the book begins with a guide to the analysis of tissue submitted for appraisal, after which the authors present a valuable checklist indicating the many entities to be considered when a diagnostic problem is encountered.

The scope of *Diseases of Bones and Joints* is immense with its consideration of imaging procedures by an internationally known authority in the field. Most of the discussion of imaging concerns ordinary X-rays, but the roles of special studies, including ultrasonography, computed tomography, bone scintigraphy, and magnetic resonance imaging are not neglected. The necessity of correlating those images with the histopathologic diagnosis is emphasized. The book then deals with the pathological entities, beginning with congenital and developmental abnormalities and continuing with injuries, inflammation, arthritis, circulatory disorders, and metabolic conditions. A large and important section discusses neoplasia and includes non-neoplastic lesions that may mimic bone tumours.

The section on congenital and developmental anomalies details this complicated field and indicates the complexities of these problems. The wide variety of responses to injury is indicated, along with a recognition that the basic reparative processes have an overlapping similarity.

In the discussion of neoplasms of bone, the importance of staging as it relates to the assessment of results of treatment and 'the furtherance of therapeutic advance' is given an appropriately prominent place. The section on neoplasms is divided into two groups: osteoblastic and cartilaginous neoplasms and a miscellaneous group. This type of division is useful and readily separates neoplasms into two main categories based on the presence or absence of matrix or ground substance produced by the cells of the tumour. The non-neoplastic lesions that may mimic bone tumours are prominently discussed in a separate section.

Finally, the authors consider the cellular biology of bone, a knowledge of which is necessary to the understanding of advances in the field of lesions of the skeleton. In this section, they briefly discuss the handling of bone specimens, decalcification, and special stains.

Diseases of Bones and Joints, encompassing a total discussion of the many complex pathological entities, represents a landmark among medical works.

D.C. Dahlin MD
Emeritus Professor of Pathology
Mayo Clinic and Mayo Foundation
Rochester, Minnesota 55905

ACKNOWLEDGEMENTS

It is our pleasure to acknowledge the assistance of our clinical and radiological colleagues in all the different hospitals with which we are associated. The advice of Professor Peter Thorogood, Eastman Dental School, on aspects of skeletal embryology was greatly appreciated.

Some members of the staff of King's College School of Medicine and Dentistry deserve special thanks. Mr Ken Davies and Mr Ron Senkus were responsible for the production of the large majority of the photographic prints. Mr Barry Pike and Dr Mark Deverell gave help with the computer software. The Medical Laboratory Scientific Officers of the Department of Histopathology cut and stained many of the sections illustrated in this book, and Ms Christine Hogg and the staff of the School Library provided assistance on many occasions. To all of these, we extend our thanks.

The line drawings were skilfully executed by Mr Maurice Murphy. Mr Paul Cooper of the Photographic Department of the Nuffield Orthopaedic Centre provided assistance with a number of the photographs.

INTRODUCTION 1

Jonathan R. Salisbury and Paul D. Byers

The subject matter of this volume is the diagnostic histopathology and morbid anatomy of osteoarticular disease in man. Animal experimental pathology is included infrequently and only where its findings particularly illuminate some aspect of diagnostic pathology. The boundaries of osteoarticular disease are traditionally defined as (1) bone including the periosteum, (2) joint including the capsule, and (3) those structures, lying outside bone and joint, whose reactions become the concern of orthopaedic pathology. Examples would include tendons, tendon sheaths and retinacula and, in some circumstances, soft tissues.

The aim is to be a reference text of osteoarticular disease. The book is arranged in four parts. Part One provides an organized framework for making a pathological diagnosis. These chapters discuss the recognition and assessment of bone in the laboratory, its histopathological examination, and the radiological features of orthopaedic disease. Part One includes a diagnostic checklist, a schema based on histological tissue patterns, which provides a means of establishing, and reviewing, a given diagnosis. Whereas the expertise of histopathology has in it a large measure of building and maintaining a memory bank of the patterns presented by tissues in histological sections, the person who sees little of osteoarticular disease is, *a priori*, at a disadvantage. A book can do little to rectify that want of opportunity, but it can give guidance in the analysis of the patterns of those tissues and of the background against which they arise.

Parts Two and Three form the major diagnostic components of the book and discuss the individual disease processes and disease entities that constitute orthopaedic pathology. These descriptions of osteoarticular disease are segregated according to the underlying disease process:

- Congenital and developmental abnormalities
- Injury
- Inflammation
- Arthritides and related conditions
- Circulatory disorders
- Metabolic bone disease
- Bone tumours

Most osteoarticular diseases are readily classifiable, according to aetiology or pathogenesis, but some, such as osteoarthritis, are not. This book uses a conventional disease classification as a method of arranging and discussing the entities but some compromises have been made to accommodate all the entries. Those excluded joint entities can be found via the index.

Part Four discusses the cell biology of bone, and comprises chapters on the embryology of the skeleton, the histology of connective tissues, the growth, architecture and structure of bone, and the reactions of bone. Such material is often lacking from standard textbooks and its inclusion here is intended to provide a compendium of background information on basic bone biology.

The chapters on practical guidance in tissue handling and preparation, analysis and interpretation will be of particular interest to practising pathologists and trainee pathologists. It is our intention, however, that the bulk of the book, particularly Parts Two, Three and Four, should be valuable not just to pathologists but also to others desiring an understanding of orthopaedic pathology. It is our hope that it will prove of value to orthopaedic surgeons (particularly those in training), radiologists, metabolic physicians, rheumatologists and also to any involved in the diagnosis of skeletal dysplasias.

The understanding of disease processes, that is the sequence of events in organs or tissues that constitute disease, evolves with the growth of knowledge. What is now regarded as the traditional classification evolved with discoveries made with the aid of the light microscope. Increasingly, as was predicated by Virchow, cells and tissues, organs and the body, are being seen in terms of biochemical function. This growth in knowledge can be seen to have deepened and strengthened understanding of disease processes, and their classification has had to be adapted to the new knowledge. In any case there is no single rigid classification of disease processes that is correct. Our knowledge and understanding is based as much on conceptualization as it is on observation. It is very difficult to know objectively what we see; easier to know what we think we see. Thus, we tell stories about the world around us. A particular classification of disease processes is drawn from a particular story. It need not necessarily be in conflict with another; the two can run parallel to arrive at the same destination.

The classification of disease processes that served until recent times is:

- Congenital/developmental
- Traumatic
- Inflammatory
- Degenerative
- Circulatory

- Metabolic/nutritional/toxic
- Neoplastic

The advance of knowledge notwithstanding, most of the foregoing classification well serves a consideration of osteoarticular diseases. Some idea of their occurrence and relative importance can be gained from the contents of a textbook of orthopaedics aimed at budding practitioners, in which the hierarchical structure is likely to be determined by the nature of ordinary clinical practice. Such a book is Apley and Solomon's *Concise System of Orthopaedics, and Fractures* (1988).

Patients' complaints are one or more of pain, swelling, stiffness, disability or deformity referable to a locality or a region, which might be the body as a whole. The authors list the causes as follows:

- congenital and developmental
- infection and inflammation
- injury and mechanical derangement
- metabolic dysfunction and degeneration
- arthritis and rheumatic disorders
- sensory disturbance and muscle weakness
- tumours and imitators

Clearly these are very similar to the disease processes listed above, with the exception that circulatory disorders have not been mentioned, and two classes of disease have been singled out – arthritis and rheumatic disorders, sensory disturbance and muscle weakness – whose members can be allocated to disease categories.

The weakest unit is degeneration. The concept of degenerative processes is based on ideas from earlier times when theories of disease were often quite different, and tissue changes in the absence of a clear aetiology or pathogenesis were regarded as degenerations. In any case not many of the conditions listed above are relevant to osteoarticular disease.

The following is taken from Anderson and Scott's *Synopsis of Pathology* (1980) where the term retrogressive cellular changes and infiltration was used.

Atrophy
  General
  Local disuse, ischaemic, pressure, endocrine, idiopathic
Degeneration
  Cloudy swelling
  Hydropic degeneration
  Fatty metamorphosis
  Interstitial fatty infiltration
  Hyaline degeneration and extracellular hyaline
    Hyaline droplets
    Mallory bodies
    Councilman bodies
    Acidophilic bodies
    Crooke's hyaline change
    Russell bodies
    Zenker's waxy degeneration
  Amyloid
  Mucinous degeneration
  Disturbances of purine metabolism
  Disturbances of glycogen metabolism
Necrosis
  Coagulative
  Caseous
  Gummatous
  Liquefactive
  Fat
  Gangrene
Calcification
  Dystrophic
  Metastatic
  Calcinosis
Pigmentation
  Endogenous
    Melanin
    Haemoglobin
      Haemosiderosis
      Haemochromatosis
      Bilirubin/haematoidin
      Malarial pigment
    Porphyrins
    Lipochromes
    Aluminium
  Exogenous
    Silver
    Lead
    Carotene

The two important conditions that are often thought of as degenerative are the age-related alterations of cartilage leading to osteoarthritis, and the reduction in bone mass, osteopaenia, and the associated disease, osteoporosis. The bone mass problem can be found a home in metabolic disorders of bone on the basis that much knowledge has been gained in understanding how the changes in bone come about in many conditions. The nature of the deposition of aluminium in bone also makes it a candidate. But after some thirty or more years of intensive study the understanding of osteoarthritis seems as obscure as ever, and although the appellation degenerative joint disease comes easily to hand, it is considered in a chapter devoted to arthritides. And that chapter also accommodates gout, which provides the logic for placing calcium pyrophosphate deposition disease, and that in turn drags along other forms of calcification by association. This chapter also gives room to tendon and tendon sheath problems.

Despite the advances in knowledge, the gaps in it must be wide and deep. Working on the principle espoused here, that knowledge grows and the gaps are filled by conjecture and tests of its predictions, then such conjectures should be available to all. However, detailed stories are extremely rare, for on the whole scientists are very cautious about admitting to conjectures, and dismissive of them, whether their own or others, as mere speculations. But it adds very considerably to the interest of pathology if it is appreciated that, in the first place, many facts are currently accepted conjectures and concepts, and are liable to change when they are found inadequate, and in the second place, a new concept, extending beyond those in current use, alerts one to possibilities and new observations. Nevertheless, there is a danger for the practice of a discipline such as diagnostic histopathology, that one forsakes the accepted model for the allure and excitement of the new at a time before this has been tried, tested and found acceptable. To acquire the ability to recognize these distinctions is part of becoming expert, and not a reason for avoidance.

REFERENCES

Anderson, W.A.D. and Scott, T.M. (1980) *Synopsis of Pathology*. C.V. Mosby, St Louis, MO.

Apley, A.G. and Solomon, L. (1988) *Concise System of Orthopaedics and Fractures*. Butterworths, London.

PART ONE

Diagnosis

A GUIDE TO THE ANALYSIS OF TISSUE SUBMITTED FOR HISTOPATHOLOGICAL EXAMINATION

Jonathan R. Salisbury, Colin G. Woods and Paul D. Byers

2.1 THE RECOGNITION AND ASSESSMENT OF BONE

Although these stages are usually a continuous process, they can be better understood if considered separately.

2.1.1 RECOGNITION

Bone is recognized in the laboratory because of information that may be:

clinical —
    statement of source of tissue
radiological –
    demonstration of source of tissue
pathological –
    analysis of specimen –
        inspection, palpation
        fine detail X-ray
        microscopy: undecalcified
                : decalcified

Large amounts of bone are easily recognized. As the volume of bone decreases relative to other tissues present so the difficulties develop, and the importance of clinical and radiological support increases. The characteristics of bone whereby it can be identified in these circumstances are:

macroscopic –
    hardness
    architecture
radiological –
    mineral content (density and distribution)
microscopic –
    intercellular matrix (pattern and quality)
    associated cells

The usefulness of these characteristics varies as one moves down the scale from abundant to minimal bone. With large bone specimens and isolated fragments the problem is one of assessment rather than of recognition. Small fragments incorporated in soft tissue can be especially difficult and specimen X-ray is often helpful here. Deposited mineral which is not bone, e.g. tumoral calcinosis, dystrophic calcification, mineralization of cartilage or tophi, usually forms amorphous deposits which do not present problems in sectioning.

Histological recognition of bone depends on the identification of intercellular material; this is not a problem when abundant, nor if the architecture and collagen organization are typically osteonal or trabecular. When they are not typical, or the number and size of units of the intercellular material diminish, the difficulties increase, as can occur in bone tumours. The differentiation that must then be made is from a number of intercellular substances which may assume a trabecular or pseudotrabecular pattern (Table 2.1). Identification turns on collagen content and organization of the suspect trabecula, and the probable nature of the forming cells. Not everything that contains collagen is bone; nevertheless, polarization light microscopy allows a reasonable judgement about the matrix in terms of bone versus not bone.

Evaluating the cells that are judged to have produced the bone (i.e. the cells which are surrounded by matrix), and the cells which are currently producing the matrix (i.e. those cells that are contiguous with the surfaces) is clearly important. This evaluation will be both an identification (e.g. osteocyte, osteoblast) and a classification (e.g. normal, reactive, neoplastic). Initially, the evaluation will be by conventional histological criteria (see below) but enzyme histochemistry for alkaline phosphatase (Bancroft and Stevens, 1990) may be needed to identify osteoblasts (either non-neoplastic or neoplastic) with certainty. Frozen sections or imprints are required for this as the enzyme is inactivated by processing into paraffin wax. The technique is quick and can be done as part of an intraoperative assessment, if required, e.g. to assess clearance during osteosarcoma resection.

In non-neoplastic bone, the cells surrounded by bone matrix are called osteocytes; they maintain the extracellular matrix components of bone. Osteocytes are osteoblast cells that have become incorporated into the bone matrix. They lie in lacunae within the bone matrix (the size of the lacunae seen in formalin-fixed sections is made larger by cytoplasmic shrinkage during fixation) and possess long cytoplasmic processes which lie in narrow channels (canaliculi) in the surrounding matrix. Visualization of these processes can be enhanced by silver techniques. Adjacent osteocytes can communicate with each other by their cytoplasmic processes and transport enough nutrients to survive.

The cells on the surface of non-neoplastic bone are called osteoblasts. They are mesenchymal cells derived from osteoprogenitor cells, derived in turn from pluripotent mesenchymal stem cells. Inactive osteoblasts and osteoprogenitor cells are flattened spindle cells closely applied to the bone surface. Actively synthesizing osteoblasts appear cuboidal in section. The hypertrophy accommodates increased quantities of rough endoplasmic reticulum and mitochondria. Osteoblasts have the ability to synthesize type 1 collagen polypeptides, glycosaminoglycans and proteoglycans, and to secrete them into the extracellular space. Osteoblasts do this on bone surfaces (or on calcified cartilage surfaces in the case of the primary spongiosa, see section 19.1) building up a layer of collagen, glycosaminoglycans and proteoglycans called osteoid. Osteoblasts can also produce matrix in sheets, variously called sheet osteoid or chondro-osteoid. The same rules about collagen content and organization and the putative parent cell apply. The mechanisms by which osteoblasts become activated and synthesize new osteoid are incompletely understood. In bone turnover, both osteoclasts and locally synthesized prostaglandins are thought to be involved.

Table 2.1 The amount and organization of collagen determines whether or not a tissue is bone

Collagen	Quantity	Organization	Conclusion
No			Not bone
Yes	Little		Not bone*
	Moderate	Woven	Bone
		Lamellar	Bone
	Much	Parallel strands	Not bone

* Fibrogenesis imperfecta osseum is an exception to this statement.

Addition of bone minerals, primarily hydroxyapatite, to the osteoid forms bone. Hydroxyapatite is a crystalline complex of calcium and phosphate hydroxides with the chemical formula $Ca_{10} (PO_4)_6 (OH)_2$. It is laid down when the combined local concentrations of Ca^{2+} and PO_4^{2-} ions exceed the solubility product. Three factors combine to bring this about:

1. Matrix vesicles are round membrane-bound vesicles produced by osteoblasts from their cell membranes and shed into the matrix. They accumulate Ca^{2+} and PO_4^{2-} ions, contain alkaline phosphatase and pyrophosphate, and act as the nidus for the precipitation of hydroxyapatite. Matrix vesicles are the most important factor controlling the mineralization of osteoid.
2. Alkaline phosphatase is abundant in osteoblasts and helps raise local Ca^{2+} and PO_4^{2-} ion concentrations.
3. Osteonectin (synonym osteocalcin), a glycoprotein present in osteoid, also binds extracellular Ca^{2+} ions.

Osteoid may be a significant component of some extraskeletal neoplasms, particularly childhood tumours, e.g. hepatoblastomas. Immunohistochemical stains can be used to demonstrate that neoplastic cells, rather than osteoblasts and osteocytes, are present on the surface and within the osteoid matrix of these neoplasms. It is thought that, as part of the transformation to a malignant phenotype, the genes for osteoid synthesis in the neoplastic cells become de-suppressed.

2.1.2 ASSESSMENT OF BONE

Histopathology is complementary to imaging for the assessment of bone pathology. X-ray studies can include the whole skeleton; histopathology, including specimen radiography, can provide much greater detail, but only of a limited sample of bone. The relative importance of the X-ray and the histopatho-logical findings will vary from case to case and must be judged within the context of the case.

(a)   Stages in the assessment of bone

Clinical
  history of patient
  source of tissue

Radiological
  morbid anatomy of lesion/s
  site of tissue

Pathological
  analysis of specimen
  macroscopic: naked eye ± X-rays of intact specimen and/or slabs cut from it
  microscopic: light microscopy of histological sections, decalcified and/or undecalcified

In order to classify bone its features must be assessed.

(b)   Macroscopic and microscopic features in the assessment of bone

Architecture:
  anatomy –
    normal
    abnormal
      – developmental
      – reactive neoformation/resorption
      – neoplastic
  volume –
    cortical
    trabecular

Structure:
  collagen content –
    normal
    reduced
  collagen organization –
    lamellar
    woven
  reversal line pattern –
    normal
    mosaic
    pseudomosaic
    appositional

Mineral deposition:
  normal
  impaired
  distribution –
    normal
    perilacunar deficiency

Surfaces:
  resorption –
    active osteoclasts
    no osteoclasts
  formation –
    active osteoblasts
    inactive osteoblasts, surface osteo-
    cytes or envelope cells
    inert

Cells:
  osteoclasts
  osteoblasts (surfaces)
  osteocytes –
    present
    reduced
    absent

Marrow space content –
  normal
  abnormal

Some details about these follow.

(c)   Architecture

This means the form into which the structural material is organized: a whole bone, cortical or cancellous portions, reactive tissue (periosteal, callus), osseous tissue of tumours (some of which may be primary osteoblastic neoplasms; others may be cartilage tumours undergoing ossification). As one moves along the scale from physical examination through imaging/morbid anatomy to histology there is more and more to be seen of less and less; and the context in which it is viewed diminishes. It behoves one in the examination of bone to establish the context of the sample, otherwise one is operating on guesswork.

The typical pattern of reactive bone formation is distinctive both in fine detail X-ray and histological section, but there is a range of variation, usually brought about by contiguity with other pathological tissues, whereby this distinguishing quality is diminished. At its best there is a background of fibrovascular tissue, perhaps with a few infiltrating round cells, in which trabeculae of woven structure form a regular open trellis-work pattern. The trabeculae contain osteocytes, and plump, cuboidal osteoblasts are prominent as a unicellular layer at the surface. Osteoclasts may or may not be found. The trabeculae mineralize to become bone (and may become visible on X-ray when sufficiently numerous). An additional component of this tissue may be islands of cartilage which grow and ossify.

Neoplastic bone has a comparable structure, i.e. woven collagen but the architectural pattern and organization are different. The size and distribution of the trabeculae may be dissimilar in that they can be smaller, more delicate, and spaced more closely. The character of the tissue in the spaces is also different; it is not granulation tissue, but the tissue of the neoplasm. It is necessary to emphasize the considerable variability that can occur from cellular tissue, with minimal or doubtful evidence of bone formation, to sheets of matrix with cells in lacunae. The latter may be difficult to distinguish from cartilage. A high collagen content favours a notion of bone, whereas metachromasia favours cartilage. Alkaline phosphatase activity in cells is indicative of osteoblasts (see above) and may be helpful here.

A difficult problem that sometimes arises in the assessment of bone tumours is the presence of small amounts of immature bone (or osteoid) within otherwise cellular neoplasms. It is often arguable as to whether or not this should be regarded as being formed by tumour cells or by reacting osteoblasts. There are no hard and fast rules for making this distinction, which is very much a matter of experience and judgement.

(d) Collagen content

This is mentioned because of the extremely rare acquired condition of bone, fibrogenesis imperfecta ossium, in which the collagen content of the osteoid is greatly reduced. Unless the tissue is examined in polarized light this reduction will not be noticed.

(e) Collagen organization

In normal mature bone the collagen fibres in each bone structural unit are parallel in one lamella but not in adjacent ones – the lamellar pattern (Table 2.1). This is indicative of osteoblasts working at a normal rate. The alternative to this structure is a disorderly arrangement of the fibres, generally referred to as woven or basketwork, produced by osteoblasts rapidly synthesizing collagen. Assessment of the pattern of collagen organization, i.e. whether it is lamellar or woven, is an important part of the histopathological assessment. Although the pattern can sometimes be seen by ordinary light microscopy, it is considerably easier to see when viewed by polarized light and microscopic study of a section containing bone should almost always include examination by polarized light. If the pattern is lamellar, then it suggests normality. If the pattern is woven, then one is beholden to hypothesize why this should be so. There may be evidence from other areas of the section that enables one to start formulating a differential diagnosis.

(f) Reversal line pattern

Cement lines appear at the interfaces between existing surfaces and the new bone laid on them. Mostly, this bone apposition is preceded by resorption (hence 'reversal' lines) but there are circumstances where the apposition occurs without preceding resorption, and a succession of appositional layers, each marked off by a cement line, is observed. This is found under circumstances where one supposes that buttressing of the existing trabecular structure is required. Cement lines thus demarcate units of bone modelling (BMUs) (Chapter 14); normally they are smooth and sweeping; in the cortex they denote osteonal boundaries. Reactive sclerosis of trabeculae (as in osteoarthritis) does not require previous resorption. This process has nothing to do with BMUs. The osteoporosis of the inferior segment of the femoral head in osteoarthritis also negates the concept of BMUs (Chapter 8).

Increased rates of turnover are associated with both irregularity in cement line contour and decrease of modelling unit size. In discussing both collagen structure and cement lines, the changes of pattern with rate have been pointed out. This is a matter of degree, not of kind. Thus the reactive changes are non-specific, and on strict histological criteria a specific diagnosis cannot be made without other evidence. Some cases of Paget's disease can show the most marked reactive changes; but to make the diagnosis solely by histology is to do so on the basis of probability, because the same patterns can be the consequence of any condition, local or general, which affects bone turnover.

(g) Mineralization (see also Chapter 10)

In reactive bone, mineralization is usually not an important consideration. However, Looser's zones in osteomalacia show the effect of inadequate mineralization. Undecalcified sections are necessary for histological demonstration of the distinction between bone and osteoid, unless the Tripp and MacKay (1972) technique of silver staining of bone prior to decalcification is used. The site of mineral deposition at the bone osteoid interface may stain in undecalcified sections; many staining procedures will show this, but solochrome cyanine (Page, 1965) or toluidine blue are the best for decalcified sections. For undecalcified sections, tetracycline labelling is the best way of demonstrating the mineralization front. Undecalcified sections are necessary to observe the tetracycline labels (see Chapter 10). Large reductions in periosteocytic mineral can be judged from stained undecalcified sections, and are an indication of osteomalacia. A useful, if specialized, technique is microradiography – literally an X-ray of a thick (70 + μm) undecalcified section. Much valuable information about bone was gained with this method in the 1950s and 1960s but it has now been superseded (Chapter 21).

(h)   Surfaces and cells

In decalcified sections active formation can be judged by the presence of plump compacted osteoblasts on bone surfaces. Resorption is indicated by crenated surfaces – Howship's lacunae with or without osteoclasts. It can be difficult to distinguish artefactual disruption of the surface. In normal bone only a proportion of surfaces show cellular activity; in reactive bone this rises considerably, and osteoblasts and osteoclasts are much in evidence. Osteocytes are used mainly as an indicator of bone viability. When they die they disappear over a period of up to 3 weeks (Cohen *et al.*, 1990) but pyknotic remnants in lacunae can be hard to assess. This nuclear material can be present from a few days after the necrosis to about one month. For practical purposes, for two weeks or so from the moment of injury one cannot delineate with any certainty the limits of the dead bone by histological assessment of sections.

2.2   A GUIDE TO THE ANALYSIS OF TISSUE SUBMITTED FOR HISTOPATHOLOGICAL EXAMINATION

No histopathological diagnosis should be approached without a context. In practical terms the context means all the information about the patient that is necessary and sufficient for diagnostic purposes. This implies the exercise of judgement in each case as to what information will be gathered. A purpose of this guide is to indicate what that is. Attention will be given to focal lesions of bone and related soft tissues which present diagnostic problems to the solution of which morbid anatomy and histopathology can contribute. Different classes of problem are constituted by the diagnosis of generalized metabolic bone disease, and the assessment of lesions already diagnosed, in terms of severity, response to therapy, or the presence of complications. Thus, what is considered here is the material submitted for purposes of diagnosis from infections, neoplasias, local reactions to trauma, and from focal manifestations of generalized disorders.

2.2.1   ASSESSMENT OF TISSUE SITE

The tissue sites in which these disease processes occur can be separated as: in bone, on bone, in soft tissue (extraosseous), in joint.

It is of prime importance to establish the site of the sample(s) to be studied. Given the importance attached to site it is necessary to know exactly what the terms 'in bone', 'on bone', 'in joint' and 'in soft tissue' are intended to imply. The concept can be applied in two ways. It can be used to identify the tissue plane in which it is thought the lesion originated, or, alternatively, it can identify where the lesion is, in the material available to the pathologist.

An amputation/resection specimen may enable the question to be answered in both senses; a biopsy may, or may not, of itself, provide an answer in any context. A biopsy may display the surrounding normal tissue and that will tell you where the biopsy came from (but not necessarily where the lesion originated).

(a)   In bone

The term 'in bone' is defined as anything which is deep to the periosteal surface of the cortex. This means that the periosteum is 'on bone'. A bone (anatomical) is a unit within a system, e.g. a limb, which contains portions of other systems. There is a choice in naming the system to which the bone belongs: osseous, skeletal, osteoarticular, musculoskeletal. In the context, the first is most suitable. The contained systems are

- Haemopoietic (normally, all of it is in bone)
- Lymphoreticular
- Vascular
- Soft tissue

(b)   On bone

'On bone' is defined as anything which is based on and projecting from the normal line of the periosteal surface of the cortex, regardless of whether the lesion is presumed or proved to arise deep to or within the fibrous layer of the periosteum.

(c)   In joint

The category 'in joint' encompasses the synovium, joint capsule and cartilage. The subchondral bone plate is an integral part of the joint embryologically, and forms a biological unit with the cartilage, but for our purposes is arbitrarily considered as 'in bone' rather than 'in joint'.

(d)   In soft tissue

'In soft tissue' means outside the fibrous periosteum (can also be called extraosseous).

2.2.2   ASSESSMENT OF THE SPECIMEN

For purposes of the analytical procedure that is outlined here the unit sample is a histological section – from one block of tissue. This means that there may be one or many sections for a single case. Although it may seem that a lot of information will accumulate in more complex cases there is a simple means to reduce it.

In principle, and when practical in the laboratory, the best procedure is to use the macroscopic examination to record the anatomy of large specimens by drawing or photography, and to enter on the illustration the location of the tissue slabs taken (see also Chapter 21. Even if the specimen is not sufficiently large or complex to merit drawing or photography, the importance of the macroscopic examination should never be underrated. Cases can be made to appear more difficult than need be, just because enough thought has not been given to the macroscopic evaluation, and the tissue blocks have been taken quickly. Trying to extract information from histological sections in such circumstances can be a fruitless exercise and it is often best to revisit the gross specimen.

2.2.3   ASSESSMENT OF THE HISTOLOGY SECTION

Tissue pattern is the primary operative category in the diagnostic process here outlined. The terms employed are purely descriptive of the appearances of tissues viewed with a scanning or low power lens. They serve as a starting point for picking out individual entities from others of similar histological appearance.

To each tissue pattern the following subcategories can be applied, although not all will be applicable in every instance:

1.   Normal
2.   Reactive (in the very broadest context of the term)
3.   Neoplastic
     (a)   Benign
     (b)   Malignant

Higher magnification, with more attention to cytological detail, will be required to make these distinctions. The following discussion introduces the tissue patterns and their sub-categories.

(a) Inflammatory

The tissue pattern may be pyogenic at various stages, or non-specific granulo-matous.

(b) Osteoblastic

Osteoblastic tissue implies the property to form bone, i.e. the cells of which it is composed have the ability to form osteoid. Failure to express the potential may mean that the observer never suspects the possibility; cytological features might suggest osteo-blasts, but it is more probable that radiographs would do so. More usually it will be evident that bone formation is, or has been, active. This is a very broad categorization and can include bone tissue which is

1. Normal
2. Reactive (includes enhanced surface activity or other signs of excessive activity as well as bone genesis)
3. Neoplastic –
   (a) Benign
   (b) Malignant

Descriptions and criteria for recognition are given for normal and reactive osteoblasts in 'Recognition of bone' (section 2.1.1) and for neoplastic osteoblasts in section 13.4.4. In the context of diagnosis, the marrow spaces in normal bone must be searched for the presence of abnormal tissues or cells which have not caused a bone reaction. Moreover, since the abnormality of metabolic bone disease may not be apparent in decalcified sections this possibility must receive attention, either on the basis of clinical, biochemical and imaging information, or by preparation of undecalcified sections. Identification of reactive bone calls for similar attention to a search for a cause, whether within the specimen or by other available information. The

latter task can be undertaken by, or in consultation with, the clinician. In the case where the amounts of bone in the section are small relative to other pathological bone-free tissue, the problem is to assess whether the bone has been included by invasion of, or is reactive to, a non-osteoblastic tissue, or if it indicates that the whole sample is osteoblastic and is merely forming a limited amount of matrix.

Given that the tissue is categorized as an osteoblastic neoplasm, the assessment of benign versus malignant may be readily apparent in the section on cytological grounds or tissue pattern. But reference to the clinical/imaging information must be made as a test of the choice or, in cases of doubt, for a guide as to the probabilities.

(c) Chondroid tissue

Chondroid tissue implies the property to form cartilage, i.e. the cells of which it is composed have the ability to form that matrix. Failure to express the potential may mean, again, that the observer never suspects the possibility; cytological features, or, in some cases, tissue pattern might suggest chondroblasts, but it is probable that radiographs would help. More usually it will be evident that cartilage formation is, or has been active. This broad categorization can include cartilaginous tissue which is

1. Normal
2. Reactive
3. Neoplastic
   (a) Benign
   (b) Malignant

Descriptions of these and criteria for recognition are given in the diagnostic schema which follows.

(d) Chordoid tissue

Chordoid tissue is included as a category because it can present a problem in the identification of tissue from the axial skeleton. There is a reasonably specific tissue pattern that identifies chordoma or ecchordosis physaliphora. But the range of the pattern is such that some examples are difficult to distinguish from metastatic carcinoma, and others from cartilage neoplasia.

(e) Giant-celled tissue

Giant-celled tissue is a very loose term. Giant cell in this context means any multinucleated cell of the osteoclast type. Multinucleated giant cells of the inflammatory type may, of course, be present in granulomatous inflammations. Taken at its broadest, the term is not very useful since most osteoarticular tissues contain osteoclasts, even if only few in number. As in the case of tissue with spaces, attention must be paid to the stroma which bears the multinucleated cells. Most tissues bearing giant cells will be found a home in one of the other operative categories, on the grounds of both histology and morbid anatomy (i.e. radiographs); this statement would apply to most benign neoplasms (which can contain osteoclast giant cells in considerable numbers), osteosarcoma, non-ossifying fibroma, malignant fibrous histiocytoma, aneurysmal bone cyst, pigmented villonodular synovitis, and cherubism. Those tissues that remain in this category will be giant cell tumour, giant cell reparative granuloma and hyperparathyroidism. In the more general terms of the subcategories the lesions will be

- Reactive (metabolic or inflammatory)
- Neoplastic

(f) Round cell tissue

Round cell tissue can be applied where the material is composed of a single type of cell of roundish morphology. Like 'giant cell tissue' the term has been long in use and has the connotation of those primary or secondary malignant tumours in bone which are difficult to diagnose.

(g) Spindle cell tissue

Spindle cell tissue is a broad term embracing any tissue whose cells are spindled. Such cells are commonly fibroblasts; but smooth muscle and Schwann cells, histiocytes at some stages of their activities and some malignant epithelial cells also qualify. Cytological features are described which are said to be characteristic for some of these. The patterns formed by the arrangement of the cells within the tissues are also used as indicators of tissue type and criteria for recognition. These patterns are affected by:

1. Cell aggregations, e.g. various fascicular arrangements, whorled relations of several types.
2. Collagen content and organization.
3. Included cells: inflammatory cells, phagocytic cells (incorporating lipids or haemosiderin), multinucleated giant cells (osteoclasts) (section 2.2.3e).

Various alternative names are available to describe spindle cell tissue according to the recognition of specific features: fibrous (normal, reactive, neoplastic), smooth muscle, neural, epithelial. The subcategories (normal, reactive, neoplastic) apply more widely to fibrous and neural tissues in the context of orthopaedic pathology, being the only ones to occur normally in sufficient bulk and to present as reactive tissues. Thus, whereas an initial inspection leads to the categorization spindle cell, continued study may indicate that there is an underlying feature leading to the use of one of the more specific categories or subcategories of spindle cell tissue.

(h) Tissues composed of vacuolated or clear cells

The classes of tissue which can be included here are:

- Adipose
- Chondroid
- Chordoid
- Epithelial
- Histiocytic

In the subcategorization normal would only be applicable to the first two (and to ecchordosis physaliphora in the third), and reactive to them and histiocyte-rich tissue. The main issue here will be neoplasia.

(i)   Tissue with spaces

There are two elements to be categorized in tissues in which spaces are prominent: the supporting tissue and the spaces. Both elements can be subcategorized according to the scheme

1. Normal
2. Reactive
3. Neoplastic
   (a) Benign
   (b) Malignant

Both might be normal in structure, the spaces being dilated vascular channels, either lymph or blood vessels. This could constitute a normal physiological response, and the 'normal' subcategory would apply. However, this is an unlikely situation; it is more probable that the response is reactive, and as in all reactive situations a cause should be sought. Reactive dilatation of blood vessels can be very impressive, and on occasion the only finding in a small sample

of tissue. The more usual reactive tissue in which the vessels catch the attention of the eye is granulation tissue. Here and in the subcategory 'neoplasia' decisions will depend on the assessment of both tissue pattern and cytology of the supporting tissue, and of the cytology of the lining cells. If the analysis favours the supporting tissue as the important element and the spaces as subsidiary, then further investigation might be undertaken according to the tissue pattern of the former. Otherwise the determination of the type of lining cell comes to the fore, and the rules for distinguishing between types must be applied. The categories of cell involved are:

- Epithelial
- Endothelial
- Synovial
- No lining (cystic degeneration in mesenchyme)

REFERENCES

Bancroft, J.D. and Stevens, A. (1990) *Theory and Practice of Histological Techniques*, 3rd edn, Churchill Livingstone, Edinburgh.

Cohen, J., Bonfiglio, M. and Campbell, C.J. (1990) Aseptic necrosis, in *Orthopedic Pathophysiology in Diagnosis and Treatment*, Churchill Livingstone, New York, p. 260.

Page, K.M. (1965) A stain for myelin using solochrome cyanin. *J. Med. Lab. Technol.*, **22**, 224–5.

Tripp, E.J. and MacKay, E.H. (1972) Silver staining of bone prior to decalcification for quantitative determination of osteoid in sections. *Stain Technol.*, **47**, 129–36.

DIAGNOSTIC CHECKLIST 3

Jonathan R. Salisbury and Paul D. Byers

3.1 INTRODUCTION

The object of the checklist is to provide a means to check or to review a diagnosis; it is not designed as a means to arrive at a diagnosis on the basis of raw data. However, there would be reason in using it to consider alternative diagnoses for the observations already made.

In drawing up the checklist it was envisaged that the following information was used in making the diagnosis to be checked, or that it could be made available to assist in reaching a conclusion:

- The basic information about the case: age, sex, relevant clinical details.
- The basic conclusions about the morbid anatomy of the lesion(s) (this implies the examination of the radiographs; see Chapter 4 on use of radiographs for details).
- Which of the categories 'in bone', 'on bone', 'in joint', 'in soft tissue' are appropriate to the lesion.
- The relevant tissue category(ies) (section 2.2.3).

The conclusions about the last two points determine the point of entry into the scheme, which is subdivided as follows:

Table 3.1

1. Preliminary section
   - criteria for normal and reactive bone

2. Entities in bone
   - osteoblastic tissue
   - chondroid tissue
   - giant celled tissue
   - spindle celled tissue
   - vacuolated or clear cells
   - tissues with spaces
   - epithelial tissues
   - reactive tissues

3. Entities on bone

4. Entities in joint

5. Entities in soft tissue
   - of tendons
   - of tendon sheaths
   - of connective tissues
   - calcifying lesions

The features (radiological, histological or clinical pathological) which serve as criteria for the diagnosis of the focal disease entities which are considered in the book are summarized under the headings essential (mandatory), optional or acceptable features, and those whose presence would exclude the diagnosis.

Brevity, which is the essence of such a scheme, imposes limitations on the qualifications and provisos that can be employed. But these are already in the text, to which reference can be made in the event of doubt or uncertainty. Nevertheless, that there is no syntax of the scheme is an actual source of unease and uncertainty, and a potential source of confusion or error. An assembly of nouns and clauses, organized under headings, is presented without any operative connections, although these are implied by the headings. The following syntactical formula will overcome these difficulties.

In order to check his diagnosis, or to substantiate the presence of a feature in the pathological material, the pathologist must locate the term in the first column. In the second column will be listed the features that are essential if the diagnosis is to stand. In the third column there will be other relevant features, which need not necessarily be present, but which will add to the weight of evidence in favour if they are. A fourth column contains features whose presence excludes the diagnosis in question.

Nothing in Nature is straightforward which means that some qualifications have had to be introduced, as follows. Thus there are exceptions to the requirement that some mandatory features be present. It is acknowledged that this makes them optional in strict terminology. But since the feature is 'classical', and nearly always present it is thought to be better to preserve its weight by keeping it in the mandatory column and to put the onus on the pathologist to double check his observations.

Under the optional column there are features noted as acceptable. These are those which, if present (and in this sense they are optional) might be taken to preclude the diagnosis or even to demand another one altogether. The fact of being annotated as being acceptable carries a warning that vigilance is necessary to ensure that nothing is being overlooked. An example is bone formation in giant cell tumour.

Finally, in the exclusion column attention has been drawn to some features which do not exclude, but which are so uncommon as to demand double checking before being allowed to pass.

3.2 PRELIMINARY SECTION

3.2.1 NORMAL AND REACTIVE BONE
(TABLE 3.2)

Table 3.2

Diagnosis	Mandatory (*exceptions)	Optional
BONE, normal		
Structural, viable	Lamellar collagen (polarized light) *woven: only in child's primary formation Viable osteocytes	Surface osteoblasts Active/inactive Howship's lacunae +/− osteoclasts
Structural, necrotic	As above but osteocytes absent or pyknotic (see p.12)	+/− Surface cells depending on marrow
Architectural	As above but in the context of compact or trabecular architecture	
BONE, reactions		
Structural, normal Viable or necrotic: active bone cell response	Lamellar collagen +/− osteocytes Either osteoclast and/or osteoblast drifts Or intense osteoclast/osteoblast focal activity (BMUs)	Marrow fibrosis or other pathology
result, in time	Either parallel cement lines, lamellar collagen Or mosaic cement lines, lamellar and woven collagen	
Architectural	As above but in the context of compact or trabecular architecture	Thick trabeculae
REACTIVE genesis		
Structural	Fibrovascular tissue supporting membrane genesis, woven collagen +/− cartilage metaplasia +/− enchondral ossification	
Architectural	As above but in form of trabecular architecture ranging from isolated trabeculum to regular open network with osteoblastic mantling	Nodular cartilage component +/− its ossification

3.3 ENTITIES IN BONE

3.3.1 OSTEOBLASTIC TISSUES (TABLES 3.3 AND 3.4)

Table 3.3

Diagnosis	Mandatory (*exceptions)	Optional (*acceptable)	Exclusion (*reconsider)
Fibrous dysplasia **(common)**	Fibrous component – collagen and cells; benign, stellate Osteoblastic component – woven bone, curved and interconnecting trabeculae (range of appearances)	Cysts; fluid Cartilage; nodules, may be major feature 'Myxoid' areas Active osteoclast collections, related to cysts Foam cells may be abundant	*If in jaws (consider primary dental tumours – may need dental pathologist's opinion)
Ossifying fibroma **(rare)**	'Mantling' by osteoblasts of most bone surfaces		*If site not skull or tibia

'Benign fibro-osseous lesion' is a term which encompasses fibrous dysplasia, ossifying fibroma and similar lesions of the jaws and is useful in those cases where lesions that are clearly benign but do not fully meet the published criteria of any particular category and may, for treatment purposes, be a perfectly adequate diagnosis.

Table 3.4

Diagnosis	Mandatory (*exceptions)	Optional (*acceptable)	Exclusion (*reconsider)
Bone island **(uncommon)**	Island of dense lamellar bone in cancellous space: morbid anatomy (radiograph) sufficient for diagnosis		
Paget's disease **(uncommon)**	Increased bone turnover *Age 40+ Porotic phase = 'cyst' Sclerotic phase = coarse enlarged bone Biochemistry: Alk phos ↑ Others normal		Other causes of increased turnover: Hyperparathyroidism Adjacent focal lesion
Hyperparathyroidism **(uncommon)**	Increased bone turnover Appropriate clinical, radiological and biochemical observations		
Leontiasis ossea **(very rare)**	Prominence of maxillae See Leontiasis ossea (section 10.5.10)		
Reparative giant cell granuloma	See reparative giant cell granuloma in section 3.3.4		
Osteoid osteoma **(uncommon)**	Size <15(20)mm Benign osteoblastic tissue Osteoclasts +/++	Pain and aspirin Radiology: small hole, variable reaction, typically substantial*	Growth of lesion Inflammation: pyogenic, chronic non-specific, granulomatous
Benign osteoblastoma **(rare)**	Size >15(20)mm X-ray: benign, moderate size, reactive bone +/− Benign osteoblastic tissue Osteoclasts +/−	Growth, few symptoms*	Features of agressive osteoblastoma: radiological − qv histological − qv
Aggressive osteoblastoma **(rare)**	X-ray: demarcated, sclerotic reaction +/−; or large, variable density, reaction +/− Mixed 'blastic tissues Variable density Fibrovascular tissue Osteoclasts +/++ No overt cytological malignancy	Long history Recurrences	Unequivocal cytological malignancy = osteosarcoma
Giant cell tumour	See giant cell tumour in section 3.3.4		

Table 3.4 *contd*

Diagnosis	Mandatory (*exceptions)	Optional (*acceptable)	Exclusion (*reconsider)
Osteosarcoma - unqualified **uncommon**	'Malignant' X-ray Malignant osteoblastic tissue Neoplastic cells +ve for alkaline phosphatase		*Age > 20
Osteosarcoma variants Chondroblastic variant **(uncommon)**	Findings of osteosarcoma as above Predominance of malignant chondroblastic tissue Malignant osteoblastic component Appropriate age and morbid anatomy		
Fibroblastic variant **(uncommon)**	Findings of osteosarcoma as above Malignant spindle cell tissue Malignant osteoblastic component Appropriate age and morbid anatomy		
Osteoclast-rich variant **(rare)**	Findings of osteosarcoma as above Malignant osteoblastic tissue Abundant osteoclasts Appropriate age and morbid anatomy		* Neoplasm centred on epiphysis
Telangiectatic variant **(rare)**	Findings of osteosarcoma as above Malignant osteoblastic tissue Telangiectasia: vascular component substantial, may suggest angiosarcoma Appropriate age and morbid anatomy		
Paget's sarcoma i.e. sarcoma in Paget's disease of bone **(rare)**	Findings of osteosarcoma as above Malignant connective tissue tumour Paget's disease at site Appropriate age and morbid anatomy	Osteoblastic Chondroblastic Fibroblastic Osteoclastic	* Age < 40 Metastatic carcinoma

Table 3.4.

Diagnosis	Mandatory (*exceptions)	Optional (*acceptable)	Exclusion (*reconsider)
Multicentric variant; synchronous **(very rare)**	Findings of osteosarcoma as above Malignant osteoblastic tumour at two or more sites appearing synchronously	More convincing if more than one bone	Pulmonary metastases
Multicentric variant; metachronous **(very rare)**	Findings of osteosarcoma as above Malignant osteoblastic tumour at two or more sites appearing sequentially	More convincing if more than one bone	Pulmonary metastases
Central variant **(very rare)**	Findings of osteosarcoma as above Well differentiated malignant osteoblastic tissue Intramedullary lesion		High grade cytological malignancy Cortical erosion Periosteal reaction *Very rare; refer to aggressive osteoblastoma
Malignant fibrous histiocytoma	See malignant fibrous histiocytoma in section 3. 3.6		

3. 3.2   CHONDROID TISSUES (TABLE 3.5)

Table 3.5

Diagnosis	Mandatory (*exceptions)	Optional (*acceptable)	Exclusion (*reconsider)
Chondroma **(very common)**	Benign chondroblastic tissue	*Pronounced cellularity (benign) in multifocal lesions	*Age > 20 *Site: in adult - axial skeleton, shoulder girdle, pelvic girdle
Benign chondroblastoma **(uncommon)**	*Epiphyseal Radiologically benign Round discrete cells *Calcified intercellular matrix (chicken wire) *Chondroid lobules	Osteoclasts Occasional mitoses	*Clear cell chondrosarcoma (see text)

Table 3.5 *contd*

Diagnosis	Mandatory (*exceptions)	Optional (*acceptable)	Exclusion (*reconsider)
Chondromyxoid fibroma **(uncommon)**	Metaphyseal Radiologically benign Chondromyxoid tissue Interlobular tissue	Interlobular tissue can be: 1. Fibrovascular +/– osteoclasts +/– haemosiderin +/– bone +/– cartilage 2. Benign chondroblastoma type (see CMF/BC text)	*Clear cell chondrosarcoma (see text)
Fibrous dysplasia	See fibrous dysplasia in section 3.3.1		
Chondrosarcoma high grade **(uncommon)**	Cytological malignancy: cellularity, plump cells, bi-nucleate cells, pleomorphism	Mitoses	Malignant osteoblastic tissue (distinguish from 1. included normal/reactive bone 2. enchondral ossification)
Chondrosarcoma low grade **(common)**	No obvious cytological malignancy Signs of growth: histological, imaging, clinical viz. invasion of bone tissue endosteal erosion periosteal apposition pathological fracture	Recurrence	*Site – hands and feet Metastases
Chondrosarcoma variants Clear cell chondrosarcoma **(rare)**	Lobulated tissue with malignant clear cells (comprising up to 100%)	Areas of conventional chondrosarcoma *Osteoclasts *Bone	
Dedifferentiated chondrosarcoma **(rare)**	Undifferentiated spindle celled sarcoma and (low grade) chondrosarcoma		Malignant osteoblastic tissue
Mesenchymal chondrosarcoma **(rare)**	Undifferentiated round cells and lobulated cartilage	Mineralization of cartilage *Vascularity ++	(See round cells)
Chondroblastic osteosarcoma	See osteosarcoma variants in section 3.3.1		

3.3 CHORDOID TISSUES (TABLE 3.6)

Table 3.6

Diagnosis	*Mandatory (*exceptions)*	*Optional (*acceptable)*	*Exclusion (*reconsider)*
Chordoma **(uncommon)**	Axial skeleton Round cells in chords Mucinous matrix +/+++	Physaliphorous cells (see text) *Chondroid areas	*Known primary carcinoma (IHC see section 14.1) *Chondrosarcoma (especially in base of skull) Notochord rest (see section 14.1)

3.3.4 GIANT CELLED TISSUES (TABLE 3.7)

Most benign neoplasms can contain osteoclast giant cells, often in considerable numbers, and should be considered in the differential diagnosis.

Table 3.7

Diagnosis	*Mandatory (*exceptions)*	*Optional (*acceptable)*	*Exclusion (*reconsider)*
Reparative giant cell granuloma **(rare)**	Benign X ray Jaws, hands and feet[a] Osteoclasts Benign spindle cells	Haemosiderin Immature bone	Epiphyseal lesion Abnormal biochemistry
'Brown' tumour of hyperparathyroidism	See hyperparathyroidism in section 10.4.5.		
Pigmented villonodular synovitis	See pigmented villonodular synovitis Section 3.5		
Aneurysmal bone cyst	See aneurysmal bone cyst in section 3.3.8		
Non-ossifying fibroma	See non-ossifying fibroma in section 3.3.6		
Histiocytosis X	See histiocytosis X in section 3.3.5		
Cherubism	See cherubism in section 15.6		

Table 3.7 *contd*

Diagnosis	Mandatory (*exceptions)	Optional (*acceptable)	Exclusion (*reconsider)
Giant cell tumour **(uncommon)**	*Site: epiphysis *Age > 20 < 40 Stromal component	Osteoclasts (other things being equal, diagnostic confidence is directly proportional to no. of osteoclasts) *Variable amount of immature bone	Abnormal biochemistry (signs of HPT) *If not juxta-articular *If in jaws
Malignant fibrous histiocytoma	See malignant fibrous histiocytoma in section 3.3.6		
Osteosarcoma	See osteosarcoma and osteosarcoma variants in section 3.3.1		

[a]Four cases (of varying credibility) of reparative giant cell granuloma were reported at sites other than jaws, hands and feet for the 5-year period 1985–1989. These sites were temporal bone (Lin and Huang 1989), pituitary fossa (Siqueira *et al.*, 1989), humerus (Thomas *et al.*, 1988) and thoracic vertebra (Inoue *et al.*, 1986).

3.3.5   ROUND CELLED TISSUES (TABLE 3.8)

Table 3.8

Diagnosis	Mandatory	Optional	Exclusion
Benign chondroblastoma	See benign chondroblastoma in section 3.3.2		
Ewing's sarcoma **(uncommon)**	Permeated pattern of bone destruction Periosteal reaction +/+++ (variety of patterns, lamellar most common) Small to medium round cells, PAS +ve	Mitoses	+ve leucocyte common antigen VMA +ve
Atypical Ewing's sarcoma **(rare)**	As above but PAS –ve Pleomorphism +		+ve leucocyte common antigen VMA +ve
Primitive neuroectodermal tumour of bone (+ Askin tumours) (rare)	Ewing's radiology as above Rosettes Nuclear pleomorphism + IHC +ve neural markers		Strongly PAS +ve +ve leucocyte common antigen VMA +ve

Table 3.8 *contd*

Diagnosis	Mandatory	Optional	Exclusion
Primary malignant lymphoma	Malignant round cells in clinical context of lymphoma Leucocyte common antigen +ve		Neural markers +ve Evidence of extraosseous lymphoma excludes primary
Histiocytosis X	Lytic defect(s) Langerhans cells	Eosinophils Plasma cells Histiocytes	
Mesenchymal chondrosarcoma	See mesenchymal chondrosarcoma in section 3.3.2		
Metastases	See epithelial tissues, section 3.3.9	VMA +ve	

3.3.6 SPINDLE CELLED TISSUES (TABLE 3.9)

Table 3.9

Diagnosis	Mandatory (*exceptions)	Optional (*acceptable)	Exclusion (*reconsider)
Fibrous dysplasia	See fibrous dysplasia in section 3.3.1		
Reparative giant cell granuloma	See reparative giant cell granuloma in section 3.3.4		
Cherubism	See cherubism in section 15.6		
Neurofibromatosis **(very rare)**	See Hunt and Pugh (1961) for review. Doubtful if neurofibroma has been identified in bone (see section 14.4.7)		
Non-ossifying fibroma (including metaphyseal fibrous cortical defect) **(common)**	Benign X-ray Benign spindle cells	Storiform pattern Foam cells Haemosiderin Osteoclasts	*Age > 25 Epiphyseal lesion
Desmoplastic fibroma **(rare)**	Benign radiologically Benign spindle cells Abundant (amyanthoid) collagen		Bone Cytological features of malignancy (see text)
Chondromyxoid fibroma	See chondromyxoid fibroma in section 3.3.2		

Table 3.9 *contd*

Diagnosis	Mandatory (*exceptions)	Optional (*acceptable)	Exclusion (*reconsider)
Benign neural tumours **(very rare)**	Spindle cells S100 protein +ve See de la Monte *et al.* (1984) for review	Antoni A and B areas	*Neurofibroma
Giant cell tumour	See giant cell tumour in section 3.3.4		
Haemangiopericytoma **(rare)**	Plump, short, spindle cells	Staghorn vessels	Known primary tumour
Malignant fibrous histiocytoma and fibrosarcoma **(uncommon)**	Cytologically malignant spindle cells	Storiform pattern Inflammatory cells Osteoclasts Immature bone formation	Other sarcomas from this section
Leiomyosarcoma **(very rare)**	Malignant tumour on X-ray Malignant spindle cells on histology No matrix Cigar shaped nuclei + Appropriate IHC See Berlin *et al.* (1987) and Kameda *et al.* (1987) for reviews of this tumour		
Fibroblastic osteosarcoma	See osteosarcoma variants in section 3.3.1		
Dedifferentiated chondrosarcoma	See dedifferentiated chondrosarcoma in section 3.3.2		
Mesenchymal chondrosarcoma	See mesenchymal chondrosarcoma in section 3.3.2		
'Malignant' spindle cells	See epithelial tissues in section 3.3.9		

3.3.7   VACUOLATED OR CLEAR CELLS
(TABLE 3.10)

Table 3.10

Diagnosis	Mandatory (*exceptions)	Optional (*acceptable)	Exclusion (*reconsider)
Lipoma **(very rare)**	Benign X-ray Mature fat		
Non-ossifying fibroma	See non-ossifying fibroma in section 3.3.6		
Fibrous dysplasia	See fibrous dysplasia in section 3.3.1		
Epithelioid haemangioendothelioma **(rare)**	IHC for factor VIII +ve in cells with intracellular lumina Features of cytological malignancy	Multiple sites	*Primary carcinoma Granulation tissue
Giant cell tumour	See giant cell tumour in section 3.3.4		
Liposarcoma **(very rare)**	Ill defined, expanding, lytic lesion Straightforward liposarcoma See Catto and Stevens (1963) Goldman (1964) and Schwartz *et al.* (1970) for reviews of this tumour	*2nd component[a]	
Chondrosarcoma	See chondrosarcoma and chondrosarcoma variants in section 3.3.2		
Chordoma	See chordoma in section 3.3.3		
Malignant fibrous histiocytoma	See malignant fibrous histiocytoma in section 3.3.6		
Metastatic carcinoma	See epithelial tissues, section 3.3.9		

[a] Occasional cases of liposarcoma mixed with another component have been reported, e.g. osteoliposarcoma (Ross and Hadfield, 1968) and liposarcoma with osteosarcomatous foci (Downey *et al.*, 1982).

3.3.8   TISSUES WITH SPACES (TABLE 3.11)

Table 3.11

Diagnosis	Mandatory (*exceptions)	Optional (*acceptable)	Exclusion (*reconsider)
Angioma **(common)**	Clusters of thin-walled vessels Benign radiology	Size variable	* Other component
Simple bone cyst **(common)**	'Simple cyst' morbid anatomy Unicameral (Usually) delicate fibrous lining Unsatisfactory histology		*If age > 20
Intraosseous ganglion **(rare)**	Fibrous walled 'cyst' Mucinous fluid		
Pigmented villonodular synovitis	See pigmented villonodular synovitis in section 3.5		
Aneurysmal bone cyst **(uncommon)**	*'Aneurysmal' morbid anatomy 1. Large spaces. 2. Thin septae of fibrovascular tissue containing immature bone Osteoclasts	*Into old age Small to no spaces Thick septae to solid tissue Other pre-existing benign lesions: fibrous dysplasia, benign neoplasia Solid ABC (Sanerkin *et al.*, 1983)	*If age > 20 Telangiectatic osteosarcoma
Vanishing bone disease **(rare)**	Morbid anatomy - focal bone osteolysis without local swelling	Scanty amount of loose vascular or fibrovascular tissue	*Substantial tissue
Angiosarcoma **(uncommon)**	Abnormal lining Cuboidal cells +	Cytological features of malignancy	Other neoplastic component Granulation tissue
Telangiectatic osteosarcoma	See osteosarcoma variants in section 3.3.1		
Metastatic carcinoma	See epithelial tissues, section 3.3.9		

3.3.9 EPITHELIAL TISSUES (TABLES 3.12 AND 3.13)

Table 3.12

Diagnosis	Mandatory	Optional	Exclusion
Metastases to bone **(very common)**	Cytological malignancy Appropriate radiology	Cell morphology: round[a], spindle[b], clear[c], spaces[d] Appropriate special stains[e]	

[a] Cells with round morphology could be:
1. Metastatic carcinoma – IHC stains for cytokeratins +ve. Metastatic adenocarcinomas are usually mucin +ve (i.e. +ve diastase-PAS, +ve alcian blue).
2. Metastatic neuroblastoma – IHC stains for neural antigens +ve (i.e. neurone-specific enolase +ve, neurofilament +ve), +ve VMA in urine.
3. Metastatic embryonal rhabdomyosarcoma – IHC stains for muscle antigens +ve (i.e. +ve desmin, myoglobin +ve in some).

[b] Cells with spindle shaped morphology could be:
1. Metastatic spindle celled carcinoma, e.g. from a primary renal cell carcinoma – epithelial markers such as keratins +ve.
2. Metastatic soft tissue sarcoma – Strong IHC +vity for vimentin may be helpful but is not diagnostic.

[c] Cells with clear cytoplasm could be metastatic carcinoma – perform IHC for cytokeratins, establish whether clear appearance is caused by glycogen (PAS with and without diastase).

[d] Cells surrounding spaces could be metastatic carcinoma – perform IHC for cytokeratins, establish whether appearance is caused by the presence of mucins in the spaces (PAS with diastase predigestion, alcian blue stains).

[e] *Special stains*
Techniques that may help in distinguishing the nature of bone metastases include histochemistry and immunohistochemistry. For all types of cell morphology, metastatic carcinomas are a possibility and so immunohistochemical staining with epithelial markers is appropriate. The two commonest types of epithelial markers are those that recognize the intermediate filaments (IF) known as cytokeratins (e.g. pan-cytokeratin, CAM 5.2, LP 34) and those that recognize human polymorphic epithelial mucin (e.g. EMA, E29, HMFG-1, HMFG-2). For spindle and round-celled tumours, metastatic sarcomas are a possibility and immunohistochemistry for vimentin (IF of mesenchymal cells), desmin (IF of muscle cells), myoglobin (oxygen carrier of muscle) or S100 protein (calcium-binding protein) may be appropriate. Vimentin may be positive in metastatic carcinoma and stains for cytokeratins may appear negative. Very rare cases of osteosarcoma can contain cytokeratin positive cells. For clear cells, periodic acid-Schiff (PAS) stains with and without diastase predigestion are required to identify glycogen which is commonly present in metastases from renal cell carcinomas. For cells with spaces, mucin stains (e.g. PAS with diastase pre-digestion, alcian blue) aid in identifying metastases from adenocarcinomas.

Table 3.13

Diagnosis	Mandatory (*exceptions)	Optional (*acceptable)	Exclusion (*reconsider)
Adamantinoma (of long bones) **(very rare)**	Variable (size, pattern) epithelial collections in a fibrous stroma IHC epithelial markers +ve	Morbid anatomy Fibrous dysplasia	Jaw (consider primary dental tumour)
Epidermoid cyst **(very rare)**	Terminal phalanges (*occur very rarely) Epidermoid cyst		

3.3.10 REACTIVE TISSUES

- Granulation tissue
- Reactive osteoblastic tissues
- Reactive cartilage (incl. malunion)
- Reactive fibrous tissue (incl. malunion)
- Reactive bone marrow
- Reactive vascular tissue
- Reactive muscle tissue
- Reactive adipose tissue

3.4 ENTITIES ON BONE (TABLE 3.14)

'On bone' = lesion contiguous with cortex, ?relationship to periosteum, no grounds for an origin within the bone or soft tissues: (see Chapter 4 on radiology).

Table 3.14

Diagnosis	Mandatory (*exceptions)	Optional (*acceptable)	Exclusion (*reconsider)
Congenital entities **(rare, very rare in laboratory)**	e.g. melorheostosis, Camurati-Englemann disease See text and Smith *et al.* (1977) and Sparkes and Graham (1972)		
Callus **(very common but rarely seen in laboratory)**	Trauma Reactive osteoblastic tissue (section 3.3.10) *Cartilage (see text)	Invasive	If trauma inappropriate *underlying cause
Avulsion fracture **(common but rare in laboratory)**	Trauma Reactive osteoblastic tissue Resolution over time (3/12) *Cartilage		If progressive *parosteal osteosarcoma
Myositis ossificans	See myositis ossificans in section 3.6		

Table 3.14 *contd*

Diagnosis	Mandatory (*exceptions)	Optional (*acceptable)	Exclusion (*reconsider)
Periosteal reaction (= periostitis) **(idiopathic = rare, others common)**	Reactive osteoblastic tissue Involves periosteum (see text)	Underlying cause (inflammatory incl. syphilis, trauma, neoplasia, varicose veins, polyarteritis) Unknown cause	Leontiasis ossea Hyperostosis frontalis interna Metabolic diseases Cherubism Hypertrophic pulmonary osteoarthropathy
Hyperostosis frontalis interna **(very rare)**	Thickening of internal table of frontal bone	Virilism Obesity Neuropsychiatric problems Underlying tumour: meningioma, angioma Vertebral hyperostosis	
Hypertrophic pulmonary osteoarthropathy **(uncommon, very rare in laboratory)**	Diaphyses Symmetrical periosteal new bone formation	Neoplastic and non-neoplastic diseases of the lung Less commonly other organs	
Subperiosteal abscess **(uncommon)**	Site X-ray (abscess) 'cavity' and reactive periostitis Histology inflammatory tissue = abscess		
Periosteal ganglion **(very rare)**	Mucoid degneration of periosteal tissue		
Osteoid osteoma **(rare)**	See osteoid osteoma in section 3.3.1		
Parosteal lipoma **(very rare)**	Major long bones and metacarpal shafts Well defined soft tissue mass adjacent to bone with periosteal bone reaction Encapsulated mature fat	Dystrophic calcification	
Osteochondroma **(common)**	Continuity of cortex and medulla Cartilage cap (*mature lesions of adults – see text) Cytologically benign cartilage		Other tumours in this section

Table 3.14 *contd*

Diagnosis	Mandatory (*exceptions)	Optional (*acceptable)	Exclusion (*reconsider)
Chondrosarcoma arising in the cartilage cap of an osteochondroma **(very rare)**	Pre-existing osteochondroma Criteria of 'conventional' chondrosarcoma (see text)		
Juxtacortical cartilage tumours			
Chondroma **(rare)**	Site Benign cartilage		
Chondrosarcoma **(rare)**	Site Malignant cartilage (see text)		
Surface osteosarcomas (see text)			
Parosteal osteosarcoma **(rare)**	Early: Site – Fibro-osteoblastic tissue *NO* cytological features of malignancy Maturation of tissue towards periosteum (i.e. tissue remodelling) Late: Malignant tumour of varied differentiation (bone, cartilage, fibrous)	Benign (not cytologically malignant) cartilage nodules	*As age exceeds 40 years *If *recent* history of trauma (see avulsion fracture) *IF cytological features of malignancy (see text)
Periosteal osteosarcoma **(rare)**	Site Osteoblastic and chondroid tissues with some features of malignancy (see text)		*As age exceeds 40 years
Conventional osteosarcoma **(very rare)**	See osteosarcoma unqualified in section 3.3.1		

3.5 ENTITIES IN JOINTS (TABLE 3.15)

Table 3.15

Diagnosis	Mandatory (*exceptions)	Optional (*acceptable)	Exclusion (*reconsider)
Non-specific synovitis **(common)**	Inflamed synovium (see text)		*Numerous polymorphs
Granulomatous synovitis including sarcoid **(uncommon in UK)**	Granulomatous inflammation		
Septic arthritis **(very rare in laboratory)**	Non-specific synovitis and polymorphs		
Pannus **(common)**	Hypertrophic inflamed synovium		
Pigmented villonodular synovitis (Giant cell tumour of tendon sheath) (Benign synovioma) **(uncommon)**	*Pigmented tissue Haemosiderin Lipid *Variable lymphocyte and plasma cell infiltrate Spaces Osteoclasts, variable numbers	*Villous or nodular or both	Haemophilia
Synovial chondromatosis **(rare)**	Cartilage nodules in synovium	Ossification of nodules Free cartilage nodules in joint space	Attached loose body
Loose body **(common)**	Fragment(s) of articular cartilage	Mineralization May become or remain attached Bone which may or not be necrotic	Rice bodies Melon seed bodies
Rice bodies and melon seed bodies **(common)**	Fibrin		
Osteoarthritis **(common)**	Progressive articular cartilage loss in the weight bearing area of a joint (see text) Bone sclerosis and marrow fibrosis after bone exposure	Osteophytes Subchondral bone cysts Necrosis	Non-progressive cartilage lesions (see text)
Rheumatoid arthritis **(common)**	Non-specific synovitis and destruction of joint surface in association with fibrovascular tissue	Multisystem disease	

Table 3.15 *contd*

Diagnosis	Mandatory (*exceptions)	Optional (*acceptable)	Exclusion (*reconsider)
Synovial haemangioma **(very rare)**	Clusters of thin-walled vessels	Can have prominent endothelial cells	
Synovial chondrosarcoma **(very rare)**	Cytologically malignant cartilage		Not originating from bone

3.6 ENTITIES IN SOFT TISSUES (TABLE 3.16)

Table 3.16

Diagnosis	Mandatory (*exceptions)	Optional (*acceptable)	Exclusion (*reconsider)
Lesions of tendons			
Ruptured tendon **(uncommon, very rare in laboratory)**	Disruption of tendon architecture	History spontaneous, rheumatoid arthritis Necrosis	
Xanthoma **(very rare)**	Clear cells (Fat stains +ve, see text)	Lipid biochemistry abnormalities	
Calcific tendinitis **(uncommon)**	Subacromial bursa and tendons of the short rotator shoulder muscles *Granulomatous inflammation (see tumoral calcinosis also)		
Lesions of tendon sheaths			
Pigmented villonodular synovitis	See pigmented villonodular synovitis in section 3.5		
Fibroma of tendon sheath **(rare)**	Anatomy: attached to tendon sheath Cytologically benign fibrocollagenous tissue Circumscribed non-infiltrative	Myxoid change Chondroid or osseous metaplasia	Foamy macrophages Osteoclasts Haemosiderin
Synovitis **(common)**	See non-specific synovitis and granulomatous synovitis in section 3.5		

Table 3.16 *contd*

Diagnosis	Mandatory (*exceptions)	Optional (*acceptable)	Exclusion (*reconsider)
'Sausage finger' (Macrodystrophia lipomatosa) **(very rare)**	Finger(s) All tissues hyperplastic Nerves enlarged		Neurofibromatous elements
Lesions in soft tissues			
Calcifying or ossifying haematoma **(rare)**	See myositis ossificans below		
Myositis ossificans **(uncommon, rare in adults < 40 years)**	Reactive fibro-osteoblastic tissue Limited progression (< 3/12)	History Morbid anatomy	
Fibrodysplasia (myositis) ossificans progressiva **(very rare)**	Chronic progressive benign fibro-osteoblastic tissue in muscle, tendon, aponeurosis and ligaments	Malformation of digits	
Tumoral calcinosis **(rare)**	Anatomical site Amorphous material in soft tissues with granulomatous reaction		Abnormal calcium biochemistry *If > 50 years
Calcinosis circumscripta **(very rare)**	Solitary dystrophic calcification	Middle-aged women Anatomical site Raynaud's phenomenon Scleroderma Sclerodactyly	Abnormal biochemistry
Calcinosis universalis **(very rare)**	Multiple foci of dystrophic calcification	Children Scleroderma Dermatomyositis	
Mineralizing neoplasms of soft tissue origin			
Calcifying aponeurotic fibroma **(very rare)**	Benign fibro-collagenous tissue with focal mineral deposition *Hands and feet	Cartilaginous metaplasia Ossification (rare)	* If > 16 years Fibromatosis Soft part chondroma

Table 3.16 *contd*

Diagnosis	Mandatory (*exceptions)	Optional (*acceptable)	Exclusion (*reconsider)
Cavernous haemangioma **(uncommon)**	Large dilated blood filled vessels lined by endothelium	Dystrophic calcification within thrombi (common) Syndromes: Maffucci's, Kasabach-Merritt, blue rubber bleb nevus	
Lipoma **(very common)**	Encapsulated mature fat	Dystrophic calcification (rare)	
Schwannoma	Spindle cells S100 +ve	Dystrophic calcification (common) Antoni A and B area	
Synovial sarcoma	Biphasic tissue pattern or monophasic tissue and appropriate immunohistochemistry	Dystrophic calcification (about 50% of tumours)	Joints
Extraskeletal bone tumours			
Osteosarcoma **(very rare)**	Anatomy See osteosarcoma - unqualified, section 3.3.1		
Soft part chondroma **(rare)**	Anatomy Benign cartilage	Adults Hands and feet Osteoclasts Stromal cells	Aponeurotic fibroma
Chondrosarcoma (conventional) **(very rare)**	Anatomy Malignant cartilage (see text)	Mineralization (common)	
Mesenchymal chondrosarcoma **(rare)**	Anatomy Undifferentiated (common) round cells and lobules of cartilage	Mineralization	
Ewing's sarcoma	Appropriate morbid anatomy Small to medium cells, PAS +ve	Mitoses	+ve leucocyte common antigen VMA +ve

REFERENCES

Berlin, O., Angervall, L., Kindblom, L.-G., Berlin, I.C. and Stener, B. (1987) Primary leiomyosarcoma of bone. A clinical, radiographic, pathologic-anatomic, and prognostic study of 16 cases. *Skeletal Radiol.*, **16**, 364–76.

Catto, M. and Stevens, J. (1963) Liposarcoma of bone. *J. Pathol. Bacteriol.*, **86**, 248–53.

de la Monte, S.M., Dorfman, H.D., Chandra, R. and Malawer, M. (1984) Intraosseous schwannoma: histologic features, ultrastructure, and review of the literature. *Hum. Pathol.*, **15**, 551–8.

Downey, E.F. Jr, Worsham, G.F. and Brower, A.C. (1982) Liposarcoma of bone with osteosarcomatous foci: case report and review of the literature. *Skeletal Radiol.*, **8**, 47–50.

Goldman, R.L. (1964) Primary liposarcoma of bone. Report of a case. *Am. J. Clin. Pathol.*, **42**, 503–8.

Hunt, J.C. and Pugh, D.G. (1961) Skeletal lesions in neurofibromatosis. *Radiology*, **76**, 1–20.

Inoue, H., Tsuneyoshi, M., Enjoji, M., Shinohara, N. and Yokoyama, K. (1986) Giant-cell reparative granuloma of the thoracic vertebra. *Acta Pathol. Jpn*, **36**, 745–50.

Kameda, N., Kagesawa, M., Hiruta, N., Akima, M., Ohki, M. and Matsumoto, T. (1987) Primary leiomyosarcoma of bone. A case report and review of the literature. *Acta Pathol. Jpn*, **37**, 291–303.

Lin, C.L. and Huang, T.S. (1989) Giant cell reparative granuloma in temporal bone – Report of a case. *Chang Keng I Hsueh*, **12**, 62–6.

Ross, C.F. and Hadfield, G. (1968) Primary osteoliposarcoma of bone (malignant mesenchymoma). Report of a case. *J. Bone Joint Surg.*, **50B**, 639–43.

Sanerkin, N.G., Mott, M.G. and Roylance, J. (1983) An unusual osseous lesion with fibroblastic, osteoclastic, osteoblastic, aneurysmal and fibromyxoid elements. 'Solid' variant of aneurysmal bone cyst. *Cancer*, **51**, 2278–86.

Schwartz A., Shuster, M. and Becker, S.M. (1970) Liposarcoma of bone. Report of a case and review of the literature. *J. Bone Joint Surg.*, **52A**, 171–7.

Siqueira, E., Tsung, J.S., Al-Kawi, M.Z. and Woodhouse, N. (1989) Case report: Idiopathic giant cell granuloma of the hypophysis: An unusual cause of hypopituitarism. *Surg. Neurol.*, **32**, 68–71.

Smith, R., Walton, R.J., Corner, B.D. and Gordon, I.R.S. (1977) Clinical and biochemical studies in Engelmann's disease (progressive diaphyseal dysplasia). *Q. J. Med.*, **46**, 273–94.

Sparkes, R.S. and Graham, C.B. (1972) Camurati-Engelmann disease. Genetics and clinical manifestations with a review of the literature. *J. Med. Genet.*, **9**, 73–85.

Thomas, I.H., Chow, C.W. and Cole, W.G. (1988) Giant cell reparative granuloma of the humerus. *J. Pediat. Orthop.*, **8**, 596–8.

IMAGING PROCEDURES IN ORTHOPAEDIC PATHOLOGY

Dennis J. Stoker

A variety of ways exists in which the skeletal pathologist can make use of X-ray films and other images to provide information which can be an invaluable complement to histopathological interpretation. This aid can be classified into anatomical location, pathological information and radiological experience.

4.1 THE CHOICE OF IMAGING METHODS

Now, almost a century since the discovery of X-rays, imaging techniques have changed dramatically. Nevertheless, in orthopaedics, in both clinical work and in pathological practice, the plain radiograph still provides the essential information required for management of the patient's disorder. The average pathologist is rarely going to gain access to more than a radiograph of the part from which tissue has been removed, so that other information, such as the presence of subtle abnormality or further lesions will usually have to be communicated through the radiologist's report or by a specific request; it is clearly also important that an expert radiological opinion is provided as to whether other lesions which may be found are likely to be of the same nature as that under primary examination.

The **radiograph** still remains the chief means of determining the rate of growth of a lesion, by reason of its ability to record subtle destruction of the cortex and, to a lesser degree, the medulla as well as the zone of transition between normal and abnormal bone – a feature that indicates the aggressive character of the pathological process.

Nevertheless, the metabolic activity of bony destruction and renewal is best demonstrated by bone **scintigraphy** because the uptake of the radionuclide is related both to the vascularity and to the metabolic activity in the bone and the adjoining soft tissues. Unfortunately scintigraphy, although highly sensitive, is also very non-specific. Further, the activity shown may not coincide with the pathologist's assessment of histological activity; for example, an apparently indolent region of fibrous dysplasia may show a moderate increase in scintigraphic activity.

The introduction of the various methods of computed transaxial imaging has enabled the portrayal of further anatomical features for the radiologist. Because a radiograph is simply a two-dimensional reproduction of a three-dimensional object, such tomographic methods as computed tomography (CT) and magnetic resonance imaging (MRI) have proved invaluable in demonstrating the changes occurring deep within the bone and differentiating them from overlying surface change. Thus it may be important for establishment of the diagnosis to know whether the matrix of a tumour is partially mineralized or not; this can be demonstrated by CT.

All current magnetic resonance (MR) imaging is dependent upon the imaging of hydrogen nuclei. As hydrogen in the body is predominantly contained in water and over 70% of our bodies are composed of water, to all intents and purposes the signal provided will reflect the water content; biochemical changes of disease, which often alter the water content, can hence be identified by this technique.

4.2 MECHANISMS OF IMAGING METHODS

It is fortunate that the various methods for imaging the body tissues function through different physical processes as this ensures that in the main they are complementary. Because of the adverse effects of ionizing radiation, the exposure of patients to X-rays at any time cannot be viewed with equanimity; indeed, if the medical applications of ultrasound and magnetic resonance had been discovered before X-rays, the additional implementation of X-ray diagnosis might well have been regarded as an unjustifiably hazardous step, in terms of irradiating the patient.

X-rays, including those employed in CT, produce an image by the attenuation of a beam of rays as it passes through the body in proportion to the density and depth of the tissue; thus cortical bone absorbs a maximal amount of X-rays and air a minimal amount. Most of the body's soft tissues are of water density and therefore cannot be distinguished on their characteristics of attenuation alone. Muscular bundles therefore are only identified by the presence of intervening adipose tissue; such fatty interposition also provides the means whereby we can determine the margins of tumoural extension from bone on the plain radiograph. CT differs only in its potential to quantify the attenuation and thereby sometimes to differentiate tumour from normal muscle; the margins may not, however, be clearly depicted as inflammatory or peritumoural oedema and compression of normal tissue often also coexists.

Most X-ray examinations are mediated through the use of a phosphor contained on a screen or screens within a light-tight cassette. This makes possible a reduction in the amount of radiation to expose the film; the disadvantage is that the phosphor crystal produces a greater amount of silver blackening and hence fine detail is lost to some degree. For the pathologist producing a radiograph of a specimen, control of radiation to the subject is not a matter of importance (and neither is the time of exposure as patient movement is negligible!) and a fine detail industrial film can therefore be used with improvement of the quality of reproduction.

Ultrasound also involves transmission of waves through soft tissue but these are of longer wavelength and do not penetrate bone; hence its use is mainly to demonstrate the presence of a soft tissue mass rather than its character. The margins of bones can be shown in particular circumstances, enabling the relationship of certain soft tissues to the deeper bony structure to be established; however, the accuracy of appositional relationship by this technique cannot be as accurate as that of computed tomography or magnetic resonance imaging.

Skeletal **scintigraphy** necessitates the intravenous injection of a bone-seeking radionuclide (usually technetium-99m labelled with a phosphorus-containing compound, e.g. methylene diphosphonate).

Uptake depends upon:

1. increased vascularity permitting greater concentration of the agent in the extracellular fluid of the bone;
2. osteoblastic activity within the bone or its environs.

Thus the concentration of the tracer within the skeleton can be recorded by a gamma camera revealing normal, increased or even reduced uptake in any particular region or bone.

Radionuclide scintigraphy differs from all other imaging techniques mentioned here in that it is a reflection of cellular activity; it can thus be of value in differentiating a latent lesion from one that is active. Scintigraphy is an extremely sensitive method but has poor spatial resolution. It also shows poor specificity in that it is not possible to distinguish between the vascularity of infection and neoplasia, nor between the reactive osteoblastic changes of trauma or healing disease.

In a similar way to scintigraphy **magnetic resonance imaging** (MRI) depends on a signal emanating from the tissues and not a transmitted wave or ray. As mentioned above, at the present time in clinical practice, only the hydrogen nucleus is imaged, so that it can be said that it is the variation in water content within a tissue or region that is being studied. The production of an image requires a strong magnetic field, an intermittent radiofrequency pulse and a period of relaxation after terminating the radiofrequency pulse, during which a signal can be recorded from the energized hydrogen ions. Many different MR pulse sequences can be used to emphasize the differences in the relaxation curves of different tissues. Computation of the multiple signals produced within a slice of tissue enables an image to be made. MRI therefore records the chemical milieu of the protons in the volume of tissue that is being imaged; as indicated, the signal can be varied by using and manipulating a variety of predetermined sequences.

MRI is measuring and recording different attributes of the tissues compared to CT. Although it is both sensitive and has great contrast resolution for the soft tissues, it is, however, not able to produce a tissue diagnosis except in the most limited of situations. Initially, it was thought to have only a limited application in orthopaedics because of the fact that cortical bone and dense fibrous tissue, e.g. tendons, give virtually no signal; this has not proved to be a restriction to any significant degree, because of the definitive and generally brighter signal of the adjoining tissues.

4.3 PROVISION OF ANATOMICAL INFORMATION

In the case of small biopsies of osseous lesions, radiographs generally provide the osteoarticular histopathologist with a sound indication of the gross anatomy of the bony and soft tissue features and the relation of the pathological lesion to them. This information can be enhanced if the surgeon can advise about the location from where he obtained the tissue so that this can be related to the radiograph or perhaps even demonstrated on a post-biopsy radiograph. This information would certainly be available where the biopsy had been undertaken under some form of imaging control. However, if the histology of the tissue obtained bears no relationship to the radiological appearance, then it is quite possible that a different region has been sampled; for example, if the lesion is shown to be uniformly mineralized and yet neither calcification nor tissue with potential for mineralization is found, then it is clear that a representative sample cannot have been obtained. In these circumstances the pathologist is entitled to recommend a further biopsy.

Further anatomical information can be obtained when the whole operative specimen becomes available. In-house X-rays by the pathologist's team can prove useful in recording the location and disposal of sections from a large specimen.

4.3.1 GENERAL CONSIDERATIONS ABOUT THE RADIOLOGICAL DIFFERENTIAL DIAGNOSIS

When, during the course of examining and interpreting a section, the pathologist turns to the patient's X-ray film, he will need to consider the differential diagnosis, as he has throughout his medical career. The use of an appropriate 'surgical sieve' will not necessarily provide a diagnosis, but it will ensure that all possibilities are considered. The presence of multiple lesions offers a smaller number of options than the solitary lesion even though one must remember that the presence of other lesions in the skeleton is not always known or broadcast.

4.4 INFORMATION ABOUT THE PATHOLOGICAL PROCESS

Considering that the natural contrast on a radiograph is dependent on three tissue elements – calcium (bone), soft tissue and fat – with a fourth (air) being rarely of any importance in skeletal practice, the amount of information provided on a plain X-ray film is remarkable. Fortunately, the information provided by the disciplines of pathology and radiology are complementary. Imaging can rarely provide a histologically accurate diagnosis with confidence although this can often be inferred by the accuracy with which the rate of growth is apparent to the experienced skeletal radiologist (Figure 4.1). Conversely, the histopathologist cannot always directly determine the rate of growth of the lesion,

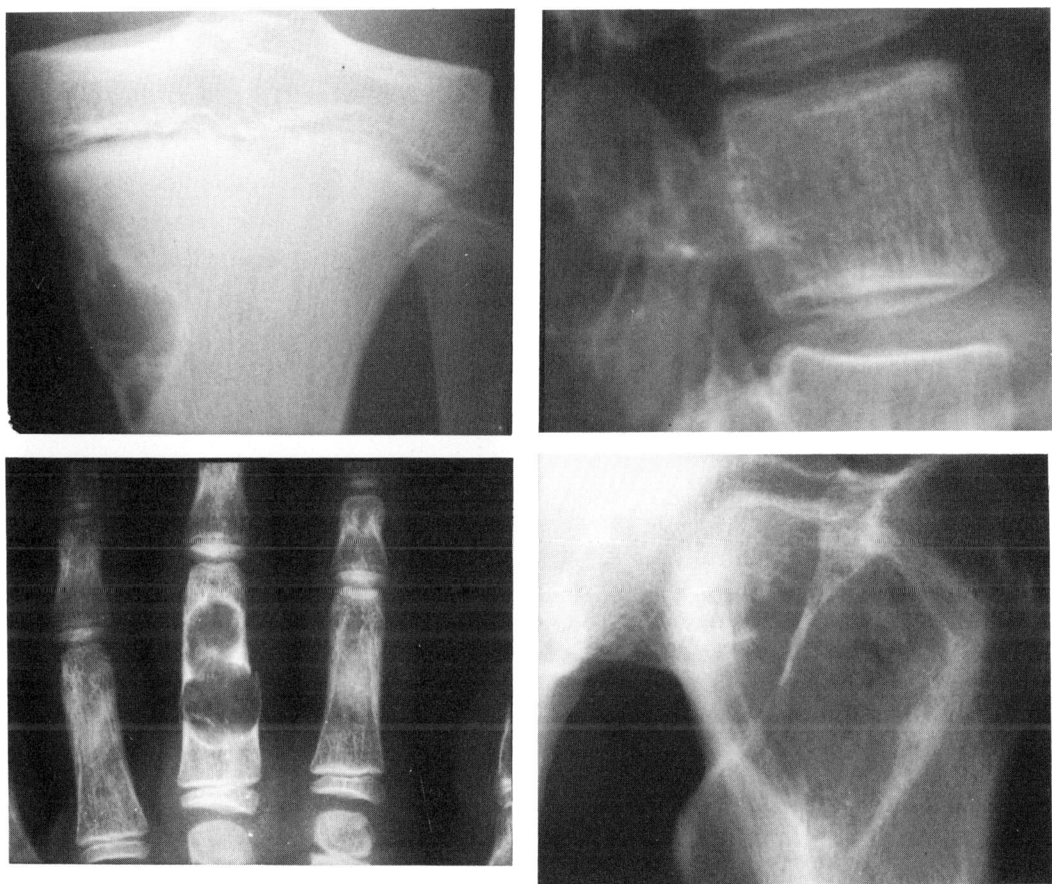

Figure 4.1 Leave me alone lesions. The radiologist can be expected to make a confident diagnosis of all these lesions and indicate that they are latent or extremely slowly growing benign disorders. Biopsy would not be required unless there were to be evidence of complication or unexpected pain, i.e. not due to evident injury.

but can infer it from the cell type seen under the microscope.

4.4.1   CONGENITAL AND DEVELOPMENTAL LESIONS

Such lesions are often generalized, multifocal or regionally located. The systemic osteochondrodysplasias, such as achondroplasia, can only be diagnosed radiologically and need a full skeletal study tailored for bone dysplasias; in the newborn or stillborn infant, this involves an X-ray film of the whole child, preferably in the AP (anteroposterior) and lateral projections. The need for routine radiography of all stillborn infants in this group cannot be overemphasized as correct genetic counselling may depend upon it. In certain disorders, such as the mucopolysaccharidoses, biochemical information is necessary for the final diagnosis; in others, refinement of the diagnosis may depend on chromosomal studies. Although radiological information constitutes the primary database for diagnosis of bone dysplasias, even experts in this narrow field have considerable difficulties and subdivisions of syndromes may depend primarily on the pattern of inheritance.

A number of developmental conditions have diagnostic features in their distribution in the skeleton and even within an affected bone. For example, in enchondromatosis (Ollier's disease) the disorder usually affects the limbs on one side of the body and one side of the affected bone; also, because the anarchic chondroid response occurs within the period of metaphyseal growth, the lytic cartilaginous lesion becomes extended and flame-shaped.

Solitary or regional bony dysplasias are also diagnosed in the main radiologically (Figure 4.2). The longstanding nature of the deformity and its presentation in childhood may help in the diagnosis as may the presence of features affecting other systems, such as the presence of café-au-lait spots in neurofibromatosis.

4.4.2   TRAUMA

A history of trauma is often helpful, but may be a mixed blessing. Patients often need to relate the pain or swelling they experience to some incident and give undue emphasis to a

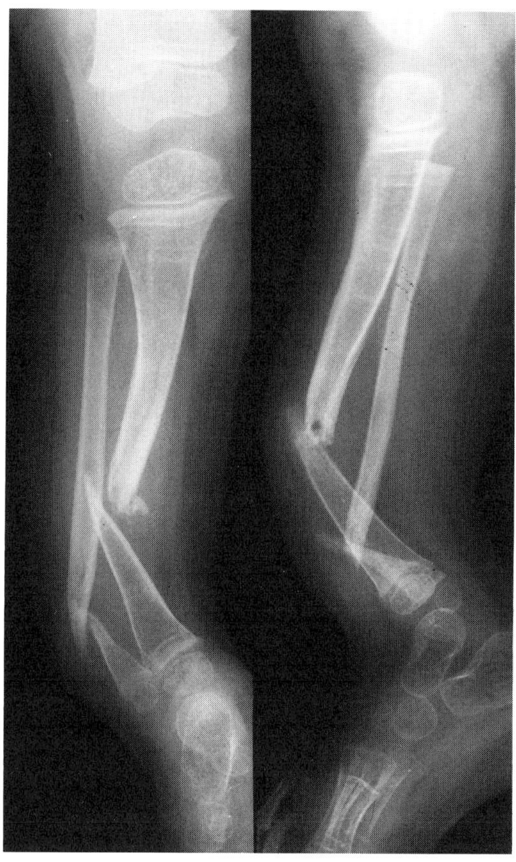

Figure 4.2 Pseudarthroses of tibia and fibula in neurofibromatosis. The discontinuity of the shafts of both bones of the leg is unlike a simple fracture as the ends are resorbed and tapered. The tibial shaft is the most common site for pseudarthrosis in this condition, the condition being brought to light by pathological fracture and failure of callus formation and healing. It should be observed that the proximal part of the shaft of the tibia is also abnormal, showing a varus inclination.

past injury. Conversely, the trauma may have been forgotten in the heat of the physical activity; this is particularly so in the case of soft tissue haematomas sustained in contact sports, which at a later date consequently may unwisely be biopsied on the basis of misinterpreted radiographic appearances (Figure 4.3). Although the pathologist may find evidence of a healing injury, all too often a limited biopsy provides evidence only of reactive change without a clear indication of the provoking cause. The radiograph, however, will often provide a clear manifestation of either a fracture within part of the lesion, or an indication that trauma is the likely cause because of the location and associated radiological features (Figure 4.4). Most fractures are easily identified, but most fractures are not the subject of biopsy so, almost by definition, the traumatic lesion the patholo-

gist receives will not have been recognized as such by the referring surgeon. Commonly therefore the pathologist will receive callus from a mineralizing lesion, misdiagnosed as a tumour, or a healing incremental fracture, perhaps of the sacrum in a postmenopausal woman, where metastasis is suspected. It may be that the clinician has not discussed the matter with the radiologist who has thus not had the opportunity to suggest a further and perhaps definitive imaging examination. Concern by the pathologist that the lesion may have a traumatic basis may lead to reappraisal of the schedule of investigations. A recurring problem is that of the stress fracture mistaken for osteosarcoma. The histopathologist should expect support from the radiologist in such a circumstance.

Particular areas of difficulty include avulsion injuries in the reparative phase when

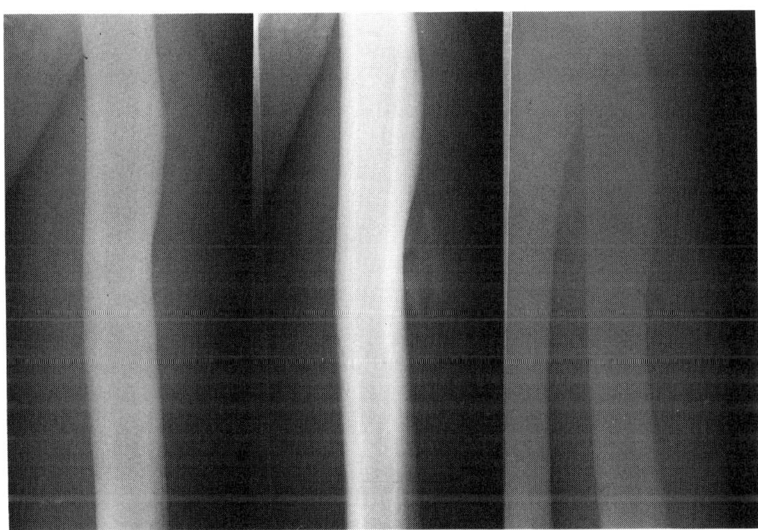

Figure 4.3 Ossifying haematoma. The initial film on the left, taken at presentation, shows only faint mineralization in the soft tissues distal to the deltoid tubercle where the patient, a young footballer, complained of a tender swelling. The other two films were taken respectively two and four weeks after the first and show maturing new bone adjacent to the humerus. This appearance is not in keeping with the alternative clinical diagnosis of a bone-forming tumour of soft tissue. It is important that this diagnosis is borne in mind and the temptation to undertake biopsy is resisted in the short term, thus avoiding anxiety and unnecessary scarring in the patient as well as unnecessary worry to the non-skeletal histopathologist.

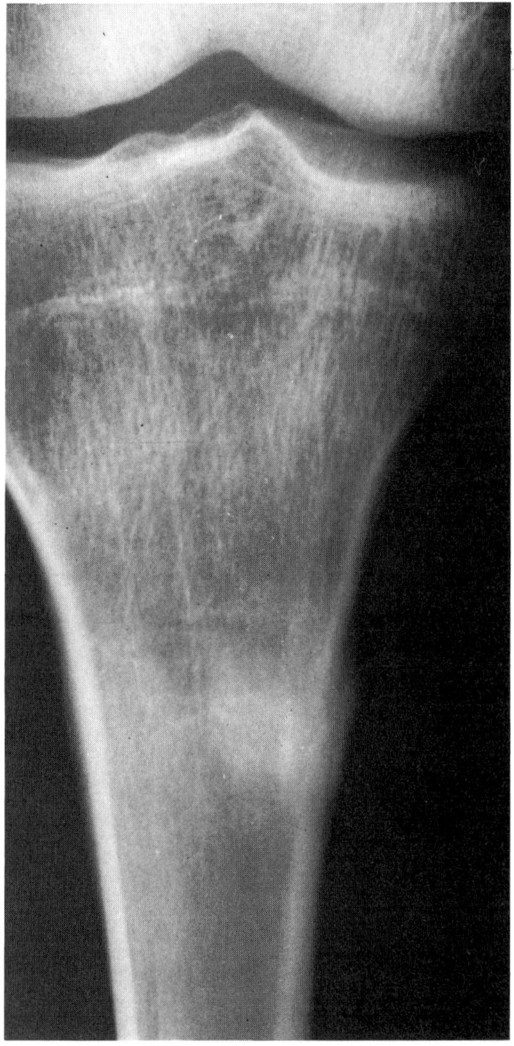

Figure 4.4 Stress fracture of proximal shaft of tibia. Stress fractures should be suspected because of characteristic locations, as in this patient. Other supportive features include simple linear periosteal reaction and a linear element to the lesion. Here the reactive endosteal change seems to be transverse and this might be supported by a similar horizontal uptake on scintigraphy or even MRI; CT is unlikely to assist as the section is in the plane of the fracture. If doubt still exists, it is entirely appropriate to defer biopsy for two weeks or so, when the repeat radiograph should show maturation rather than further destruction.

there may be considerable reactive new bone formation. Pragmatically, little adverse effect on the prognosis of a sarcoma will follow a wait of two weeks, but this may be sufficient time for the radiograph of an ossifying injury to show clear evidence of healing of a fracture or ossifying haematoma, with maturation of the reparative bone.

4.4.3 INFECTION

The problems of the traumatic lesion are mirrored in osteomyelitis when the tissue obtained contains none of the diagnostic inflammatory material necessary for a confident diagnosis of infection. Osteomyelitis is a permeative process, usually beginning in the medulla of a long bone or at the disco-vertebral junction (Figure 4.5). In children, the typical location is in the metaphysis of a long bone, from whence the infection may cross the growth plate. Radiologically, the differential diagnosis may be that of a permeating tumour. Reaction of the host bone may be similar, producing little endosteal change in the first instance, but linear periosteal reaction and often a soft tissue extension. The margins of an infective soft tissue mass, showing inflammatory oedema, are usually ill-defined whereas a tumour mass is well-defined because the peritumoural oedema is less. The radiological evidence of an inconclusive diagnosis and the absence of a causative organism may encourage the histopathologist to advise a more extensive repeat biopsy. Such a problem is most often encountered in the case of chronic sclerosing osteomyelitis (Garre); the histopathological opinion here is critical as such an infection is associated with few residual organisms and hence culture is often negative. In our experience, an unsound diagnosis of infection may be made in lymphoma of bone (Figure 4.6) either because infection coexists or, equally, because inflammatory changes alone are present in the biopsy specimen.

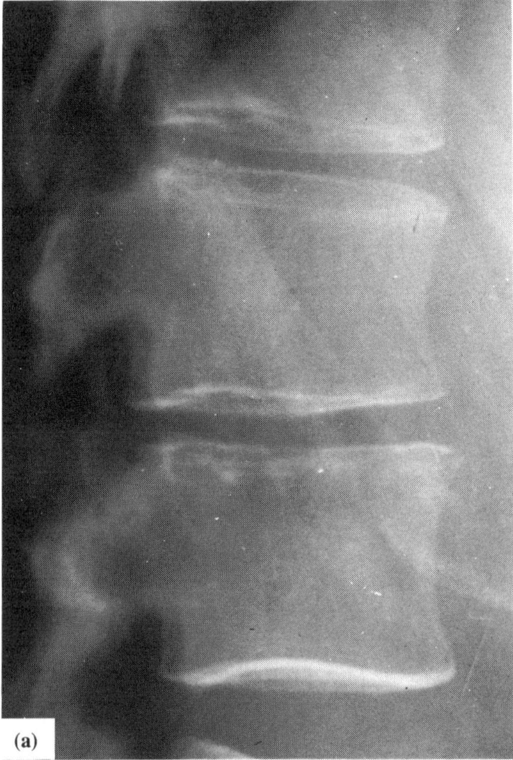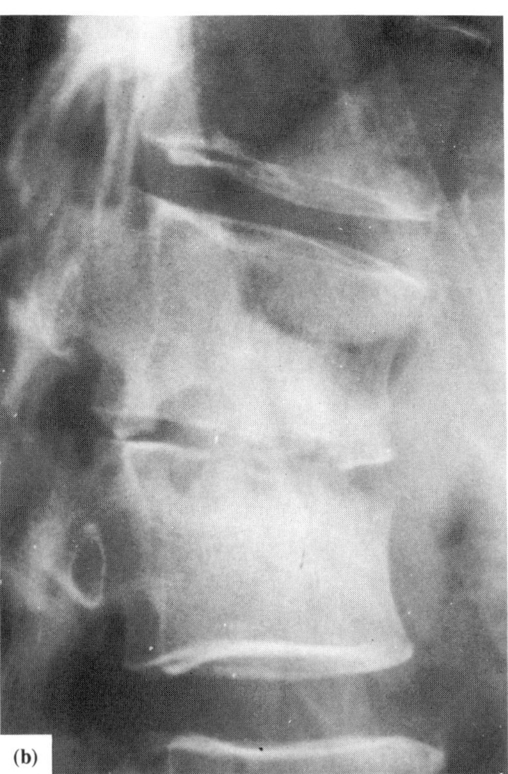

Figure 4.5 Spondylodiscitis of thoracic spine. (a) The disc space is narrowed and there is some loss of definition of the upper vertebral plate of the adjoining vertebra; this is typical of early radiological change in osteomyelitis of the spine. (b) Several weeks later further loss of discal height is complemented by erosion of the anterior two-thirds of the vertebral end-plate; this has caused some kyphotic deformity. Observe also the sclerotic reaction of the adjoining bone on both sides of the disc.

In the spine, infection generally spreads rapidly into the intervertebral disc and in so doing destroys the subchondral cortex of the centrum (Figure 4.7). Tumours usually are slower in attacking the disc and the disc spaces are therefore preserved for weeks or months, whereas the vertebral body may collapse as a consequence of the infiltration.

4.4.4 DEGENERATIVE DISORDERS AND OSTEONECROSIS

Degenerative changes in the joints and subchondral bone and the intervertebral discs and their vertebral margins rarely offer a problem to the histopathologist in differen-tial diagnosis. Occasionally the radiological appearance of a chronic degenerative disc lesion may resemble low-grade or burnt-out infective spondylodiscitis (Figure 4.8). The radiologist may need the pathologist's confirmatory support because the 'degenerative' changes with a sclerotic reaction may mask an underlying cause; this is seen in pigmented villonodular synovitis of the hip where, in contrast to response to the disorder in other locations, articular cartilage may be destroyed at an early stage with appearances resembling 'primary' osteoarthrosis.

No radiological change on the plain film is discernible at the time of bone death or for 6–8 weeks thereafter. Early confirmation of

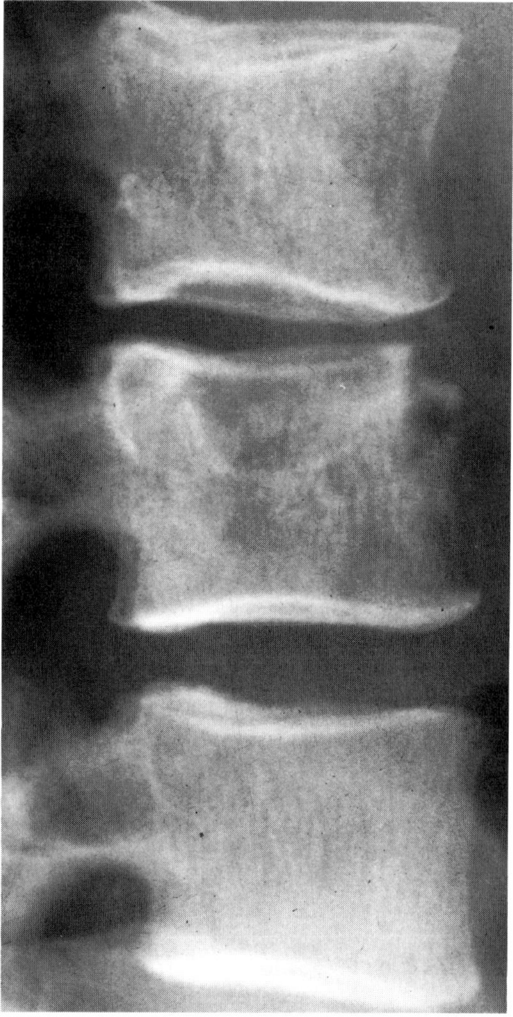

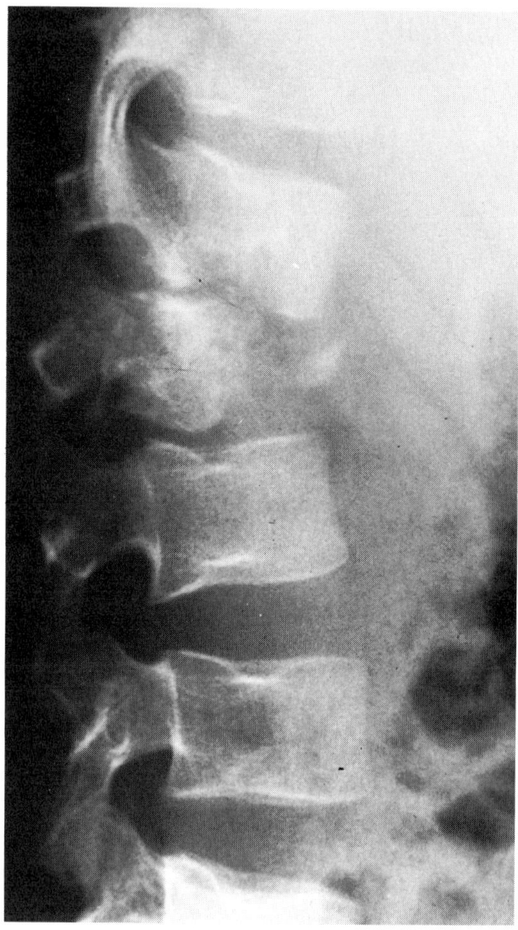

Figure 4.7 Salmonella osteomyelitis in sickle-cell disease. The changes at T12 and L1 indicate destruction of the disc and the adjoining vertebral body – a feature of infective spondylodiscitis. The presence of flat-topped indentations of the vertebral endplates at several levels indicates central infarction and is almost pathognomonic of sickle-cell disease.

Figure 4.6 Hodgkin's disease of vertebral body. A mixed lytic and sclerotic lesion affects the upper half of the affected vertebra. Observe also the anterior vertebral erosion, which is characteristic of Hodgkin's disease and may be associated with involvement of adjoining prevertebral lymph nodes. The disc space above is narrowed, but unlike in osteomyelitis, the endplate is not eroded; it is likely that the process so weakened the endplate that the nucleus pulposus prolapsed into the vertebra.

the presence of avascular necrosis requires the use of bone scintigraphy or MRI, both of which methods are accurate within the first week of discontinuation of the blood supply. Radiographic changes occur with revascularization of the bone and 'creeping substitution' of the dead trabeculae; such changes, to the radiologist, may rarely suggest reaction from other causes, e.g. infection, trauma or benign tumour. A case in point would be

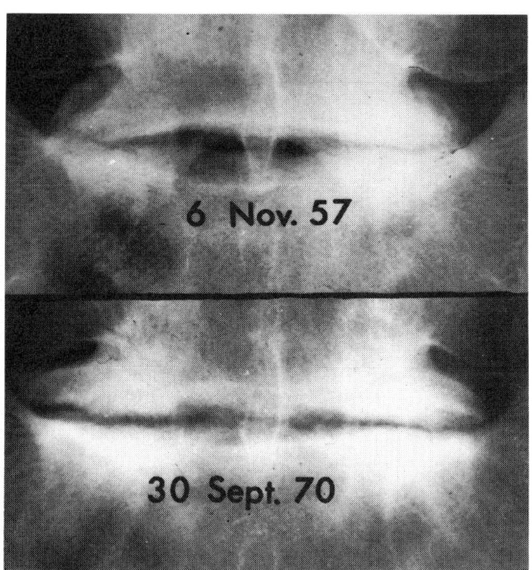

Figure 4.8 Degenerative spondylosis. Serial films show progressive reduction in height of the lumbosacral intervertebral disc space. Coupled with this, the adjoining vertebral bodies show stress sclerosis and the marginal osteophytes have increased.

when the presence of medullary infarction leads to an appearance more suggestive of a chondroid tumour than osteonecrosis and MR imaging may be needed to provide additional diagnostic information. Fortunately, in most circumstances, the location and characteristics of the sclerosis will indicate the true diagnosis.

4.4.5 METABOLIC DISEASE OF BONE

In this group of diseases, as a support for the histopathologist, radiology comes only second to biochemical assessment of the patient.

Changes are usually generalized with the presence, usually, of osteopenia. Only three major disorders exist – osteoporosis, osteomalacia and hyperparathyroidism – although these may co-exist. The plain film is notoriously inaccurate for assessing bone density,

hence the introduction of qualitative CT (QCT) and dual-energy X-ray absorptiometry (DXA) for accurate quantitative assessment of bone content, especially in **osteoporosis**, where bone mass is reduced but the bone is otherwise normal. Disorders such as myelomatosis, where the presentation may also be with generalized osteopenia, have generally to be excluded by other means, biochemical or histological.

Although assessment of osteoporosis from the plain radiograph is bedevilled by observer error and technical variation, serial complications such as incremental fractures or vertebral compression can readily be identified. These will also be demonstrated nonspecifically by bone scintigraphy.

In **osteomalacia**, in theory the reduction of bone mineralization should produce some diagnostic features; in practice the visual assessment of bony density is fraught with difficulties and has been proven in countless studies to be quite inaccurate. This results from the variations in body build and in radiographic technique that can exist. The changes that are present in osteomalacia consist of osteopenia, a diminution of the clarity of the trabecular pattern and the presence of Looser's zones (Figure 4.9). The radiological diagnosis of osteomalacia depends on the identification of these latter lesions (pseudofractures) which fortunately usually produce increased uptake on bone scintigraphy. If there is no focal symptom to indicate a particular site this should be X-rayed as the lesions are often painful, but a whole-body assessment by radionuclide scintigraphy is preferable to a radiographic skeletal survey, which constitutes a greater dosage of ionizing radiation.

Although sometimes resembling stress fractures, Looser's zones do not involve exactly the same locations and do not produce much callus, although pseudofractures can progress to true fractures and both types of lesions can heal with minimal callus formation.

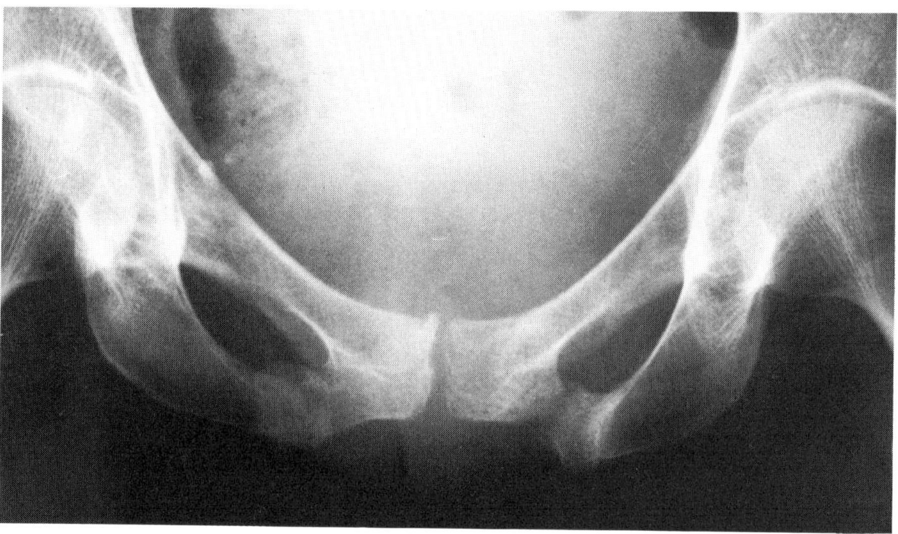

Figure 4.9 Osteomalacia. The breaks in the lower ischiopubic rami are Looser's zones and the only characteristic radiological feature of osteomalacia. That on the patient's left is the more typical, being several millimetres wide and, unlike a fracture, it shows no callus formation.

These limitations apply to the diagnosis of osteomalacia in the adult; the radiological features of osteomalacia in the child (rickets) are generally diagnostic, although it rarely is possible to suggest the cause of the disorder from X-ray appearances alone. The changes in rickets affect the metaphyses where growth is most active although skeletal growth is generally delayed. The failure of normal mineralization at the growing metaphyses causes an apparent widening of the growth plate and the consequent weakness of these structures leads to widening and cupping of the metaphyses with normal activity (Figure 4.10). Thus the earliest changes in the preschool child affect the wrist; later in childhood the knees are maximally involved. In the relatively common osteomalacia affecting the Asian adolescent and young adult arriving in the Northern hemisphere, one should look for the changes in the still open growth plates of apophyses such as those of the iliac crests.

Hyperparathyroidism of both the primary and secondary variety is characterized by osteopenia and subperiosteal erosion of the cortices. Of course generalized osteoclasis takes place in a wide number of locations, but the loss of the sharp cortical margin is easiest to discern on X-ray of the hands, especially in the phalanges where the grossest changes are usual present on the radial side of the middle phalanx of the index finger. Recognition here really only reflects the ability to produce a clear radiograph on a high definition film-screen combination because of the small size of the part and the lack of much surrounding soft tissue.

Hyperparathyroidism presents an occasional pitfall for both the pathologist and the radiologist. To the former, a focal region of active osteitis fibrosa may resemble a giant cell tumour; such a 'brown tumour' (Figure 4.11) usually does not have the radiological characteristics of a giant cell tumour and the radiologist is more likely to opt for another differential diagnosis, such as metastasis. Radiological demonstration of multiple lesions, subperiosteal erosion, generally increased skeletal uptake on scintigraphy

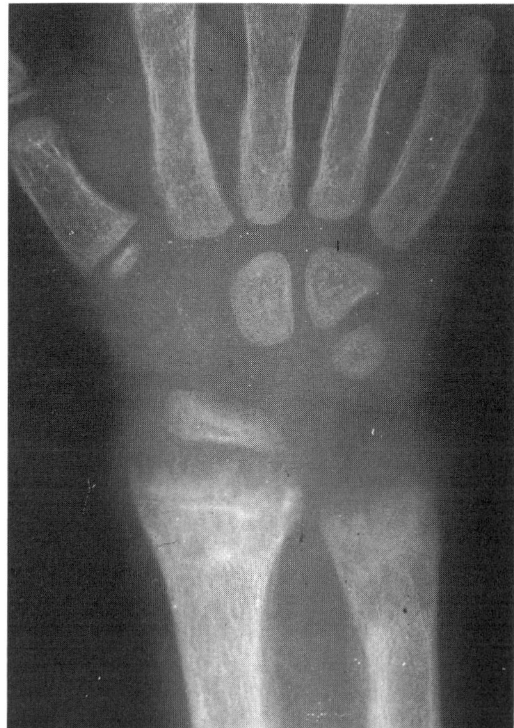

Figure 4.10 Rickets. Delayed skeletal maturation is present in this 5-year-old child. Apparent widening of the radial growth plate is due to undermineralization of the metaphysis. Both the radial and ulnar metaphyses are ragged and splayed. These features are common to all forms of rickets. The child in this case was West Indian, possibly implicating reduced exposure to sunlight, but was also epileptic and on treatment with phenytoin and other anticonvulsants which are known to induce liver enzymes that convert Vitamin D to less-active metabolites.

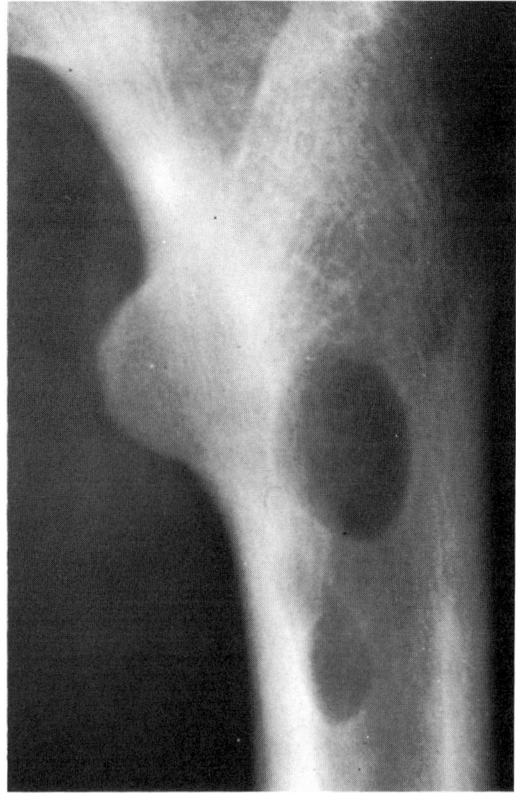

Figure 4.11 'Brown tumours' of hyperparathyroidism. Several well-demarcated cyst-like lesions are present in the femoral shaft. Perhaps unusually, no other skeletal abnormality suggests the diagnosis of osteitis fibrosa. The radiological differential diagnosis might include metastases or subacute abscesses.

and inappropriate appearance and location of the lesions will suggest the correct diagnosis and lead to a request for biochemical confirmation.

4.4.6 THE SPACE-OCCUPYING SOLITARY LESION OF BONE

In most cases the osteoarticular pathologist will need the assistance of radiology when confronted with a tumour or tumour-like disorder of bone. Apart from the pathological specimen, he or she hopefully shares with the radiologist the following valuable clinical information:

- Age of the patient
- Site of the lesion
- Presence of painful symptoms relating to the lesion
- Information about previous surgery

Usually the film or a radiological opinion will be available before the report is issued and it is important that the histopathologist should insist on the provision of a plain radiograph (Figure 4.12) and a radiological opinion. The essential task is the correlation of the radiological findings with the provisional histological diagnosis. If the radiological appearance is supportive then no problem exists; if there is a contradiction, then the radiological differential diagnosis must be compared with the pathological one, to see if common ground exists. In this way a diagnosis acceptable to both disciplines may be found, or at least, the divergences of opinion can be aired. On the relatively unusual occasion when the radiologist cannot accept the diagnosis of the pathologist, the latter must proceed with caution on the basis that the specimen provided may not be representative of the whole pathological process, as visualized by the radiologist. Such dialogues must be based on regular discussions and mutual respect between the specialists, if the end point is going to be an improvement in the management of the patient.

Faced with the plain film, the main local features are noted by the radiologist:

- Size of the lesion
- A mainly lytic or sclerotic appearance
- Marginal sclerosis and extent
- Width of transition zone between normal and abnormal bone, presence or absence of periosteal new bone formation and type
- Presence or absence of a soft tissue mass and, if present, the clarity of its definition

The radiologist's training leads to the use of these features to reach a conclusion as to the benignity or aggression of the lesion, based primarily on the well-established concepts laid down by Lodwick *et al.* (1980). Aggression is a better term than malignancy for this conclusion, because perhaps less than the pathologist, the radiologist is not able to detect a likelihood that any particular tumour will metastasize and, for example, a giant cell tumour may appear radiologically

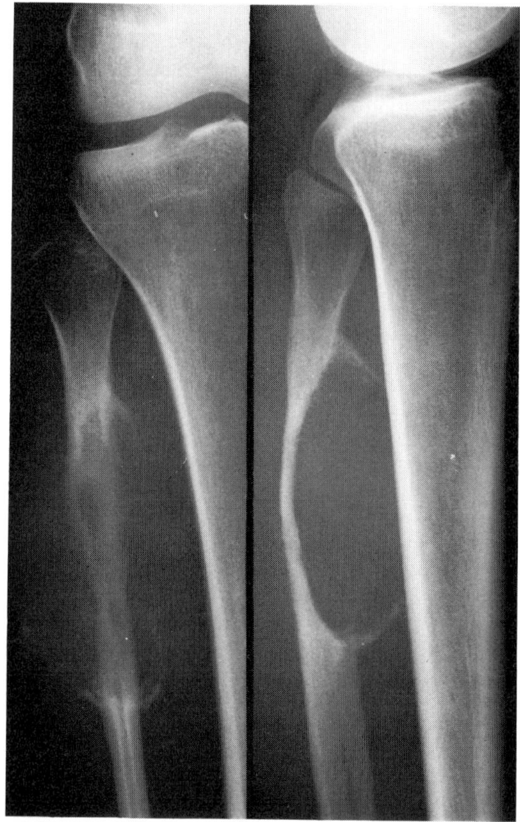

Figure 4.12 Aneurysmal bone cyst of the fibula. The eccentric expanding lesion of the proximal third of the shaft has produced a blister-like appearance with only a thin eggshell covering of residual cortex. Occurring here in a young adult this appearance is quite characteristic of an aneurysmal bone cyst although biopsy is required for confirmation.

quite as destructive as a metastatic carcinoma.

4.4.7   RATE OF GROWTH

The slower the rate of growth of a tumour, the greater the tissue response and subsequent remodelling of the host bone. Non-tumoural conditions such as infarction and perhaps certain monostotic forms of fibrous dysplasia cause sclerosis in the medulla with no effect on the cortex.

Slow but inexorable growth, such as is found in low-grade chondroid tumours (Figure 4.13), will lead to expansion of the cortex. The combination of pressure erosion on the endosteal surface and a variable amount of periosteal new bone being laid down results in either an unaltered or a thickened cortex (Figure 4.14); the more rapid the growth, the thinner the cortex will become with this grade of activity.

Because benign tumours, such as non-ossifying fibromas (Figure 4.15), are peripherally located in the bone, they may lead to thinning and expansion of the cortex but the endosteal margin has a well-defined thin sclerotic border also, suggesting the benignity of the lesion.

Moderate growth embraces an overlap between the aggressive benign and the low-grade malignant lesion, for example, the similar appearances of a giant cell tumour and a metastasis to bone from a renal carcinoma, so that the patient's age may be important although an overlap in prevalence may be evident in this element also.

With aggressive permeative destruction, the differential diagnosis includes metastatic carcinoma, primary sarcomas of bone (Figure 4.16) and infection; other features have to be taken into account in their differentiation.

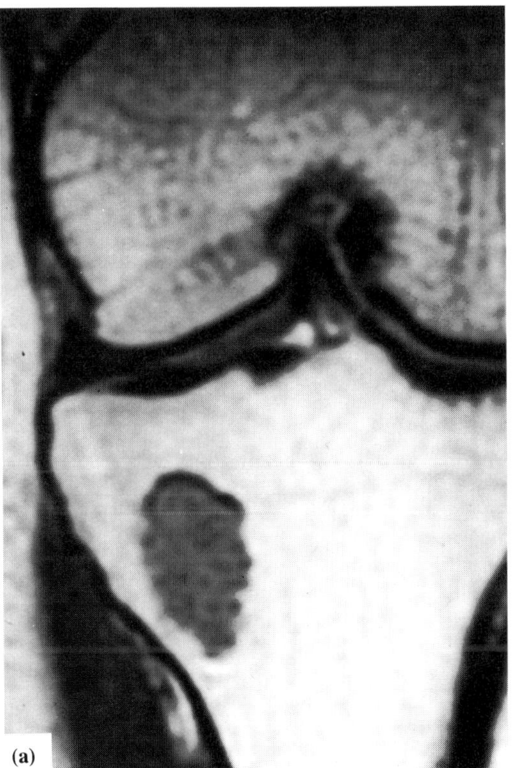

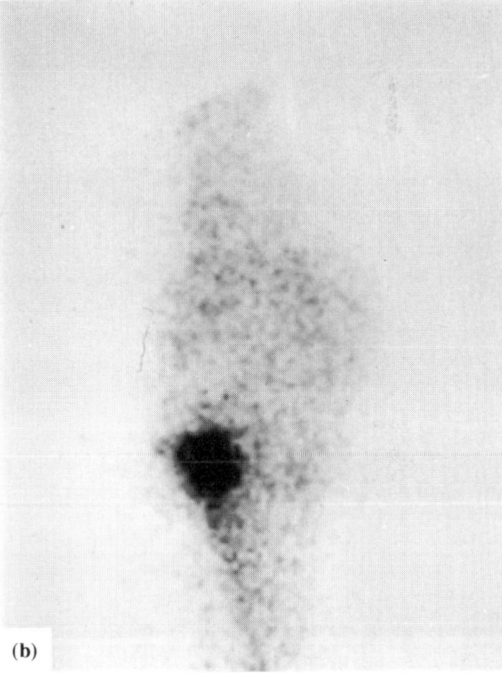

Figure 4.13 Low-grade (grade I) chondrosarcoma of proximal tibia. On this coronal T1-weighted MRI image the normal bright signal from the marrow has been replaced in the region of the medullary chondroid tumour by an intermediate signal equivalent to that of normal muscle. The lesion could not be identified on the plain radiograph (a) but showed increased uptake on bone scintigraphy (b). Such a combination is almost always an indication for CT or MRI.

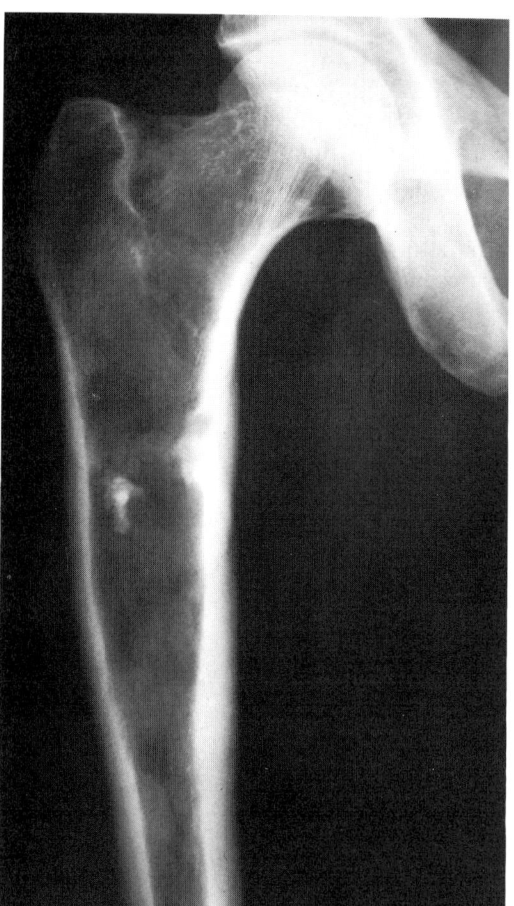

Figure 4.14 Chondrosarcoma of proximal shaft of femur. The tumour is showing a characteristic appearance in one of its most common locations. Slow growth has resulted in expansion and scalloping of the endosteal margin of the cortex. An area of popcorn-like calcification within the lytic matrix suggests the chondroid nature of the tumour. In this location the radiological differential diagnosis can often include fibrous dysplasia – another slowly growing lesion with matrix calcification.

4.4.8 SOFT TISSUE EXTENSION

Apart from distant metastasis, the main characteristic of the malignant primary, and to a lesser extent secondary, tumour of bone is spread beyond the periosteum. Such soft

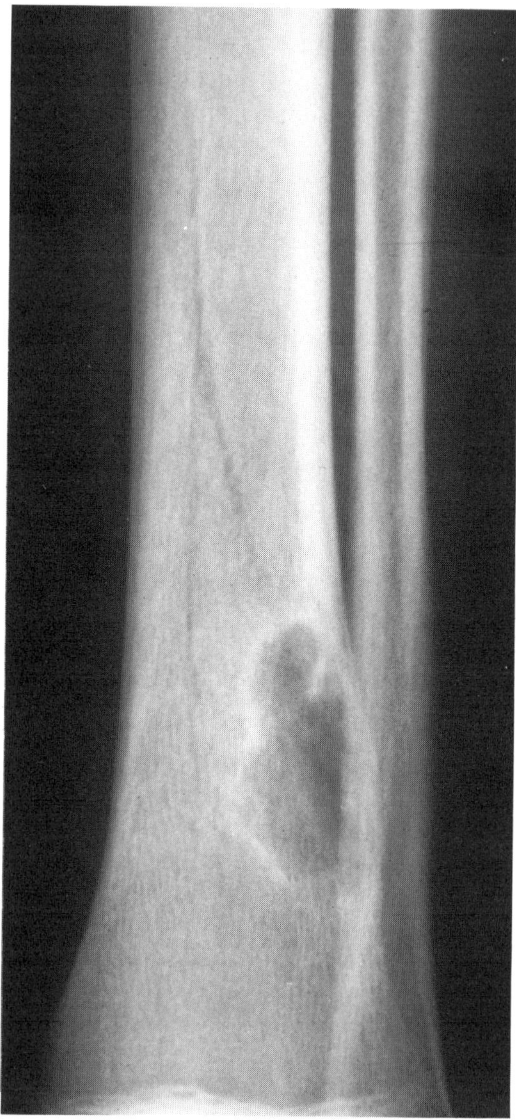

Figure 4.15 Non-ossifying fibroma of distal tibial shaft. Situated characteristically in the diametaphysis of a child or young adult, this lesion is similar to a benign cortical defect both radiologically and histologically. It is centred on the cortex and in this patient has so weakened the bone that an undisplaced spiral fracture has resulted. Note the benign feature of a lobulated sclerotic margin separating the lesion from the normal medulla.

tissue spread is characterized by a well-defined soft tissue mass outlined by the

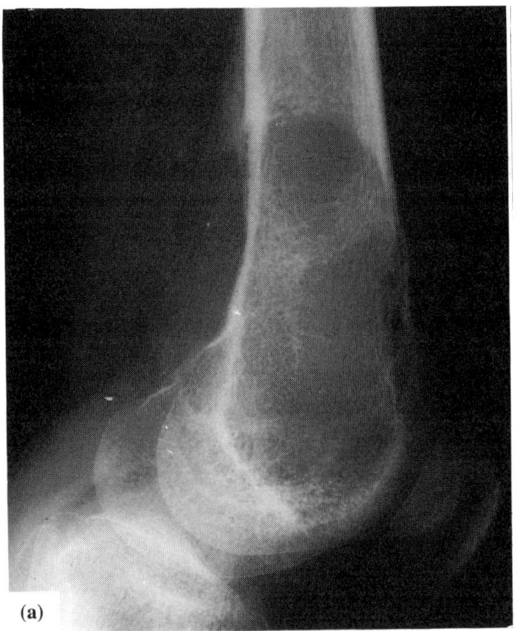
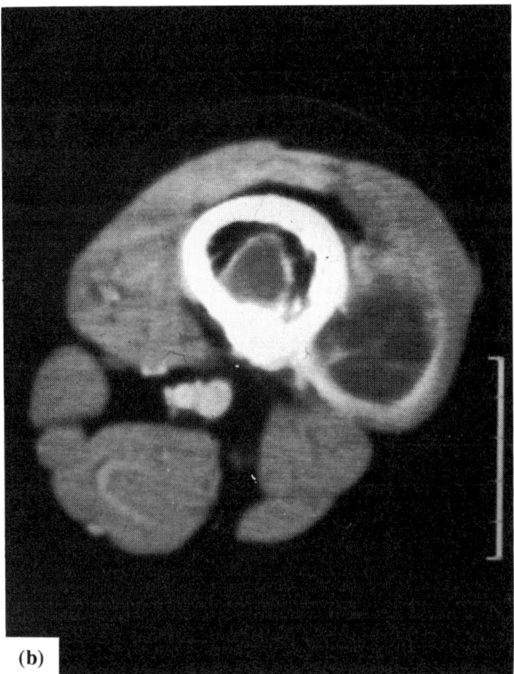

Figure 4.16 Fibroblastic osteosarcoma of distal end of femur. This 25-year-old man presented with a painful swelling above the knee. (a) The plain film shows a destructive and mainly lytic lesion with a soft tissue extension and reactive bony triangles posteriorly. (b) A CT slice at a proximal level of the lesion demonstrates that the medullary involvement is circumscribed and that the extension into the vastus lateralis has a bony margin posteriorly, it is invasive and ill-defined anteriorly. This exemplifies the increase in the spatial information that can be obtained from computed imaging.

intermuscular fat planes (Figure 4.17); because of the greater oedema, the margin of an abscess related to osteomyelitis is often ill defined. Of course, it is not possible radiologically to identify the periosteum except by inference of its relationship to the thinned cortex or to the reactive triangles at the margins of the extension from the bone.

The situation is well exemplified by the characteristics of the aneurysmal bone cyst. Although benign in nature, this lesion may enlarge rapidly; so rapidly in fact because of its expanding vascular spaces that it can be said to be growing too fast for a sarcoma that is obliged to enlarge by cellular replication. However, in most cases, the aneurysmal bone cyst retains a thin eggshell covering of bone over its bulge beyond the line of the cortex, indicating that it is still contained within the periosteum (Figure 4.18).

4.5 CONCLUSIONS ON THE USE OF OTHER IMAGING METHODS TO SUPPLEMENT THE RADIOGRAPH

4.5.1 ULTRASONOGRAPHY

The use of ultrasound is of little value in the diagnosis of a bone tumour. It has some value, on account of its instant availability and inexpensiveness, in the confirmation and location of the actual presence of a soft tissue tumour. Other imaging methods are, however, necessary for further progress.

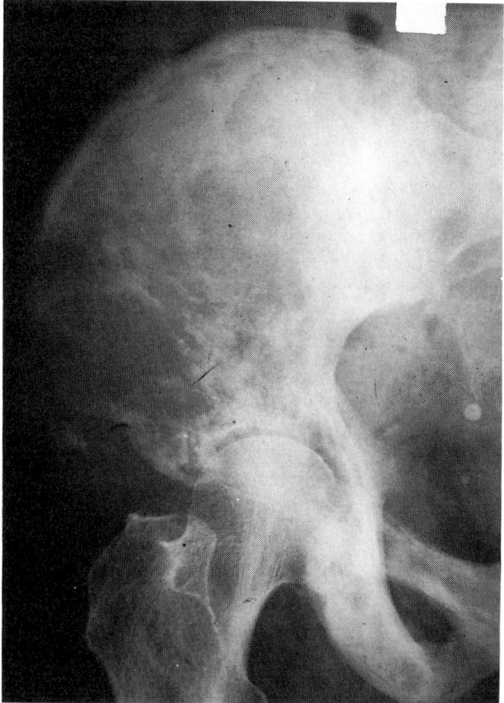

Figure 4.17 Osteosarcoma in Paget's disease. The characteristic features of Paget's disease are to be seen in the ischial ramus. A destructive lesion affects the anterior margin of the ilium. This was shown to be associated with a large soft tissue mass and was correctly assumed to be a Paget's sarcoma.

4.5.2 COMPUTED TOMOGRAPHY (CT)

CT has virtually replaced linear tomography in this field. Its great advantage lies in the demonstration of the spatial anatomy (Figure 4.19), with particular value in complex regions such as the facial skeleton and the bony pelvis. Because cortical bone gives no signal with magnetic resonance images, changes in the fine trabecular pattern can only be shown successfully by CT. Equally, although the periosteum cannot be demonstrated by any imaging method, CT can show the finest eggshell ossification produced by the periosteum displaced by a tumour (Figure 4.18), and thus indicate that the tumour

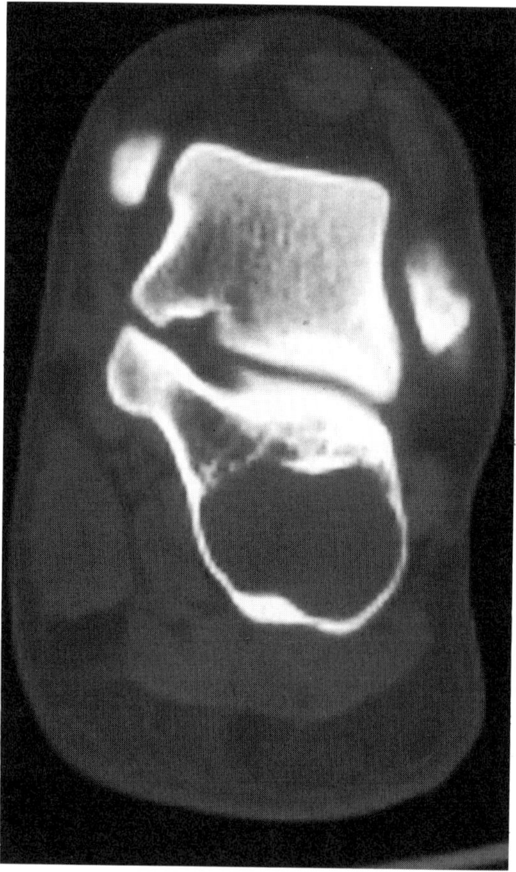

Figure 4.18 Aneurysmal bone cyst of calcaneus. The CT scan clearly shows the expansion of the bone with an 'eggshell' type of residual cortex. In complex regions like the foot, only computed imaging can demonstrate the anatomical extension of such a lesion with clarity.

remains within the membrane and hence does not present the overtly aggressive characteristic of malignancy, spread from the bony envelope in to the surrounding soft tissues. The use of CT in lesions lying deep within the body, e.g. an aneurysmal cyst extending into the pelvic cavity, can be invaluable in terms of future management (Figure 4.19).

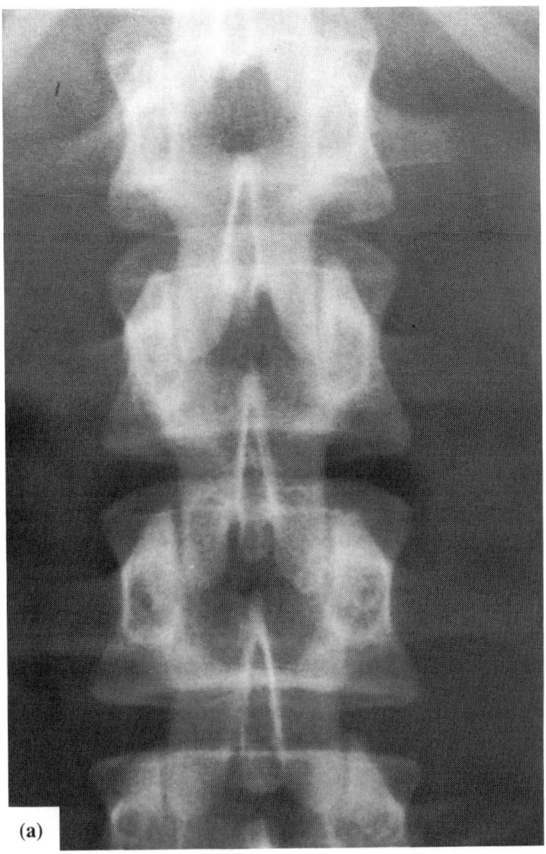

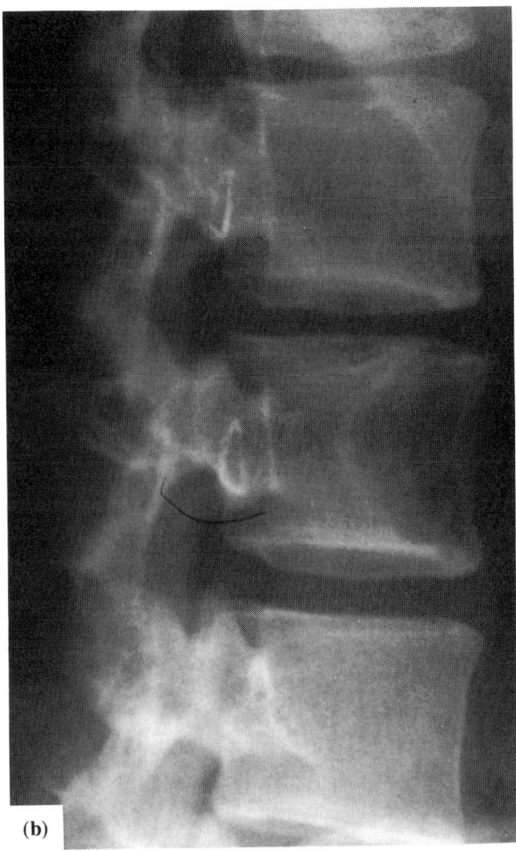

Figure 4.19 'Solid' aneurysmal bone cyst of L3. (a) Little abnormality is shown on the AP projection. (b) On the lateral view, the anterior half of the vertebral body is scalloped with a sclerotic endosteal margin; this is a feature of benignity.

4.5.3 BONE SCINTIGRAPHY

This is a highly sensitive method of assessing bony activity but very non specific. Certain relatively non-reactive tumours such as myeloma, will not necessarily produce any discernible alteration of uptake and the method therefore is then unreliable. Bone necrosis at an early stage is likely to show reduced activity, progressing to increased activity as revascularization and reossification occur. A positive scintigraphic scan calls for a plain radiograph of the region to identify the cause. A positive radionuclide scan and a negative radiograph necessitates clarification by a more sensitive technique, e.g. CT or MRI.

4.5.4 MAGNETIC RESONANCE IMAGING

This imaging technique is the most recent and the most complex; it is likely that its full potential is far from being achieved yet. It provides a high resolution and the ability to image in multiple planes, so that a comparison with the usual sectional plane of a pathological specimen can usually be anticipated prior to surgical removal. Although a very intricate method, it does not lead to very intuitive interpretation as its signals in fact represent the chemical milieu and especially, at its present level of development, the presence or absence of water. Thus although a disease process with tissue oedema may be present (Figure 4.20), MRI usually cannot

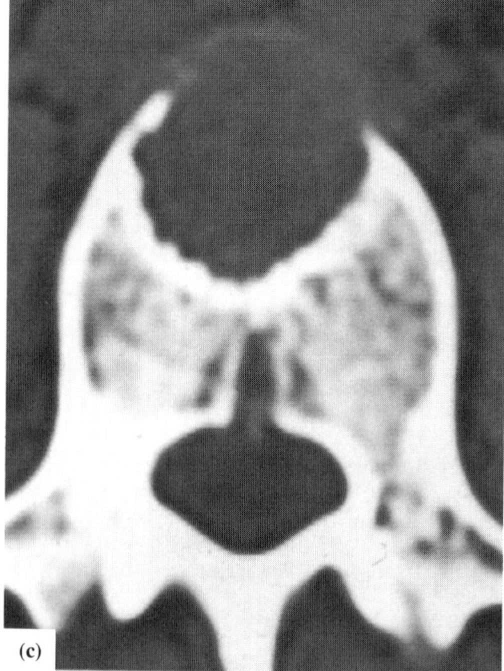

Figure 4.19 'Solid' aneurysmal bone cyst of L3. (c) The CT examination confirms the sclerotic posterior margin, indicative of slow growth and reaction of the host bone. Although more aggressive anteriorly, the thin blister-like bulge also suggests that the lesion is benign and has not extended beyond the periosteum.

indicate whether the increased local hydration is due to trauma, infection or tumour and, if the latter, what cell type it might be. There are certain exceptions to this statement in that the signals of blood (haematoma) and fat are usually readily assessable, particularly with the use of specifically selected sequences. Fortunately the evidence of MRI does not have to be taken in isolation and together with the testimony of the plain radiograph and other imaging techniques a composite picture can often be presented.

4.6   RADIOLOGICAL EXPERIENCE

Clearly, the osteoarticular pathologist who accepts the complementary value of radiographic information will gain some expertise

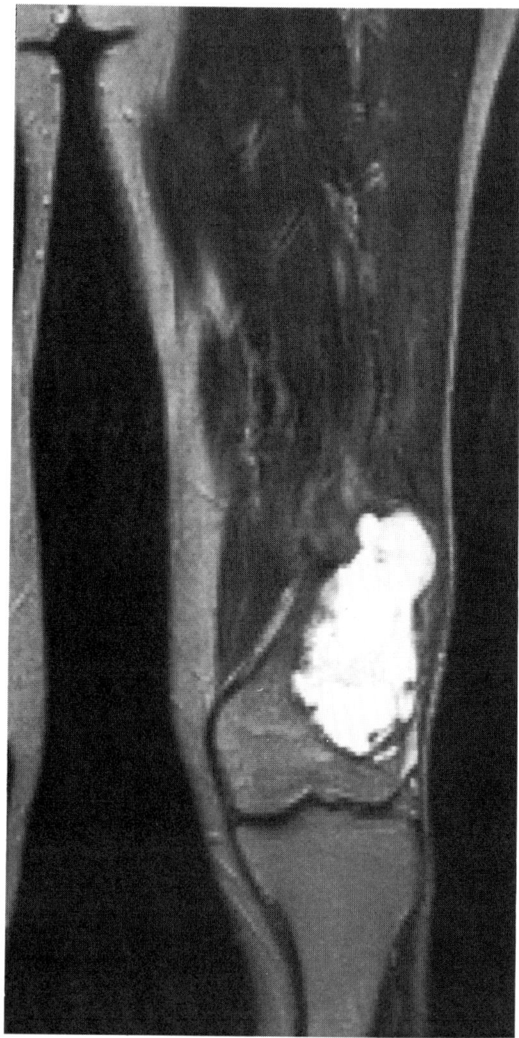

Figure 4.20 Osteosarcoma of distal end of femur. The MR image obtained with T2 weighting makes the tumour appear bright compared with the surrounding bone and muscle. This type of sequence is extremely valuable to supplement the anatomical information of standard T1 weighting with information about homogeneity and marginal activity or oedema.

in the interpretation of these images. However, it must be said, the same is true of the radiologist who takes the opportunity to use a microscope to study pathological preparations. In both cases, the diagnostic experience is likely to relate to the more typical presentations only. On most occasions, and particularly when there is a particular problem of interpretation, a dialogue is invaluable and should be encouraged. It goes without saying that both must be experienced in the orthopaedic field if the maximum benefit is to be achieved; an osteoarticular pathologist and a general radiologist would be as much a mismatch as the opposite combination. As a radiologist, I do not believe that the object is for the pathologist to make a definitive radiological diagnosis at the start, although after making a working diagnosis, it is entirely appropriate, and indeed entertaining, to hazard a specific diagnosis. It is important to remember under these circumstances the percentage accuracy and not just the diagnoses that were correct!

It is much more important to consider whether the radiological pattern is compatible with the histopathological diagnosis made on material received. Thus:

- If the primary radiological diagnosis is the same as the histological one, the chance of error is remote.
- If the primary diagnosis is wrong but one of the stated alternatives is correct, the histological diagnosis is probably safe.

Sometimes, particularly in the case of rarer disorders, the definitive histological diagnosis was not even considered by the radiologist, perhaps because the information provided and imaging procedures undertaken were limited. It is then necessary to review the radiological information in full and specifically address the question of compatible diagnoses.

Finally, the radiologist cannot perhaps accept that the radiological and histopathological diagnoses are sufficiently well-suited to be compatible in any way. It is then a question of whether the specimen viewed by the histopathologist is adequate and representative or whether there might be different appearances in different regions of the lesion. In this circumstance, a further biopsy may be needed or, where the entire lesion has been resected, further examination of the tissue blocks may need to be made.

4.7 CONCLUSION

The diagnostic processes of radiology and histopathology are complementary. Radiology provides the histopathologist with information about the extent of the lesion, its homogeneity, features of the reaction of the host bone that are mainly related to rate of growth and, depending upon the type of imaging procedure, additional information about activity, soft tissue spread, calcification and necrosis.

The ideal method for acquiring such information is through personal contacts between the radiologist and pathologist. However, the pathologist, particularly when giving a second opinion, must gain some expertise in the interpretation of X-ray films and consequently insist, in osteoarticular cases, on the provision of radiographic images in addition to the pathological material.

REFERENCE

Lodwick, G.S., Wilson, A.J., Farrell, C., Virkamma, P. and Dittrich, F. (1980) Determining growth rates of focal lesions of bone from radiographs. *Radiology*, **134**, 577.

PART TWO

Disease Processes and Disease Entities (excluding Neoplasia)

CONGENITAL AND DEVELOPMENTAL DISORDERS

5

Alan J. Darby and Paul D. Byers

About 7% of paediatric admissions are for single gene and chromosomal disorders, and 15–20% for congenital malformations of various types. Aetiologically these conditions can be classed as:

1. Genetic
   (a) Chromsome anomalies
   (b) Mutant genes of large effect
   (c) Polygenic predisposition (numerous genes of individual small effect)

2. Non-genetic: intrinsic and extrinsic teratogenic factors.

There are problems in discussing congenital disorders arising out of the confusing and changing terminology. These changes are a reflection of growing knowledge and developing concepts. In 1974 Smith proposed a classification which he hoped would provide a useful basis for discussion, and lead to a generally adopted classification. By 1982 he and other specialists, an international working party, further developed the terms and definitions (Spranger *et al.*, 1982).

The term congenital literally means present at birth. Variations from the norm at that time can collectively be referred to as congenital anomalies, or more loosely as birth defects. Some of these are errors of morphogenesis, some of metabolism, and possibly of other classes: Warkany (1971) points to errors of behaviour and function as members of the overall class of anomalies.

The concepts and terminology of Spranger (1982) and his associates are as follows:

1. Malformation: a defect of an organ, part of an organ, or larger region of the body, resulting from an intrinsically abnormal developmental process. It is emphasized that an organ or region is involved, and that the causal defect has been from the beginning within the site affected. The time of the appearance of the malformation is immaterial to the concept.

2. Disruption: a morphologic defect of an organ or part of an organ, or a larger region of the body, resulting from the extrinsic breakdown of, or interference with an originally normal developmental process.

3. Deformation: an abnormal form or shape or position of a part of the body caused by mechanical forces.

4. Dysplasia: an abnormal organization of cells into tissues, and its morphological results; it is the process and consequence of dyshistogenesis.

Multiple anomalies may be based on the same cause, or pathogenesis, or may occur together statistically or by chance. A number of explanations for these phenomena are possible:

1. Polytopic field defect: disturbances of a single developmental field giving rise to a pattern of anomalies.

2. Sequence: a pattern of multiple anomalies derived from a single known, or

presumed, prior anomaly or mechanical factor.

3. Syndrome: a pattern of multiple anomalies thought to be pathogenetically related and not known to represent a single sequence or a polytopic field defect.
4. Association: a non-random occurrence in two or more individuals of multiple anomalies not known to be a polytopic field defect, sequence, or syndrome.

Important to these definitions is the concept of the developmental field: a region or part of an embryo which responds as a co-ordinated unit in embryonic interaction, and results in complex or multiple anatomic structures. Embryonic interaction implies a reciprocal influence of one developing tissue on one or more others. Thus an intrinsic disturbance in a developmental field can lead to multiple anatomically related manifestations.

Regulatory mechanisms control growth, development and organization of tissues. Cells are in part self-regulating, and interactive. The chromosomes are a key feature. Functionally, the extremely long chromosomal structure, composed of sequences of small molecules of the nucleotide class, has regional divisions, identified as genes, each responsible for the first step in the production of a particular protein. The number of regions on one chromosome is many thousands, making possible complex and variable cell activities, i.e. differentiation. This implies mechanisms for switching on and off the activities of portions of chromosomes.

The chromosomal structure, sensitive to external forces, physical or chemical, is in constant need of maintenance. The pairing of chromosomes serves this end, in that each provides a model for the other, which can be followed by the reparative process. Irreparable modification in the local structure of a gene represents a mutation, which may be of greater or less consequence to the individual or his progeny.

Chromosomal anomalies arise spontaneously in several ways: mutations; and translocations, deletions, or additions during cell division; they may be transmissible. Such anomalies are present in 4% or more of zygotes; the majority result in abortion, accounting for around 60% of those in the first trimester. Nevertheless, it is estimated that the health of 1 in 200 live births will be affected. Four syndromes account for the majority: Down's, Klinefelter's, XXY, XXX; together they occur once in 250 live births (each 1 in 1000).

Many of the genetic abnormalities of large effect express themselves as metabolic disorders, often based on the failure of an enzyme or the structural abnormality of molecule. These can be summarized as follows:

- Amino acid metabolism
- Amino acid transport
- Purine and pyrimidine metabolism
- Carbohydrate metabolism
- Sphingolipidoses
- Lipid and lipoprotein metabolism
- Mucopolysaccharides, glycoproteins, mucolipids
- Porphyrias
- Metal metabolism – copper, zinc, iron

Genetic skeletal dysplasias are disorders of pre- and postnatal skeletal growth, characterized by some or all of:

- Short stature
- Bodily disproportion
- Deformity
- Functional abnormality

These arise primarily as the result of an abnormality of the physeal plate, which is responsible for growth in length. But periosteal function may be abnormal, affecting the girth of bone; and the remodelling activity may also be abnormal. If only the last two are affected, then it is possible to have dysplasia with little or no effect on stature.

The genetic skeletal dysplasias contrast with the proportionate short stature due to endocrine, nutritional or maturational causes, or chronic disease. Of these last some primary metabolic disorders are notable:

1. Calcium or phosphorus
    Hypophosphataemic rickets
    Pseudodeficiency rickets
    Late rickets
    Idiopathic hypocalcuria
    Hypophosphatasia
    Pseudohypoparathyroidism
2. Carbohydrates
    Mucopolysaccharidoses (including Hurler syndrome)
    Mucolipidoses
    Others
3. Lipids
    Niemann–Pick disease
    Gaucher disease
4. Nucleic acids
5. Amino acids
6. Metals

The skeletal dysplasias must also be differentiated from dysostoses in which malformations of individual bones, or regional constellations, occur as a result, it is believed, of an extrinsic or intrinsic factor acting during organogenesis, and hence are non-genetic. The more common of these are the following congenital disorders:

- Muscular torticollis
- High scapula
- Pseudarthrosis of the clavicle
- Radio-ulnar synostosis
- Radial hemimelia
- Abduction contracture of the hip and pelvic obliquity
- Dislocation of the hip
- Developmental coxa vara
- Dislocation of the knee
- Deficiency of the fibula
- Absence of the tibia
- Talipes equinovarus
- Metatarsus varus
- Talipes calcaneovalgus
- Convex pes valgus
- Pes planovalgus
- Torsional deformities of the lower limb

These are best recognized and understood at the macroscopic level. At the microscopic level the tissues present no specifically recognizable abnormality.

The final group of major developmental disorders involving the skeleton are the dysplasias of the spinal cord and vertebral column. Embryologically, the former arises from the folding of the neural crest to form a closed tube; the vertebrae are paired mesodermal/ectodermal derivatives which eventually fuse before and behind the cord.

The opposing folds of the neural crest first fuse in the destined thoracic region. Closure extends up and down. The envelopment by the protoskeletal structures follows at a time distance. But the whole process is intricately related, and degrees of failure are possible. Anencephaly is the more serious at the head end; and total spina bifida without neuralation, in the spinal region. These are, of course, incompatible with life, but lesser degrees of involvement are, and children with spina bifida, usually sacral but sometimes cervical, survive. There are degrees in both the vertebral defect and the intermingling of neural, mesodermal, and ectodermal derivatives in the soft tissue at the site. The smallest defects in these regions are diastematomyelia, in which the cord is divided longitudinally over a short distance, usually in the lumbar segment. Occasionally a bony outgrowth from the vertebral body will project through it.

Another lesser defect can arise from the fact that the neural tube is longer in the embryo than the destined spinal cord, and the distal segment atrophies to become the filum terminale. It can happen that the atrophic process is incomplete, with the result that the cord becomes tethered.

The manner of formation of vertebral

bodies – midline fusion of lateral masses, and fusion in the horizontal plane with the mass above (or below) – opens the way to a range of developmental failures in their formation. All these lesser anomalies of the cord and vertebrae may come to light as incidental findings, or because they give rise to symptoms and signs.

Genetic disorders may be either heritable or sporadic. In the former class there are in the order of 3000 defined or suspected entities, about 500 of which relate to the skeleton. As already mentioned, the classification of these has been problematic. An international working group produced in 1972 a classification of constitutional disorders of bone (the 1972 Paris Classification). This was revised in 1983, and again in 1992 (see Appendix, section 5.10). The latest revision differs from the earlier ones in being restricted to developmental disorders of chondro-osseous tissue, the osteochondrodysplasias. Revision of the dysostoses, developmental disorders of single bones, although necessary, was beyond the resources of the Working Group (Beighton *et al.*, 1992). In the appendix are to be found the 1992 classification and the part of the 1983 classification that was not revised in 1992.

There follows here a discussion of the more common osteochondrodysplasias. In the appendix (section 5.10) are references to entities that have not been touched on.

5.1   THE SKELETAL DYSPLASIAS

5.1.1   INTRODUCTION

In practice, congenital and developmental disorders present to the pathologist in two groups: as a biopsy from a child or adult; or as an autopsy examination following termination of pregnancy, because of abnormalities detected by ultrasound, or death in the perinatal or neonatal periods. Most of the biopsies relate either to metabolic disorders of bone or to tumours or tumour-like disorders and these are described elsewhere in this volume. This chapter will concentrate on the post-mortem examination of the dysplasias. The check list in Table 5.1 may act as a useful aide memoire.

Relevant to the interpretation of the pathology are the clinical data, including a detailed family history. The presence of maternal factors such as diabetes, alcoholism, drugs and infections should be noted.

5.1.2   THE EXTERNAL EXAMINATION

Unlike most autopsies, the greater part of the diagnostic process precedes taking up the scalpel. A picture, or in this case several pictures, is worth a thousand words. Photographs, preferably with a scale, are an essential part of the autopsy report. They provide a record of abnormalities that may be difficult to describe or even missed in the initial examination and are available for later objective analysis for research or diagnosis. Full frontal and lateral photographs are a minimum requirement. Close ups of the head, hands and feet may confirm such abnormalities as the hitchhiker thumbs of diastrophic dysplasia or the polydactyly found in many of the short rib polydactyly syndromes. Other anatomical abnormalities may be photographed as required.

5.1.3   RADIOLOGICAL EXAMINATION

High quality radiographs are the single most important requirement for the diagnosis of skeletal dysplasias. Time taken in positioning the fetus and obtaining well-exposed X-rays will be repaid many times over. An anteroposterior view with straightened arms and legs (held in position with tape if necessary) and a true lateral are the absolute minimum for diagnostic purposes. The lateral view is particularly useful for evaluating vertebral abnormalities. Specific views of the hands and feet are also useful if they are not well seen in the full skeletal X-rays.

Table 5.1 Check list for skeletal dysplasia autopsy

Clinical data – including family history

Photographs

Whole body: anterior
posterior
lateral
Close up: lateral head
hands and feet
specific abnormalities

Radiographs
Anteroposterior
Lateral
Hands and feet

Histology
Parietal bone
Humerus and femur
Lumbar vertebrae (sagittal)
Costochondral junction
Laryngeal or tracheal cartilage

Special investigations
Epiphyseal and growth plate cartilage for electron microscopy
Skin for chromosomal analysis
Spleen and cartilage for DNA and/or histochemical analysis

Several excellent accounts of the radiological features of the dysplasias are available (Wynne-Davies *et al.*, 1985; Spranger, 1989; Spranger and Maroteaux, 1990).

5.1.4 PATHOLOGICAL EXAMINATION

The rest of the autopsy follows the normal routine. However, as well as taking skin for chromosomal analysis, the spleen and samples of cartilage should be frozen at $-70°C$ for future DNA and biochemical studies.

In addition, skeletal tissues must be taken for microscopy. Because histological appearances may vary from one site to another, a standardized protocol is recommended (Yang *et al.*, 1986). A minimum of proximal femur, tibia and humerus, costochondral junction and a sagittal block of lumbar vertebrae should be examined. As changes in extraskeletal cartilage may also be present, a block of tracheal or laryngeal cartilage should

be added if not already taken. Finally, spare tissue should always be retained in case referral to a specialist centre is required. For fetuses terminated early in pregnancy, the whole bone may be embedded after careful trimming to aid orientation. With larger specimens, the bone may need dividing longitudinally to ensure adequate fixation. Care is needed to avoid damage to the fragile growth plate. Gentle slicing through most of the cartilage with a fresh scalpel blade, followed by division of the bone using a slow speed diamond saw is recommended.

After 24 to 48 hours in buffered formol saline, blocks for paraffin embedding should be decalcified in either EDTA or 10% formic acid in formalin. Strong acids are not recommended. Embedding in paraffin is adequate for most purposes, but undecalcified resin sections may provide additional information in some cases. Tissue processed for electron microscopy may also be useful for both diagnostic and research purposes. The staining of sections is partly a matter of personal preference but a variety of special stains will often aid diagnosis and is recommended as a routine. In addition to haematoxylin and eosin, periodic acid – Schiff (PAS) with diastase aids identification of cytoplasmic inclusions and toluidine blue, alcian blue and trichrome stains are all useful in detecting various matrix abnormalities.

Interpretation of sections requires a knowledge of the normal appearances at various ages (Ornoy *et al.*, 1988). Attention must be given to both cells and matrix in the resting cartilage, all layers of the growth plate and the metaphyseal bone (Table 5.2). The orientation of chondrocytes (columnation) and of bone trabeculae is also important. Several reviews of the histology of the dysplasias have appeared in recent years (Sillence *et al.*, 1979; Stanescu *et al.*, 1984; Gilbert *et al.*, 1987). However, readers of these and other papers should be warned that the histopathological terms used are not always well-defined or equivalent to similar terms in other fields. Further sources of confusion are the continuing controversies and changes in the nomenclature of the dysplasias.

5.1.5 CLASSIFICATION

With over a hundred types of dysplasia described, some form of classification is essential for diagnostic purposes. As men-

tioned above, radiographs are the lynch pin of diagnosis although histological criteria are becoming increasingly useful. The diagnostic groups listed in Table 5.3, modified from the recent international classification (Beighton *et al.*, 1992), may be of use.

The remainder of this chapter will be devoted to describing various features of the entities in these groups of disorders.

5.2 PLATYSPONDYLY GROUP

Thanatophoric dysplasia
  Type I

Thanatophoric dysplasia
  Type II (Cloverleaf skull)

Thanatophoric 'variants':
  Torrance
  San Diego
  Luton
  Shiraz
  Glasgow

Achondroplasia

Opsismodysplasia

Skeletal dysplasias with significant platyspondy (flattening of the vertebral bodies) as a major diagnostic feature include thanatophoric dysplasia (TD) and its so-called variants, achondroplasia and opsismodysplasia.

Table 5.2 Histological analysis

Type of abnormality
1. No abnormality
2. Cellular abnormality
3. Matrix abnormality
4. Abnormality of chondro-osseous transformation zone

Site of abnormality
1. Resting cartilage
2. Growth plate
3. Chondro-osseous transformation zone
4. Metaphysis

Table 5.3 Diagnostic groups

Platyspondyly group
Achondrogenesis group
Short rib polydactyly group
Diaphyseal group
Metatropic group
Kniest-like group
Stippled epiphyses group
Bone density and mineralisation group

5.2.1 THANATOPHORIC DYSPLASIA TYPE I

This is the commonest lethal skeletal dysplasia with an incidence of about 1:42 000 births. It occurs sporadically, probably as an autosomal dominant mutation. Its distinctive features were first described by Maroteaux in 1967.

Clinically it presents as severe short-limbed dwarfism. The head is large with a prominent forehead and hypoplastic mid-face bearing a superficial resemblance to achondroplasia. Often the shortening of the limbs is not accompanied by a corresponding reduction of soft tissue mass giving rise to a 'Michelin Man' appearance of the limbs.

Radiographs show marked platyspondyly, best seen in the lateral view. On the antero-posterior projection, the lumbar vertebral bodies and pedicles form U-shaped structures and there is a reduction of the interpedicular distances. The long bones are short and bowed with broad, slightly irregular, cupped metaphyses. The combination of broad metaphyses and curved shafts is most pronounced in the femora where it gives rise to the characteristic 'telephone receiver' appearance.

The histological appearances have been extensively reported (Horton *et al.*, 1979a, 1988; Langer *et al.*, 1987), but sections from several sites may be needed to see the full picture. The resting cartilage is normal. The growth plate shows a variable degree of disorganization, relatively normal areas alternating with regions lacking zones of proliferation and hypertrophy and without column formation. Vascularization of the growth plate is reduced and cartilage abuts directly on to bone forming transverse trabeculae rather than the vertically oriented trabeculae resulting from normal enchondral ossification. Periosteal bone formation extends a variable distance around the epiphyses correlating with the marginal metaphyseal spurs that contribute to the cupping seen radiologically. Bands of fibrous tissue invaginate the margin of the growth plate extending in from the groove of Ranvier. Further in from the periphery, well circumscribed areas of fibrous tissue are present at the chondro-osseous junction, referred to variously as 'tufts' (Ornoy *et al.*, 1985; Horton *et al.*, 1988) and as 'ossifying cartilage canals' (Langer *et al.*, 1987). These abnormal zones of fibrous tissue possess ultrastructural and histochemical features of both membranous and endochondral ossification (Horton *et al.*, 1988).

5.2.2 THANATOPHORIC DYSPLASIA WITH CLOVERLEAF SKULL (TD TYPE II)

The cloverleaf skull anomaly was described in 1960 by Holtermuller and Wiedemann as an isolated finding in one patient. They found 12 other cases in the literature, eight of which had chondrodysplasia. Since Maroteaux's description of thanatophoric dysplasia in 1967, it has become accepted that the chondrodysplasias referred to by Holtermuller and Wiedemann were in fact cases of TD type II. The cloverleaf deformity is produced by premature fusion of the sutures of the skull base and the coronal, lambdoid and sagittal sutures. The result is lateral bulging of the temporal regions and a towering prominence centred on the anterior fontanelle.

Justification for separating TD type II (with cloverleaf skull) from TD type I is based on subtle radiological and histological differences, the most obvious of which is the presence of straight femora in most cases of TD type II. More detailed accounts of the differences may be found in Gilbert *et al.* (1987) and Langer *et al.* (1987).

5.2.3 THANATOPHORIC VARIANTS

A number of dysplasias have been reported where the radiological features are indistinguishable from, or closely related to, thanatophoric dysplasia. These include those known as: 'San Diego' (Horton *et al.*, 1979a), 'Torrance' (Horton *et al.*, 1979a; Kaibara *et al.*, 1983), 'Shiraz' (Sedaghatian, 1980), 'Luton' (Winter and Thompson, 1982) and 'Glasgow' (Connor *et al.*, 1985; Maroteaux *et al.*, 1988). Whether or not these all deserve to stand alone as distinct entities awaits more detailed analysis.

5.2.4   ACHONDROPLASIA

Achondroplasia is one of the commonest forms of skeletal dysplasia affecting approximately 1 in 26 000 live births. In the common heterozygous form, despite the striking clinical and radiological findings, histological changes are minimal. By light microscopy, the growth plate in achondroplasia may be indistinguishable from normal. Histochemical and ultrastructural abnormalities have been reviewed by Maynard *et al.* (1981). Now that antenatal diagnosis may be offered to achondroplastics, it should be remembered that the changes do not become recognizable by ultrasound until about week 16.

Homozygous achondroplasia is extremely rare but has been the subject of a number of detailed case reports (Aterman *et al.*, 1983; Stanescu *et al.*, 1990). Affected infants usually die at or shortly after birth. The radiology may closely resemble, and the histology may be indistinguishable from, thanatophoric dysplasia. The family history is essential to avoid diagnostic embarrassment for the pathologist.

5.2.5   OPSISMODYSPLASIA

In 1984 Maroteaux *et al.* described three patients who died from cardiorespiratory failure in early childhood. Clinically they had rhizomelic dysplasia, short hands and a narrow thorax. Facial abnormalities including a short nose and depressed bridge of nose were present.

Radiologically there was extreme platyspondyly. Bone maturation was retarded and there was marked shortening of the bones of the hands and feet.

Histology showed a wide hypertrophic zone with poor columnation and irregular vascularization. The zone of provisional calcification was absent and unmineralized fibrous tissue and osteoid was in direct contact with the hypertrophic cartilage. Tongues of cartilage extended into the metaphyseal trabeculae.

5.3   ACHONDROGENESIS GROUP

Achondrogenesis IA (Houston–Harris)
Achondrogenesis IB (Fraccaro)
Achondrogenesis II (Langer–Saldino)
Hypochondrogenesis
Spondyloepiphyseal dysplasia congenita

5.3.1   ACHONDROGENESIS TYPE I

Lethal achondrogenesis was traditionally divided into groups: type I (Parenti–Fraccaro) and type II (Langer–Saldino). However, in 1988 Borochowitz *et al.* clearly delineated two subdivisions of type I and suggested the new nomenclature for types I and II as given above. This has been widely accepted and both subdivisions are still regarded as autosomal recessive.

(a)   Type IA (Houston–Harris)

Clinically there is no distinction between types I and II. The affected fetuses are very short with severe micromelia. The head appears relatively large, with a round face and small mouth, and the neck is often barely discernible.

Radiologically there is poor skull ossification and absent ossification of the vertebral bodies. The ribs are short with multiple fractures. The ilia are short and almost crescentic. The limb bones are extremely short and deformed.

Histologically the cartilage is hypervascular but the matrix is normal. The resting zone is hypercellular and the chondrocytes sit in large lacunae with a round central 'bull's eye' nucleus. The cytoplasm contains PAS-positive, diastase-resistant, inclusion bodies (Yang *et al.*, 1976a). Similar changes are seen in the respiratory tract cartilage. The growth plate is disorganized with poor columnation and cellular cartilage extends into irregular broad metaphyseal bony trabeculae.

(b)   Type IB (Fraccaro)

As mentioned, the clinical features are the same as type IA. Likewise, radiologically there is poor ossification of the calvarium and vertebral bodies. However, the posterior pedicles are usually present and the thoracic vertebral bodies may be visible in some cases. The long bones are short and stellate or trapezoid in form and ossification of the fibula is absent.

Histology of the cartilage shows a weakly staining and vacuolated matrix with slit-like vascular canals. The chondrocytes are surrounded by a more darkly staining ring which appears to represent collagen fibrils within the lacunar space. The appearances are similar in the respiratory tract cartilage. No cytoplasmic inclusions are present. The growth plate is disorganized and in some areas appears to abut directly onto the metaphyseal bone.

5.3.2   ACHONDROGENESIS TYPE II (LANGER – SALDINO)

This is a milder form of achondrogenesis. Unlike type I it is now thought to be inherited in an autosomal dominant fashion as are the other two members of this group, hypochondrogenesis and spondyloepiphyseal dysplasia congenita (SEDC). These three dysplasias are further related by their common link to a defect in collagen type II formation (Godfrey *et al.*, 1988; Godfrey and Hollister, 1988; Murray *et al.*, 1989). Furthermore, the milder forms of achondrogenesis

type II appear to merge radiologically with hypochondrogenesis and SEDC.

The radiographic appearances include marked underossification of the vertebral bodies, pubic and ischial bones. The calvarium is better ossified than in achondrogenesis type I. The long bones are short with cupped and flared metaphyses.

Histologically there is increased vascularity of the cartilage, often with prominent perivascular fibrosis. The cartilage is hypercellular with deficient matrix and large chondrocytic lacunae in all zones. Under high magnification a loose fibrillar material can be seen in the lacunar spaces. Chondrocyte column formation is disturbed and the chondro-osseous transformation zone is irregular. Cellular cartilage persists in the metaphyseal bony trabeculae which are abnormally orientated and wide.

5.3.3   HYPOCHONDROGENESIS

It is debatable whether this is a separate entity. Radiologically it appears to be a mild form of achondrogenesis type II with which it forms a continuous spectrum (Borochowitz *et al.*, 1986a). The histology is also similar to achondrogenesis type II. The severity of the histological changes also varies but does not always correlate with the radiology. It has been suggested that these changes are seen more consistently in the vertebral bodies than in the long bones.

5.3.4   SPONDYLOEPIPHYSEAL DYSPLASIA CONGENITA

In the newborn period SEDC may be indistinguishable from mild cases of achondrogenesis type II and hypochondrogenesis. Usually it is compatible with life but a few patients die in the neonatal period.

Histologically the growth cartilage may be normal after infancy, but in the newborn shows slight disorganization most obvious in the hypertrophic zone. An important distinguishing feature is the presence of small, sometimes multiple, PAS-positive, diastase-resistant, cytoplasmic inclusion bodies in the resting and hypertrophic cartilage (Yang *et al.*, 1980). At the light microscopic level these are similar to the inclusions seen in achondrogenesis type II, short rib polydactyly syndrome type III and Kniest dysplasia.

5.4　SHORT RIB POLYDACTYLY GROUP (SRP)

SRP Type I (Saldino–Noonan)
SRP Type II (Majewski)
SRP Type III (Verma–Naumoff)
SRP Type IV (Beemer–Langer)
Asphyxiating thoracic dysplasia (Jeune)
Ellis–van Creveld (chondroectodermal) dysplasia

The nomenclature of the short rib polydactyly (SRP) syndromes is very confusing and still evolving. Not all patients have polydactyly and some authors now refer simply to the short rib syndromes. Various numbering systems have been used and eponymous syndromes do not always correspond as closely as one might wish with the authors' original accounts. To avoid confusion it is probably best to conform to the 1992 international classification (Beighton *et al.*, 1992) and to use both numbers and eponyms when giving a diagnosis.

The international classification names six types as listed above. All types of SRP appear to be autosomal recessive. Most cases are stillborn or lethal in the neonatal period. Patients with SRP III or ATD who survive infancy frequently develop severe renal problems.

5.4.1　SRP I (SALDINO–NOONAN)

This lethal dysplasia usually results in premature birth and is associated with congenital heart defects and anomalies of the urogenital and alimentary tracts.

Radiologically the ribs are very short. The vertebral bodies are small and round with irregular outlines. The long bones are extremely short, broad and underremodelled. The humeri and femora often have pointed ends.

Histologically (Gilbert *et al.*, 1987; Erzen *et al.*, 1988), there is mild disorganization of the growth plate. Tongues of cartilage extend from its margins into the metaphysis. In the proximal femur and humerus, disordered chondrocytes converge on a large central area of fibrosis.

5.4.2　SRP II (MAJEWSKI)

Radiologically there are short ribs but the vertebrae and long bones are comparatively normal except for the tibiae which are short and oval.

Histologically (Chen *et al.*, 1980b), the resting cartilage is unremarkable but the growth plate is stunted and disorganized with minimal columnation. The proliferative zone is barely discernible and there are only a few haphazardly arranged hypertrophic cells. The changes are most severe in the ribs (Gilbert *et al.*, 1987).

5.4.3　SRP III (VERMA–NAUMOFF)

Clinically this is similar to SRP I. Radiographs show very short ribs with a narrow cylindrical thorax. The ilia are short with medial and lateral spurs forming an inverted V. Limb bones are very short with metaphyseal spurs.

Histology shows an irregular chondro-osseous junction. The growth plate is disorganized with little hypertrophic change except at the periphery where there is a periosteal spur of bone corresponding to the X-ray appearance.

5.4.4　SRP IV (BEEMER–LANGER)

Only seven cases of this probably autosomal recessive condition have been described (Yang *et al.*, 1991). The radiographic findings are similar to SRP II (Majewski) except that the tibiae are more normal and the ilia smaller. In addition there is bowing of the radii and ulnae.

Histologically there is a prominent albeit disorganized hypertrophic zone. Large irregular islands of cartilage are seen in the metaphysis of the proximal humerus and femur.

5.4.5 ASPHYXIATING THORACIC DYSPLASIA (ATD) (JEUNE)

Radiographs show short horizontal ribs and a narrow bell-shaped thorax. The ilia are short with a lateral spur at the border of the sciatic notch. The long bones are short, and sometimes bowed, with smooth bulbous ends.

Histologically the proliferating and hypertrophic chondrocytes are reduced in number and arranged in groups. The chondro-osseous junction is smooth. A lattice-like pattern of cartilage columns is seen in the metaphyses of the long bones but not in the vertebrae. Yang *et al.* (1987) have attempted to split ATD into two types: ATD type II is said to correspond to classical Jeune form of ATD whereas ATD type I bears many similarities to SRP III (Verma–Naumoff) and the two conditions may represent different points on a spectrum.

5.4.6 ELLIS–VAN CREVELD (CHONDRO-ECTODERMAL) DYSPLASIA (CED)

Ellis–van Creveld (CED) appears similar to ATD both clinically and radiologically. Distinguishing features include skin lesions and nail dysplasia in CED. Congenital heart defects are common in CED but rare in ATD. Polydactyly is always present in at least one limb in CED but is rare in ATD.

Histologically (Yang *et al.*, 1987; Erzen *et al.*, 1988) the appearances may resemble SRP I (Saldino–Noonan) or may be barely distinguishable from normal.

5.5 DIAPHYSEAL ABNORMALITY GROUP

Campomelic dysplasia
Boomerang dysplasia
Atelosteogenesis type I
Atelosteogenesis type II (de la Chapelle)
Diastrophic dysplasia

5.5.1 CAMPOMELIC DYSPLASIA

This is one of the commonest skeletal dysplasias although its pathogenesis is unknown (Houston *et al.*, 1983). Most patients are stillborn or die in early infancy. They have relatively large heads, short trunks and short limbs. The thighs are anteriorly bowed and there may be talipes equinovarus.

Radiographs confirm the bowing of the femurs and often other long bones. In addition the scapulae are small, as are the pedicles of the thoracic vertebrae.

Abnormalities of the brain, heart, respiratory and urogenital tracts are common. Histology shows no abnormality of resting cartilage, growth plate or metaphyseal bone.

5.5.2 BOOMERANG DYSPLASIA

A rare sporadic lethal dysplasia (Kozlowski *et al.*, 1985). Patients have relatively large heads, short trunks and short limbs. The major radiographic features are in the severely shortened limbs. The bones show variable and often absent ossification. Some, particularly the tibiae, are misshapen and curved resembling a boomerang.

Histology shows absence of growth plates and failure of ossification except for a few bony trabeculae arising from loose fibrous tissue. The cartilage exhibits variable cellularity and contains scanty giant, sometimes multinucleated, chondrocytes similar to those seen in atelosteogenesis.

5.5.3 ATELOSTEOGENESIS TYPE I

This dysplasia was described simultaneously by Sillence *et al.* and Maroteaux *et al.* in 1982. It is a rhizomelic dysplasia with club feet and normal hands.

Radiographs show absence or hypoplasia of the distal humerus and femur, hypoplasia of the thoracic vertebral bodies and bowing of the tibia and forearm bones. The metacarpals and phalanges are underossified or absent.

Histology reveals cystic spaces throughout the resting cartilage and growth plate. Relatively acellular areas are present in the resting cartilage and these areas contain scanty, irregularly shaped, multinucleated giant cells. The growth plate shows moderately good columnation with an excess of matrix in the hypertrophic zone.

5.5.4 ATELOSTEOGENESIS TYPE II (DE LA CHAPELLE)

Clinically this is similar to type I with the addition of respiratory tract abnormalities and small digits (Whitley *et al.*, 1986). Radiographic differences include small vertebral bodies with irregular contours and an anterior tongue-like projection. The ulnae and fibulae are small and almost triangular in shape. The proximal femoral and humeral metaphyses are irregular compared to their smooth outlines in type I. Histologically the most striking feature is the presence of multiple concentric rings (lacunar halos) around the chondrocytes of the resting cartilage. The growth plate is only slightly disorganized with better columnation than type I.

5.5.5 DIASTROPHIC DYSPLASIA

Diastrophic dwarfism is a generalized disorder of cartilage leading to short stature, degenerative arthritis, tracheomalacia, cauliflower ear and joint laxity. It is a non-lethal disorder but several histological studies are available (Horton *et al.*, 1979b; Stanescu *et al.*, 1984). The resting cartilage contains large irregularly distributed chondrocytes with concentric rings similar to those seen in atelosteogenesis type II (de la Chapelle). Small acellular areas containing thickened irregular collagen fibres are present. The growth plate is narrow with short regular columns separated by wide septa with a fibrillar appearance.

Unfortunately, although antenatal diagnosis is now available the histological appearances in the fetus have not been reported.

5.6 METATROPIC GROUP

Metatropic dysplasia
Fibrochondrogenesis
Schneckenbecken dysplasia

5.6.1 METATROPIC DYSPLASIA

The term metatropic derives from the Greek word *metatropos* meaning changing patterns. This reflects the evolution from short-limbed dwarfism in infancy to short-trunk dwarfism and kyphoscoliosis with increasing age.

At present it is a poorly defined and probably heterogeneous disorder (Beck *et al.*, 1983). There are probably three types of patient: a non-lethal autosomal recessive type, a non-lethal dominant form with less severe spinal and pelvic changes and a lethal type, probably autosomal recessive. The clinical features have often been confused with Morquio's syndrome in surviving patients.

Radiographically there is marked shortening of long bones with a 'dumb-bell like' enlargement of the metaphyses. Severe platyspondyly is present and there is flaring of the iliac crest.

Pathologically the epiphyses of the long bones are enlarged to such an extent that they are obvious both clinically and at autopsy and the term 'hyperchondrogenesis' has been applied to the disorder. Histological studies are conflicting, possibly reflecting both the genetic heterogeneity and the different ages of patients studied. The cells of the resting cartilage contain metachromatic inclusions (Gilbert *et al.*, 1987). Growth plate maturation appears normal but vascular invasion is irregular and bone formation may be decreased. An uncoupling of endochondral and perichondral growth has been suggested (Boden *et al.*, 1987).

5.6.2 FIBROCHONDROGENESIS

This is a rare but histologically and radiologically well-defined entity. Since the first report (Lazzaroni-Fossati *et al.*, 1978), a further six cases have been described (Eteson *et al.*, 1984; Whitley *et al.*, 1984; Bankier *et al.*, 1991).

Clinically there is severe rhizomelic shortening, a short neck and narrow chest. The face is round with protuberant eyes and there is a cleft palate. Like metatropic dwarfism the ends of the long bones are palpably enlarged.

Radiographs show platyspondyly and on the lateral view the vertebral bodies are pear shaped. The ilia are small. The long bones are short with very broad and slightly irregular metaphyses with small marginal spurs.

Histology shows hypercellular resting cartilage with spindle-shaped chondrocytes. Cells are often arranged in clusters with a fibrous margin. In some areas there is variable cellularity and foci of cystic degeneration. Respiratory tract cartilage is normal. The growth plate lacks columnation, the cells being clustered in nests within a fibrous matrix. The trabecular pattern in the metaphysis is disordered.

5.6.3 SCHNECKENBECKEN DYSPLASIA

This entity was described independently by two groups (Borochowitz *et al.*, 1986b; Knowles *et al.*, 1986). Its somewhat bizarre name reflects the snail like configuration of the ilia. The family described by Knowles is the same as that reported by Laxova *et al.* (1973) as probable achondrogenesis. It is a severe short-limbed dwarfism with normal hands and feet and a relatively large head.

Radiographs show hypoplastic vertebral bodies. On a lateral view the small punctate body contrasts strikingly with the well-developed posterior arch. The clavicles are handlebar shaped and the ribs are short and curved. The ilia are hypoplastic with an unusual medial projection giving them a characteristic snail-like outline. The long bones are short with metaphyseal flaring and cupping.

Histology shows hypercellular resting cartilage with some clustering of chondrocytes. The cells are round with a large central nucleus. The growth plate is short with a relative paucity of proliferative cells but good columnation. The chondro-osseous junction is smooth and the metaphyseal trabeculae are normally orientated. At the margins of the growth plate there are small spicules of hypercellular bone.

5.7 KNIEST-LIKE GROUP

Kniest dysplasia
Dyssegmental dysplasia
   (Silverman-Handmaker type)
Dyssegmental dysplasia
   (Rolland-Desbuquois type)

5.7.1 KNIEST DYSPLASIA

This dysplasia is characterized clinically by short-limbed dwarfism with kyphoscoliosis. The eyes are prominent, and often myopic, the mid-face flat, and there is deafness. The joints are prominent with restricted movement. The condition is usually compatible with life but lethal cases have been reported (Chen *et al.*, 1980a; Spranger and Maroteaux, 1990).

Radiographs show platyspondyly with vertical clefts in the vertebral bodies. The long bones are short with broad metaphyses and large epiphyses.

The resting cartilage is hypercellular with spindle-shaped cells frequently arranged in a storiform pattern and superficially resembling fibrochondrogenesis. The growth plate is also hypercellular with poor columnation.

The matrix contains small foci of myxoid change, and PAS-positive, diastase-resistant, cytoplasmic inclusions are present, in both growth plate and resting cartilage.

5.7.2 DYSSEGMENTAL DYSPLASIA

This is a lethal short-limbed dwarfism with a short trunk and short thick bowed long bones. A vertebral segmentation defect is evident radiologically, whence the name of the condition. Histological features resemble Kniest dysplasia with prominent lakes of mucoid degeneration.

Radiological and histological features distinguishing between the more severe Silverman–Handmaker type and the milder Rolland–Desbuquois form have been described (Aleck *et al.*, 1987).

5.8 STIPPLED EPIPHYSES GROUP (CHONDRODYSPLASIA PUNCTATA)

Rhizomelic type
Conradi–Hunermann type
X-linked recessive type
Tibia-metacarpal type
Mild Sheffield type

This is a heterogeneous group of disorders also known as chondrodysplasia punctata. The term Conradi–Hunermann dysplasia is often applied indiscriminately to all such disorders but should be restricted to the X-linked dominant form. As well as the entities listed above, there are a number of disorders with so-called secondary punctate calcification. These disorders include Zellweger's syndrome and other peroxisomal disorders, vitamin K-epoxide reductase deficiency, trisomies 18 and 21, prenatal rubella syndrome and fetal exposure to warfarin, phenytoin and alcohol. Other rare forms of chondrodysplasia punctata include dappled diaphysis dysplasia (Carty *et al.*, 1989; Nairn and Chapman, 1989), and Greenberg dysplasia (Greenberg *et al.*, 1988).

5.8.1 RHIZOMELIC CHONDRODYSPLASIA PUNCTATA

This rare autosomal recessive disorder is commonly lethal in the first few months of life. It is one of the peroxisomal group of disorders and is associated with deficient synthesis of dihydroxyacetone phosphate acyltransferase (DHAP-AT). Diagnosis is possible prenatally by enzyme assay in amniotic cells and postnatally in fibroblasts and platelets. Plasma phytanic acid levels are also raised (Poulos *et al.*, 1988).

Patients have severe limb shortening, cataracts and facial deformities giving them a 'chipmunk' appearance. Surviving patients show severe mental retardation and icthyotic skin lesions. Radiographs at birth show short humeri and femora with irregular metaphyses and punctate calcification in the region of the epiphyses. The vertebral bodies have coronal clefts. In surviving patients the punctate calcification and coronal clefts disappear but platyspondyly and kyphoscoliosis develop.

Histology shows foci of cystic degeneration, fibrosis and calcification of resting cartilage. The growth plate is usually within normal limits (Gilbert *et al.*, 1976, 1987; Poulos *et al.*, 1988).

5.8.2 CONRADI–HUNERMANN CHONDRODYSPLASIA PUNCTATA

This is a genetically heterogeneous group of predominantly X-linked dominantly inherited disorders with a relatively good prognosis. It is an asymmetric epiphyseal dysplasia. There is epiphyseal and spinal punctate calcification which disappears with age. It is sometimes associated with cataracts and skin changes. Histologically there is focal myxoid degeneration and calcification of resting cartilage, particularly near the proliferative zone, but the growth plate itself is normal.

A lethal form of X-linked dominant chondrodysplasia also exists. Whether this is a separate entity or a severe manifestation of the Conradi–Hunermann dysplasia is uncertain (Spranger and Maroteaux, 1990).

5.8.3   X-LINKED RECESSIVE CHONDRODYSPLASIA PUNCTATA

This rare, usually non-lethal, dysplasia is due to an inherited chromosomal deletion. Several types of chromosomal abnormality have been reported and are often associated with mental retardation and icthyotic skin changes (Wulfsberg *et al.*, 1992).

5.8.4   TIBIA-METACARPAL AND MILD SHEFFIELD TYPES

These two milder types are delineated on radiographic and clinical grounds (Rittler *et al.*, 1990; Sheffield *et al.*, 1976) and as yet lack clear pathological descriptions.

5.9   BONE DENSITY AND MINERALIZATION GROUP

Osteogenesis imperfecta
Osteopetrosis
Melorheostosis
Diaphyseal dysplasia
    (Camurati-Engelmann)
Hypophosphatasia

5.9.1   OSTEOGENESIS IMPERFECTA

Osteogenesis imperfecta (OI) is a group of disorders with increased bone fragility leading to fractures and deformity. They have varying forms of inheritance. All cases have defects of collagen type I formation of one sort or another. Four major syndrome groups have been identified (Sillence, 1990) but these may well be superseded by advances at the molecular genetics level.

(a)   Osteogenesis imperfecta type I

This is autosomal dominant and is the commonest variety of OI. It is sometimes subdivided into those with and without dentinogenesis imperfecta (DI). The sclerae are usually deep blue. Fractures occur with minimal trauma. Patients with OI type I and DI tend to have an earlier onset and more severe disease than those with normal teeth. Early onset deafness is a common complication. Juvenile osteoporosis is the main differential diagnosis.

(b)   Osteogenesis imperfecta type II

This group of patients suffers from severe bone fragility leading to stillbirth or early death. Several forms of inheritance have been described. The patient is usually short and radiographs show thin, poorly ossified bones with multiple fractures. The long bones are often short and crumpled. Histology shows hypercellular bone, often with areas having a curious blue spiculation, and fracture callus. The growth plate is normal but the metaphyseal trabeculae are reduced and delicate in appearance.

(c)   Osteogenesis imperfecta type III

This is an autosomal recessive severe, but usually non-lethal, syndrome. The sclerae are pale blue or normal. Fractures are usually present at birth and lead to progressive deformity. Occasionally fractures may be associated with exuberant callus formation simulating osteosarcoma.

(d)   Osteogenesis imperfecta type IV

This is autosomal dominant. The sclerae are light blue at birth but this fades by adulthood. It may be associated with dentinogenesis imperfecta. Severity is variable but, like type I, the number of fractures tends to decrease with increasing age.

5.9.2   OSTEOPETROSIS

Several forms of osteopetrosis have been described. Those presenting early are often fatal. Milder cases presenting later are sometimes known as osteopetrosis tarda or Albers – Schönberg disease. The early onset form of the disease is usually autosomal recessive. Radiologically there is increased density of bones. Modelling is abnormal, sometimes leading to a 'bone within a bone' appearance. Histology shows crowding out of the marrow space by abnormally thick bony trabeculae, some of which retain a cartilaginous core. This is because osteoclasts, although present, fail to resorb bone adequately.

The milder late onset form is usually autosomal dominant. Recently a form of osteopetrosis associated with carbonic anhydrase II deficiency has been described (Sly *et al.*, 1983).

5.9.3   MELORHEOSTOSIS

This is a rare form of sporadic hyperostosis with a linear distribution along long bones (Campbell *et al.*, 1968). Not uncommonly, changes in the overlying skin and subcutaneous tissue, and joint contractures and stiffness may occur before changes in the bone are appreciated. Radiologically, the area of abnormal sclerotic bone appears to flow down the bone like wax dripping down the side of a candle. One or more bones may be involved. Histology shows a mixture of lamellar and woven bone with marrow fibrosis.

5.9.4   DIAPHYSEAL DYSPLASIA (CAMURATI–ENGELMANN)

A rare autosomal dominant condition. Severity may vary considerably between different members of the same family. Symptoms start with bone pain and any bone can be involved. Radiographs show symmetrical fusiform enlargement of the diaphyses with normal metaphyses and epiphyses. The diaphyseal cortex enlarges by both endosteal and periosteal appositional new bone formation. Histology shows unremarkable woven bone formation (Hundley and Wilson, 1973).

5.9.5   HYPOPHOSPHATASIA

This group of disorders has a variety of clinical manifestations and modes of inheritance and includes a congenital lethal form. It is caused by a deficiency of the tissue-non-specific alkaline phosphatase isoenzyme.

The lethal form is inherited as an autosomal recessive. Patients have short deformed limbs and a round soft head. Radiologically there is severely deficient ossification of all bones. Radiolucent tongues may extend from the epiphysis into the metaphysis. Fractures may be present. Histological changes are those of rickets with a broad growth plate, a deficient zone of provisional calcification and undermineralized trabeculae lined by osteoid (Fallon *et al.*, 1984) (see Chapter 10).

REFERENCES

Aleck, K.A., Grix, A., Clericuzio, C. *et al.* (1987) Dyssegmental dysplasias: clinical, radiographic, and morphologic evidence of heterogeneity. *Am. J. Med. Genet.*, **27**, 295–312.

Aterman, K., Welch, J.P. and Taylor, P.G. (1983) Presumed homozygous achondroplasia. A review and report of a further case. *Pathol. Res. Pract.*, **178**, 27–39.

Bankier, A., Fortune, D., Duke, J. *et al.* (1991) Fibrochondrogenesis in male twins at 24 weeks. *Am. J. Med. Genet.*, **38**, 959–98.

Beck, M., Roubicek, M., Rogers, J.G. *et al.* (1983) Heterogeneity of metatropic dysplasia. *Eur. J. Pediatr.*, **140**, 231–7.

Beighton, P., Giedion, A., Gorlin, R. *et al.* (1992) International classification of osteochondrodysplasias. *Am. J. Med. Genet.*, **44**, 223–9.

Boden, S.D., Kaplan, F.S., Fallon, M.D. (1987) Metatropic dwarfism: uncoupling of endochondral and perichondral growth. *J. Bone Joint Surg.*, **69A**, 174–84.

Borochowitz, Z., Ornoy, A., Lachman, R. *et al.* (1986a) Achondrogenesis II – Hypochondrogenesis: variability versus heterogeneity. *Am. J. Med. Genet.*, **24**, 273–88.

Borochowitz, Z., Jones, K.L., Silbey, R. *et al.* (1986b) A distinct lethal neonatal chondrodysplasia with snail-like pelvis: schneckenbecken dysplasia. *Am. J. Med. Genet.*, **25**, 47–59.

Borochowitz, Z., Lachman, R., Adomian, G.E. *et*

al. (1988) Achondrogenesis type I: delineation of further heterogeneity and identification of two distinct subgroups. *J. Pediatr.*, **112**, 23–31.

Byers, P.H. (1989) Invited editorial: molecular heterogeneity in chondrodysplasias. *Am. J. Hum. Genet.*, **45**, 1–4.

Campbell, C.J., Papademetriou, T. and Bonfiglio, M. (1968) Melorheostosis. A report of the clinical, roentgenographic and pathological findings in fourteen cases. *J. Bone Joint Surg.*, **50A**, 1281–303.

Carty, H., Kozlowski, K. and Sillence, D. (1989) Dappled diaphyseal dysplasia. *Fortschr. Roentgenstr.*, **150**, 228–9.

Chen, H., Yang, S.S. and Gonzalez, E. (1980a) Kniest dysplasia: neonatal death with necropsy. *Am. J. Med. Genet.*, **6**, 171–8.

Chen, H., Yang, S.S., Gonzalez, E. *et al.* (1980b) Short rib-polydactyly syndrome, Majewski type. *Am. J. Med. Genet.*, **7**, 215–22.

Connor, J.M., Connor, R.A.C., Sweet, E.M. *et al.* (1985) Lethal neonatal chondrodysplasias in the west of Scotland 1970–1983 with a description of a thanatophoric dysplasia like, autosomal recessive disorder, Glasgow variant. *Am. J. Med. Genet.*, **22**, 243–53.

Erzen, M., Stanescu, R., Stanescu, V. *et al.* (1988) Comparative histopathology of the growth cartilage in short-rib polydactyly syndromes I and III and in chondroectodermal dysplasias. *Ann. Genet.*, **31**, 144–50.

Eteson, D.J., Adomian, G.E., Ornoy, A. *et al.* (1984) Fibrochondrogenesis: radiologic and histologic studies. *Am. J. Med. Genet.*, **19**, 277–90.

Eteson, D.J., Beluffi, G., Burgio, G.R. *et al.* (1986) Pseudodiastrophic dysplasia: a distinct newborn skeletal dysplasia. *J. Pediatr.*, **109**, 635–41.

Fallon, M.D., Teitelbaum, S.L., Weinstein, R.S. *et al.* (1984) Hypophosphatasia: clinicopathologic comparison of the infantile, childhood and adult forms. *Medicine*, **63**, 12–24.

Gilbert, E.F., Opitz, J.M., Spranger, J.W. *et al.* (1976) Chondrodysplasia punctata – rhizomelic form. Pathologic and radiologic studies of three infants. *Eur. J. Pediatr.*, **123**, 89–109.

Gilbert, E.F., Yang, S.S., Langer, L. *et al.* (1987) Pathologic changes of osteochondrodysplasia in infancy. *Pathol. Annu.*, **22 (2)**, 283–345.

Godfrey, M. and Hollister, D.W. (1988) Type II achondrogenesis–hypochondrogenesis: identification of abnormal type II collagen. *Am. J. Hum. Genet.*, **43**, 904–13.

Godfrey, M., Keene, W.R., Blank, E. *et al.* (1988) Type II achondrogenesis–hypochondrogenesis: morphologic and immunohistopathologic studies. *Am. J. Hum. Genet.*, **43**, 894–903.

Greco, M.A., Alvarez, S.P., Genieser, N.B. *et al.* (1984) Dyssegmental dwarfism: a histological study of osseous and non-osseous cartilage. *Hum. Pathol.*, **15**, 490–3.

Greenberg, C.R., Gruber, H.E., DeSa, D.J.B. *et al.* (1988) A new autosomal recessive lethal chondrodystrophy with non-immune hydrops. *Am. J. Med. Genet.*, **29**, 623–32.

Holtermuller, K. and Wiedemann, H.R. (1960) Kleeblattschadel-Syndrom. *Med. Monatsschr.*, **14**, 439–46.

Horton, W.A., Rimoin, D.L., Hollister, D.W. *et al,* (1979a) Further heterogeneity within lethal neonatal short-limbed dwarfism: the platyspondylic types. *J. Pediatr.*, **94**, 736–42.

Horton, W.A., Rimoin, D.L., Hollister, D.W. *et al.* (1979b) Diastrophic dwarfism: a histochemical and ultrastructural study of the enchondral growth plate. *Pediatr. Res.*, **13**, 904–9.

Horton, W.A., Hood, O.J., Machado, M.A. *et al.* (1988) Abnormal ossification in thanatophoric dysplasia. *Bone*, **9**, 53–61.

Horton, W.A., Campbell, D., Machado, M.A. *et al.* (1989) Tissue and cell studies of the growth plate in the chondrodysplasias. *Am. J. Med. Genet.*, **34**, 91–5.

Houston, C.S., Opitz, J.M., Spranger, J.W. *et al.* (1983) The campomelic syndrome. *Am. J. Med. Genet.*, **15**, 3–28.

Hundley, J.D. and Wilson, F.C. (1973) Progressive diaphyseal dysplasia. *J. Bone Joint Surg.*, **55A**, 461–74.

Kaibara, N., Yokoyama, K. and Nakano, H. (1983) Torrance type of lethal neonatal short-limbed platyspondylic dwarfism. *Skeletal Radiol*, **10**, 17–19.

Knowles, S., Winter, R. and Rimoin, D. (1986) A new category of lethal short-limbed dwarfism. *Am. J. Med. Genet.*, **25**, 41–6.

Kozlowski, K., Sillence, D., Cortis-Jones, R. *et al.* (1985) Boomerang dysplasia. *Br. J. Radiol.*, **58**, 369–71.

Langer, L.O., Yang, S.S., Hall, J.G. *et al.* (1987) Thanatophoric dysplasia and cloverleaf skull. *Am. J. Med. Genet.*, **Suppl 3**, 167–79.

Laxova, R., O'Hara, P.T., Ridler, M.A.C. *et al.* (1973) Family with probable achondrogenesis and lipid inclusions in fibroblasts. *Arch. Dis. Child.*, **48**, 212–16.

Lazzaroni-Fossati, F., Stanescu, V., Stanescu, R. *et*

al. (1978) La fibrochondrogenese. *Arch. Fr. Pediatr.*, **35**, 1096–104.

Lee, B., Vissing, H., Ramirez, F. *et al.* (1989) Identification of the molecular defect in a family with spondyloepiphyseal dysplasia. *Science*, **244**, 978–80.

Maroteaux, P., Lamy, M. and Robert, J.M. (1967) Le nanisme thanatophore. *Presse Med.*, **75**, 2519–24.

Maroteaux, P., Spranger, J., Stanescu, V. *et al.* (1982) Atelosteogenesis. *Am. J. Med. Genet.*, **13**, 15–25.

Maroteaux, P., Stanescu, V., Stanescu, R. *et al.* (1984) Opsismodysplasia: a new type of chondrodysplasia with predominant involvement of the bones of the hand and the vertebrae. *Am. J. Med. Genet.*, **19**, 171–82.

Maroteaux, P., Stanescu, R., Stanescu, V. *et al.* (1988) Recessive lethal chondrodysplasia: 'round femoral inferior epiphysis type'. *Eur. J. Pediatr.*, **147**, 408–11.

Maynard, J.A., Ippolito, E.G., Ponseti, I.V. *et al.* (1981) Histochemistry and ultrastructure of the growth plate in achondroplasia. *J. Bone Joint Surg.*, **63A**, 969–79.

Molz, G. and Spycher, M.A. (1980) Achondrogenesis type I: light and electron-microscopic studies. *Eur. J. Pediatr.*, **134**, 69–74.

Murray, L.W., Bautista, J., James, P.L. *et al.* (1989) Type II collagen defects in the chondrodysplasias. I. Spondyloepiphyseal dysplasias. *Am. J. Hum. Genet.*, **45**, 5–15.

Nairn, E.R. and Chapman, S. (1989) A new type of lethal short-limbed dwarfism. *Pediatr. Radiol.*, **19**, 253–7.

Ornoy, A., Adomian, G.E., Eteson, D.J. *et al.* (1985) The role of mesenchyme-like tissue in the pathogenesis of thanatophoric dysplasia. *Am. J. Med. Genet.*, **21**, 613–30.

Ornoy, A., Borochowitz, Z., Lachman, R. *et al.* (1988) *Atlas of Fetal Skeletal Radiology*. Year Book Medical Publishers, Chicago.

Ponseti, I.V. (1970) Skeletal growth in achondroplasia. *J. Bone Joint Surg.*, **52**, 101–16.

Poulos, A., Sheffield, L., Sharp, P. *et al.* (1988) Rhizomelic chondrodysplasia punctata: clinical, pathologic, and biochemical findings in two patients. *J. Pediatr.*, **113**, 685–90.

Rimoin, D.L. and Lachman, R.S. (1990) The chondrodysplasias. In: *Principles and Practice of Medical Genetics*, 2nd edn (eds A.E.H. Emery and D.L. Rimoin), Churchill Livingstone, London, pp. 895–932.

Rimoin, D.L. and Sillence, D.O. (1981) Chondro-osseus morphology and biochemistry in the skeletal dysplasias. *Birth Defects*, **XVII** (1), 249–65.

Rimoin, D.L., Hughes, G.N.F., Kaufman, R.L. *et al.* (1970) Endochondral ossification in achondroplastic dwarfism. *N. Engl. J. Med.*, **283**, 728–35.

Rittler, M., Menger, H. and Spranger, J. (1990) Chondrodysplasia punctata, tibia-metacarpal (MT) type. *Am. J. Med. Genet.*, **37**, 200–8.

Sedaghatian, M.R. (1980) Congenital lethal metaphyseal chondrodysplasia: a newly recognized complex autosomal recessive disorder. *Am. J. Med. Genet.*, **6**, 269–74.

Sheffield, L.J., Danks, D.M., Mayne, V. *et al.* (1976) Chondrodysplasia punctata – 23 cases of a mild and relatively common variety. *J. Pediatr.*, **89**, 916–23.

Sillence, D.O., Horton, W.A. and Rimoin, D.L. (1979) Morphologic studies in the skeletal dysplasias. *Am. J. Pathol.*, **96**, 813–60.

Sillence, D.O. (1990) Disorders of bone density, volume and mineralisation. In: *Principles and Practice of Medical Genetics*, 2nd edn (eds A.E.H. Emery and D.L. Rimoin), Churchill Livingstone, London, pp. 933–51.

Sillence, D.O., Lachman, R.S., Jenkins, T. *et al.* (1982) Spondylohumerofemoral hypoplasia (giant cell chondrodysplasia): a neonatally lethal short-limb skeletal dysplasia. *Am. J. Med. Genet.*, **13**, 7–14.

Sly, W.S., Hewett–Emmett, D., Whyte, M.P. *et al.* (1983) Carbonic anhydrase deficiency identified as the primary defect in the autosomal recessive syndrome of osteopetrosis with renal tubular acidosis and cerebral calcification. *Proc. Natl. Acad. Sci. USA*, **80**, 2752–6.

Spranger, J. (1989) Radiologic nosology of bone dysplasias. *Am. J. Med. Genet.*, **34**, 96–104.

Spranger, J. and Maroteaux, P. (1990) The lethal osteochondrodysplasias. *Adv. Hum. Genet.*, **19**, 1–103.

Spranger, J., Benirchke, K., Hall, J.G. *et al.* (1982) Errors of morphogenesis: concepts and terms. Recommendations of an international working group. *J. Pediatr.*, **100**, 160–5.

Stanescu, V., Stanescu, R. and Maroteaux, P. (1984) Pathogenic mechanisms in osteochondrodysplasias. *J. Bone Joint Surg.*, **66A**, 817–36.

Stanescu, R., Stanescu, V. and Maroteaux, P. (1990) Homozygous achondroplasia: morphologic and biochemical study of cartilage. *Am. J. Med. Genet.*, **37**, 412–21.

Warkany, J. (1971) *Congenital Malformations. Notes and Comments.* Year Book Medical Publishers, Chicago.

Whitley, C.B., Langer, L.O., Ophoren, J. *et al.* (1984) Fibrochondrogenesis: lethal, autosomal recessive chondrodysplasia with distinctive cartilage histopathology. *Am. J. Med. Genet.*, **19**, 265–75.

Whitley, C.B., Burke, B.A., Granroth, G. *et al.* (1986) De la Chapelle dysplasia. *Am. J. Med. Genet.*, **25**, 29–39.

Winter, R.M. and Thompson, E.M. (1982) Lethal, neonatal, short-limbed platyspondylic dwarfism. A further variant? *Hum. Genet.*, **61**, 269–72.

Wulfsberg, E.A., Curtis, J. and Jayne, C.H. (1992) A boy with X-linked recessive chondrodysplasia punctata due to an inherited X-Y translocation with a current classification of these disorders. *Am. J. Med. Genet.*, **43**, 823–8.

Wynne–Davies, R., Hall, C.M. and Apley, A.G. (1985) *Atlas of Skeletal Dysplasias.* Churchill Livingstone, Edinburgh.

Yang, S.S., Heidelberger, K.P. and Bernstein, J. (1976a) Intracytoplasmic inclusion bodies in the chondrocytes of type I lethal achondrogenesis. *Hum. Pathol.*, **7**, 667–73.

Yang, S.S., Heidelberger, K.P., Brough, A.J. *et al.* (1976b) Lethal short-limbed chondrodysplasia in early infancy. In: *Perspectives in Pediatric Pathology*, Vol 3, (eds H.S. Rosenberg and R.P. Bolande), Year Book Medical Publishers, Chicago, pp. 1–40.

Yang, S.S., Chen, H., Williams, P. *et al.* (1980) Spondyloepiphyseal dysplasia congenita. *Arch. Pathol. Lab. Med.*, **104**, 208–11.

Yang, S.S., Kitchen, E., Gilbert, E.F. *et al.* (1986) Histopathologic examination in osteochondrodysplasias. Time for standardisation. *Arch. Pathol. Lab. Med.*, **110**, 10–2.

Yang, S.S., Langer, L.O., Cacciarelli, A. *et al.* (1987) Three conditions in neonatal asphyxiating thoracic dysplasia (Jeune) and short rib-polydactyly syndrome spectrum: a clinicopathologic study. *Am. J. Med. Genet.*, **Suppl 3**, 191–207.

Yang, S.S., Roth, J.A. and Langer, L.O. (1991) Short rib syndrome Beemer–Langer type with polydactyly: a multiple congenital anomalies syndrome. *Am. J. Med. Genet.*, **39**, 243–6.

5.10 APPENDIX

With increasing interest in genetic disorders, and the need to maximize the utility of resources and data, Skeletal Dysplasia Groups are being established as a means of pooling information. The United Kingdom group under the chairmanship of Dr Alan Darby seeks to ensure that the maximum amount of data becomes available for increasing the understanding of these conditions by offering advice and forming a central collection of case material.

A comprehensive collection of information about birth defects is to be found in the Birth Defects Encyclopedia published by the Centre for Birth Defects Information Services in the USA. This voluntary organization operates international data collecting as well as processing and disseminating services. The information is presented in the form of illustrated articles. These are stored on computer and are accessible by Fax from anywhere in the world, given the appropriate Fax system. Since the Centre is continually acquiring information the data base is under constant revision, and the revised material is put into the computer data bank as soon as it is completed. The articles are also available on CD-ROM and published in the form of an encyclopedia, a volume of almost 2000 pages. The information is organized so as to facilitate diagnosis using the data from a case, working with either the encyclopedia or a computer program.

5.10.1 THE 1992 REVISION OF THE INTERNATIONAL CLASSIFICATION OF OSTEOCHONDRODYSPLASIAS BY THE INTERNATIONAL WORKING PARTY ON CONSTITUTIONAL DISEASES OF BONE

Members of the Working party:
P. Beighton, Cape Town; A. Giedion, Zurich; R. Gorlin, Minneapolis; J. Hall, Vancouver; B. Horton, Houston; K. Kozlowski, Sydney; R. Lachman, Los Angeles; L.O. Langer, Minneapolis; P. Maroteaux, Paris; A. Poznanski, Chicago; D.L. Rimoin, Los Angeles; D. Sillence, Sydney; J. Spranger, Mainz.

(a) Osteochondrodysplasias

A. *Defects of the tubular (and flat) bones and/or axial skeleton*

1. Achondroplasia group
Thanatophoric dysplasia	AD	Langer *et al.*, 1969
Thanatophoric dysplasia-straight femur/clover leaf skull type	AD	Langer *et al.*, 1987
Achondroplasia	AD	Langer *et al.*, 1967
Hypochondroplasia	AD	Hall and Spranger, 1979a

2. Achondrogenesis
Type IA	AR	Houston *et al.*, 1972
Type IB	AR	Weidemann *et al.*, 1974

3. Spondylodysplastic group (Perinatally lethal)
San Diego type	Sp	Horton *et al.*, 1979
Torrance type	Sp	Kaibara *et al.*, 1983
Luton type	Sp	Winter and Thompson, 1982

4. Metatropic dysplasia group
Fibrochondrogenesis	AR	Lazzaroni–Fossati *et al.*, 1978
Schneckenbecken dysplasia	AR	Borochowitz *et al.*, 1986
Metatropic dysplasia	AD	Beck *et al.*, 1983

5. Short rib dysplasia group (with/without polydactyly)
SR(P) type I (Saldino–Noonan)	AR	Saldino and Noonan, 1972
SR(P) type II (Majewski)	AR	Majewski *et al.*, 1971
SR(P) type III (lethal thoracic dysplasia)	AR	Naumoff *et al.*, 1977
SR(P) type IV (Beemer-Langer)	AR	Beemer *et al.*, 1983
Asphyxiating thoracic dysplasia	AR	Jeune *et al.*, 1955
Ellis–van Creveld dysplasia	AR	McKusick *et al.*, 1964

6. Atelosteogenesis/diastrophic dysplasia group
Boomerang dysplasia	Sp	Tenconi *et al.*, 1983
Atelosteogenesis type I	Sp	Maroteaux *et al.*, 1982
Atelosteogenesis type 2 (de la Chapelle)	AR	Whitley *et al.*, 1986
Omodysplasia I (Maroteaux)	AD	Maroteaux *et al.*, 1986
Omodysplasia II (Borochwitz)	AR	Borochowitz *et al.*, 1991
Oto-palatal-digital syndrome type 2	XLR	Fitch *et al.*, 1983
Diastrophic dysplasia	AR	Lamy and Maroteaux, 1960
Pseudodiastrophic dysplasia	AR	Eteson *et al.*, 1986

7. Kniest–Stickler dysplasia group
Dyssegmental dysplasia–Silverman Handmaker type		
Dyssegmental dysplasia–Rolland–Desbuquois type	AR	Aleck *et al.*, 1987
Kniest dysplasia	AD	Kim *et al.*, 1975
Oto-spondylo-megaepiphyseal dysplasia	AR	Giedion *et al.*, 1982
Stickler dysplasia (heterogeneous, some not linked to Col2A1)	AD	Herrmann *et al.*, 1975

8. Spondylo-epiphyseal dysplasia congenita group   AD   Saldino, 1971
    Langer–Saldino dysplasia (Achondrogenesis type II)
Hypochondrogenesis	AD	Maroteaux *et al.*, 1983
Spondyloepiphyseal dysplasia congenita	AD	Spranger and Langer, 1970

9. Other Spondylo epi-(meta)-physeal dysplasias
    X-linked Spondylo-epiphyseal dysplasia tarda   XLD   Maroteaux *et al.*, 1957
    Other late onset spondyloepi-(meta)-physeal   Beighton *et al.*, 1984
    dysplasias (Namaqualand d, Irapa D)   Hernandez *et al.*, 1980
    Progressive pseudo-rheumatoid dysplasia   AR   Spranger *et al.*, 1983
    Dyggve–Melchior–Clausen dysplasia   AR   Spranger *et al.*, 1975
    Wolcott–Rallison dysplasia   AR   Stoss *et al.*, 1982
    Immunoosseous dysplasia   AR   Spranger *et al.*, 1991
    Pseudo-achondroplasia   AD   Maroteaux and Lamy, 1959
    Opsismodysplasia   AR   Maroteaux *et al.*, 1984 a, b

10. Dysostosis multiplex group   Spranger, 1987
    Mucopolysaccharidoses: Hopwood and Morris, 1989
    I-H   AR
    I-S   AR
    II   XLR
    III-A   AR
    III-B   AR
    III-C   AR
    III-D   AR
    IV-A   AR
    IV-B   AR
    VI   AR
    VII   AR
    Fucosidosis   AR
    α-Mannosidosis   AR
    β-Mannosidosis   AR
    Aspartylglucosaminuria   AR
    gM1-Gangliosidosis, several forms   AR
    Sialidosis, several forms   AR
    Sialic storage disease   AR
    Galactosidosis, several forms   AR
    Mucosulfatidosis   AR
    Mucolipidosis II   AR
    Mucolipidosis III   AR
    Mucolipidosis IV   AR

11. Spondylometaphyseal dysplasias
    Spondylometaphyseal dysplasia–Kozlowski type   AD   Kozlowski *et al.*, 1967
    Spondylometaphyseal dysplasia-corner fracture   AD   Langer *et al.*, 1990
    type (Sutcliffe)
    Spondyloenchondrodysplasia   AR   Schorr *et al.*, 1976

12. Epiphyseal dysplasia
    Multiple epiphyseal dysplasia Fairbanks/Ribbing   AD   Hulvey and Keat, 1969

13. Chondrodysplasia punctata (stippled epiphyses) group
    Rhizomelic type   AR   Spranger *et al.*, 1971
    Conradi–Hunnermann type   XLD   Happle, 1979
    X-linked recessive type   XLR   Maroteaux, 1989
    MT-type   Sp   Rittler *et al.*, 1990
    Others including CHILD syndrome;   Happle *et al.*, 1980
    Zellweger syndrome; Warfarin embryopathy,   Poznanski *et al.*, 1970
    chromosomal abnormalities;   Hall *et al.*, 1980
    fetal alcohol syndrome   Maroteaux *et al.*, 1984a

14. Metaphyseal dysplasia		
type Jansen	AD	Charrow and Poznanski, 1984
type Schmid	AD	Lachman *et al.*, 1988
type Spahr	AR	Spahr and Spahr-Hartmann, 1961
type McKusick (CHH)	AR	McKusick *et al.*, 1965
Metaphyseal anadysplasia	XLR?	Maroteaux and Badoual 1990
type Schwachman	AR	Schmerling *et al.*, 1969
Adenosine deaminase deficiency	AR	Cedarbaum *et al.*, 1976
15. Brachyrachia (short spine dysplasia)		Shohat *et al.*, 1989
Brachyolmia, several types		Horton *et al.*, 1983
16. Mesomelic dysplasia	AD	Langer, 1965
Dyschondrosteosis		
Langer type	AR	Kunze and Klemm, 1980
Nievergelt type	AD	Hess *et al.*, 1978
Robinow type	AD	Butler and Wadlington, 1987
17. Acro/acromesomelic dysplasia		
Acromicric dysplasia	Sp	Maroteaux *et al.*, 1986
Geleophysic dysplasia	AR	Spranger *et al.*, 1984
Acrodysostosis	AD	Maroteaux and Malamut, 1968
Tricho-rhino-phalangeal dysplasia type 1	AD	Giedion *et al.*, 1973
Tricho-rhino-phalangeal dysplasia type 2	AD	Langer *et al.*, 1984
Saldino–Mainzer dysplasia	AR	Mainzer *et al.*, 1970
Pseudohypoparathyroidism	AD	Fitch, 1982
Several types	AR? XLD?	Levine *et al.*, 1988
Cranioectodermal dysplasia	AR	Levin *et al.*, 1977
Acromesomelic dysplasia	AR	Langer *et al.*, 1977
Grebe dysplasia	AR	Grebe, 1952
18. Dysplasias with significant (but not exclusive) membraneous involvement		
Cleido-cranial dysplasia	AD	Jensen, 1990
Osteodysplasty, Melnick–Needles	XLD	Melnick and Needles, 1966
19. Bent bone dysplasia group		
Campomelic dysplasia	AR	Houston *et al.*, 1983
Kyphomelic dysplasia	AR	Hall and Spranger, 1979
Stuve–Wiedemann dysplasia	AR	Stuve and Wiedemann, 1971
20. Multiple dislocations with dysplasia		
Larsen syndrome	AD	Larsen *et al.*, 1950
Desbuquois	AR	Le Merrer *et al.*, 1991
Spondylo-epi-metaphyseal dysplasia with joint laxity	AR	Beighton and Kozlowski, 1980
21. Osteodysplastic primordial dwarfism group		
Type I	AR	Majewski and Spranger, 1976
Type II	AR	Majewski *et al.*, 1982

22. Dysplasias with decreased bone density	AD	Sillence *et al.*, 1979
Osteogenesis imperfecta (several types)	AR,AD	
Osteoporosis with pseudo-glioma	AR	Frontali *et al.*, 1985
Idiopathic juvenile osteoporosis	Sp	Dent and Friedman, 1965
Bruck syndrome	AR	Viljoen *et al.*, 1989
Homocystinuria	AR	Mudd *et al.*, 1985
Singleton–Merten syndrome	Sp	Singleton and Merten 1973
Geroderma osteodysplastica	AR	Hunter *et al.*, 1978
Menkes syndrome	XLR	Menkes, 1988
23. Dysplasias with defective mineralization		
Hypophosphatasia (several types)	AR	Machler *et al.*, 1986
Hypophosphataemic rickets	XR	
Pseudo-deficiency rickets, several types	AR	Liberman *et al.*, 1983
		Barsony *et al.*, 1980
Neonatal-hyperparathyroidism	AR	Spiegel *et al.*, 1977
24. Dysplasia with increased bone density		
Osteopetrosis		
(a) precocious type	AR	Loria-Cortes *et al.*, 1977
(b) delayed type	AD	Johnston *et al.*, 1968
(c) intermediate type	AR	Kahler *et al.*, 1984
(d) with renal tubular acidosis	AR	Sly *et al.*, 1985
Dysosteosclerosis	AR	Spranger *et al.*, 1968
Pycnodysostosis	AR	Maroteaux and Lamy, 1962
Osteosclerosis type Stanescu	AD	Dipieri and Gutman, 1984
Axial osteosclerosis including		
(a) Osteomesopycnosis		
(b) with Bamboo hair (Netherton syndrome)	AR	Porter and Starke, 1968
(c) Trichothiodystrophy	AR	Happle *et al.*, 1984
Osteopoikilosis	AD	Melnick, 1959
Melorrheostosis	Sp	Campbell *et al.*, 1968
Osteopathia striata	Sp	Gehweiler *et al.*, 1973
Osteopathia striata with cranial sclerosis	AD	Horan and Brighton, 1978
Diaphyseal dysplasia, Camurati–Engelmann	AD	Sparkes and Graham, 1962
Craniodiphyseal dysplasia	AD	Schaefer *et al.*, 1986
	AR	Tucker *et al.*, 1976
Lenz–Majewski dysplasia	Sp	Gorlin and Whitley, 1983
Craniometaphyseal dysplasia	Sp	Langer *et al.*, 1991
Endosteal hyperostoses		
(a) van Buchem disease	AR	van Buchem *et al.*, 1962
(b) Sclerosteosis	AR	Beighton, 1988
(c) Worth disease	AD	Worth and Wollin, 1966
(d) with cerebellar hypoplasia	AR	Charrow *et al.*, 1991
Pachydermoperiostosis	AD	Rimoin, 1965
Frontometaphyseal dysplasia	XLR	Gorlin and Wintes, 1980
Craniometaphyseal dysplasia		
(a) severe type	AR	Penchaszadeh *et al.*, 1980
(b) mild type	AD	Holt, 1966
Pyle (disease) dysplasia	AR	Beighton, 1987
Osteo-ectasia with hyperphosphatasia	AR	Fanconi *et al.*, 1964
Oculo-dento-osseous dysplasia		
(a) severe type	AR	Traboulsi *et al.*, 1986
(b) mild type	AD	Patton and Lawrence, 1985

Familial infantile cortical hyperostosis Caffey	AD	MacLachlan *et al.*, 1984

B. Disorganized development of cartilage and fibrous components of skeleton

Dysplasia epiphysealis hemimelica	Sp	Wiedemann *et al.*, 1981
Multiple cartilaginous exostoses	AD	Shapiro *et al.*, 1979
Enchondromatosis (Ollier)	Sp	Mainzer *et al.*, 1971
Enchondromatosis with haemangioma (Maffucci)	Sp	Loewinger *et al.*, 1977
Metachondromatosis	AD	Maroteaux, 1971
Osteoglophonic dysplasia	Sp	Beighton, 1989
Fibrous dysplasia (Jaffe–Lichenstein)	Sp	Firat and Stutzman, 1968
Fibrous dysplasia with skin pigmentation and precocious puberty (McCune–Albright)		
Cherubism	AD	Peters, 1979
Myofibromatosis (generalized fibromatosis)	AR	Modi, 1982

C. Idiopathic Osteolyses

1. Predominantly phalangeal

Hereditary acro-osteolysis, several forms		Spranger *et al.*, 1974
Hajdu–Cheney type	AD	Udell *et al.*, 1986

2. Predominantly carpal/tarsal

Carpal-tarsal osteolysis with nephropathy	AD	Carnevale *et al.*, 1987
Francois syndrome (dermo-chondral-corneal dystrophy)	AR	Caputo *et al.*, 1988

3. Multicentric

Winchester syndrome	AR	Winchester *et al.*, 1969
Torg type	AR	Torg *et al.*, 1969
Mandibulo-acral dysplasia	AR	Tenconi *et al.*, 1986

4. Other

Familial expansile osteolysis	AD	Osterberg *et al.*, 1988

5.10.2   THOSE PARTS OF THE 1983 REVISION OF THE INTERNATIONAL CLASSIFICATION OF CONSTITUTIONAL DISEASES OF BONE NOT REVISED IN 1992

(a)   Dysostoses

Malformation of individual bones, singly or in combination

Dysostoses with cranial and facial involvement

1. Craniosynostosis (several forms)

2. Craniofacial dysostosis (Crouzon)

3. Acrocephalo-syndactyly

(a) type Apert	AD
(b) type Chotzen	AD
(c) type Pfeiffer	AD
(d) other types	

4. Acrocephalo-polysyndactyly (Carpenter and others)   AR

5. Cephalo-polysyndactyly (Grieg)   AD

6. First and second branchial arch syndromes
    (a) mandibulo-facial dysostosis (Treacher–   AD
    Collins-Franceschetti)
    (b) acro-facial dysostosis (Nager)
    (c) oculo-auriculo-vertebral dysostosis (Goldenhar)   AR
    (d) others

7. Cerebro-costo-mandibular syndrome
    (Hallermann–Streiff–Francois)

Dysostoses with predominant axial involvement
1. Vertebral segmentation defects (including Klippel-Fiel)

2. Cervico-oculo-acoustic syndrome (Wildervanck)

3. Sprengel anomaly

4. Spondylo-costal dysostosis
    (a) dominant form   AD
    (b) recessive forms   AR

5. Oculo-vertebral syndrome (Weyers)

6. Osteo-onychodysostosis   AD

7. Cerebro-costo-mandibular syndrome   AR

Dysostoses with predominant involvement of extremities
1. Acheiria

2. Apodia

3. Tetraphocomelia syndrome (Roberts)   AR
    (SC pseudothalidomide syndrome)

4. Ectrodactyly
    (a) Isolated
    (b) Ectrodactyly-ectodermal dysplasia cleft palate   AD
    syndrome
    (c) Ectrodactyly with scalp defects   AD

5. Oro-acral syndrome (aglossia syndrome, Hanhart
    syndrome)

6. Familial radio-ulnar synostosis

7. Brachydactyly, types A,B,C,D,E (Bell's classification)   AD

8. Symphalangism   AD

9. Polydactyly (several forms)

10. Syndactyly (several forms)

11. Polysyndactyly (several forms)

12. Camptodactyly

13. Manzke syndrome

14. Poland syndrome

15. Rubinstein–Taybi syndrome

16. Coffin–Siris syndrome

17. Ancytopenia–dysmelia syndrome (Fanconi) — AR

18. Blackfan–Diamond anaemia with thumb anomalies (Aase syndrome) — AR

19. Thrombocytopenia-radial aplasia syndrome — AR

20. Oto-digital-facial syndrome
    (a) type Papillon–Leage (lethal in male) — XLD
    (b) type Mohr — AR

21. Cardiomelic syndromes (Holt–Oram and others) — AD

22. Femoral focal deficiency (with or without facial anomalies)

23. Multiple synotoses (includes some forms of symphalangism) — AD

24. Scapulo-iliac dysostosis (Kosenow-Sinois) — AD

25. Hand foot genital syndrome — AD

26. Foot dermal hypoplasia (Goltz) (lethal in male) — XLD

Miscellaneous disorders with osseous involvement
1. Early acceleration of skeletal maturation
   (a) Marshall–Smith syndrome
   (b) Weaver syndrome
   (c) other types

2. Marfan syndrome — AD

3. Congenital contractural arachnodactyly — AD

4. Cerebro-hepato-renal syndrome (Zellweger)

5. Coffin–Lowry syndrome — SLR

6. Cockayne syndrome — AR

7. Fibrodysplasia ossificans congenita — AD

8. Epidermal nevus syndrome (Solomon)

9. Nevoid basal cell carcinoma syndrome

10. Multiple congenital fibromatosis

11. Neurofibromatosis — AD

Chromosomal aberrations
   Lipids
1. Niemann–Pick disease (sphingomyelinase deficiency) (several forms) — AR

2. Gaucher disease (beta-glucosidase deficiency) (several forms) — AR

3. Farber disease lipogranulomatosis (ceraminidase deficiency) — AR

REFERENCES

Aleck, K.A., Clericuzio, C., Kaplan, P. *et al.* (1987) Dyssegmental dysplasias: clinical, radiographic and morphologic evidence of heterogeneity. *Am. J. Med. Genet.*, **27**, 295–312.

Barsony, J., McKoy, W., DeGrange, D.A. *et al.* (1989) Selective expression of a normal action of the 1,25-dihydroxy-vitamin D3 receptor in human skin fibroblasts with hereditary severe defects in multiple actions of that receptor. *J. Clin. Invest.*, **83**, 2093–101.

Beck, M., Roubicek, M., Rogers, J.G. *et al.* (1983) Heterogeneity of metatropic dysplasia. *Eur. J. Pediatr.*, **140**, 231–7.

Beemer, F.A., Langer, L.O., Klep-de-Pater, J.M. *et al.* (1983) A new short rib syndrome; report of two cases. *Am. J. Med. Genet.*, **14**, 115–23.

Beighton, P. (1987) Pyle disease (metaphyseal dysplasia). *J. Med. Genet.*, **24**, 321–4.

Beighton, P. (1988) Sclerosteosis. *J. Med. Genet.*, **25**, 200–3.

Beighton, P. (1989) Osteoglophonic dysplasia. *J. Med. Genet.*, **26**, 572–6.

Beighton, P. and Kozlowski, K. (1980) Spondylo-epi-metaphyseal dysplasia with joint laxity and severe, progressive kyphoscoliosis. *Skeletal Radiol.*, **5**, 205–12.

Beighton, P., Christy, G. and Learmonth, D. (1984) Namaqualand hip dysplasia. An autosomal dominant entity. *Am. J. Med. Genet.*, **19**, 161–9.

Borochowitz, Z., Jones, K.L., Silbey, R. *et al.* (1986) A distinct lethal neonatal chondrodysplasia with snail-like pelvis: Schneckenbecken dysplasia. *Am. J. Med. Genet.*, **25**, 45–59.

Borochowitz, Z., Barak, M. and Hershkowitz, S. (1991) Familial micromelic dysplasia with dislocation of radius and distinct face. A new skeletal dysplasia syndrome. *Am. J. Med. Genet.*, **39**, 91–6.

Butler, M.G. and Wadlington, W.B. (1987) Robinow syndrome: report of two cases and review of the literature. *Clin. Genet.*, **31**, 77–85.

Campbell, C.J., Papademetriou, T. and Bonfiglio, M. (1968) Melorheostosis: a report of the clinical, roentgenographic and pathological findings in fourteen cases. *J. Bone Joint Surg.*, **50A**, 1281–99.

Caputo, R., Sambvani, N., Monti, M. *et al.* (1988) Dermochondrocorneal dystrophy (Francois syndrome). Report of a case. *Arch. Dermatol.*, **124**, 424–8.

Carnevale, A., Canun, S., Mendoza, L. and del

Castillo, V. (1987) Idiopathic multicentric osteolysis with facial anomalies and nephropathy. *Am. J. Med. Genet.*, **26**, 877–86.

Cedarbaum, S.D., Kaitila, J., Rimoin, D.L. *et al.* (1976) The chondroosseous dysplasia of ADA deficiency with severe combined immunodeficiency. *J. Pediatr.*, **89**, 737–47.

Charrow, J. and Poznanski, A.K. (1984) The Jansen type of metaphyseal chondrodysplasia: confirmation of dominant inheritance and review of radiographic manifestations in the newborn and adult. *Am. J. Med. Genet.*, **18**, 321–7.

Charrow, J., Poznanski, A.K., Unger, F.M. *et al.* (1991) Autosomal recessive cerebellar hypoplasia and endosteal hyperostosis. *Am. J. Med. Genet.*, **41**, 464–8.

Dent, C.E. and Friedman, M. (1965) Idiopathic juvenile osteoporosis. *Q. J. Med.*, **34**, 177–210.

Dipieri, J.E. and Gutman, J.D. (1984) A second family with autosomal dominant osteosclerosis, Type Stanescu. *Am. J. Med. Genet.*, **18**, 13–8.

Eteson, D.J., Beluffi, G., Burgio, G.R. *et al.* (1986) Pseudodiastrophic dysplasia: a distinct newborn skeletal dysplasia. *J. Pediatr.*, **109**, 635–41.

Fanconi, G., Moreira, G., Uehlinger, E. *et al.* (1964) Osteochalasia desmalis familiaris: hyperostosis corticalis deformans juvenilis, chronic idiopathic hyperphosphatasia and microcranium. *Helv. Paediatr. Acta*, **19**, 279–95.

Fasanelli, S., Kozlowski, K., Reiter, S. *et al.* (1985) Dyssegmental dysplasia. *Skeletal Radiol.*, **14**, 173–7.

Firat, D. and Stutzman, L. (1968) Fibrous dysplasia of bone: Review of twenty four cases. *Am. J. Med.*, **44**, 421–9.

Fitch, N. (1982) Albright's hereditary osteodystrophy: a review. *Am. J. Med. Genet.*, **11**, 11–29.

Fitch, N., Jequier, S. and Gorlin, R. (1983) The oto-palatal syndrome, proposed type II. *Am. J. Med. Genet.*, **15**, 655–64.

Frontali, M., Stomeo, C. and Dallapiccola, B. (1985) Osteoporosis-pseudoglioma syndrome: report of three affected sibs and an overview. *Am. J. Med. Genet.*, **22**, 35–47.

Gehweiler, J.A., Bland, W.R., Carden, T.S. *et al.* (1973) Osteopathia striata – Voorhoeve's disease: review of the roentgen manifestations. *Am. J. Radiol.*, **113**, 450–8.

Giedion, A., Burdea, M., Fruchter, Z. *et al.* (1973) Autosomal dominant transmission of the tricho-rhino-phalangeal syndrome: report of 4 unrelated families, review of 60 cases. *Helv. Paediatr. Acta*, **28**, 249–59.

Giedion, A., Brandner, M., Lecanellier, J. *et al.* (1982) Oto-spondylo-megaepiphyseal dysplasia (OSMED). *Helv. Paediatr. Acta*, **37**, 361–80.

Gorlin, A. and Winter, R.B. (1980) Frontometaphyseal dysplasia: Evidence for X-linked inheritance. *Am. J. Med. Genet.*, **5**, 81–4.

Gorlin, R.J. and Whitley, C.B. (1983) Lenz– Majewski syndrome. *Radiology*, **149**, 129–31.

Grebe, H. (1952) Die Achondrogenesis: Ein einfach rezessives Erbmerkmal. *Folia Hered. Pathol.*, **2**, 23–8.

Hall, B.D. and Spranger, J. (1979) Familial congenital bowing with short bones. *Radiology*, **132**, 611–4.

Hall, B.D. and Spranger, J. (1979a) Hypochondroplasia. *Radiology*, **133**, 95–100.

Hall, J.G., Pauli, R.M. and Wilson, K.M. (1980) Maternal and fetal sequelae of anticoagulation during pregnancy. *Am. J. Med.*, **68**, 122–40.

Happle, R. (1979) X-linked dominant chondrodysplasia: review of literature and report of a case. *Hum. Genet.*, **53**, 65–73.

Happle, R., Koch, H. and Lenz, W. (1980) The CHILD syndrome. *Eur. J. Pediatr.*, **134**, 27–33.

Happle, R., Traupe, H., Grobe, H. *et al.* (1984) The Tay syndrome (congenital ichthyosis with trichothiodystrophy). *Eur. J. Pediatr.*, **141**, 147–52.

Hernandez, A., Ramirez, M.L., Nazara, Z. *et al.* (1980) Autosomal recessive spondylo-epi-metaphyseal dysplasia (Irapa type) in a Mexican family: Delineation of the syndrome. *Am. J. Med. Genet.*, **5**, 179–88.

Herrmann, J., France, T.D., Spranger, J.W. *et al.* (1975) The Stickler syndrome (hereditary arthro-ophthalmopathy). New York Excerpta Medica for the National Foundation-March of Dimes. Birth Defects **XI** (2), 76–103.

Hess, O.M., Goebel, N.H. and Streuli, R. (1978) Familliarer mesomeler Kleinwuchs (Nievergelt Syndrom). *Schweiz Med. Wschr.*, **108**, 1202–6.

Holt, J.F. (1966) The evolution of cranio-metaphyseal dysplasia. *Ann. Radiol.*, **9**, 209–14.

Hopwood, J.J. and Morris, C.P. (1989) The mucopolysaccharidoses. *Mol. Biol. Med.*, **7**, 381–404.

Horan, F.T. and Beighton, P.H. (1978) Osteopathia striata with cranial sclerosis: an autosomal dominant entity. *Clin. Genet.*, **13**, 201–6.

Horton, W.A., Rimoin, D.L., Hollister, D.W. *et al.* (1979) Further heterogeneity within lethal neonatal short limbed dwarfism: the plato-spondylic types. *J. Pediatr.*, **94**, 736–42.

Horton, W.A., Langer, L.O., Collins, D.L. *et al.* (1983) Brachyolmia, recessive type (Hobaek): a clinical, radiographic and histochemical study. *Am. J. Med. Genet.*, **16**, 201–11.

Houston, C.S., Awen, C.F. and Kent, H.P. (1972) Fatal neonatal dwarfism. *Can. Assoc. Radiol.*, **23**, 45–61.

Houston, C.S., Opitz, J.M., Spranger, J.W. *et al.* (1983) The campomelic syndrome: review, report of 17 cases and follow-up on the currently 17-year-old boy first reported by Maroteaux *et al.* in 1971. *Am. J. Med. Genet.*, **15**, 3–28.

Hulvey, J.T. and Keats, T. (1969) Multiple epiphyseal dysplasia. *Am. J. Roentgenol.*, **106**, 170–7.

Hunter, A.G.W., Martsolf, J.T., Baker, C.G. *et al.* (1978) Gerogerma osteodysplastica: a report of two families. *Hum. Genet.*, **40**, 311–25.

Jensen, B.L. (1990) Somatic development in cleidocranial dysplasia. *Am. J. Med. Genet.*, **35**, 69–74.

Jeune, M., Beraud, C. and Carron, R. (1955) Dystrophie thoracique asphyxiante de caractere familial. *Arch. Fr. Pediatr.*, **12**, 1886–91.

Johnston, C.C., Lavy, N., Lord, T. *et al.* (1968) Osteopetrosis: a clinical, genetic, metabolic and morphologic study of the dominantly inherited, benign form. *Medicine*, **47**, 149–67.

Kahler, S.G., Burns, J.A. and Aylsworth, A.S. (1984) A mild autosomal recessive form of osteopetrosis. *Am. J. Med. Genet.*, **17**, 451–64.

Kaibara, N., Yokoyama, K. and Nakano, H. (1983) Torrance type of lethal neonatal short-limbed platyspondylic dwarfism. *Skeletal Radiol.*, **10**, 17–9.

Kim, H.J., Beratis, N.G., Brill, P. *et al.* (1975) Kniest syndrome with dominant inheritance and mucopolysacchariduria. *Am. J. Hum. Genet.*, **27**, 755–64.

Koslowski, K., Maroteaux, P. and Spranger, J. (1967) La dystostose metaphysaire. *Presse Med.*, **75**, 2769–74.

Kunze, J. and Klemm, T. (1980) Mesomelic dysplasia, type Langer: a homozygous state for dyschondrosteosis. *Eur. J. Pediatr.*, **134**, 269–72.

Lachman, R.S., Rimoin, D.L. and Spranger, J. (1988) Metaphyseal chondrodysplasia, Schmid type: Clinical and radiographic delineation with a review of the literature. *Pediatr. Radiol.*, **18**, 93–102.

Lamy, M. and Maroteaux, P. (1960) Le nanisme diastrophique. *Presse Med.*, **68**, 1977–80.

Langer, L.O. (1965) Dyschondrosteosis, a heritable bone syndrome with characteristic roentgenographic features. *Am. J. Roentgenol.*, **95**, 178–88.

Langer, L.O., Baumann, P.A. and Gorlin, R.J. (1967) Achondroplasia. *Am. J. Roentgenol.*, **100**, 12–26.

Langer, L.O., Spranger, J.W., Greinacher, I. *et al.* (1969) Thanatophoric dwarfism. *Radiology*, **92**, 285–94.

Langer, L.O., Beals, R.K., Solomon, I.L. *et al.* (1977) Acromesomelic dwarfism: manifestations in childhood. *Am. J. Med. Genet.*, **1**, 87–100.

Langer, L.O., Krassikof, N., Laxova, R. *et al.* (1984) The tricho-rhino-phalangeal syndrome with exostoses (or Langer–Giedion syndrome): four additional patients without mental retardation and review of the literature. *Am. J. Med. Genet.*, **19**, 81–111.

Langer, L.O., Yang, S.S., Hall, J.G. *et al.* (1987) Thanatophoric dwarfism and cloverleaf skull. *Am. J. Med. Genet.*, **Suppl. 3**, 167–79.

Langer, L.O., Brill, P.W., Ozonoff, M.B. *et al.* (1990) Spondylometaphyseal dysplasia, corner fracture type: a heritable condition associated with coxa vara. *Radiology*, **175**, 761–6.

Langer, L.O., Brill, P.W., Afshani, E. *et al.* (1991) Radiographic features of craniometadiaphyseal dysplasia wormian bone type. *Skeletal Radiol.*, **20**, 37–41.

Larsen, L.J., Schottstaedt, E.R. and Bost, F.C. (1950) Multiple congenital dislocations associated with characteristic facial abnormality. *J. Pediatr.*, **37**, 574–81.

Lazzaroni-Fossati, F., Stanescu, V., Stanescu, R. *et al.* (1978) La fibrochondrogenese. *Arch. Fr. Pediatr.*, **35**, 106–104.

Le Merrer, M., Young, I.D., Stanescu, V. *et al.* (1991) Desbuquois syndrome. *Eur. J. Pediatr.*, **150**, 793–6.

Levin, L.S., Perrin, J.C.S., Ose, L. *et al.* (1977) A heritable syndrome of craniosynostosis, short thick hair, dental abnormalities, and short limbs. Cranioectodermal dysplasia. *J. Pediatr.*, **90**, 55–61.

Levine, M.A., Ahn, T.G., Klupt, S.F. *et al.* (1988) Genetic deficiency of the alpha subunit of the guanidine nucleotide-binding protein G(s) as the molecular basis for Albright hereditary osteodystrophy. *Proc. Natl. Acad. Sci. USA*, **85**, 617–21.

Liberman, U.A., Eil, C. and Marx, S.J. (1983) Resistance to 1,25-dihydroxy-vitamin D: association with heterogeneous defects in cultured skin fibroblasts. *J. Clin. Invest.*, **71**, 192–200.

Loewinger, R.J., Lichtenstein, J.R., Dodson, W.E. *et al.* (1977) Mafucci's syndrome: a mesenchymal dysplasia and multiple tumour syndrome. *Br. J. Dermatol.*, **96**, 317–22.

Loria-Cortes, R., Quesada-Calvo, E. and Cordero-Chaverri, E. (1977) Osteopetrosis in children: a report of 26 cases. *J. Pediatr.*, **91**, 43–7.

MacLachlan, A.K., Gerrard, J.W., Houston, C.S. *et al.* (1984) Familial infantile cortical hyperostosis in a large Canadian family. *Can. Med. Assoc. J.*, **130**, 1172–4.

Machler, M., Frey, D., Gal, A. *et al.* (1986) X-linked dominant hypophosphatemia is closely linked to DNA markers DXS41 and DXS43 at Xp22. *Hum. Genet.*, **73**, 271–5.

Mainzer, F., Saldino, R.M., Ozonoff, M.B. *et al.* (1970) Familial nephropathy associated with retinitis pigmentosa, cerebellar ataxia and skeletal abnormalities. *Am. J. Med.*, **49**, 556–62.

Mainzer, F., Minagi, H. and Steinbach, H.L. (1971) The variable manifestations of multiple enchondromatosis. *Radiology*, **99**, 377–88.

Majewski, F., Pfeiffer, R.A., Lenz, W. *et al.* (1971) Polysyndaktylie, verkurzte Gliedmassen und Genitalfehlbildungen: Kennzeichen eines selbstandigen Syndroms. *Z. Kinderh.*, **111**, 118–38.

Majewski, F. and Spranger, J. (1976) Uber einen neuen Typ des primordialen Minderwuchses: Der brachymele primordiale Minderwuchs. *Z. Kinderh.*, **124**, 499–503.

Majewski, F., Ranke, M. and Schinzuel, A. (1982) Studies of microcephalic primordial dwarfism. II. The osteodysplastic type II of primordial dwarfism. *Am. J. Med. Genet.*, **12**, 23–5.

Maroteaux, P. (1971) La metachondromatose. *Z. Kinderh.*, **109**, 246–61.

Maroteaux, P. (1980) L'osteomesopycnose: une nouvelle affection condensante de transmission dominante autosomique. *Arch. Fr. Pediatr.*, **37**, 153–7.

Maroteaux, P. (1989) Brachytelephalangic chondrodysplasia punctata: a possible X-linked recessive form. *Hum. Genet.*, **82**, 167–70.

Maroteaux, P. and Badoual, J. (1990) La chondrodysplasie microcephalique sublethale. Syndrome de Taybi–Linder, nanisme microcephalique primordial de types I et III. *Arch. Fr. Pediatr.*, **47**, 103–6.

Maroteaux, P., Lamy, M. and Bernard, J. (1957) La dysplanie spondylo-epiphysaire tardive. *Presse Med.*, **65**, 1205–8.

Maroteaux, P. and Lamy, M. (1959) Les formes pseudo-achondroplastiques des dysplasies spondylo-epiphysaires. *Presse Med.*, **67**, 383–6.

Maroteaux, P. and Lamy, M. (1962) La pycnodysostose. *Presse Med.*, **70**, 999–1002.

Maroteaux, P. and Malamut, G. (1968) L'acrodysostose. *Presse Med.*, **76**, 2189–92.

Maroteaux, P., Spranger, J, Stanescu, V. *et al.* (1982) Atelosteogenesis. *Am. J. Med. Genet.*, **13**, 15–25.

Maroteaux, P., Stanescu, V. and Stanescu, R. (1983) Hypochondrogenesis. *Eur. J. Pediatr.*, **141**, 14–22.

Maroteaux, P., Lavollay, B., Bomsell, F. *et al.* (1984a) Chondrodysplasie ponctué et intoxication alcoolique maternelle. *Arch. Fr. Pediatr.*, **41**, 547–50.

Maroteaux, P., Stanescu, V., Stanescu, R. *et al.* (1984b) Opsismodysplasia: a new type of chondrodysplasia with predominant involvement of the bones of the hand and the vertebrae. *Am. J. Med. Genet.*, **19**, 171–82.

Maroteaux, P., Stanescu, V., Stanescu, R. *et al.* (1986) Acromicric dysplasia. *Am. J. Med. Genet.*, **24**, 447–59.

Maroteaux, P., Sauvegrain, J., Christpin, A. *et al.* (1989) Omodysplasia. *Am. J. Med. Genet.*, **32**, 371–5.

Maroteaux, P., Verloes, A., Stanescu, V. *et al.* (1991) Metaphyseal anadysplasia: a metaphyseal dysplasia of early onset with radiological regression and benign course. *Am. J. Med. Genet.*, **39**, 4–10.

McKusick, V.A., Egeland, J.A., Eldridge, R. *et al.* (1964) Dwarfism in the Amish. I. The Ellis–van Creveld syndrome. *Bull. Johns Hopkins Hosp.*, **113**, 306–36.

McKusick, V.A., Eldridge, R., Hostetler, J.A. *et al.* (1965) Dwarfism in the Amish. II. Cartilage-hair hypoplasia. *Bull. Johns Hopkins Hosp.*, **116**, 285–326.

Melnick, J.C. (1959) Osteopathia condensans disseminata (osteopoikilosis): study of a family of 4 generations. *Am. J. Roentgenol.*, **82**, 229–38.

Melnick, J.C. and Needles, C.F. (1966) An undiagnosed bone dysplasia: a two family study of 4 generations and 3 generations. *Am. J. Roentgenol.*, **97**, 39–48.

Menkes, J.H. (1988) Kinky hair disease: twenty five years later. *Brain Dev.*, **10**, 77–9.

Modi, N. (1982) Congenital generalised fibromatosis. *Arch. Dis. Child.*, **57**, 881–2.

Mudd, S.H., Skovby, F., Levy, H.L. *et al.* (1985) The natural history of homocystinuria due to cystathionine beta-synthetase deficiency. *Am. J. Hum. Genet.*, **37**, 1–31.

Naumoff, P., Young, L.W., Mazer, J. *et al.* (1977) Short rib-polydactyly syndrome type III. *Radiology*, **122**, 443–7.

Osterberg, P.H., Wallace, R.G.H. *et al.* (1988) Familial expansile osteolysis: a new dysplasia. *J. Bone Joint Surg.*, **70**, 255–60.

Patton, M.A. and Laurence, K.M. (1985) Three new cases of oculodentodigital (ODD) syndrome: development of the facial phenotype. *J. Med. Genet.*, **22**, 386–9.

Penchaszadeh, V.B., Gutierriz, E.R. and Figueroa, E.P. (1980) Autosomal recessive craniometaphyseal dysplasia. *Am. J. Med. Genet.*, **5**, 43–55.

Peters, W.J.N. (1979) Cherubism: a study of twenty cases from one family. *Oral Surg.*, **47**, 307–11.

Porter, P.S. and Starke, J.C. (1968) Netherton's syndrome. *Arch. Dis. Child.*, **43**, 319–22.

Poznanski, A.K., Nosanchuk, J.S., Baublis, J. *et al.* (1970) The cerebro-hepato-renal syndrome (CHRS). *Am. J. Roentgenol.*, **109**, 313–22.

Rimoin, D.L. (1965) Pachydermoperiostosis (idiopathic clubbing and periostosis). Genetic and physiologic considerations. *N. Engl. J. Med.*, **272**, 923–31.

Rittler, M., Menger, H. and Spranger, J. (1990) Chondrodysplasia punctata, tibia-metacarpal (MT) type. *Am. J. Med. Genet.*, **37**, 200–8.

Saldino, R.M. (1971) Lethal short-limbed dwarfism, achondrogenesis and thanatophoric dwarfism. *Am. J. Roentgenol.*, **112**, 185–97.

Saldino, R.M. and Noonan, C.D. (1972) Severe thoracic dystrophy with striking micromelia, abnormal osseous development, including the spine, and multiple visceral abnormalities. *Am. J. Roentgenol.*, **114**, 257–63.

Schaefer, B., Stein, S., Oshman, D. *et al.* (1986) Dominantly inherited craniodiaphyseal dysplasia: a new craniotubular dysplasia. *Clin. Genet.*, **30**, 381–91.

Schorr, S. Legrum, C. and Ochshorn, M. (1976) Spondyloenchondrodysplasia: enchondromatosis with severe platyspondyly in two brothers. *Radiology*, **118**, 133–9.

Schmerling, D.H., Prader, A., Hitzig, W.H. *et al.* (1969) The syndrome of exocrine pancreatic insufficiency, neutropenia, metaphyseal dysostosis and dwarfism. *Helv. Paediatr. Acta*, **24**, 547–75.

Shapiro, F., Simon, S. and Glimcher, M.J. (1979) Hereditary multiple exostoses: anthropometric, roentgenographic and clinical aspects. *J. Bone Joint Surg.*, **61A**, 815–24.

Shohat, M., Lachman, R., Gruber, H.E. *et al.* (1989)

Brachyolmia: radiographic and genetic evidence of heterogeneity. *Am. J. Med. Genet.*, **33**, 209–19.

Sillence, D.O., Senn, A. and Danks, D.M. (1979) Genetic heterogeneity in osteogenesis imperfecta. *J. Med. Genet.*, **16**, 101–16.

Singleton, E.B. and Merten, D.F. (1973) An unusual syndrome of widened medullary cavities of the metacarpals and phalanges, aortic calcification and abnormal dentition. *Pediatr. Radiol.*, **1**, 2–7.

Sly, W.S., Whyte, M.P., Sundaram, V. *et al.* (1985) Carbonic anhydrase II deficiency in 12 families with the autosomal recessive syndrome of osteopetrosis with renal tubular acidosis and cerebral calcification. *N. Engl. J. Med.*, **313**, 139–45.

Spahr, A. and Spahr-Hartmann, I. (1961) Dysostose metaphysaire familiale: Etude de 4 cas dans une fratrie. *Helv. Paediatr. Acta*, **16**, 832–49.

Sparkes, R.S. and Graham, C.B. (1972) Camurati–Englemann disease. Genetics and clinical manifestations with a review of the literature. *J. Med. Genet.*, **9**, 73–85.

Spiegel, A.M., Marx, S.J., Brown, E.M. *et al.* (1977) Neonatal primary hyperparathyroidism with autosomal dominant inheritance. *J. Pediatr.*, **90**, 269–72.

Spranger, J.W. (1987) Mini Review: inborn errors of complex carbohydrate metabolism. *Am. J. Med. Genet.*, **28**, 489–99.

Spranger, J.W. and Langer, L.O. (1970) Spondyloepiphyseal dysplasia congenita. *Radiology*, **94**, 313–22.

Spranger, J.W., Albrecht, C., Rohwedder, H.J. *et al.* (1968) Die Dysosteosklerose: Eine Sonderform der generalisierten Osteoskleroses. *Fortschr. Roentgenstr.*, **109**, 504–12.

Spranger, J.W., Opitz, J.M. and Bidder, U. (1971) Heterogeneity of chondrodysplasia punctata. *Humangenetik*, **11**, 190–212.

Spranger, J.W., Langer, L.O. and Wiedemann, H.R. (1974) *Bone Dysplasias.* Fischer/Saunders, Stuttgart/Philadelphia, p. 211.

Spranger, J.W., Maroteaux, P. and Der Kaloustian, V.M. (1975) The Dyggve–Melchior–Clausen syndrome. *Radiology*, **114**, 415–22.

Spranger, J.W., Albert, C., Schilling, F. *et al.* (1983) Progressive pseudorheumatoid arthropathy of childhood (PPAC): a hereditary disorder simulating rheumatoid arthritis. *Eur. J. Pediatr.*, **140**, 34–40.

Spranger, J.W., Gilbert, E.F., Arya, S. *et al.* (1984)

Geleophysic dysplasia. *Am. J. Med. Genet.*, **419**, 487–99.

Spranger, J.W., Hinkel, G.K., Stoss, H. *et al.* (1991) Schimke immuno-osseous dysplasia: a newly recognized multi-system disease. *J. Pediatr.*, **119**, 64–72.

Stoss, H., Pesch, H.J., Pontz, B. *et al.* (1982) Wolcott–Rallison syndrome: diabetes mellitus and spondyloepiphyseal dysplasia. *Eur. J. Pediatr.*, **138**, 120–9.

Stuve, A. and Weidemann, H.R. (1971) Congenital bowing of the long bones in two sisters. *Lancet*, **i**, 495.

Tenconi, R., Kozlowski, K. and Largaiolli, G. (1983) Boomerang dysplasias. *Fortschr. Roentgenstr.*, **138**, 378–80.

Tenconi, R., Miotti, F., Miotti, A. *et al.* (1986) Another Italian family with mandibuloacral dysplasia. Why does it seem more frequent in Italy? *Am. J. Med. Genet.*, **24**, 357–64.

Torg, J.S., DiGeorge, A.M., Kirkpatrick, J.A. *et al.* (1969) Hereditary multicentric osteolysis with recessive transmission: a new syndrome. *J. Pediatr.*, **75**, 243–52.

Traboulski, E.K., Faris, B.M. and Der Kaloustian, V.M. (1986) Persistent hyperplastic primary vitreous and recessive oculo-dento-osseous dysplasia. *Am. J. Med. Genet.*, **2**, 95–100.

Tucker, A.S., Klein, L. and Anthony, G.J. (1976) Craniodiaphyseal dysplasia: evolution over a five year period. *Skeletal Radiol.*, **1**, 47–53.

Udell, J., Schumacher, J.R., Kaplan, F. and Fallon, M.D. (1986) Idiopathic familial acroosteolysis: histomorphometric study and literature review of the Hajdu–Cheney syndrome. *Arthritis Rheum.*, **29**, 1032–8.

van Buchem, F.S.P., Halders, H.N., Hansen, J.F. *et al.* (1962) Hyperostosis corticalis generalisata: a report of seven cases. *Am. J. H. Med.*, **33**, 387–97.

Viljoen, D., Versfeld, G. and Beighton, P. (1989) Osteogenesis imperfecta with congenital joint contractures (Bruck syndrome). *Clin. Genet.*, **36**, 122–6.

Weinstein, L.S., Shenker, A., Gejman, P.V. *et al.* (1991) Activating mutations of the simulatory G protein in the McCune–Albright syndrome. *N. Engl. J. Med.*, **325**, 1688–95.

Whitley, C.B., Burke, B.A., Granroth, G. *et al.* (1986) De la Chapelle dysplasia. *Am. J. Med. Genet.*, **25**, 229–39.

Weidemann, H.R., Remagen, W., Hienz, H.A. (1974) Achondrogenesis within the scope of the conatally manifested generalized skeletal dysplasias. *Z. Kinderh.*, **116**, 223–51.

Weidemann, H.R., Mann, M. and Kreudenstein, P.S. (1981) Dysplasia epiphysealis hemimelica-Trevor disease with severe manifestations in a child. *Eur. J. Pediatr.*, **136**, 311–16.

Winchester, P. Grossman, H., Lim, W.N. *et al.* (1969) A new acid mucopolysaccharidosis with skeletal deformities simulating rheumatoid arthritis. *Am. J. Roentgenol.*, **106**, 121–8.

Winter, R.M. and Thompson, E.M. (1982) Lethal, neonatal, short-limbed platyspondylic dwarfism: a further variant? *Hum. Genet.*, **61**, 269–70.

Worth, H.M. and Wollin, D.G. (1966) Hyperostosis corticalis generalisata congenita. *J. Can. Assoc. Radiol.*, **17**, 67–74.

INJURY

6

Paul D. Byers

6.1 INTRODUCTION

Injury is a broad term covering the effect of agents extrinsic or intrinsic to the body.

6.1.1 EXTRINSIC AGENTS

These can be animate or inanimate. In the first case the reactions to which they give rise are discussed under infection, infestation and inflammation. The inanimate agents of injury are (Pounds *et al.*, 1991; Klein, 1991):

1. Chemical
   (a) Industrial chemicals
   (b) Therapeutic drugs
   (c) Ethanol
   (d) Tobacco smoke
   (e) Aflatoxins and other toxic natural products
2. Physical
   (a) Ultraviolet light
   (b) Ionizing radiation
   (c) Mechanical
   (d) Thermal

Of these, orthopaedic pathology is mainly concerned with mechanical injury to bones and joints, tendons and ligaments, and muscle attachments, but the effects of drugs (steroids and NSAIDs), ionizing radiation (internal and external sources) and of ingested heavy metals are sometimes of concern.

6.1.2 INTRINSIC AGENTS

Broadly speaking, these can be any failure of the normal function of bodily organs. Thus, the malfunction of the endocrine glands, the failure of parenchymatous organs or of the heart or the vascular system are examples. Many of these have effects on bone but are discussed under rubrics other than injury. However, deprivation of its blood supply can cause serious injury to bone, and is considered under the heading of avascular or, alternatively, aseptic necrosis.

An important aspect of injury is the two levels of reaction to it: at the site of injury, and a more general response regionally or throughout the body.

6.2 THE REGIONAL AND GENERALIZED REACTIONS

Two phases have been recognized in the generalized reaction to injury, 'ebb' and 'flow' (Cuthbertson, 1942, 1976). The first is characterized by depressed energy production, manifested in part as a lowering of body temperature and the state of shock. This is reversed within 24 hours and the metabolic processes are increased. The magnitude of the reaction is related to the severity of the injury rather than to its cause. There are levels of severity below which the reaction is not observed. When injury is sufficient to induce reaction, there is also a reduced intake of exogenous fuel leading to activation of anabolic and catabolic hormones which mobilize and utilize fat and protein to provide energy to drive the body's metabolic processes to sustain life and effect healing. This calls on depot fat and, mainly, muscle protein. Some of the ensuing changes

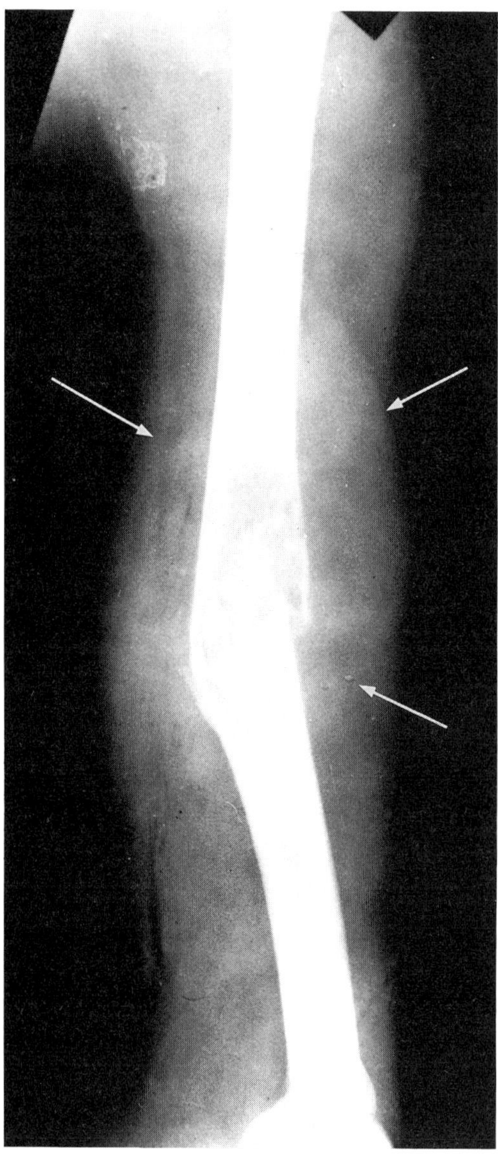

Figure 6.1 10-year-old female. Pathological fracture 10 days previously at the site of a simple bone cyst. Fracture callus has formed a large, smooth, firm swelling (arrows) encasing the ovoid well-delineated osteolytic lesion. This was biopsied as a potentially malignant neoplasm. The fact of such massive growth in so short a time precludes that possibility.

in body composition are loss of solids (=weight loss), of potassium and magnesium. Potassium is lost from cells through failure of the sodium pump; sodium is retained and causes cellular swelling, which may have serious consequences, especially for renal and cerebral function. The intricacies of the metabolic pathways which are involved are described in the relevant literature (Smith, 1980).

In addition to the foregoing, there is increased urinary excretion of calcium and hydroxyproline derived from resorption of bone. This can be induced in healthy subjects by immobilization alone (Howard *et al.*, 1944, a,b; Howard, 1945; Hulley *et al.*, 1971). However, the loss is less than that following fracture (Dietrich *et al.*, 1948). In both categories the excretion was maximal after about 4 weeks, and was at a time when urinary nitrogen was falling. The mean maximal excretions were: fracture 500 mg/day; bed rest 340 mg/day (normal adult male 180 mg/day). Thus post-injury bone loss is due to more than immobilization. This has been referred to by Frost (1983, 1986) as the Regional Acceleratory Phenomenon (RAP; Chapter 15). Whereas there may be no generalized reaction to minor injuries, there is, according to Frost, a regional one, although in a very minor injury this might be no more than the inflammatory reaction to it.

Trauma causes cell and tissue damage, incites inflammation, and leads to reactive changes, and repair and healing. These lack specificity as to cause, so that if features in this sequence are imputed to trauma, then there must be adequate evidence that this has occurred and is of appropriate kind and of sufficient degree. If there is any doubt on this point then the possibility of underlying pathology must be considered. But equally it is necessary to be alert to the possibility that the history of trauma is being suppressed, as in cases of battering, particularly of children. Caffey (1945) was early in the recognition of this.

6.3   INJURY (TRAUMA): HEALING AND REPAIR

6.3.1   FRACTURE

Fractures do not present clinical problems which require the aid of histological analysis unless there is an underlying disorder to be investigated. In pathological fracture the reactive tissue may be substantial and comprise part or all of a biopsy (Figures 6.1–6.5). The pathologist must be alert to the distinguishing features of reactive tissues discussed in Chapter 14 where some reference is made to the literature on the biology of fracture repair (Hall, 1992).

Delayed union and non-union of fractures sometimes lead to biopsy in a quest for assessment of progress in healing or of a cause for failure to heal. The steps in the normal course of fracture repair are well known, but within those there is a good deal of variation in time scale, quantities of reparative tissue formed and its evolution (Sevitt, 1981). Knowledge of the course of fracture repair is needed for this evaluation.

Fracture healing is affected by the effectiveness of reduction and the means and success of stabilization. Ashhurst (1992) has studied these in experimental animals. For didactic description of fracture healing, the usual assumptions are an uncomplicated diaphyseal fracture, good reduction and reasonable stability by plaster cast. Topics which also need to be addressed are fractures of predominantly cancellous bone, effects of avascular necrosis, healing with the use of compression devices and mobility at the fracture site. These are discussed after the description of repair and healing in a diaphyseal fracture in which the periosteum has also been parted. The descriptions of details of the process vary according to the dynamic interpretation of static appearances in histological sections (McKibbin, 1978). But the basic pattern of developments are agreed.

Several stages in the process have been identified (McKibbin, 1978; Sevitt, 1980, 1981):

1. Immediately, haemorrhage and inflammation.
2. In a few days, proliferation of repair (granulation) tissue and formation of a collar of callus around the shaft of each fragment. McKibbin has called this primary callus.
3. After 7–10 days, bridging of the gap

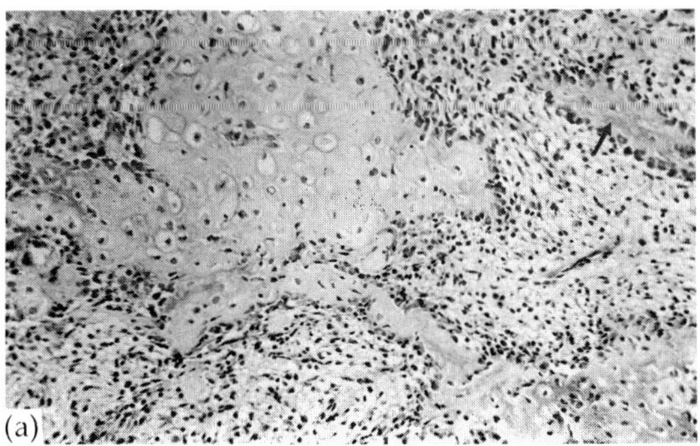
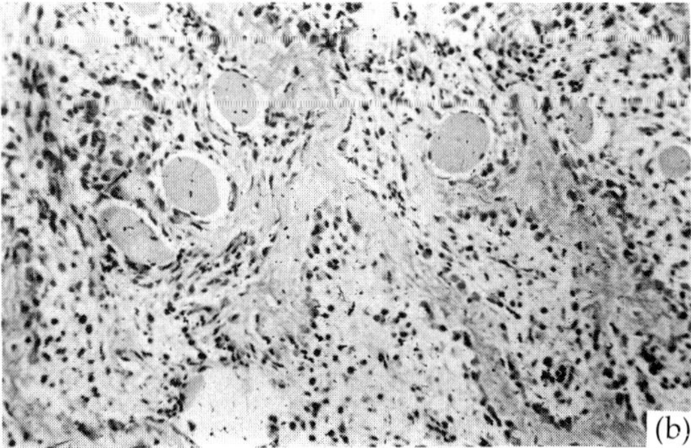

Figure 6.2 Photomicrographs of the fracture callus from Figure 6.1. The basic structure is moderately cellular fibrovascular tissue with evenly dispersed trabeculae of woven bone, some of which are mineralized. The trabeculae are outlined by a single layer of plump osteoblasts ('osteoblastic rimming'). In (a) there is a nodule of cartilage undergoing mineralization and ossification. In (b) there are included muscle fibres as a result of the invasiveness of callus.

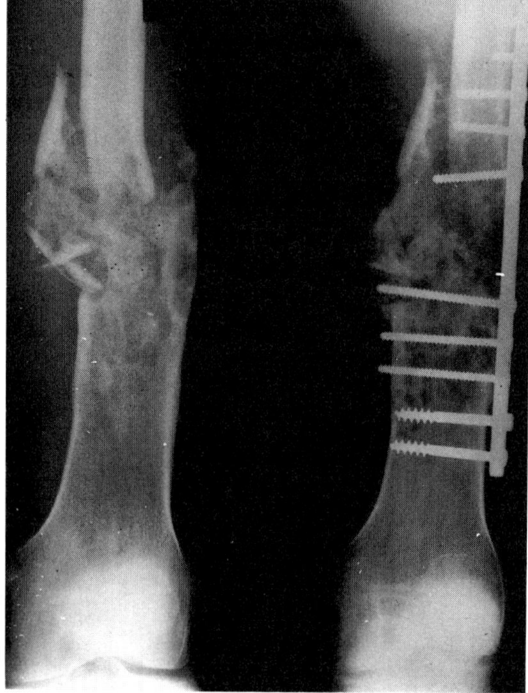

Figure 6.3 Male, 53-years old. Pathological fracture through central chondrosarcoma. The outline of the main tumour mass is visible proximally and distally. Despite the sharp margin, tumour growth is indicated by endocortical erosion and expansion of the distal fragment. There is an enormous amount of fracture callus which is surrounding and obscuring the lesion. Biopsy of the lesion consisted mainly of fracture callus with some small tumour fragments.

between the collars by a further bout of callus formation: the bridging callus.
4. Days later, callus formation in the medullary cavities of the fragments: the late medullary callus.
5. Over many months, remodelling of the accumulated callus.

(a) Haemorrhage

This is proportional to the damage to blood vessels. The role of the blood clot has been disputed (McKibbin, 1978). Sevitt (1981),

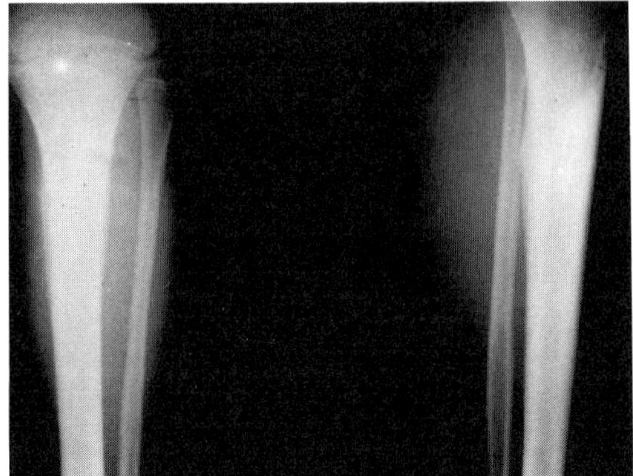

Figure 6.4 Male, 11-years old. Radiograph following a period of recurrent pain brought on by exercise. A focus of periosteal reaction is present in the upper tibial metaphysis posteriorly. Biopsy undertaken to exclude neoplasia (Figure 6.5 (a)–(d)).

with an extensive experience of fracture material from humans, maintained that the blood clot played no part in healing and was removed. However, with progress in the discovery and understanding of peptide control factors, the blood clot is recognized as one potential repository for them.

(b) Necrosis

This is proportional to the loss of blood supply, and at the least affects the marrow, trabecular and cortical bone immediately adjacent to the fracture. The topic is discussed further below.

(c) Inflammation

This is aseptic, with vascular dilatation, exudation of fibrin-rich fluid and infiltration by small numbers of mixed inflammatory cells – mononuclear cells including macrophages, lymphocytes, and mast cells – and polymorphs and probably bone cell precursors. The precipitated fibrin provides the support for reparative tissue. The inflammatory exudate, both serous and cellular, is a source of factors influencing the course of events (Hulth, 1989; Cornell and Lane, 1992). Phagocytic cells begin the removal of debris; but necrotic bone at the fracture is not resorbed.

(d)   Formation of repair tissue

Fibroblasts and endothelial cells of viable tissues – periosteum, adjacent soft tissues, and marrow – proliferate to create granulation tissue which advances towards the fracture gap.

(e)   Formation of callus

This results from the differentiation, within the granulation tissue, of precursor cells into osteoblasts, and sometimes chondrocytes, with the formation of matrices in the granulation tissue. The granulation tissue, and the following callus differentiation surrounding the two bone ends, advance towards each other. In favourable circumstances, they may bridge the gap, but leave the space between the bone ends filled by serofibrinous material.

(f)   Bridging the fracture gap (Figure 6.6)

It is evident that local conditions will do much to determine outcome: the difficulty that the primary callus has in bridging the gap will be closely proportional to the damage at the time of fracture and the difficulties in reduction and stabilization. It is the more usual sequence for a second bout of callus formation to occur, which is thought to be derived by inductive influences on pluripotent cells in surrounding soft tissues (Cornell and Lane, 1992). The proportion of cartilage in this tissue is determined in part by the stability of the fragments: within limits, more movement = more cartilage. In due time, the cartilage undergoes ossification.

Beginning a little later and proceeding more slowly, the medullary callus bridges the gap internally, establishing the continuity

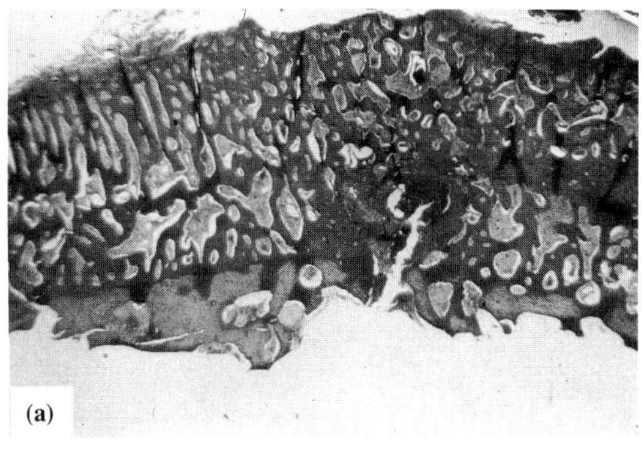

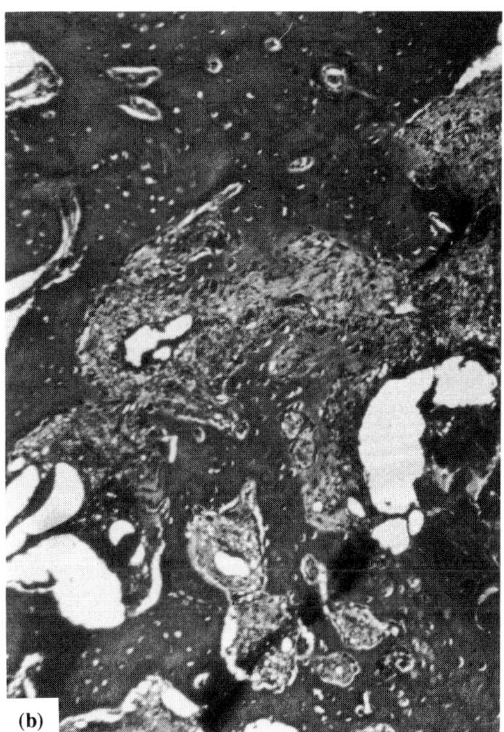

Figure 6.5 Photomicrographs of biopsy from Figure 6.4. (a) low power view; the periosteal surface is at the top overlying a broad band of reactive tissue resting on an osteoporotic cortex bearing a stress fracture. All the bone marrow spaces are replaced by fibrous tissue. The fracture site is bounded by dense reactive bone. The fracture gap has not been bridged and is lined by fibrovascular tissue undergoing some limited osseous and chondroid differentiation (b).

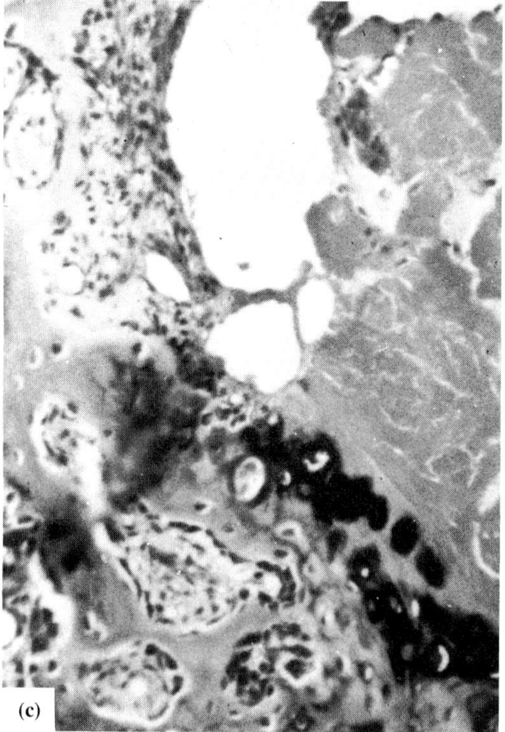

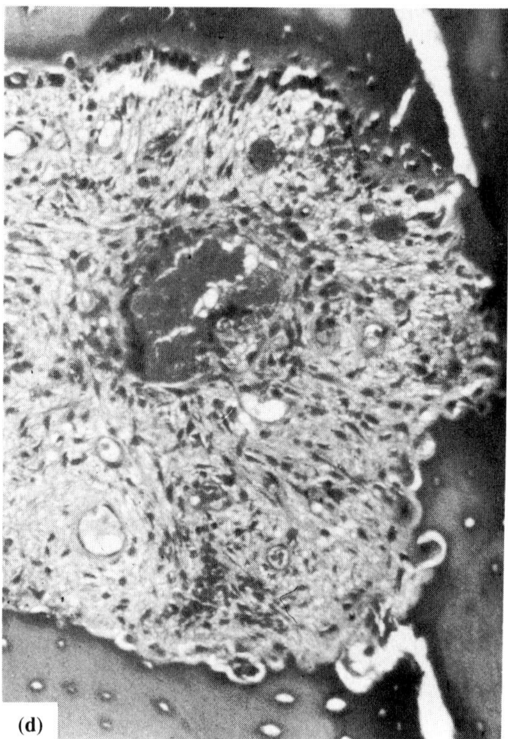

Figure 6.5 Photomicrographs of biopsy from Figure 6.4. (c) The space is filled by serofibrinous exudate. Throughout the specimen there is active remodelling of viable and necrotic bone, as in (d), where a cavity in necrotic bone (empty osteocytic lacunae) filled by fibrovascular tissue is undergoing resorption at most surfaces but with osteoblastic rimming in part.

between the cortices and the marrow cavities.

6.3.2 RESTRUCTURING THE FRACTURE SITE

It will be seen that there are two means of altering bone (Chapter 20). The remodelling process, functional throughout life, is based on the 'bone multicellular unit' (BMU) in which, at a single site, bone is resorbed by a wave of osteoclastic activity and is replaced by a following wave of osteoblasts: the difference between the amounts removed and replaced determine the volume and morphology of the site; for a region these will be determined by the number of BMUs that are activated over time. In contrast, modelling is active during growth and only to a limited extent later. In this the bone cells are not coupled, although their activity must be co-ordinated: they work at different surfaces, frequently opposed, and are able, relatively quickly, to change the disposition of large volumes of bone, such as correcting the angulation of a healed, mal-aligned fracture. According to age, these processes serve to restructure the callus and to revitalize the necrotic bone.

Modelling and remodelling of the callus and of the bone at the site of injury are directed toward restoring the normal anatomy and the lamellar structure of the site. The callus between cortices will be built up little by little into cortical tissue. The

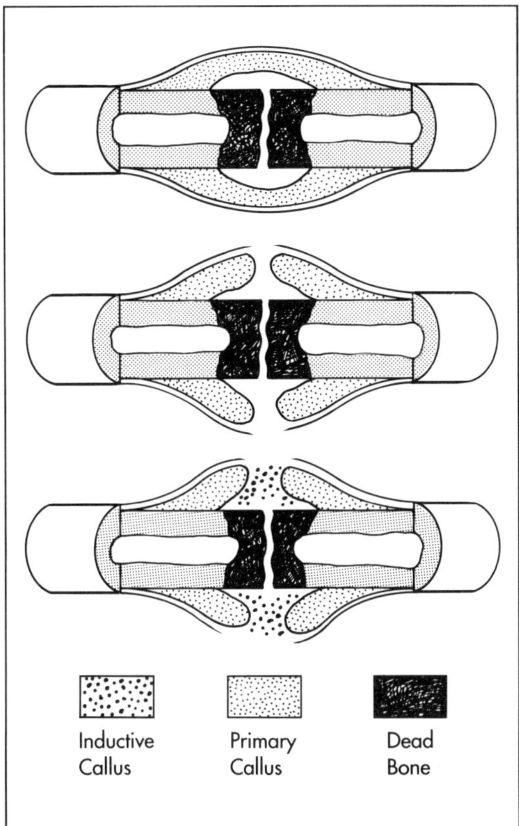

Figure 6.6 A schematic representation of alternative means of forming external bridging callus. Top: Intact periosteum leads to a callus bridge. Middle and bottom: periosteum ruptured; if the primary callus response cannot bridge the gap callus induced in soft tissues may. Reproduced from McKibbin (1978) with permission.

medullary callus, in the case of diaphyseal fractures, will be removed; in the case of metaphyseal/epiphyseal fractures it will be remodelled into cancellous tissue. The time scale is a function of the variables: age, severity, reduction and stabilization. At the optimum, it is weeks to months; with adverse variables it is months to years. The rate of progress slows over time, so that restoration to normal recedes as the variables move away from the optimum, and may never be complete.

As vascular regeneration penetrates the osteonal canals of the necrotic cortex, or supports osteoclasts in the creation of new osteons, turnover will commence replacing the dead tissue. This is a long-term project which, in severe fractures, can extend for years beyond the final healing of the fracture.

In addition, as a manifestation of the reaction to injury, the regional acceleratory phenomenon (RAP; Frost, 1983, 1986), can lead to an increase of remodelling space on cortical endosteal, osteonal and trabecular surfaces and a reduced mineralized tissue volume detectable in radiographs. Younger patients will recover from this in due course, but it is more persistent in older people.

6.3.3 DELAYED UNION AND NON-UNION, AND PSEUDARTHROSIS

These conditions arise from a failure adequately to bridge the fracture gap. There may be difficulties in the management of a case that account for this. But there are also unexplained instances, and hypotheses to match. In delayed union the gap is bridged by slowly ossifying fibrous or fibrocartilaginous tissue. If ossification ceases altogether then there is non-union, which might be qualified as fibrous.

Milgram (1991) has studied the pathology of 95 fractures which failed to heal; 41 of these were extra-articular. He concluded that these were fibrous unions, in some of which small coalescing clefts formed, and in a few these clefts were sufficiently extensive to qualify as a pseudarthrosis. None were lined by synovium, but some contained small amounts of clear fluid. The remaining 54 specimens were intra-articular, mainly femoral necks. In some there was fibrous union, with and without cleft formation, and sometimes full-blown pseudarthrosis, as above. But in others, pseudarthrosis had been present from the beginning. These were all femoral neck fractures with necrosis of the head. There had been reaction in the distal segment but this had never bridged the gap. However arrived at, some long-standing pseudarthroses will have regions of bone exposure; if viable this bone will be of increased density, possibly more pronounced than the condensation of the bone underlying the dense fibrous or fibrocartilaginous tissue.

(a) Compression devices (Figures 6.6 and 6.7)

Mobility at the fracture site results in formation of cartilage in callus. The complete absence of mobility, such as can be achieved by compression plates, results in minimal callus. Given that there is close apposition of the fracture surfaces, healing is effected by cortical remodelling (Olerud and Danckwardt-Lilliestrom, 1968). As soon as there is an osteonal blood supply reaching the end of at least one fragment, the activity of bone cells can be supported and the remodelling process can be set in motion. At some points the osteoclast cutting cone will cross the fracture gap and continue in the other fragment. The formative phase will do likewise, and the cylinder of new lamellar bone filling the resorption cavity will unite the two parts. Over time the number of such events will increase with a proportionate increase in the strength of the union.

(b) Avascular necrosis following fracture

Every fracture results in some degree of vascular disruption and bone necrosis. To this may be added the effects of plates and screws and of intramedullary nails. The blood supply of bones is discussed in Chapter 14, and of the femoral head below (Figure 6.8). Diaphyseal fracture may interrupt blood flow at three levels (Sevitt, 1981): osteonal, transverse cortical, nutrient. The first gives rise to the least necrosis; in a rib, for example, a few millimetres. Transverse cortical vessels, carrying blood from the medulla through the

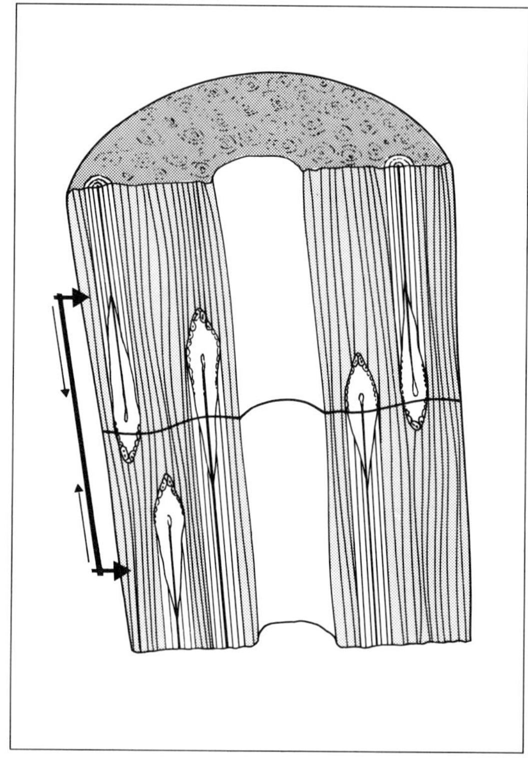

Figure 6.7 A schematic representation of fracture healing with compression plate. Success depends on a close approximation of the fracture surfaces. Cutting cones, the resorption phase of basic multicellular units, starting in either fragment, resorb a cavity across the fracture line. The formation phase then fills it in, which, in effect, creates a tie rod between the fragments. The strength of the union at any time is proportional to their number. Given time, the whole of the fracture site will be remodelled.

cortex, supply a number of osteonal vessels so that larger zones are involved by their interruption. They are vulnerable to stripping of the periosteum, accidental or surgical, which will compound intraosseous disruption. Tearing of the nutrient artery has the most serious effect, proportional to the level, and is greater in the distal fragment where it can involve many centimetres of cortex. Sevitt (1981) found that marrow necrosis was more or less co-extensive with that of the cortex. The effect of medullary nails varies between cortical and cancellous bone, tight and loose fits, and reaming or not. Cancellous vasculature is not so extensively disrupted by a nail, necrosis is restricted and gives rise around the nail to bone resorption and an enclosing fibrous membrane. In the cortical medulla the degree of nutrient artery damage is related to reaming and fit. Sevitt's (1981) experience of 17 human cases indicates that the necrosis is widespread but patchy. The immediate response is thought to be reversal of flow through transverse cortical vessels which will maintain some osteonal vessels, or later, support their regeneration.

There follows widespread extraosseous vascular proliferation, vascular penetration of the cortex (aided by osteoclastic resorption) and periosteal osteogenesis. Gradually there is revascularization of the osteons and the medulla. The time scale for this is measured in weeks. In the medulla, osteoclasts widen the canal to allow formation of a fibrous membrane around the nail; in the cortex, remodelling slowly (over years) replaces the necrotic bone; but in addition the balance of the remodelling leads to cortical osteoporosis.

The arrangement of the vasculature makes some bones prone to avascular necrosis following fracture. The carpal navicular is one, but the most common is the femoral head following fracture of the neck (Figure 6.8). A superior group of retinacular arteries is the main supply. This is augmented by a minor contribution from inferior retinacular vessels and in some instances from vessels entering through the ligamentum teres. These groups of vessels anastomose, but it is uncommon for this to sustain the viability of heads following fractures which tear the superior retinacular vessels. From a review of reports of the incidence of avascular necrosis of femoral heads following cervical fracture, Sevitt (1981) concludes that one-third remain viable, one-third become totally necrotic,

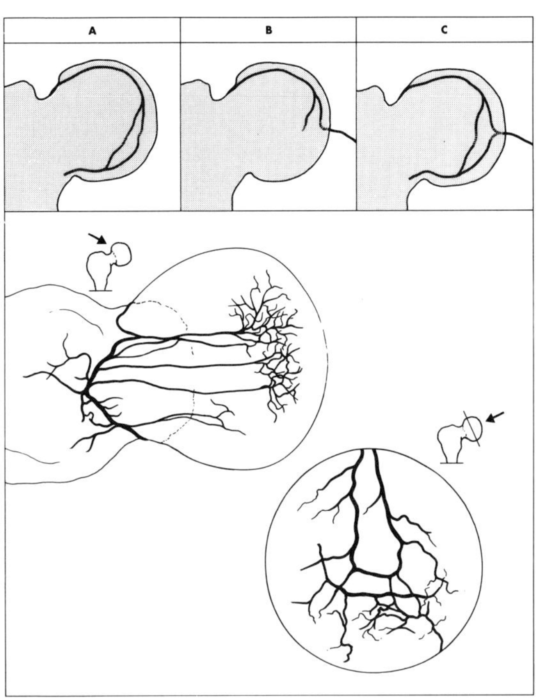

Figure 6.8 Schematic representation of the vascular supply to the femoral head after Wertheimer and Fernandes-Lopes (1971) injection studies (see text). Top row: three sources of supply: superior and inferior epiphyseal (each with a number of entering branches), and ligamentum teres combine in several arcades: A, superior/inferior (68%); B, superior/ligamental (15%); C, the three sources (17%). Bottom row: two of the arterial anastomotic distribution patterns within femoral heads. Only the main vessels are shown; numerous finer branches spread throughout the head to reach the subchondral zone.

and one-third develop some degree of partial necrosis. The consequences to fracture healing are discussed below, and the outcome of the infarct in Chapter 9.

(c)   Healing of cancellous bone

The cycle of events is no different here from that described above. But healing is influenced by the thin cortex at cancellous bone sites, and by the absence of an osteoblastic layer (cambium) in the periosteum at some. Examples of the latter are the carpal bones, the patella and the femoral neck. Good reduction and firm apposition are essential to good union. Under favourable conditions there is vascular sprouting and granulation tissue formation within a few days on both sides of the fracture. The two fronts, with their following osteogenesis, approach and bridge the gap. Trabecular necrosis in favourable situations is minimal, and is taken care of by resorption, or provides surfaces for apposition so that some trabecula near the fracture line have a necrotic core. If one fragment is necrotic, e.g. a femoral head, healing can take place from the viable fragment alone, given good reduction and stability. However, the reparative tissue extends only a little way into the necrotic fragment.

With progressively less favourable conditions, bridging is difficult and the granulation tissue becomes fibrous and forms the initial union, which may later ossify. Otherwise fibrous- or non-union results.

(d) Healing of amputation stumps

Sevitt (1981) remarks on the paucity of data about the healing of amputated bone in man. His own experience was also very limited, but sufficient to illustrate the earlier stages of the response. This is similar to fracture healing but at a somewhat slower rate. The proliferation of vessels starts within a few days, taking place in periosteal, extra periosteal and medullary tissues. The level of amputation, above or below the entry of the nutrient artery, affects the extent of loss of medullary and cortical supply (Brookes, 1971; Hansen-Leth, 1979) and will influence the time required for regeneration. The new medullary vessels fan out towards the cut ends, and extend beyond them to the limiting soft tissue cover, where they meet and mingle with the periosteal vessels and whatever vessels grow from the exposed osteonal canals. Osteogenic tissue develops in the medulla, and on the endosteal and periosteal surfaces, the equivalent of callus without cartilage. As it develops the new bone extends to close the medulla with an osseous plate. Remodelling takes place, which leads to cortical osteoporosis, and possibly some reshaping of the stump.

(e) Slipped femoral capital epiphysis

This condition affects a small number of adolescents, about 9–16 years of age, male:female=6:4. Burrows (1957) reported an assessment of 100 cases, some of whom tended to be tall, obese and sexually underdeveloped. But there was a high proportion of normal children and no classification of disease pattern emerged. The slip takes place in the physis. There is no histological evidence that it is abnormal (Jaffe, 1972), and avascular necrosis is not part of the pathogenesis, although it may be a complication of treatment, as documented by Hall (1957) who included the 100 cases of Burrows' (1957) report. Pain and disability are mild during the slow progress of chronic slipping, which takes place posteriorly in the direction of force at maximum load (i.e. when the hip is flexed as in mounting stairs). In its early stages the posterior displacement of the epiphysis may not be so obvious as in a lateral view. Recognition may be obscured by pain referred to the knee. The time scale of the process is months, extending to a year or more, during which the neck remodels with buttressing posteriorly and rounding down of the projecting anterior face of the metaphysis. However, events may be precipitated by even a mild trauma with acute displacement of the epiphysis – so-called acute on chronic slip.

It should be realized that opportunities to examine specimens have been few, and are from cases of some duration. The changes in the physis have not been uniform over its whole extent: buckling, reduplication, fragmentation, and displacement of fragments into the epiphysis or metaphysis are reported by Jaffe (1972) in patients with symptoms of 6–12 months. One must suppose that there are less pronounced alterations at earlier times, a deflection of the axis of the cell columns. Since growth does not cease during the course of the slip it must constitute part of the mechanism for the gradual shift. Throughout the chronic phase the epiphysis has the support of the periosteal tissue which links with the periphery of the physis. The acute slip is a fracture through the physis, with tearing of the supporting collagen fibres from the periosteum.

The stage which the condition reaches before it is arrested, ultimately by closure or synostosis of the physis, will determine the degree of deformity. Remodelling of the femoral neck can restore conditions towards normal (Angel, 1982). However, there remains some risk of osteoarthritis in early adult life.

The complications of avascular necrosis and chondrolysis lead to more severe derangement. The pathology of the former is as described under circulatory disorders. The cause of chondrolysis is unknown; it can follow any treatment including prolonged immobilization, which speaks for the value of passive motion in the preservation of joints (Akeson *et al.*, 1992).

(f)   Physeal fracture

Also unlikely to be seen by histopathologists are fractured physes. Dale and Harris (1958), and Salter and Harris (1963) correlated animal and clinical studies of this condition. The blood vessels supplying most epiphyses enter through the periosteum at the sides. In a few, notably the femoral head, articular cartilage overlaps the physeal plate and the nutrient vessels must enter through the cartilage. In the event of a physeal fracture the latter arrangement exposes the vessels to damage and puts the epiphysis at risk of necrosis. Since the epiphyseal vessels supply

the reserve zone of the physis, its growth is also at risk. Most physes are under compression; a few, such as the trochanters are tensioned. The latter are fractured by avulsion; the former by shearing, splitting or crushing. Avulsion and shearing forces fracture the physis through the hypertrophic zone at the interface with the calcified zone. Since the growth mechanism of the epiphyseal fragment is undisturbed, and there is no vascular penetration to support calcification and ossification, the physis becomes greatly thickened at 10 days in rabbits. At that time callus, originating from the periosteum and the metaphyseal segment, which remains viable following the fracture, is starting to bridge the gap. By three weeks healing has been effected, the ossification process restored and the physis is normal in its appearance. Thus careful reduction can lead to normality.

Fracture of the physis has been used clinically as a means of leg lengthening. Turner and Anderson (1992) review the effects of trauma on the physis, and discuss experimental and clinical experience of distraction epiphysolysis, in which the physis is fractured through the calcified zone by distraction apparatus, and chondrodiastasis, where distraction forces are not sufficient to cause fracture but can stimulate the physis. Positive results have been obtained, but there can be difficulties and complications, and there is still more to be learned about the procedures.

(g)   Joints: injury to articular cartilage

Accidental or experimental injuries that affect only the cartilage do not heal. There is minimal response of adjacent chondrocytes, either necrosis or some proliferation, but virtually no reparative tissue is produced (Nevo *et al.*, 1992). Most observers have found that experimental incisions of cartilage, either partial or full thickness do not heal; there is only one report to the contrary (Calandruccio and Scott Gilmer, 1962). However, when the lesion extends through the subchondral plate, as in osteochondral fracture, fibrovascular tissue, developing in the marrow, advances to fill the gap. Given no great displacement, it attaches to the fractured cartilage surfaces, and may proliferate and extend over the articular surface. Chondroid differentiation can take place, but there are no good data as to how common this is. Sevitt (1981) illustrates a few cases. However, substantial reformation of cartilage at surfaces with full thickness loss, and some exposure of the underlying marrow, does occur as seen in osteoarthritis, sometimes as a spontaneous event, sometimes as a result of treatment by osteotomy (Byers, 1974). Where fractures are near the articular margin, pannus from the synovium may extend over the cartilage gap. Resorption of cartilage by the fibrous tissue can take place. Healing of the underlying subchondral fracture is determined by the same factors that influence cancellous bone fracture healing elsewhere.

(h)   Neuropathic arthropathy: Charcot joint

Loss of deep joint sensation is generally regarded as leading to loss of protective mechanisms during load bearing activity, and a joint so affected may in time disintegrate. In many such joints subchondral fractures are an initiating event, but not in others. Nevertheless, even in the latter, mechnical damage seems to play a part (Johnson, 1967). Charcot was not the first to record cases, but it was he who associated the neuropathy and joint failure. Tabes was the first recognized neurological disorder, but over time many conditions came to be recorded: syringomyelia, congenital sensory neuropathy, diabetic and other peripheral neuropathies, paraplegia and other traumatic and compressive lesions (Brown *et al.*, 1992). The joints principally affected are knees and feet, but hip, shoulder, vertebral joints and others can be affected. The fact that some joints show bone loss and others bone sclerosis and osteophytosis in the course of disintegration suggests there may be more to the pathogenesis than sensory deprivation (Johnson, 1967; Key, 1932). The progress of the joint failure can be followed radiographically, but pathological observations are at a late stage, either at post-mortem or following amputation. Cartilage and bone fractures, and grinding down of opposing bones, result in abundant debris free within the joint and incorporated in synovium (Jaffe, 1972). This is suggestive of the diagnosis, as is the extensive tissue disorder and the associated fibro-osseous reaction in the form of fibrosis, modelling and remodelling and callus. Ultimately the diagnosis depends on the demonstration (usually clinical) of neuropathy. Late stages of some joints bear a resemblance to osteoarthritis.

6.3.4   OSTEOCHONDRITIS DISSECANS

The condition known as osteochondritis dissecans is now generally accepted to be a traumatic subchondral fracture (Aichroth, 1971 a, b) (Figure 6.9). The many theories about it have been summarized by Nagura (1960). Conceivably it might be the result of stress. Nevertheless, it is also a topic bound by history to avascular necrosis and its consequences, and thereby allied to many eponymous conditions thought to be of that causation, which are discussed in section 9.3.

Osteochondritis dissecans is a condition in which there is a partial or complete separation of a segment of articular cartilage and subchondral bone from the joint surface. The lesion has been recognized since the studies by Konig, published in 1888. Many of the separated fragments are necrotic, which has been responsible for inclusion in the category of avascular necrosis, although there has been much controversy over trauma versus necrosis as the primary event (Nagura, 1960). At the present time, the weight of opinion favours trauma on the basis of epidemiological and experimental evidence (Aichroth, 1971a, b).

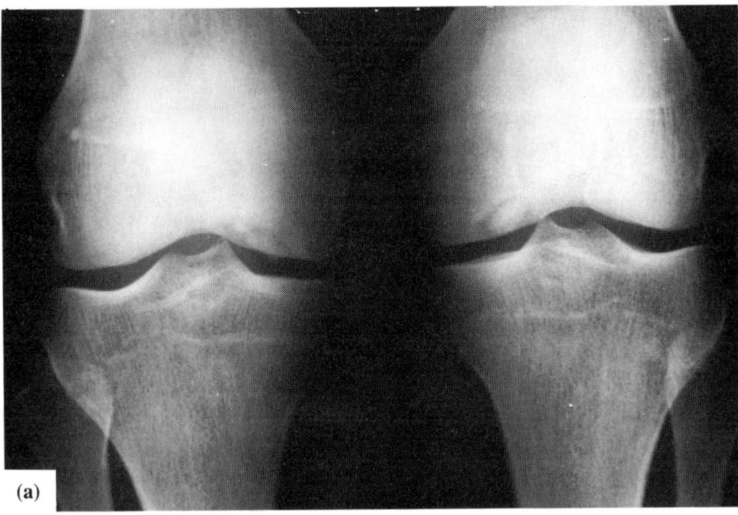

Figure 6.9 Osteochondritis dissecans. (a) Radiograph of young adult male with lesions bilaterally in the medial femoral condyles. There is a clear-cut separation of a crescent of bone from the subchondral osseous tissue. The profile of the subchondral plate is uniform suggesting that the articular cartilage is intact.

The age range is 5–50 (mean 18) years. The usual site is the lower end of the femur (85% medial femoral condyle, 15% lateral). Other sites much less commonly affected are patella, tibial plateau, the convex surfaces of metatarsals (Freiberg's disease; usually the second is involved), ankle, elbow and hip. Attention is drawn to the lesion by pain and/or instability, usually following trauma. The radiograph shows a semilunar defect in the articular surface; the separated fragment may be *in situ*. Most *in situ* fragments will heal, particularly in children, provided they are stable. If not, the crater fills with fibrous tissue, which, over time will mature to chondroid tissue and may after many years be difficult to identify. The fragment may remain partially attached, or detach completely. In the former instance, the bone component may remain viable, otherwise it becomes necrotic. The cartilage remains viable in any case. Loose in the joint, the fragment acquires a mantle of viable cells with the

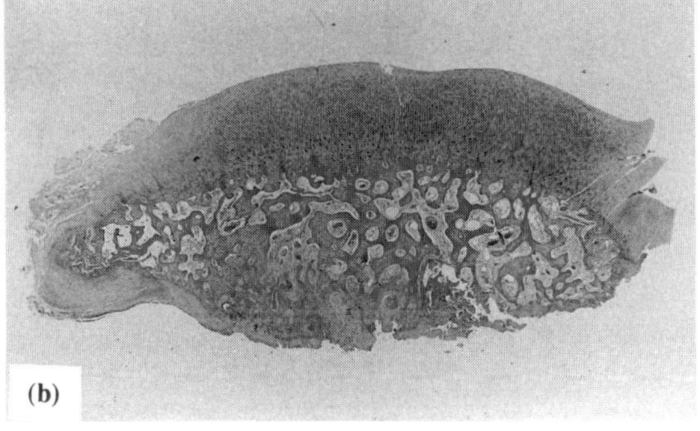

Figure 6.9 Osteochondritis dissecans. (b) The osteochondral fragment which was still partially attached by articular cartilage and fibrous tissue to the crater in the femoral condyle. Essentially normal articular cartilage, apart from thinning and fraying at one edge. At this site, reactive chondroid tissue has overgrown the free margin and extended to the undersurface. The bone architecture is basically intact except in the central region where there is dense fibrous tissue and extensive bone remodelling. The tissues are viable throughout.

capacity to produce chondroid mineralizing matrix which gradually encases the fragment.

Macroscopically, a well-seated lesion, over which the cartilage has not been disturbed, will not be detectable. Less well-lodged lesions may be detected by giving under pressure, or may be seen because the cartilage has acquired a ridge or cleft around the margin of the fracture; it will be more obvious if the cleft is sufficient for the fragment to lift from its bed. Marginal lesions may be retained *in situ* only by a fibrous strand arising from the adjacent synovium. The crater will have a soft tissue covering, which in the course of time can come to fill it and to differentiate to chondroid tissue which blends in with the articular cartilage.

The fragment consists of viable articular cartilage, and subchondral bone which is usually necrotic; viable tissue in the marrow, or viable bone comes about through persistent attachment by a vascularized pedicle, or through revascularization while *in situ*, possibly with attendant episodes of bone apposition. The bone may have fragmented from the trauma of weight bearing. The length of time the fragment has remained loose in the joint will determine other features: calcium deposition in the necrotic marrow and the acquisition of a connective tissue mantle. The latter is spindle celled at the outset but undergoes chondroid differentiation, and increases in amount so as to entomb the fragment in calcified cartilage (Milgram, 1977a, b, 1978).

6.3.5 STRESS FRACTURES

The diagnostic histopathologist sees tissue from stress and avulsion fractures when, clinically, the possibility of neoplasia arises (Figures 6.4 and 6.5) (Linscheid and Coventry, 1962; Davies and Bradley, 1991; Meaney and Carty, 1992). This usually occurs with children, and in adults with multiple stress fractures. What is required of him is to recognize the reactive tissue and the absence of neoplasia. The latter fact does not exclude the possibility of its presence elsewhere, but the observation can calm a tense situation long enough for the reactive nature of the lesion to declare itself clinically and by imaging (section 4.4.2). The following résumé sets out the framework in which this problem can arise.

Devas (1975, 1963) writing from his experience in control of the Stress Fracture Bureau at the Middlesex Hospital from 1957 to 1975 defined the fracture as occurring in normal bones of healthy people doing everyday activities and with no injury. The activity might be unusual for the individual, but not of itself an exceptional one, as for example a walking holiday by an office worker. Training and performance of athletes and entertainers are customary activities for them and as often as not the fracture develops in the normal course of the individual's activity. Devas stressed the fact that the quality of bone changed with age, and that this affected the incidence and nature of the fracture.

However, the difficulty of defining normal bone has increased as growing attention has been focused on osteoporosis, leading to increased use of the qualifying terms insufficiency and fatigue (Hansson, 1938; Hullinger, 1944; Pentecost *et al.*, 1964; Daffner and Pavlov, 1992). Moreover, Looser zones of osteomalacia have long been recognized as stress fractures. Since the fractures in these conditions in many instances are without antecedent trauma, they meet the criterion for a stress fracture.

It is not proposed to discuss the mechanics that cause the damage. Various observations of microdamage to bone have been made (Lagier, 1971; Todd *et al.*, 1972; Frost, 1973; 1986 Charon *et al.*, 1982; Arlot *et al.*, 1983; Benaissa *et al.*, 1989). The damage is either clefts and splits without discontinuity, or complete fractures of individual trabeculae (Figure 6.10). The former have been demonstrated by Frost (1960) by bulk staining of bone in fuchsin before sectioning. The latter have been shown in macerated bones at low magnification, with histological confirmation. The hypothesis is that as the result of the repetitively applied forces this accumulates more rapidly than it can be repaired by modelling or remodelling in the case of incomplete lesions, or by fracture callus in complete lesions.

Freeman *et al.* (1974), using techniques they had developed earlier (Todd *et al.*, 1972) to study trabecular fractures (Figure 6.10), quantitated the number of trabecular fractures in ten post-fracture femoral heads, and in the femoral necks and heads of 15 cadavers ranging in age from 20 to 90 years, and assessed the bone density of the specimens. The specimens were macerated, dried, weighed, their volume determined, then divided into 3–5 mm slices and the number and distribution of fracture calluses counted (Figure 6.11). Some fractures were present in all, excepting one of three 20-year olds. As bone density fell, the number of fractures rose; the critical point for a steep rise was 0.5 g/cm^3. They concluded that:

1. The occasional fatigue fracture is physiological.
2. There is a critical bone density at which the number of fractures rises steeply.
3. Gross fracture of the femoral neck is a terminal event of progressive trabecular failure due to fatigue, not impact.

The controls in a study by Fazzalini *et al.* (1987) provide corroboration of the association of falling trabecular density and increasing trabecular fractures found by Freeman *et al.* (1974).

Random blocks of tissue from femoral heads of the elderly, obtained post-mortem or post-fracture are likely to contain trabecular fractures (Figure 6.10).

However, as described below, many stress fractures are cortical, in young and healthy individuals in whom there is no question of osteopenia. The microdamage described by

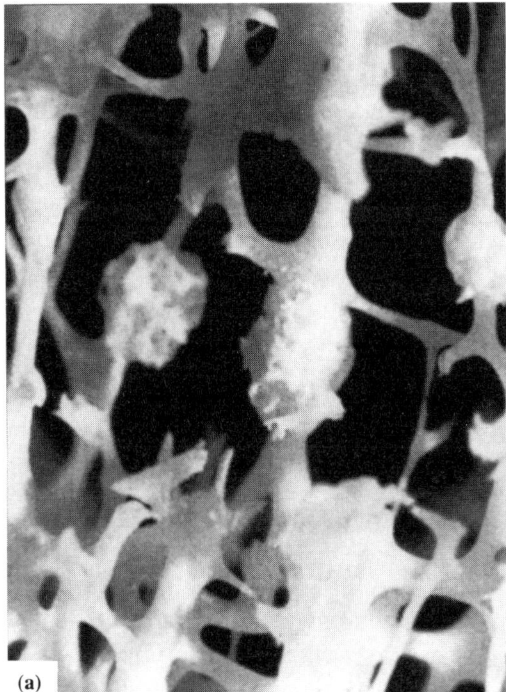

(a)

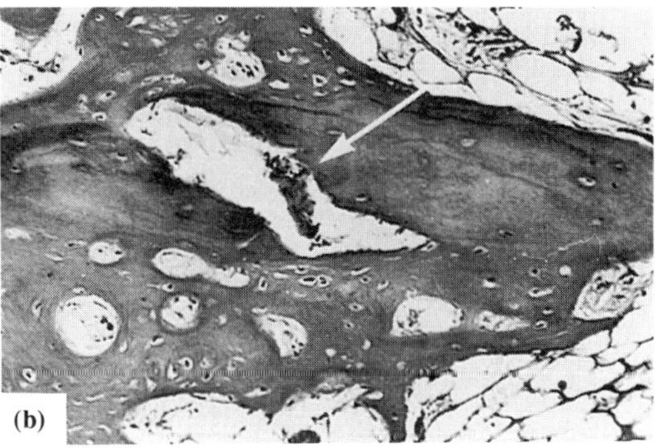

(b)

Figure 6.10 Trabecular stress fractures. (a) Macerated cancellous bone of femoral head showing three trabeculae with focal callus. The fractures appear to have occurred in a locus of osteoporosis. (b) Histological section of another fracture showing the fracture line and surrounding callus. (From Todd *et al.*, 1972 with permission of publisher and authors.)

Frost (1960) can be postulated to be applicable here. But such damage is not apparent with the techniques that would be used in a diagnostic laboratory. The features that will be observed, dependent on sampling, are callus originating in the periosteum; a fracture line in the cortical bone, usually of some width and filled with amorphous eosinophilic material, and reactive changes in the original bone: fibrovascular tissue in spaces; possibly membranous bone formation, and metaplastic cartilage, remodelling of the mature bone (Figures 6.4 and 6.5). The extent of the fracture, its duration and the degree of continuing stress to which it has been subjected, will obviously influence the make-up of the reaction.

Clinically, there is usually a period in which the symptoms develop before the patient presents himself, if indeed he does. The symptoms are pain on activity, relieved by rest. If activity is curtailed healing usually occurs without treatment. Otherwise the rate of progress is proportional to the degree of continuing activity. Some fractures will go on to complete discontinuity; transverse distraction fractures of the mid-shaft of the tibia are at greatest risk (see below).

The fractures can be classified (Devas, 1975) as:

- Distraction
    oblique
    longitudinal
    transverse
- Compression

Distraction fractures affect a segment of cortex on the convexity of a bone subjected to bending forces. The oblique is the most common; occasionally it goes on to complete fracture. Longitudinal fractures extend in the long axis of tubular bone, sometimes for considerable distances. They often take origin from an oblique fracture. The least common is the transverse fracture, usually arising in the mid-shaft of a long bone, and prone to extending to a complete fracture.

Compression fractures occur in cancellous bone, particularly of the femur, tibia and calcaneum. It is difficult to visualize

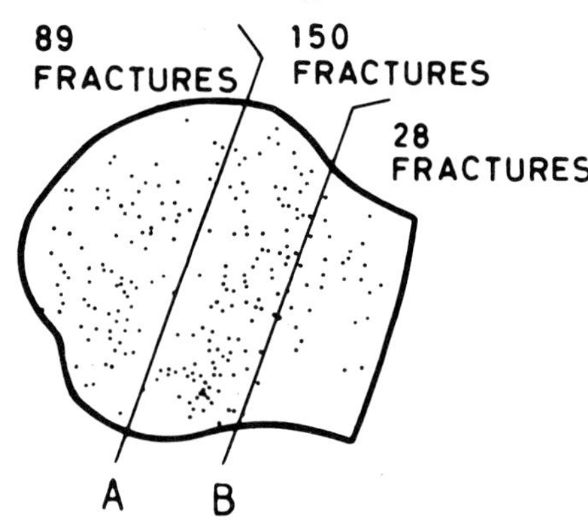

Figure 6.11 A composite map of the trabecular fractures found in 16 femoral heads obtained at autopsy and prepared by maceration and division into 3–5 mm slices. The ages ranged from 20 to 90 years, and the fractures/specimen from 0–100. The region between the lines A and B is the most common site of femoral neck fracture. (From Freeman *et al.*, 1974 with permission of publisher and authors.)

the fracture itself radiographically, but the hazy shadow of the mineralized callus marks its site. This type of fracture in the elderly, particular if multiple, may be mistaken for metastases (Davies and Bradley, 1991). Fractures of the tarsal sesamoids are of the compression type, and may be affected by avascular necrosis (Galloches, 1967).

Stress fractures occur at all ages but the patterns vary with age: children and the aged tend to have the same types.

The sites at which Devas (1975) recorded fractures are presented in Table 6.1 augmented by data from some other sources. He did not establish prevalance figures since his material was coming from an undefined population with many referred cases. However, he did give some internal comparisons, some of which are interpreted in Table 6.1

The incidence of stress fractures is difficult to establish. From the records of an American Army training base, Pester and Smith (1992)

Table 6.1 Sites of stress fractures in various age groups: 1, children to puberty; 2, to age about 30 years; 3, middle age; 4, elderly

Site	Type			
		Distraction		Compression
	Oblique	Longitudinal	Transverse	
Stress fractures				
Foot				
Calcaneus			3,4	
Calcaneal apophysis	1			
Navicular[a,b]			3,4	
Metatarsals[d]	1–4	1–4	1–4	1–4
Sesamoids, hallux			1[u]	
Fibula				
Lower third[e]	1–4			
Shaft			1[i]	
Tibia				
Metaphyses, prox	2			1[c],4
dist	2			4
Diaphysis[f]	2	1[u]–4	2	4[u]
Tubercle[g]	1,2			
Medial malleolus[u]	2,3			
Tibia + prox or dist Fibula metaphyses	4[w]			4[w]
Femur				
Shaft		1[u]–4	1[u]–4	
Neck	2–4			2–4
Head[h]				3,4
Patella				1,2
Pelvis				
Pubis inferior ramus	1,4			
superior ramus	4			
Ilium[j]				4
Trunk				
Ribs	2–4			
Vertebral body[j]				4
Pars interarticularis	1,2			
Upper limb				
Humerus	2			
Ulna	2–4			

Stress avulsions
Pelvis, iliac spines
Lesser trochanter of femur
Patella, lower pole
Tibial tubercle
(see also section on avulsions)

[a]Rare occurrence. [b]Kohler's avascular necrosis in child. [c]Common. [d]Order of incidence= 2,3,4,5,1 (rare); multiple and bilateral common. [e]Sometimes at higher levels. [f]Devas estimates 10% of tibial stress fractures are longitudinal, 5% transverse. [g]Osgood Schlatter's disease in child. [h]Devas does not record this in young adults, although Frost and others do. [i]Infants. [j]Devas does not record this category; for ilium see Davies and Bradley (1991); vertebra, Hansson *et al.* (1988). [u]Uncommon. [w]Mostly in women.

showed an incidence in the lower limb of 0.96% in male recruits on basic training, and 1.09% for females. The common sites, as a percentage of the total, were: metatarsals, 66% and 31%; calcaneus, 20% and 39% and lower leg, 13% and 27% in males and females, respectively.

A modification of the training reduced the prevalence by 16% in males and 7% in females.

Idiopathic avascular necrosis, particularly of the femoral head, is usually considered to be the result of vascular occlusion, and a variety of mechanisms for the latter are proposed (Chapter 9). All the proposed mechanisms are controversial, including the one giving a role to stress fractures. This topic is discussed further in Chapter 9 in connection with idiopathic osteonecrosis and Perthes' disease. But since Devas (1975) has figured so prominently in this section it can be mentioned that he concluded from his clinical observations that it seemed likely that stress fracture within the femoral head was responsible for necrosis in adult patients treated with steroid and was the basis for Perthes' disease.

As a final comment it seems odd that Devas did not consider osteochondritis dissecans to be the result of stress fracture. He uses the term in his book for a number of lesions, but none are that of the articular surface of the femoral condyle which are discussed here under osteochondritis dissecans. Perhaps at the time he was writing this lesion was regarded as primarily vascular, although now the traumatic hypothesis is in the ascendant.

6.4　BONE FORMATION IN SOFT TISSUES: AVULSION INJURY AND HETEROTOPIC OSSIFICATION

It is possible to mark out within the melange of ossifying lesions of soft tissue, both reactive and neoplastic, territories of interest to pathologists, radiologists, clini-cians and a variety of biologists. These overlap, although it may not be apparent from every vantage point, and the degree of coincidence of interest has varied as new knowledge has come to light. The reactive lesions are frequently referred to as myositis ossificans, but since there is often no inflammation, or involvement of muscle this term has come to be regarded by some as inappropriate, who replace it by the broader concept heterotopic ossification. This is broader in that it leaves open the aetiology/pathogenesis, and includes non-neoplastic ossification at all sites, which number most of the tissues of the body (Urist, 1989; Korhonen and Vaananen, 1992). Notwithstanding, there is still confusion in trying to compose a classification, for it seems necessary to have a category 'post-traumatic' which clearly overlaps with pseudomalignant osseous tumour of soft tissue, or alternatively, as some would have it, pseudomalignant myositis ossificans. Perhaps the explanation lies in the clinical presentation: pathologists know about lesions from those cases where there is uncertainty in clinicians' minds about the diagnosis; but other cases where there is no doubt do not arouse the same interest. Certainly, the literature on the subject goes back to the turn of the century, and turns largely on clinical and radiographic features, especially in CNS disorders and, more recently, after prosthetic joint replacement (e.g. Stover *et al.*, 1991); but, good detailed pathological descriptions are hard to find except where the subject concerns the differentiation from neoplasia (Ackerman, 1958). The following is proffered for the discussion here of the subject:

Avulsion injury

Heterotopic ossification
  Epithelial induction
    Transitional
    Gall bladder
    Established cell lines

Post-traumatic
  Single major blow
  Repeated minor blows

Lesions affecting
  Par-osseous and para-articular tissues
  Muscles
  Tendons and ligaments

Induction following
  Prosthetic replacement of bones
  and joints
  Burns
  Tetanus
  Neurological conditions
  Arthropathies

Induction by connective tissue matrices
  demineralized bone
  demineralized dentine

Pseudomalignant osseous tumour of soft
tissue

This can be extended by the concept that
proliferative fibroblastic lesions are variants of one disease process, an idea that has
been expanded by Enzinger and his colleagues (Soule *et al.*, 1986; quoted by
Dupree, 1990):

- Nodular fasciitis
- Subcutaneous pseudosarcomatous
  fasciitis
- Proliferative fasciitis
- Infiltrative fasciitis
- Pseudosarcomatous fasciitis
- Fasciitis ossificans
- Intravascular fasciitis
- Cranial fasciitis
- Proliferative myositis
- Myositis ossificans, florid phase
- Pseudomalignant myositis ossificans

The last entry of the second list is the
pseudomalignant osseous tumour of soft tissue of the first list, and forms the link. The
whole is reduced to manageable proportions
by setting on it the boundaries of diagnostic
osteoarticular pathology: only two of the
ossifying lesions in the above lists are likely
to come into consideration.

For the diagnostic pathologist these
important entities are avulsion injury, which
must be differentiated from parosteal
osteosarcoma and its variants; and pseudomalignant osseous tumour, which is not to
be confused with soft tissue osteosarcoma. A
third, rare lesion, discussed below, may be
included: a fibro-osseous pseudotumour of
the digits (Dupree and Enzinger, 1986).

The remainder in the lists are important
for their clinical relevance and/or for their
place in pathophysiology and the molecular
biology of bone formation. Although the
osteogenic potential of urinary tract epithelium first drew attention to heterotopic
ossification (Huggins, 1931; Wlodarski,
1992), the greater interest in the study of
bone induction now revolves around the
demineralized matrices of bone and dentine, from which bone morphogenetic proteins have been extracted, as briefly
discussed and referenced in Chapter 18. It
may be that the unfolding of these control
mechanisms of cell proliferation and differentiation propels the concept of commonal-
ity among the lesions and the unified
classification.

Diagnosis is not in doubt, and does not
require the aid of the pathologist in cases
where the lesion arises in association with
recognized antecedents as listed. Nor for that
matter is there difficulty when there has
been unequivocal trauma to the site such as a
blow or sufficient trauma to avulse a tendon
attachment. But a solitary lesion without
antecedent cause is a problem.

(a) Avulsion injury (Figure 6.12)

The reparative tissue induced by the avulsion is in effect fracture callus and will be a
mixture of granulation, chondroid and bony
tissue. In radiographs, the avulsed fragment
may not be visible, and the first indications
come from mineralization of the callus.
Appearing, under the given circumstances,
at a site for which parosteal osteosarcoma has

a predilection, such as the posterior aspect of the lower femoral metaphysis, a biopsy may be taken (given the differential diagnosis, biopsy could be postponed without risk to the patient, giving time for the lesion to declare itself by its progress).

The proportions of the tissues will vary, but their histological structure is benign: a regular pattern of trabeculae with a single osteoblast layer, ossifying cartilage nodules and granulation tissue with no cytological features of malignancy. If the edge of the tissue is included in the section, the tissue will be ramifying into contiguous normal tissues, as is the habit of reparative tissue, with no encapsulation.

(b) Pseudo-malignant osseous tumour of soft tissue (Figure 6.13)

This is an infrequent lesion, which occurs more in younger athletic age groups, but has a wide range; Enzinger and Weiss (1988) quote 9–84 years. It forms rapidly, usually within a muscle, but may involve subcutaneous fat or soft tissues of fingers and toes (see below). It is often associated with trauma or unaccustomed heavy labour, but may be without apparent antecedent cause. Local

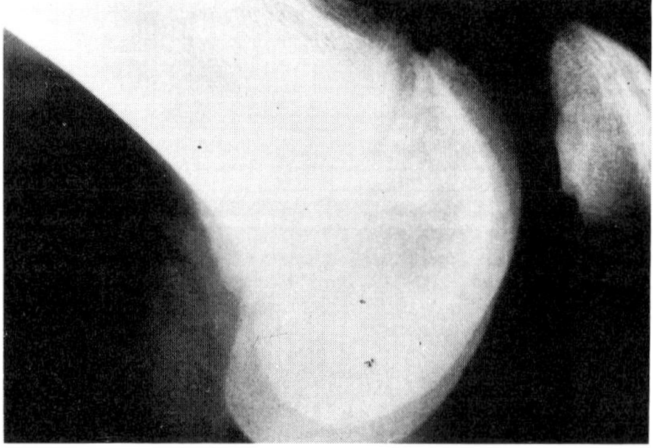

Figure 6.12 Active male teenager. Avulsion injury at the adductor magnus insertion. The callus reaction has given rise to a faintly mineralized swelling on the surface of the bone.

pain and tenderness is followed by diffuse soft swelling, which becomes firm and then hard over 2–4 weeks. It is often painful, but is not necessarily so. It occurs most often in the thigh, arm, buttock, or hand, but has been recorded in many other sites. Within a few weeks of onset it will appear in radiographs as a definable mass in soft tissue, with an irregular floccular pattern of mineral ('dotted veil'). If the lesion is left alone it will become better defined as it matures, and may then resorb, or remain stable. When available the tissue has a distinctive, specific structure. This has been described by Ackerman (1958) as zoning. At the macroscopic level, best demonstrated by fine detail radiograph of a slab cut through the specimen (Figure 6.13), there is a bony periphery and a soft tissue centre. Microscopically, the bone is graded in development from without in, and is covered by a thin layer of fibroblastic tissue, loose and myxoid according to Enzinger and Weiss (1988), which is most cellular in proximity to the bone, where the cells are osteoblastic and form the outer shell. The bone is woven in its structure, quite compact at its outer edge, diminishing internally to wispy strands, and is actively remodelled. The remodelling will, over time, convert the bone to lamellar type, or gradually remove it. The internal spaces of the bone contain fibrovascular tissue; but the central space enclosed by the bone is filled with highly cellular spindle cell tissue in which there may be found macrophages, chronic inflammatory cells, multinucleated cells, endothelial cell proliferation, entrapped muscle fibres, haemorrhage and fibrinous material (Enzinger and Weiss, 1988). The spindle cells may show mild to moderate pleomorphism, and readily observed mitoses. Without knowledge of the entity this tissue makes it hard to resist a diagnosis of malignancy. A point about this lesion that is not discussed is the activity at the interface between the bony shell and the inner spindle cell tissue: is bone formed, resorbed or remodelled?

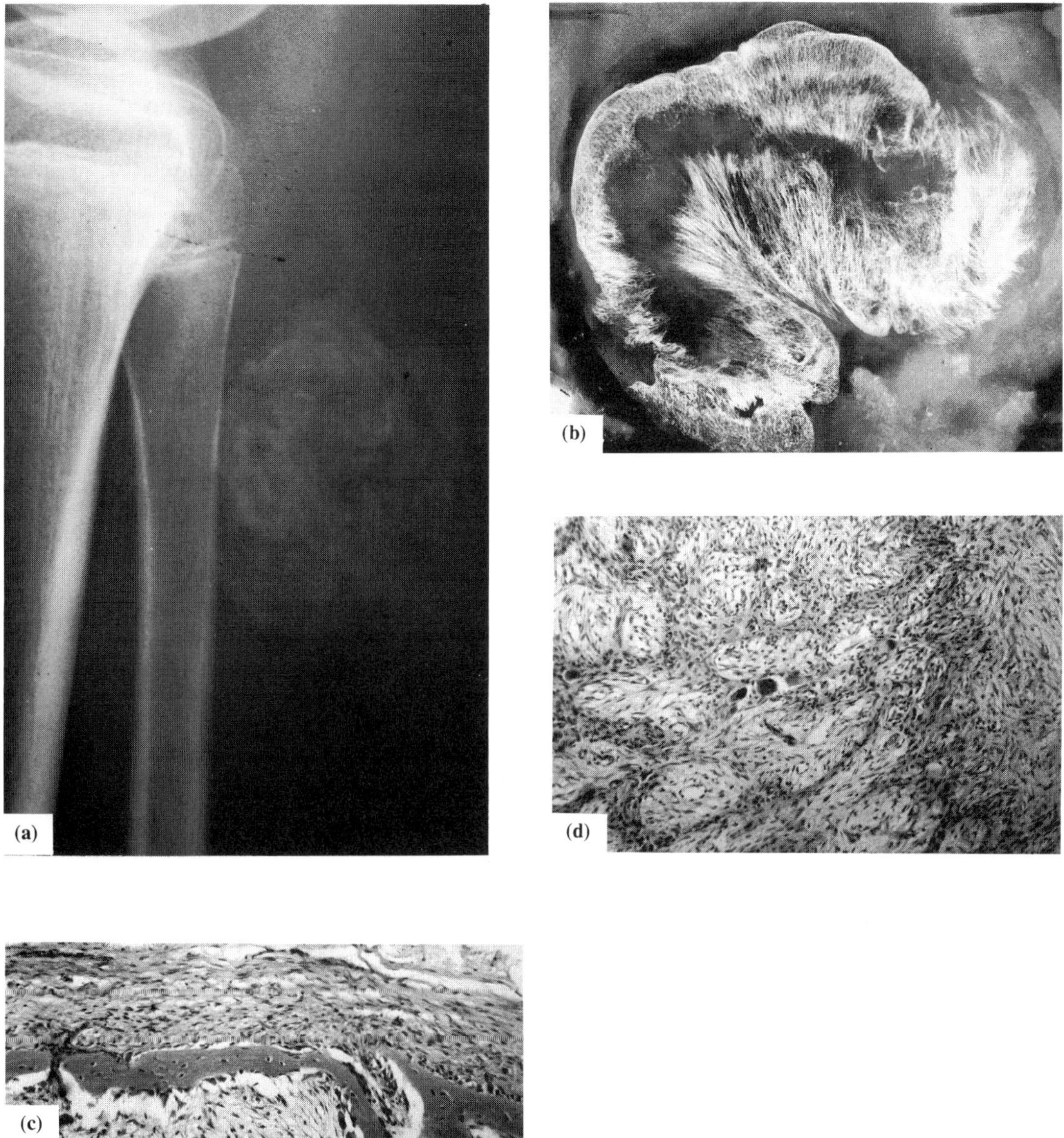

Figure 6.13 (a) Boy: myositis ossificans/pseudomaligant osseous tumour of soft tissue. Pain in the calf of short duration. A well-delineated mineralized soft tissue mass with maximum density at the periphery. (b) Fine-detail radiograph of a slab from the excised specimen shows zoning of the tissues; a thin peripheral band of densely mineralized tissue, a broad band of trabecular bone and a mineral-free centre. (c) At the top, enclosing fibrous tissue. Beneath this, a continuous band of bone with trabecular structures extending internally. Active remodelling of the internal bone surfaces is present. (d) Non-mineralized tissue from the centre of the lesion shows two tissue patterns: loose fibrovascular tissue trabeculated by denser fibrous tissue and highly cellular spindle-celled tissue. This type of tissue, in isolation, can be confused with malignancy.

Regarded as the same category of lesion is one in the soft tissues of the fingers or toes, in which the component tissues are not so well ordered, and again tempt a diagnosis of soft tissue osteosarcoma (Spjut and Dorfmann, 1981; Dupree and Enzinger, 1986) (Chapter 13).

6.5 TENDONS AND LIGAMENTS

6.5.1 TENDONS

Tendon insertions and tendon sheaths or, in their absence, peritendinous tissues sometimes give rise to symptoms after unaccustomed, persistent or strenuous use, for example, tennis elbow, etc. The pathogenesis of these is not clear, nor is the pathology since in many instances there is no need or justification to interfere surgically, nor to remove tissue. More clear cut are conditions leading to discontinuity of tendons, as the result of exertion or of laceration. The former class are either avulsions at origin or insertion, when the pathology is that of fracture (section 6.4), or a rupture of the tendon itself. Other forms of direct trauma can disrupt tendons, some causing clean cuts, others compound injuries.

Division of a tendon results in a nonpyogenic inflammatory reaction, most evident in the paratendinous tissue, and death of tenocytes. The extent of the necrosis is determined by the interference with the blood supply. The most compromising deprivation comes from stripping of the paratenous tissue through which the tendon receives an important supply. Traumatic deprivation coupled with tight suturing can quickly lead to a tendon falling apart and to the sutures pulling out (Peacock, 1959).

There is a reparative response on the part of tendon, but it is not substantial in comparison with that of the surrounding tendon sheath or paratenon, the main sources of the reparative tissues when tendons are divided. This extrinsic process is very effective, and strong union is achieved even when there is a gap between the ends. However, the outcome may be unsatisfactory because of undue lengthening of the tendon, or because of adhesions which limit gliding. The former is avoided by approximating the ends. The latter is a serious problem only in the regions of tendon enclosed in a sheath where adhesions form readily between the gliding surfaces. Much of the detailed information about tendon repair is the result of research to overcome this problem which is the major obstacle to restoration of function in tendon injuries of the hand involving ensheathed portions. Artificial sheaths made from a variety of materials had been tried without success. The reasons for this became apparent in the study of animal models (Potenza, 1964; Lindsay, 1979) in which it was shown that the reparative tissue grew into the artificial sheath and attached to any injury of the tendon surface, such as a needle track or forceps mark, as well as the site of division. The granulation tissue penetrates this, and forms an irregular collagen meshwork joining the two ends. Over time this is remodelled until at the end of four months the tendon structure is restored at full strength (Ketchum, 1977). It is difficult to form a clear idea of the remodelling mechanism. Frost (1986), acknowledging the limited information on the topic, proposes both micro- and macromodelling mechanisms operating at the molecular, cellular and tissue levels which are somewhat similar to those known in bone. As references he quotes Klein *et al.* (1977, 1982). Akeson *et al.* (1992) discussing the beneficial effect of continuous passive motion in the healing of connective tissues, including bone and cartilage, refer to the prevention, or limitation of adhesions following tendon repair in the territory of the flexor tendon sheath when this technique is employed.

6.5.2 LIGAMENTS

Frank *et al.* (1983) have recorded the natural history of the healing of experimentally induced rupture of the medial collateral ligament of rabbit knees, seeking to resolve some of the conflicting evidence about duration and effectiveness of the process. There was an immediate inflammatory reaction and granulation tissue formation in the region, with penetration between the severed ends of the ligament. The inflammation and tissue production reached its maximum at the 21-day observation and had diminished slightly by the 42-day examination. The whole of the ligament participated to some degree in the reaction, shown by increased cellularity and a degree of disorganization. There was continuing resolution of the reaction with tissue maturation and remodelling over the first year. Thereafter progress was slower but the reduction in the number and size of fibroblasts continued as did the longitudinal reorientation of the fibres to the final observation at 2.5 years. Macroscopically at that time the fascia was less adherent to the scar, which had not assumed the dense white appearance of normal tendon and was evident as a 2–3 mm band between the relatively normal ends. There had not been tissue contraction and the normal pre-strain of ligaments had not returned (i.e. they did not retract when separated from bone attachment).

6.6 INJURY BY IONIZING RADIATION

The effects of radiation on the skeleton became a subject of intense interest in the 1940s following the recognition of the extent to which radionuclides could enter bone. At the pathological level they affected the skeleton through internal irradiation of its cells, including marrow and vessels, disturbing their function and inducing neoplasia. Interest also extended to radiotherapy, since it gave rise to similar effects. The reviews by Vaughan (1962, 1968, 1971) of radiation disease are comprehensive in their coverage and references to the literature. There was also considerable interest at this time in the use of radioactive calcium and strontium as trace elements in the study of the normal mineral metabolism of bone and its alterations in metabolic bone disease.

Radiation reaches the skeleton from external or internal sources (Vaughan, 1971). The former are X-rays, gamma rays or fast neutrons. The latter are alpha, beta and gamma rays from internally deposited radionuclides. The various rays eject electrons from the atoms of the material through which they pass; the atoms become positively charged, leading to chemical change of the parent molecule. Fast neutrons lead indirectly to ionization and chemical change. The consequences may be immediate or delayed cell death, arrest of cell division, or abnormalities that persist in successive generations and cause abnormal repair or malignancy (Vaughan, 1968).

The specific ionization is the number of ionizations per micron of path length, a linear energy transfer. There is characteristic energy for every radiation emisssion, measured in million electron volt units (MeV). There are a number of units of dose: roentgen, rad, rem, rep, curie, of which the rad and the curie are most used. The rad is an expression of absorbed dose (energy): 1 rad = 100 ergs/g of tissue. One curie is 3.7 × 10^{10} atom disintegrations per second, and the specific activity of a radionuclide is the curies per unit mass.

6.6.1 BONE-SEEKING RADIONUCLIDES

Attention was drawn to the dangers of radium poisoning in watchdial painters in 1925 by Martland *et al.* Interest was intensified by recognition of the importance of bone-seeking radionuclides (Hamilton, 1947), leading to studies of exposed individuals (Evans *et al.*, 1969; Finkel *et al.*, 1969). Marshall (1969) divided nuclides into surface and volume seekers. The former are incorporated into bone at mineralizing sites. The latter are more profusely distributed because they are not only deposited in the mineralizing osteoid but also exchange with the calcium of the hydroxyapatite crystals in the bone. Table 6.2 lists the more common bone-seeking radionuclides (Vaughan, 1971).

In man only the long-term effect of radium could be studied, as a result of the use by radium dial painters of ^{226}Ra (see below). However, there have been extensive studies of many radionuclides in a variety of mammals (Vaughan, 1962). Much of this animal research was directed to determining maximum permissible levels of exposure. The problem is complex because of the many factors that determine dose, and the different distributions in the skeleton. The two tissues principally at risk are bone and marrow, giving rise to osteosarcoma and leukaemia or malignant myeloproliferative disorder. Beta radiation is more effective than alpha radiation in causing osteosarcoma; those alpha emitters that deposit only in the surface are more effective than those distributed diffusely (since that portion of the radioactivity within the bone does not reach the osteoblasts). Radioplutonium is not only a surface seeker but is also taken up by marrow cells and has the potential to cause leukaemia.^{90}Sr and its decay product are beta emitters, and the long range of these puts marrow at risk, producing a malignant myeloproliferative disorder in some animals rather than osteosarcoma.

6.6.2   EXTERNAL RADIATION

Natural environmental irradiation is common – cosmic rays, radioactive potassium, uranium and thorium and their decay products – but has never been shown to be hazardous. Fallout from atomic explosions (Liebow *et al.*, 1949; Hiroshima and Nagasaki, 1981), accidental or deliberate, and accidents involving radionuclides are also environmental hazards. There are also occupational hazards, although radiation protection regulations minimize these. In addition, the diagnostic and therapeutic use of irradiation also present some dangers.

The effects on the skeleton of internal and external irradiation are broadly similar. These can be grouped under:

- Osteodysplasia
- Fracture
- Alterations in bone volume

Table 6.2 Bone-seeking radionuclides

	Half-life	*Decay product*	*Distribution*
^{45}Ca	165 days	Stable	Volume
^{32}P	14.3 days	Stable	Volume
^{90}Sr	28 years	^{90}Y beta	Volume
^{224}Ra	3.6 days	Stable	Volume
^{226}Ra	1620 years	Ra alpha (3.8 days)	Volume
^{228}Ra	6.7 years	^{228}Ac beta and alpha (6.13 h)	Volume
^{90}Y	64 hours	Stable	Surface
^{228}Th	1.9 years	^{224}Ra	Surface
^{239}Pu	24 000 years	^{235}U	Surface
^{242}Am	458 years	^{237}Np	Surface

- Osteomyelitis
- Neoplasia
    Leukaemia
    Osteosarcoma
    Carcinoma (radium)

Osteodysplasia is a reference to the effect on cells and the subsequent changes in bone. It will come to the notice of pathologists in children and adults who have undergone radiotherapy for neoplasia. There continue to be gaps in the knowledge about this subject, leading to some uncertainty in discussing it. When bone is irradiated the exposed tissues are bone, blood vessels and marrow. These can be considered separately.

In general the consequences of irradiation may be immediate or delayed cell death, arrest of cell division, or abnormalities that persist in successive generations and cause abnormal repair or malignancy. Osteodysplasia is not the result of immediate cell death, and it is debatable if delayed cell death plays a part long term.

The dysplastic effect is, obviously, most evident during childhood. The principal source of radiation damage in this age group is the treatment of neoplasia. Technical improvements and chemotherapy (which has its own attendant risks (Tucker *et al.*, 1987)) have reduced exposure, and increased survival. Reduced exposure has lowered the risk of complications, but longer survival has increased the chance of their manifestation. The cell activity in growth plates is disturbed, resulting in reduction of cell proliferation, matrix production and ossification. As a result the plate thickens. Growth plates have the ability to recover from these effects, but they cannot make up for lost growth. The interference with growth is manifested in the irradiated regions. An indication of their nature and incidence comes from the report by Butler *et al.* (1990). A total of 143 patients out of approximately 2600 had been treated with radiotherapy (as part of multi treatment protocols) between 1970 and 1987 and sur-

vived to skeletal maturity. More than one condition was present in some cases.

Pain	51
Chest and rib deformities	51
Scoliosis/Kyphoscoliosis	50
Kyphosis	14
Leg inequality	12
Secondary sarcoma	3

The diseases which had been treated were:

Hodgkin's disease	44
Nephroblastoma	30
Acute lymphoblastic leukaemia	26
Non-Hodgkin's lymphoma	18
Ewing's tumour of bone	9
Rhabdomyosarcoma	6
Neuroblastoma	6
Ovarian teratoma	2
Renal cell carcinoma	1
Hepatoblastoma	1

6.7   DYSPLASIA IN THE BONE OF ADULTS

The event that brings radiation damaged bone to attention is fracture. This is usually the neck of femur (following pelvic irradiation in women), and less frequently the ribs or clavicle following irradiation for cancer of the breast or lungs, and the mandible in oral cancer. Although it is usual to speak of radiation necrosis as being the underlying cause, it is far from clear in pathological material that necrosis is antecedent to the fracture (Bonfiglio, 1953; Goodman and Sherman, 1963; Catto, 1976).

Damage to tissues by radiation is the same irregardless of the nature of the source (Vaughan, 1971). It is however variable; apart from tissue dosage, which is difficult to determine with precision, there are other variables, many inherent in the individual and not understood, which affect the response. Moreover the pathological changes are individually non-specific (Fajardo, 1982), but taken together are suggestive and can be confirmed by the history. They are acute (days to weeks) and delayed (months to years). Capillaries and sinusoids dilate, and actively dividing cells die in numbers relative to determining factors. The narrow responses are shown in Table 6.3.

The fate of adipose marrow tissue according to haematologists is rather insignificant (Fajardo, 1982); but, for osteoarticular pathologists there are considerable alterations (Catto, 1976). Oedematous fibrous tissue appears and in places there is dense fibrous tissue, investing blood vessels and trabecular bone, and undergoing irregular calcium deposition. Metaplastic bone formation may take place within this.

In general descriptions of radiation damage, blood vessel alterations have an important place. However, in descriptions of bone from humans (mostly femoral heads following postirradiation fracture) these are not prominent (Catto, 1976).

In bone the early (and late) changes have been studied in animals (Jee, 1971); the late changes have been studied in humans. Early on there is a diminution in the number of bone cells, osteoblasts being more sensitive, followed by a reduction in pre-osteoblasts and osteoclasts. Osteocytic death is not immediately apparent. In keeping with general observations, there is some return of the bone cells after an interval. Alterations in bone structure then begin to appear and in due course are detectible radiographically.

Remodelling is disturbed with an imbalance towards resorption. This produces thinned trabeculae, and widened osteonal canals. When the latter coalesce they form cavities detectable in radiographs as small lucent foci (Figure 6.14). But there is also appositional formation, widening the trabeculae in places. Moreover, woven bone formation built onto trabeculae, some of which are depleted of their osteocytes, in addition to metaplastic formation in the fibrous marrow and the calcium deposition referred to above, serve to increase bone density. The irregular disposition of these various activities leads to a mixed pattern of porosis and sclerosis in radiographs. Sometimes this is mistakenly referred to as radiation osteitis, for there is no inflammation, or as radiation necrosis, for the necrotic element is often minimal. A more acceptable term is radiation osteodysplasia. Microradiography shows there to be abnormalities of mineralization of bone (Vaughan, 1962), which are not by themselves sufficient to be detectable in clinical radiographs. These are normally seen in aged individuals, but not to the same degree as in radiated bone. They are mineral deposition in osteocyte lacunae, dense mineral at the inner surface of osteons and occlusion of osteons by dense calcium deposits.

The consequences of this condition, which may include effects which are not discernible

Table 6.3 Marrow responses to radiation

Time	Dose (total rads)	Response
3 days	400	Decrease in nucleated cells, marked in precursors of red and myeloid cells
8 days	1000	No blast cells; dilated sinusoids; haemorrhage
16 days	2000	Cellularity 20% of normal
35 days	5000	Extreme hypoplasia; plasma cells, histiocytes, lymphocytes remain; yellow gelatinous tissue; sinusoids less dilated
3 months		>50% patients have partial return of normoblasts, granulocytes, megakaryocytes
5–12 months		Second, permanent wave of depression in those with recovery

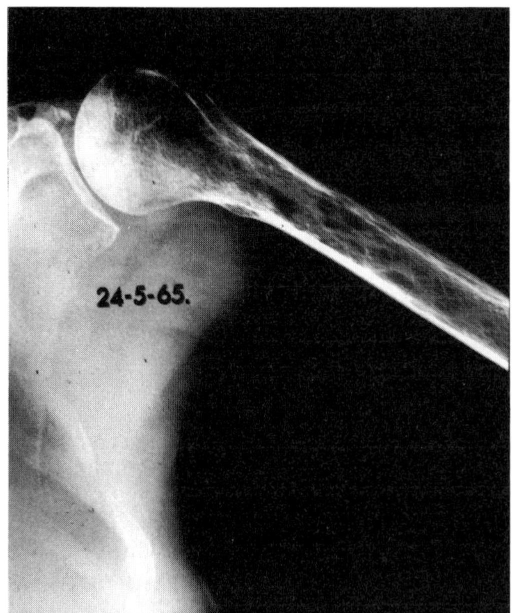

Figure 6.14 Postirradiation dysplasia of humerus.

histologically, are a liability to fracture (the most usual site is femoral neck, followed by ribs, clavicle, neck of humerus), collapse of the femoral head, or osteomyelitis (the mandible in particular).

Although fracture is widely attributed to necrosis, this is not always borne out on pathological examination. Catto (1976) examined three specimens in which necrosis was confined to a segmental collapse, which could have been the consequence of fracture In only one had there been a fracture of the neck. Other cases have been reported by MacDuogall *et al.* (1950), Bonfiglio (1953), and Goodman and Sherman (1963). In the first of these the femoral head was completely necrotic.

6.7.1   OSTEOMYELITIS

This is a complication of irradiation of oral neoplasms. The incidence is inversely proportional to the health of the teeth; it is least common in the edentulous. The inflammatory reaction is not affected by the preceding radiation.

6.7.2   INDUCED NEOPLASIA

Advances in molecular biology have clarified concepts of the pathogenesis of cancer (Alberts *et al.*, 1989) and have abetted understanding of post irradiation neoplasia. Neoplasia is the result of mutation in genes that regulate cell division. It is calculated that, in a mutagen-free environment, every single gene is likely to have undergone mutation on 10^{10} separate occasions in the lifetime of any individual human being. That death from cancer is not universal is accounted for by the ability of the cell to repair its DNA, and by the normal restrictions on cell proliferation exercised by 'social control genes'. It seems likely, therefore, that it requires several mutations of a particular set of genes in a single cell to enable its unlimited growth and clone formation. These genes are concerned with the production of proteins which stimulate or inhibit cell proliferation. There is more information about the former, the normal proto-oncogenes and their mutated oncogenes, than the latter.

In addition to the spontaneous mutations referred to above, the genes can be transformed by environmental agents, which may be chemical, physical or viral. Radiation, a physical agent, has, in common with other initiators, a latent period of some years during which, one assumes, subsequent mutations occur to free a cell from growth restraints. There is no distinguishing feature about neoplasms following upon irradiation. Therefore the decision that such an event has happened depends on establishing that:

1. it has arisen in an irradiated field
2. a tumorigenic dose has been administered
3. there has been a period of latency

4.   the neoplasm is different from any antecedent at the site

5.   it is not a metastasis

Both internal and external radiation give rise to neoplasia of bone. These are mostly osteosarcomas, but chondrosarcoma, fibrosarcoma and undifferentiated sarcoma have been reported. They are mainly in the femur, but many other sites have been involved. In children, radiation gives rise to osteochondromas. Internal radiation has been associated with carcinomas of the nasal apparatus. In bone, both internal (^{224}Ra) and external irradiation give rise to leukaemias.

REFERENCES

Ackerman, L.V. (1958) Extraosseous localised non-neoplastic bone and cartilage formation (so-called myositis ossificans). Clinical and pathological confusion with malignant neoplasms. *J. Bone Joint Surg.*, **40A**, 279–98.

Aichroth, P.M. (1971a) Osteochondritis dissecans of the knee. A clinical survey. *J. Bone Joint Surg.*, **53B**, 440–7.

Aichroth, P.M. (1971b) Osteochondral fractures and their relationship to osteochondritis dissecans of the knee. An experimental study on animals. *J. Bone Joint Surg.*, **53B**, 448–54.

Akeson, W.H., Amiel, D., Kwan, M. *et al.* (1992) Stress dependence of synovial joints. In *Bone*, Vol. 5, *Fracture Repair and Regeneration* (ed. B.K. Hall), CRC Press, Boca Raton, FL, pp. 33–60.

Alberts, A., Bray, D., Lewis, J. *et al.* (1989) *Molecular Biology of the Cell*, 2nd edn, Garland Publishing, New York and London, Chapter 21.

Angel, J.C. (1983) Slipped upper femoral epiphysis. In *Postgraduate Textbook of Clinical Orthopaedics* (ed. N.H. Harris), John Wright, Bristol, pp. 120–6.

Arlot, M.E., Bonjean, M., Chavassieux, P.M. *et al.* (1983) Bone histology in adults with avascular necrosis. Histomorphic evaluation in iliac crest biopsies of 77 patients. *J. Bone Joint Surg.*, **65A**, 1319–27.

Ashhurst, D.E. (1992) Macromolecular synthesis and mechanical stability during fracture repair. In *Bone*, Vol. 5, *Fracture Repair and Regeneration*, (ed. B.K. Hall), CRC Press, Boca Raton, FL, pp. 61–122.

Benaissa, R., Uhthoff, H.K. and Mercier, P. (1989) Repair of trabecular fractures. Cadaver studies of the upper femur. *Acta Orthop. Scand.*, **60**, 585–9.

Bonfiglio, M. (1953) The pathology of fracture of the femoral neck following irradiation. *Am. J. Roentgenol.*, **70**, 449–59.

Brookes, M. (1971) *The Blood Supply of Bone.* Butterworths, London.

Brown, C.W., Jones, B., Donaldson *et al.* (1992) Neuropathic (Charcot) arthropathy of the spine after traumatic spinal paraplegia. *Spine*, **17 (6S)**, 103–8.

Burrows, H.J. (1957) Slipped upper femoral epiphysis. *J. Bone Joint Surg.*, **39B**, 641–58.

Butler, M.S., Robertson, W.W., Rate, W. *et al.* (1990) Skeletal sequelae of radiation therapy for malignant childhood tumours. *Clin. Orthop.*, **251**, 235–40.

Byers, P.D. (1974) The effects of high femoral osteotomy on osteoarthritis of the hip. *J. Bone Joint Surg.*, **56B**, 279–90.

Caffey, J. (1957) Some traumatic lesions in growing bones other than fractures and dislocations: clinical and radiological features. *Br. J. Radiol.*, **30**, 225–38.

Calandruccio, R.A. and Scott Gilmer, W. (1962) Proliferation, regeneration and repair of articular cartilage of immature animals. *J. Bone Joint Surg.*, **44A**, 431–55.

Catto, M. (1976) Pathology of aseptic bone necrosis, in *Aseptic Necrosis of Bone* (ed. J.K. Davidson), Excerpta Medica, Amsterdam, Chapter 2.

Charon, S., Bavery, E., Malik, M.E. *et al.* (1982) Osteonecroses de la tranplantation renale. *Lyon. Med.*, **247**, 339–47.

Cornell, C.N. and Lane, J.M. (1992) Newest factors in fracture healing. *Clin. Orthop.*, **277**, 297–311.

Cuthbertson, D.P. (1976) Surgical metabolism: historical and evolutionary aspects. In *Metabolism and the Response to Injury.* (eds A. W. Wilkinson and D.P. Cuthbertson), Pitman Medical, Kent, pp. 1–34.

Daffner, R.H. and Pavlov, H. (1992) Stress fractures: current concepts. *Am. J. Roentgenol.*, **159**, 245–52.

Davies, A.M. and Bradley, S.A. (1991) Iliac insufficiency fractures. *Br. J. Radiol.*, **64**, 305–9.

Devas, M.B. (1963) Stress fractures in children. *J. Bone Joint Surg.*, **45B**, 528–410.

Devas, M.B. (1975) *Stress Fractures.* Churchill Livingstone, Edinburgh.

Dietrich, J.E., Whedon, D.G. and Shorr, E. (1948)

Effects of immobilisation upon various metabolic and physiologic functions of normal men. *Am. J. Med.*, **4**, 3–36.

Dupree, W.B. (1990) Progress in pseudosarcomatous and borderline soft tissue tumours, in *Pathobiology of Soft Tissue Tumours* (eds C.D.M. Fletcher and P.H. McKee), Churchill Livingstone, Edinburgh, p. 265.

Dupree, W.B. and Enzinger, F.M. (1986) Fibro-osseous pseudotumour of the digits. *Cancer*, **58**, 2103–9.

Enzinger, F.M. and Weiss, S.W. (1988) *Soft Tissue Tumors*, 2nd edn, C.V. Mosby, St Louis.

Evans, R.D., Keane, A.T., Kolenkow, R.J. *et al.* (1969) In *Delayed Effects of Bone Seeking Radionuclides* (eds C.W. Mays *et al.*), University of Utah Press, pp. 157–91.

Fajardo, L.F. (1982) *Pathology of Radiation Injury.* Masson Publishing USA, Inc.

Fazzalini, N.L., Vernon-Roberts, B. and Darracott, J. (1987) Osteoarthritis of the hip. Possible protective and causative roles of trabecular microfractures in the head of the femur. *Clin. Orthop.*, **216**, 224–33.

Finkel, M.P., Miller, C.E. and Hasterlik, R.J. (1969) In *Delayed Effects of Bone Seeking Radionuclides* (eds C.W. Mays *et al.*), University of Utah Press, pp. 195–224.

Frank, C., Schachar, N. and Dittrich, D. (1983) The natural history of healing in the repaired medial collateral ligament. *J. Orthop. Res.*, **1**, 179–88

Freeman, M.A.R., Todd, R.C. and Pirie, C.J. (1974) The role of fatigue in the pathogenesis of femoral neck fractures. *J. Bone Joint Surg.*, **56B**, 698–702.

Frost, H.M. (1960) Presence of microscopic cracks in vivo in bone. *Henry Ford Hosp. Med. Bull.*, **8**, 25–35.

Frost, H.M. (1964) The etiopathogenesis of aseptic necrosis of the femoral head. In *Proceedings of the Conference on Aseptic Necrosis of the Femoral Head*, St Louis, MO, pp. 393–413.

Frost, H.M. (1973) *Orthopaedic Biomechanics.* Charles C. Thomas, Springfield, IL.

Frost, H.M. (1983) The regional acceleratory phenomenon. *Henry Ford Hosp. Med. J.*, **31**, 3–9.

Frost, H.M. (1986) *Intermediary Organisation of the Skeleton.* CRC Press, Boca Raton, FL, Vol I, p. 300; Vol II, pp. 219–20.

Gallocher, J. (1967) A study of sesamoid bones and related structures of the 1st MTP joint. *Chiropodist*, **22**, 419–35.

Goodman, A.H. and Sherman, M.S. (1963) Post irradiation fractures of the femoral neck. *J. Bone Joint Surg.*, **45A**, 723–30.

Hall, B.K. (1992) *Bone*, Vol. 5: *Fracture Repair and Regeneration.* (ed. B.K. Hall), CRC Press, Boca Raton, FL.

Hall, J.E. (1957) The results of treatment of slipped upper femoral epiphysis. *J. Bone Joint Surg.*, **39B**, 655–73.

Hamilton, J.C. (1947) The metabolism of the fission products and the heaviest elements. *Radiology*, **49**, 325–43.

Hansen-Leth, C. (1979) Bone revascularisation and bone healing in the amputation stump. An experimental study. *Acta Orthop. Scand.*, **50**, 39–47.

Hansson, C.J. (1938) On insufficiency fractures of femur and tibia. *Acta Radiol.*, **19**, 554–9.

Hansson, T., Keller, T. and Jonson, R. (1988) Fatigue fracture morphology in human lumbar motion segments. *J. Spinal Disord.*, **1**, 33–8.

Hiroshima and Nagasaki (1981) The committee for the compilation of materials on damage caused by the atomic bombs in Hiroshima and Nagasaki. Iwanami Shoten, Tokyo.

Howard, J.E. (1945) Protein metabolism during convalescence after trauma. Recent studies. *Arch. Surg.*, **50**, 166–70.

Howard, J.E., Parson, W., Stein, K.E. *et al.* (1944a) Studies on fracture convalescence. I. Nitrogen metabolism after fracture and skeletal operations in healthy males. *Bull. Johns Hopkins Hosp.*, **75**, 156–60.

Howard, J.E., Winternitz, J., Parson, W. *et al.* (1944b) Studies on fracture convalescence. II. The influence of diet on post-traumatic nitrogen deficit exhibited by fracture patients. *Bull. Johns Hopkins Hosp.*, **75**, 209–24.

Huggins, C.B. (1931) The formation of bone under the influence of epithelium of the urinary tract. *Arch. Surg.*, **22**, 377–408.

Hulley, S.B., Vogel, J.M., Donaldson, C.L. *et al.* (1971) The effect of supplemental oral phosphate on bone mineral changes during prolonged bed rest. *Clin. Invest. Med.*, **50**, 2506–18.

Hullinger, C.W. (1944) Insufficiency fracture of the calcaneus similar to march fracture of metatarsal. *J. Bone Joint Surg.*, **26**, 751–7.

Hulth, A. (1989) Current concepts of fracture healing. *Clin. Orthop.*, **249**, 266–84.

Jaffe, H.L. (1972) *Metabolic, Degenerative and Inflammatory Diseases of Bone.* Lea and Febiger, Philadelphia.

Jee, W.S.S. (1971) Bone-seeking radionuclides and bones in *Pathology of Irradiation* (ed. C.C Berdjis), Williams and Wilkins, Baltimore, pp. 186–212.

Johnson, J.T.H. (1967) Neuropathic fractures and joint injuries. Pathogenesis and rationales of prevention and treatment. *J. Bone Joint Surg.*, **49A**, 1–30.

Ketchum, L.D. (1977) Primary tendon healing: a review. *J. Hand Surg.*, **2**, 428–35.

Key, J.A. (1932) Clinical observations of tabetic arthropathies (Charcot joints). *Am. J. Syph.*, **16** 429–46.

Klein, G.L. (1991) The aluminium content of parenteral solutions: current status. *Nutr. Rev.*, **49**, 74–9.

Klein, L., Dawson, M.H. and Heiple, K.G. (1977) Turnover of collagen in the rat after denervation. *J. Bone Joint Surg.*, **59A**, 1065–7.

Klein, L., Player, R.S., Heiple, K.G. *et al.* (1982) Isotopic evidence for resorption of soft tissues and bone in immobilised dogs. *J. Bone Joint Surg.*, **64A**, 223–30.

Kohler, A. (1908) Ueber eine haufige, bisher auscheinend unbekannte erkrankung einzeiner kindlicher knocken. *Munch. Med. Wochenschr.*, **55**, 1923–25.

Korkonen, L.K. and Vaananen, K. (1992) Bone inductive molecules and enhancement of repair and regeneration, in *Bone*, Vol 5; *Fracture Repair and Regeneration* (ed. B.K. Hall), CRC Press, Boca Raton, FL, pp. 209–32.

Lagier, R. (1971) Idiopathic aseptic necrosis of the femoral head. An anatomo-pathological concept. In *Idiopathic Ischaemic Necrosis of the Femoral Head in Adults* (ed. W.M. Zinn), Georg Thieme, Stuttgart, pp. 49–67.

Liebow, A.A., Warren, S. and DeCoursey, E. (1949) Pathology of atomic bomb casualties. *Am. J. Pathol.*, **25**, 853–1027.

Lindsay, W.K. (1979) Tendon healing: a continuing experimental approach. In *Tendon Surgery of the Hand* (ed. C. Verdan), Churchill Livingstone, Edinburgh, Chapter 6, pp. 35–9.

Linscheid, R.L. and Coventry, M.B. (1962) Unrecognised fractures of long bones suggesting primary bone tumours. *Proc. Mayo Clinic*, **37**, 599–606.

MacDougall, J.T., Gibson, A. and Williams, T.H. (1950) Irradiation necrosis of the femoral neck. *Arch. Surg.*, **61**, 325–45.

Marshall, J.H. (1969) In *Delayed Effects of Bone Seeking Radionuclides* (eds C.W. Mays *et al.*), University of Utah Press, pp. 7–23.

Martland, H.S., Conlon, P. and Knef, J.P. (1925) Some unrecognised dangers in the use and handling of radio-active substances: with special reference to the storage of insoluble products of radium and mesothorium in the reticulo-endothelial system. *J. Am. Med. Assoc.*, **85**, 1769–76.

McKibbin, B. (1978) The biology of fracture healing in long bones. *J. Bone Joint Surg.*, **60B**, 150–62.

Meaney, J.E. and Carty, H. (1992) Femoral stress fractures in children. *Skeletal Radiol.*, **21**, 173–6.

Milgram, J.W. (1977a) The classification of loose bodies in human joints. *Clin. Orthop.*, **124**, 282–91.

Milgram, J.W. (1977b) The development of loose bodies in human joints. *Clin. Orthop.*, **124**, 292–303.

Milgram, J.W. (1978) Radiologic and histologic manifestations of osteochondritis dissecans of the distal femur. *Radiology*, **126**, 305–11.

Milgram, J.W. (1991) Nonunion and pseudoarthrosis of fracture healing. A histopathologic study of 95 human specimens. *Clin. Orthop.*, **268**, 203–13.

Nagura, S. (1960) The so-called osteochondritis of Konig. *Clin. Orthop.*, **18**, 100–2.

Nevo, Z., Robinson, D. and Halperin, N. (1992) The use of grafts composed of cultured cells for the repair of cartilage and bone. In *Bone*, Vol. 5, *Fracture Repair and Regeneration* (ed. B K. Hall), CRC Press, Boca Raton, FL, pp. 123–52.

Olerud, S. and Danckwardt-Lilliestrom, G. (1968) Fracture healing in compression osteosynthesis. *J. Bone Joint Surg.*, **50B**, 844–51.

Peacock, E. (1959) A study of the circulation in normal tendons and in healing grafts. *Ann. Surg.*, **149**, 415–28.

Pentecost, R.L., Murray, R.A. and Brindley, H.H. (1964) Fatigue, insufficiency and pathological fractures. *J. Am. Med. Assoc.*, **187**, 1001–4.

Pester, S. and Smith, P.C. (1992) Stress fractures in the lower extremities of soldiers in basic training. *Orthop. Rev.*, **21**, 297–303.

Potenza, A.D. (1964) Prevention of adhesions to healing digital flexor tendons. *J. Am. Med. Assoc.*, **187**, 187–91.

Pounds, J.G., Long, G.J. and Rosen, J.F. (1991) Cellular and molecular toxicity of lead in bone. *Environ. Health Perspect.*, **91**, 17–32.

Salter, R.B. and Harris, W.R. (1963) Injuries involving the epiphyseal plate. *J. Bone Joint Surg.*, **45A**, 587–622.

Sevitt, S. (1980) Healing of fractures in man. In *The Scientific Foundations of Orthopaedics and Traumatology* (eds R. Owen, J. Goodfellow and P. Bullough), William Heinemann, London, pp. 258–73.

Sevitt, S. (1981) *Bone Repair and Fracture Healing in Man.* Churchill Livingstone, Edinburgh.

Smith, R. (1980) Calcium, phosphorus and magnesium metabolism. In *The Scientific Foundations of Orthopaedics and Traumatology* (eds. R. Owen, J. Goodfellow and P. Bullough), William Heinemann, London, pp. 213–23.

Soule, E.H., Lattes, R. and Enzinger, F.M. (1986) Pseudosarcomatous (proliferative) fibroblastic lesions. *ASCP Classical Teaching Collections, Soft tissue series* no. 1. American Society of Clinical Pathologists Press, Chicago, p. 2.

Spjut, H.J. and Dorfman, H.D. (1981) Florid reactive periostitis of the tubular bones of the hands and feet. A benign lesion which may simulate osteosarcoma. *Am. J. Surg. Pathol.*, **5**, 423–33.

Sykes, M.P., Savel, H., Chu, F.C.H. *et al.* (1964) Long term effects of therapeutic irradiation upon the marrow. *Cancer*, **17**, 1144–8.

Stout, A.P. (1953) Tumours of the soft tissue, in *Atlas of Tumour Pathology*, 2nd Series, Fascicle 5, Armed Forces Institute of Pathology, Washington DC.

Stover, S.L., Garland, D.E. and Nilsson, O.S. (eds) (1991) Symposium on Heterotopic ossification. *Clin. Orthop.*, **263**, 2–120.

Todd, R.C., Freeman, M.A.R. and Pirie, C.J. (1972) Isolated trabecular fatigue fractures in the femoral head. *J. Bone Joint Surg.*, **54B**, 723–8.

Tucker, M.A., D'Angio, G.J., Boice, J.D. *et al.* (1987) Bone sarcomas linked to radiotherapy and chemotherapy in children. *N. Engl. J. Med.*, **317**, 588–93.

Turner, A. and Anderson, J. (1992) Growth plate distraction and response of growth plates to trauma. In *Bone* Vol. 5, *Fracture Repair and Regeneration* (ed. B.K. Hall), CRC Press, Boca Raton, FL, pp. 233–8.

Urbaniak, J.R., Bright, D.S., Gill, L.H. *et al.* (1974) Vascularization and the gliding mechanism of free flexor-tendon grafts inserted by the silicone-rod method. *J. Bone Joint Surg.*, **56A**, 473–82.

Urist, M.R. (1989) Bone morphogenetic protein, bone regeneration, heterotopic ossification and the bone marrow consortium, In *Bone and Mineral Research*, Vol 6 (ed. W.A. Peck), Elsevier, Amsterdam.

Vaughan, J. (1962) Bone disease induced by radiation. *Int. Rev. Exp. Pathol.*, **1**, 244–369.

Vaughan, J. (1968) The effects of skeletal radiation. *Clin. Orthop.*, **56**, 283–303.

Vaughan, J. (1971) The effects of radiation on bone. In *The Biochemistry and Physiology of Bone*, 2nd edn, Vol. 3 (ed. G.H. Bourne), Academic Press, New York and London, pp. 485–534.

Wertheimer, L.G. and Fernandes-Lopes, S.D.L. (1971) Arterial supply to the femoral head. A combined angiographic and histological study. *J. Bone Joint Surg.*, **53A**, 545–56.

Wlodarski, K.H. (1992) Bone formation in soft tissues. In *Bone*, Vol. 5, *Fracture Repair and Regeneration* (ed. B.K. Hall), CRC Press, Boca Raton, FL., pp. 313–37.

Anthony J. Freemont

Inflammation is the organism's response to noxious stimuli. The latter will include: infection, radiation, extremes of temperature, chemicals and a variety of other insults. The processes of inflammation are mediated by three different types of cell: those that are native to the inflamed tissue, those that are recruited into the tissue from the bloodstream and those in distant organs that secrete mediators into the bloodstream.

Most stimuli to inflammation cause local tissue injury, and it is the cells at the locus that are the first to respond in the sequence of chemical changes that typifies inflammation. Here, four main groups of cells are responsible: tissue mast cells (Lowman *et al.*, 1988), fixed tissue macrophages or histiocytes, endothelial cells and nerve cells.

Cells recruited secondarily from the circulation include neutrophil polymorphs (Malich and Gallin, 1988), lymphocytes and cells of the monocyte macrophage lineage (Johnston, 1988).

A third group of cells, those acting at a distance, also include lymphoid cells and cells of the monocyte macrophage lineage (Johnston, 1988), and fixed cells of specific organs such as lymph nodes, spleen and liver.

An essential component in determining the activities of the cells are local environmental influences. Of particular importance are adjacent cells and the complex molecules of the extracellular fluid and tissue matrix (Alberts *et al.*, 1989). A flux of alterations in these initiate, maintain and resolve the inflammatory reaction. Notable among these are the release of metabolites from damaged cells, the local production or accumulation of bacterial endo- and exotoxins, the activation of the complement system and the presence of foreign antigens.

It is a conventional didactic simplification to consider inflammation as comprising two major types of tissue reaction, acute and chronic (Ryan and Majno, 1977). Although this is convenient, it has to be recognized that it is over-simplified and that there can be considerable overlap as the body responds to individual noxious stimuli.

7.1 ACUTE INFLAMMATION

Acute inflammation is characterized by a rapid and short-lived response. The classical signs are heat, redness, oedema, pain and loss of function (Figure 7.1), resulting from a series of major cellular and biochemical events at the tissue level. These fall into three major categories, changes in vascular flow and calibre, increased vascular permeability and leucocyte exudation.

7.1.1 CHANGES IN VASCULAR FLOW AND CALIBRE

The immediate response is a transient arteriolar vasoconstriction, rapidly followed by vasodilatation (Figure 7.2). This affects vessels which are actively carrying blood and a larger number of resting, constricted vessels in which no blood is flowing. The result is an increased volume of blood flowing into the

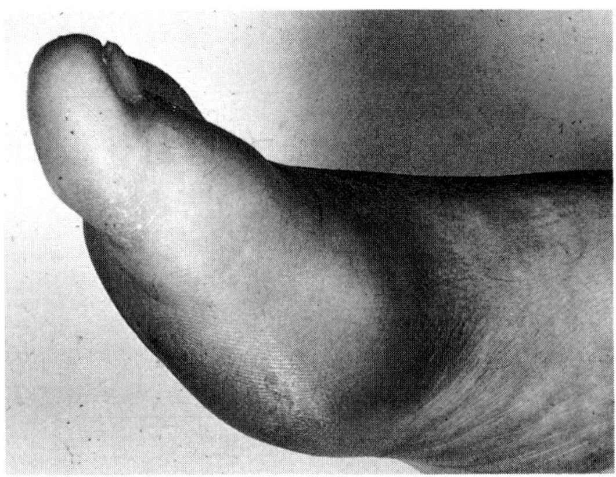

Figure 7.1 The toe of a patient with acute gout. It is red, swollen, hot and very painful.

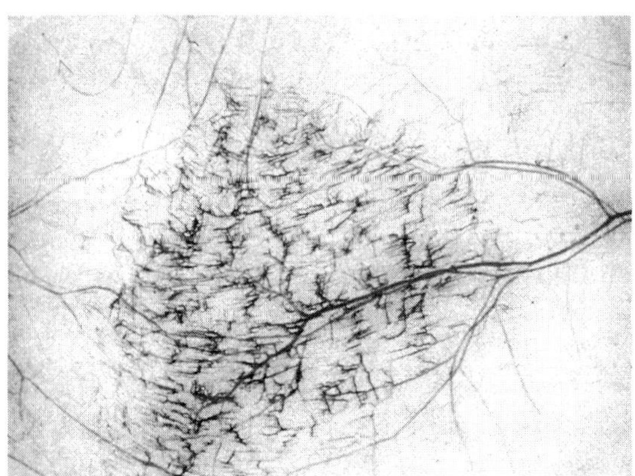

Figure 7.2 In this preparation of mesentery the central area has had a drop of histamine placed upon it 3 min before the photograph was taken. Note the increased number of vessels in comparison with the peripheral area which shows the normal vascular pattern (see vasoactive amines, p. 132)

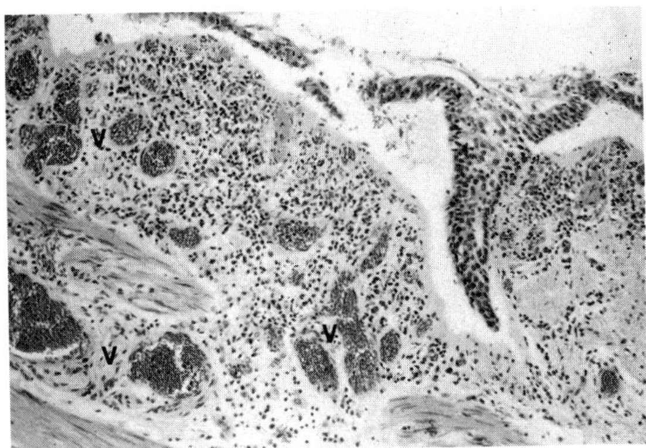

Figure 7.3 Grossly dilated venules (V) filled with red blood cells.

tissue, which accounts for the local heat and redness, and a general slowing of the flow rate, which can lead to stasis (Figure 7.3). This increases the number of leucocytes entering the lesion and promotes their margination, a prerequisite for leucocyte migration into the tissue.

7.1.2 INCREASED VASCULAR PERMEABILITY

The counter gradients of intravascular hydrostatic pressure and osmotic pressure of the proteins, together with the normal semipermeable capillary and venular walls, determine fluid flow out of and into the circulation. Imbalance of these three factors almost invariably causes an accumulation of excessive amounts of fluid within the tissue. In inflammation increased hydrostatic pressure and disruption of the normal endothelial barrier lead to oedema and the classical sign of swelling. The mechanism acting on endothelial cells is chemically mediated contraction. This results in their separation and the increased permeability of the vessel (Figure 7.4). Although the action of the chemical mediator(s) is transient, it may lead to sublethal or lethal endothelial injury, rendering the cells ineffective as a barrier to fluid exudation.

7.1.3 LEUCOCYTE EXUDATION

For blood-borne cells to enter the tissue their headlong rush through the vasculature must be halted, they must have time to change their function and the opportunity to migrate across the local vessel walls must be offered and taken.

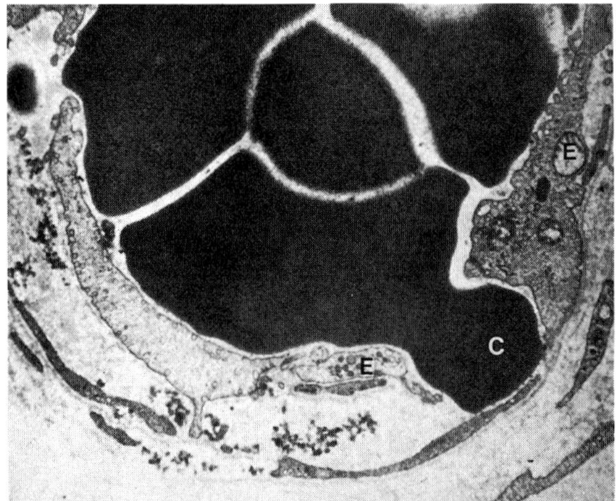

Figure 7.4 Vascular contents (C) exuding between two endothelial cells (E) separated as a consequence of inflammation. (× 5000)

Leucocytes tend, because of the laws of haemodynamics, to travel in the centre of the stream and rarely come into contact with the walls of the blood vessels, which restrict the opportunity to migrate into the tissue. The vasodilatation of acute inflammation leads to a slowing of flow and a more even distribution of leucocytes across the blood vessel, allowing greater contact with the endothelium (Figure 7.5). At the

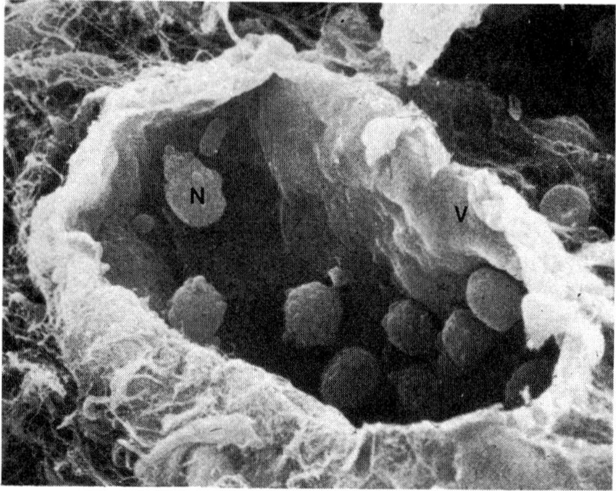

Figure 7.5 Scanning electron micrograph of neutrophils (N) adherent to the lining of a transected venule (V).

same time the inflammatory process up-regulates a series of leucocyte adhesion molecules on the endothelial cell surface (Edelman, 1986; Hynes, 1987) and generates leucocyte chemoattractants within the damaged tissue. The former enables leucocytes to adhere to the endothelium. The second directs the migration of leucocytes towards the site of inflammation. Adhesion depends upon the mutual recognition of complementary molecules on the surface of the leucocyte and the endothelial cell. There are very many of these such as the CD11 β2 integrin (LFA-1) on leucocytes, and endothelial cell ligands such as endothelial leucocyte adhesion molecule 1 (ELAM1) and the intercellular adhesion molecules (ICAM) (Figure 7.6).

Once adherent, leucocytes migrate through the interendothelial junctions (Figure 7.7), and the basement membrane into the tissue, where they follow a chemical gradient to the site of injury.

In acute inflammation the migrating cells are neutrophils and monocyte derived macrophages. The neutrophil is predominant and is the first of the cells to enter the tissue, the macrophages following a little later. Chemoattractant molecules for neutrophils include bacterial products, fragments of the complement molecules, eicosanoids and cytokines (see below). A reaction between the chemoattractant and receptor molecules on the surface of the leucocyte starts a series of intracellular reactions which activate intracellular contractile proteins (Figure 7.8). These control the local release of digestive enzymes and the mobility of the cell which allow it to pass through the structural elements of the tissue.

At the site of cellular injury polymorphs perform a number of functions (Malich and Gallin, 1988), the most important of which is phagocytosis. A complex series of chemical reactions, caused by the inflammatory mediators, coat bacteria with opsonin, which makes them more readily phago-

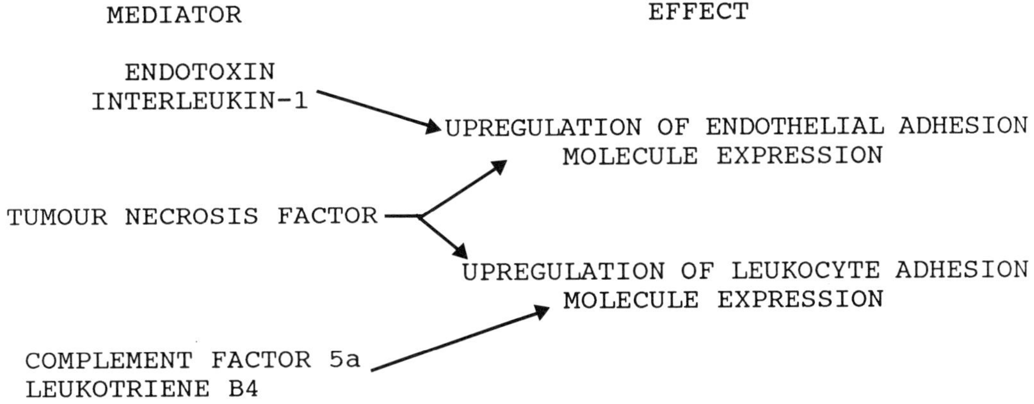

Figure 7.6 Examples of mediators and their actions on endothelial leucocyte interactions.

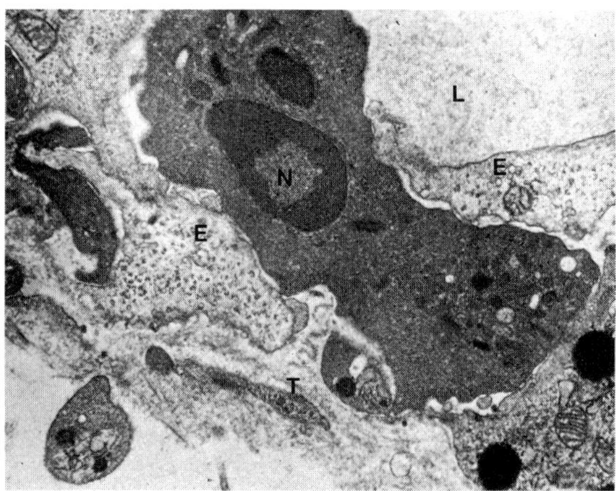

Figure 7.7 Neutrophil (N) migrating between endothelial cells (E) from the vessel lumen (L) to adjacent tissue (T). (× 25 000)

cytosed by the polymorphs. The polymorph attaches to the opsonin and by the production of pseudopodia completely surrounds and internalizes the bacterium, enclosed in cell membrane (Figure 7.9), to form a cyst-like space, a phagosome. This is then fused with lysosomes, membrane-bound packages of digestive enzymes, to form a phagolysosome within which digestion of the bacterium occurs (Figure 7.10) by chemical reactions having two major components, one dependent upon oxygen and the other not.

Oxygen-dependent mechanisms generate free oxygen radicals which exchange electrons with chemicals in the bacterial wall, leading to their lysis. The oxygen-independent mechanisms involve a variety of chemicals, including lysozyme, lactoferrin and basic and acidic proteins, which hydrolyse dead bacteria. In addition to phagocytosis and subsequent degranulation and release of killing and digesting molecules into an internalized phagosome, the polymorphs will also release into the extracellular environment such substances as lysozomal enzymes, oxygen-derived free radicals and eicosanoids which continue to mediate aspects of the inflammation.

7.1.4   CHEMICAL MEDIATORS

The control and mediation of the inflammatory reaction, even as it is currently understood, is a highly ordered chemical system about which it is possible to give here only a brief account of some major components. Some mediators are present in the circulation and in tissue cells, from where they can rapidly initiate an acute response. Others which sustain it are synthesized as part of that response (Table 7.1).

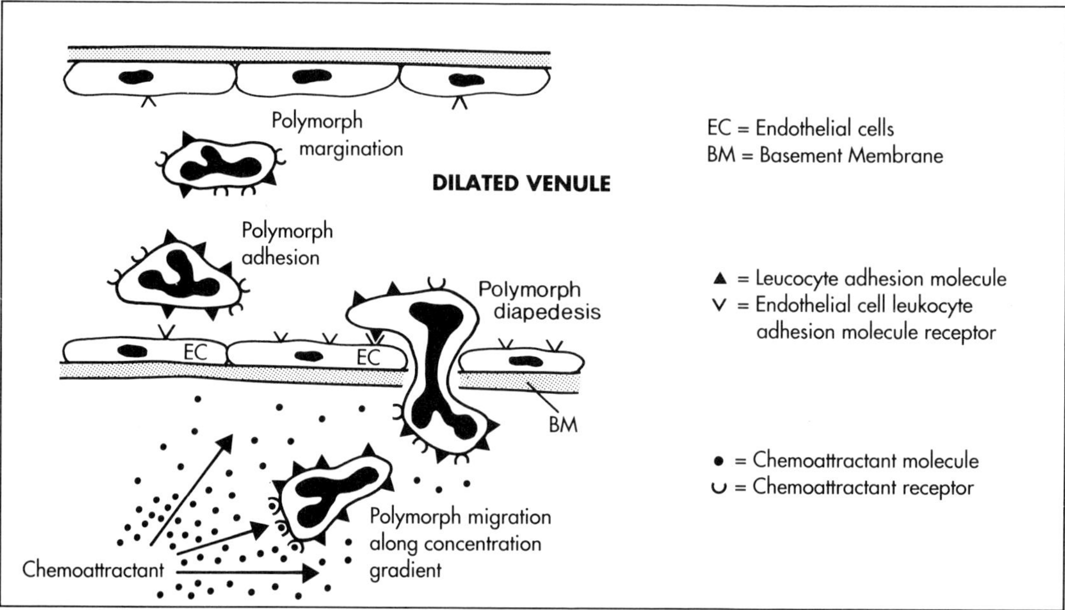

Figure 7.8 Diagram showing neutrophil migration.

Table 7.1 Examples of mediators of inflammation and their origin

Plasma factors (preformed)	Complement Clotting system Kinins

Preformed cellular products	Vasoactive amines
	  Histamine
	  5-Hydroxytryptamine
	Neutrophil products
	  Lysosomal enzymes

Newly synthesized cellular products	Neutrophil products
	  Oxygen-derived free radicals
	Arachidonic acid metabolites
	  Prostanoids
	  Leukotrienes
	Cytokines

(a)   Complement system

Complement is a series of proenzymes produced by the liver and secreted into the blood. Rather like the clotting system, complement is activated on the basis of a cascade in which the initial stimulus produces a few molecules of the first enzyme and rapidly leads to a stepwise amplification in the numbers of effector enzyme molecules. The key molecule in this cascade is complement

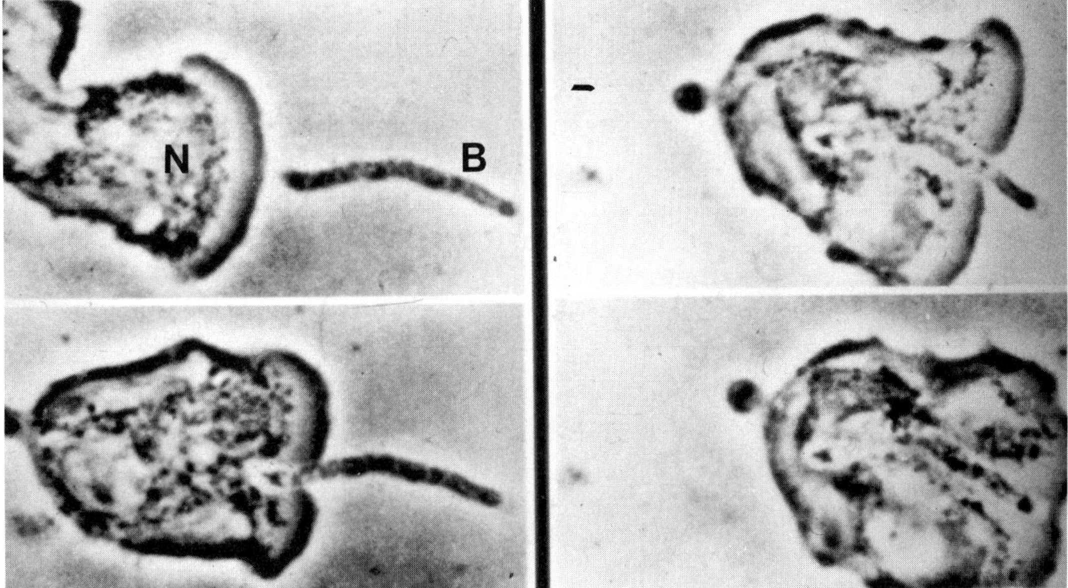

Figure 7.9 Sequence of phase-contrast photomicrographs showing engulfment and digestion of a bacterium (B) by a neutrophil (N). (× 400)

factor 3, or C3 (Figure 7.11). This is converted into its active components, C3a and C3b, by two different mechanisms. The classic pathway is initiated by antigen–antibody complexes and leads through complement components 1, 4 and 2 to the production of C3 convertase, which changes C3 to C3a and C3b. C3 convertase production can also be stimulated through the alternative pathway, activated by endotoxins, complex polysaccharides and aggregated globulins. C3b has three major effects. The first feeds back into the alternative pathway and inhibits the production of C3 convertase. The second is to activate the fifth component of complement (C5) to form C5a and C5b. Thirdly, C3b is a powerful opsonin. C3a increases vascular permeability as does C5a; the latter is also highly chemoattractive to most leucocytes. C5b initiates the action of a further four enzymes within the cascade to form a large complex, which is a powerful enzyme able to perforate the cellular membrane of bacteria.

This bypasses the sodium pump; sodium and water enter the cell, which swells and explodes.

(b) Clotting system

The clotting system is another cascade. In acute inflammation clotting factors in the bloodstream leak into the tissue or onto surfaces by virtue of the increased vascular permeability. Here they are activated and a cascade leads to the production of fibrin from fibrinogen (Figure 7.12). The fibrin may serve to wall off the site of inflammation and inhibit its spread. It may deposit on serosal surfaces. In addition, certain components produced during fibrin formation and breakdown (fibrin degradation products) increase vascular permeability and some are even chemoattractants.

(c) Kinin system

The kinin system is activated in acute

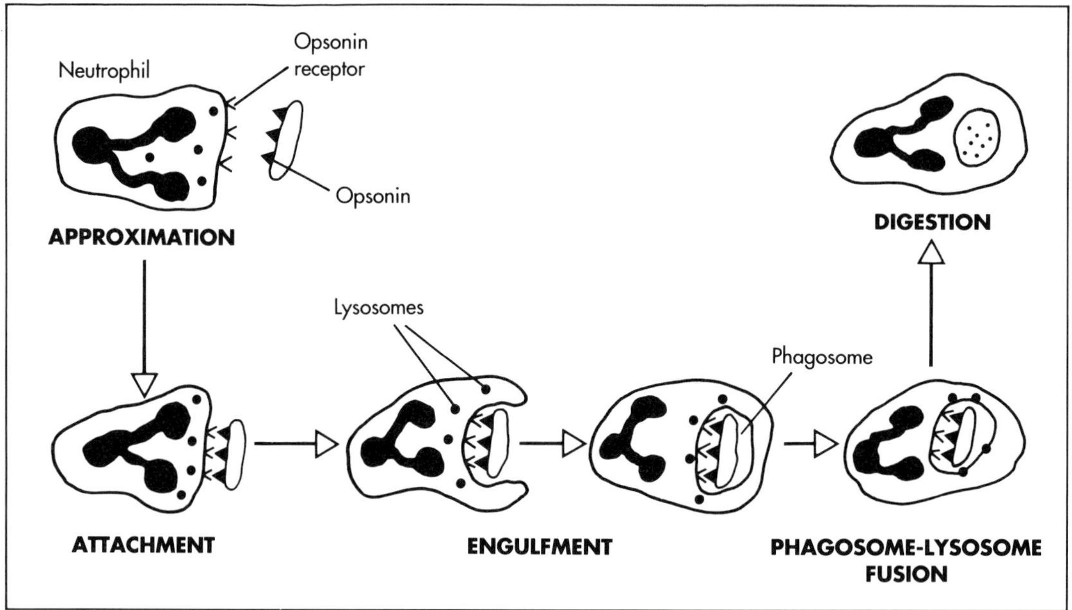

Figure 7.10 Diagram showing the events of phagocytosis.

inflammation via the clotting factor, Factor XII, which, when activated, converts pre-kallikrein, synthesized in the liver and leaked into the tissue by permeable vessels, into kallikrein. This cleaves a high-molecular-weight kininogen to produce bradykinin, a potent stimulator of vascular permeability. Kallikrein is part of a feedback mechanism that activates more Factor XII; also, it is a chemoattractant for neutrophils.

(d)   Vasoactive amines

Vasoactive amines, notably histamine and 5-hydroxytryptamine are components of the granules of mast cells (Lowman *et al.*, 1988), basophils and platelets and, as their name would suggest, by their action on blood vessels, lead to vasodilatation and increased vascular permeability. They are readily degraded molecules and their effects are relatively short lived. They are, however, believed to initiate some of the earliest vascular changes in acute inflammation. Release

of these products from the mast cells, that are a normal component of most tissues, is caused by physical agents and chemical reactions including the activation of IgE attached to the mast cell, C3a and C5a formation, and the binding of the cytokine interleukin I to its cell membrane receptor. 5-Hydroxytryptamine is released from platelets as part of the platelet release reaction.

(e)   Products of neutrophils

Neutrophils release a variety of chemicals of varying molecular complexity into their environment (Henson and Johnson, 1987; Malich and Gallin, 1988). These have a series of very elaborate direct and indirect effects on the tissue into which they are released. Some are potent enzymes leading to an exacerbation of tissue injury, whereas others act as cytokines which can be regarded as local hormones influencing the activity of other cells (Table 7.2). Similar substances are also produced by macrophages.

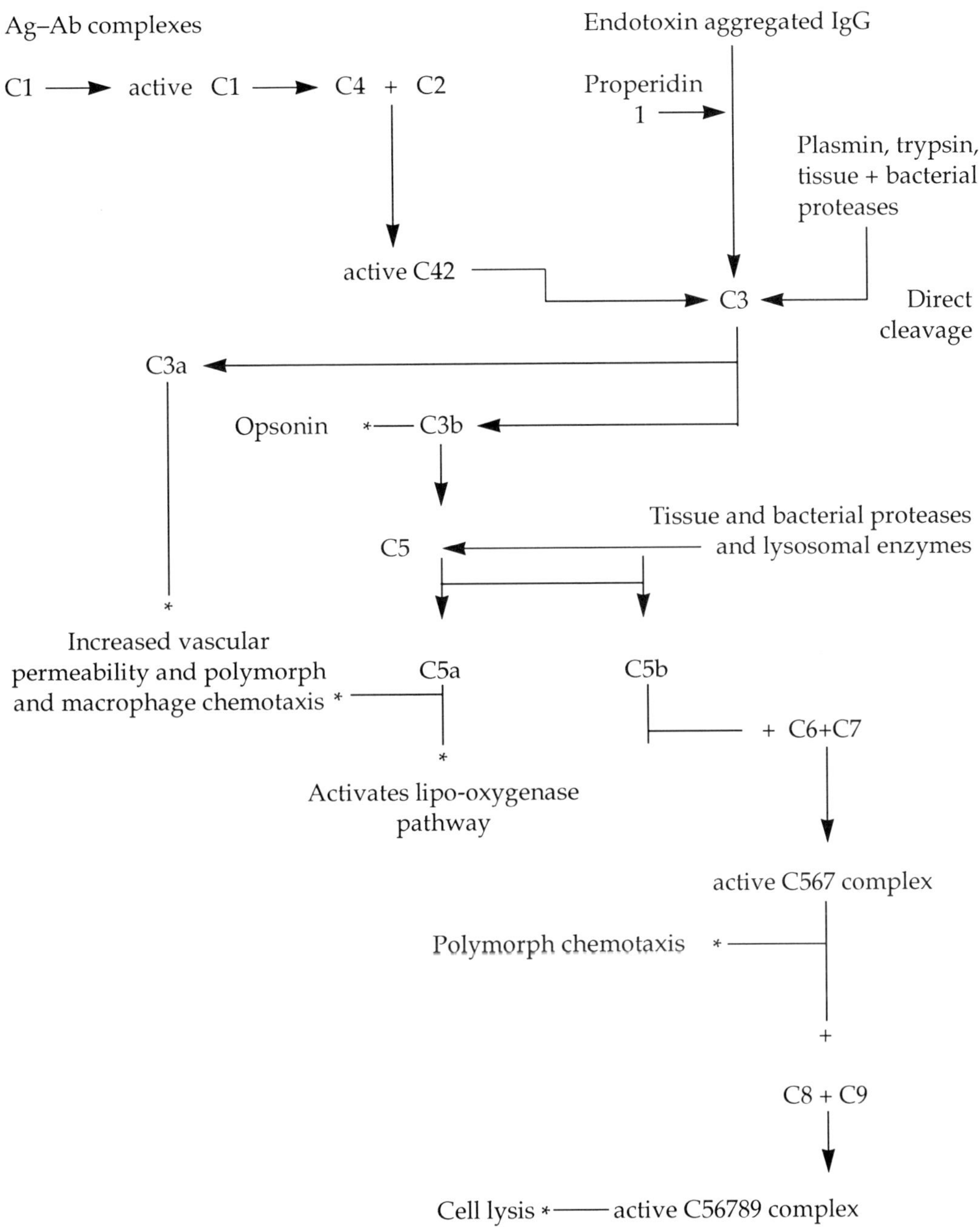

Figure 7.11 Diagram of the complement system.

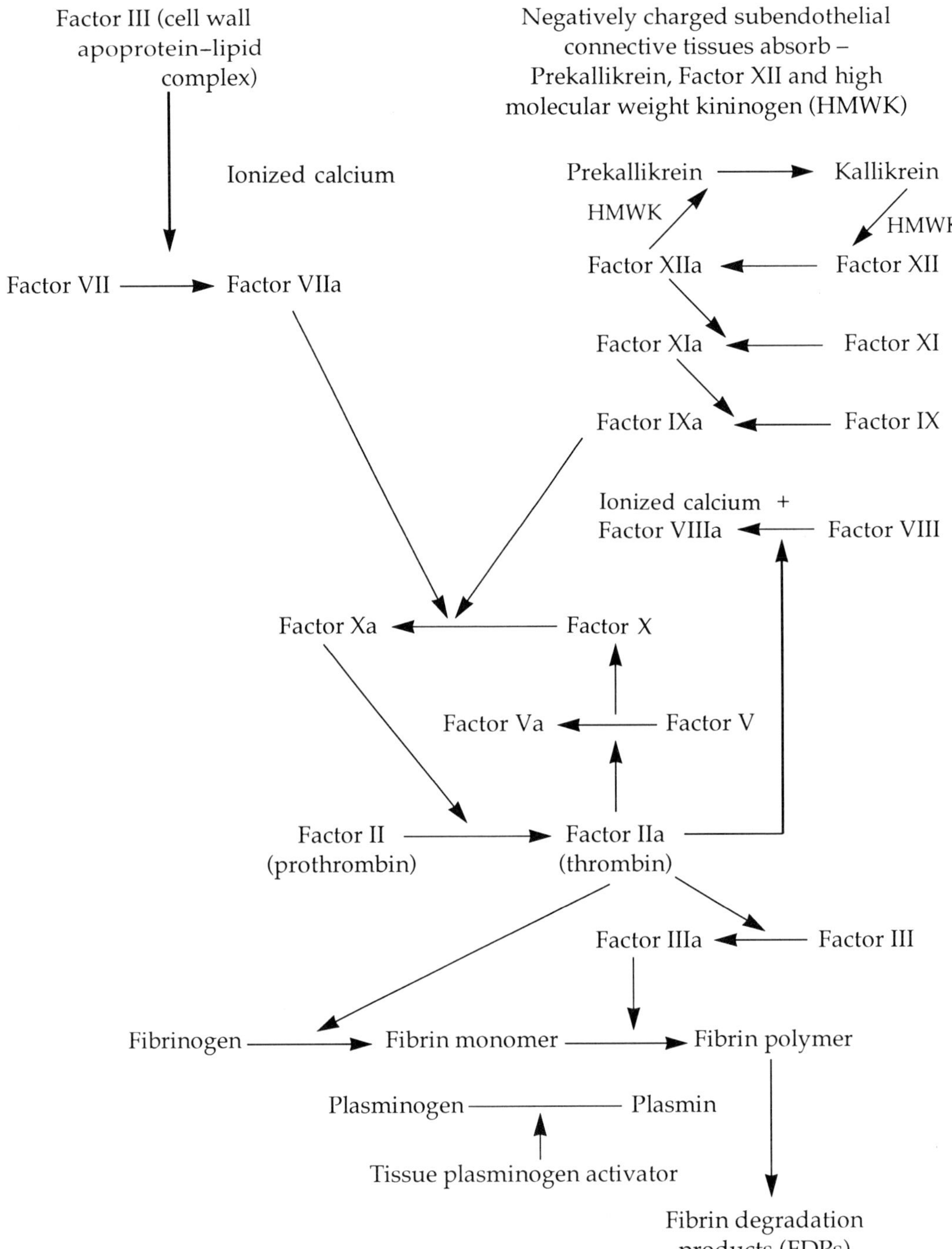

Figure 7.12 Diagrammatic representation of the clotting system.

Table 7.2 Neutrophil products with inflammatory properties

Lysozyme
Myeloperoxidase
Phospholipase A_2
Elastase
Cathepsins
Acid hydrolases
Cationic proteins
Collagenase
Lactoferrin
Alkaline phosphatase
Gelatinase

(f) The arachidonic acid metabolites

Arachidonic acid is a naturally occurring component of cell membranes (O'Flaherty, 1982). Through the actions of the enzymes cyclo-oxygenase and lipoxygenase two major groups of inflammatory chemical mediators can be produced from arachidonic acid (Figure 7.13). These substances together are known as eicosanoids, the two groups being the prostanoids (or prostaglandins) and the leukotrienes. Certain of the prostanoids, notably PGI_2 (prostacyclin), cause vasodilatation whereas others will cause vasoconstriction. Prostanoids are also responsible for the generation of the pain associated with acute inflammation. The leukotrienes, notably leukotrienes D_4 and E_4, cause increased vascular permeability and upregulated leucocyte adhesion; the leukotriene B_4 is a powerful chemoattractive agent.

(g) Oxygen-derived free radicals

Free electrons generated during the complex chemical interactions of acute inflammation may attach to a variety of atoms to form simple free radicals (Henson and Johnston, 1987). These are short-lived, unstable atoms with an unpaired electron, which they can donate to organic molecules. Consequent alterations in these molecules, particularly unsaturated lipids of cell membranes, leads to endothelial cell damage, with an increase in vascular permeability; inactivation of antiproteases, thus leading to the unopposed action of some of the enzymes released by inflammatory cells; and injury not only to cells such as bacteria, which are harmful, but also to local host cells and inflammatory cells.

Free radicals can be removed from the tissue or scavenged, by a variety of substances. These include the serum proteins ceruloplasmin and transferrin, enzymes such as superoxide dismutase and catylase and sulphydryl compounds such as cysteine.

(h) Cytokines

Cytokines are polypeptides produced by activated macrophages, lymphocytes and other inflammatory cells (Ross *et al.*, 1986; Gospodarowicz *et al.*, 1987; Sporn *et al.*, 1987). These substances react with cells within their environment, and at a distance, and cause some of the cellular changes seen in inflammation. There are many cytokines which have rather confusing names. These reflect either the function assigned to them when initially identified or, the associated group of chemicals to which they belong. They include substances such as the interleukin family and tissue necrosis factors. They act on endothelium (Mantovani and Dejana, 1989) to increase leucocyte adhesion, and stimulate clotting; they act on fibroblasts, to

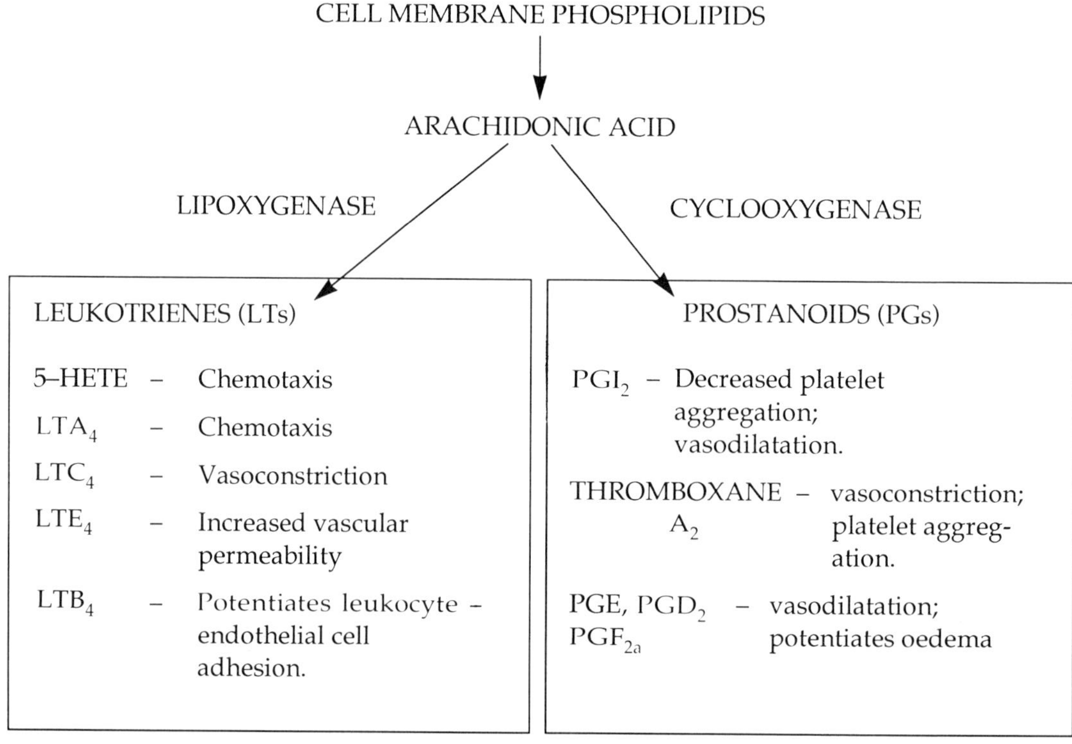

Figure 7.13 The arachidonic acid pathway.

increase collagen formation and on many other local tissue cells to change their function. They mediate effects at a distance from the tissue via the bloodstream and are responsible for the acute phase response and other systemic effects such as fever, neutrophilia, changed generalized haemodynamics and slow wave sleep (Table 7.3).

Many of the data presented here are derived from studies *in vitro*. New techniques such as immunohistochemistry and *in situ* hybridization, applicable to *in vivo* studies, are advancing the understanding of these disease mediators (Table 7.4).

7.1.5 OUTCOME

The outcome of acute inflammation depends both on the nature and extent of the inflammatory reaction and on the amount of local tissue damage.

Usually, acute inflammation resolves with complete restoration of the normal tissue architecture. This is favoured if the acute inflammation is associated with minimal cell death, rapid elimination of the initial stimulus and occurrence within an organ capable of regeneration.

It is usually only pyogenic bacteria that cause formation of pus, which commonly tracks to and is discharged from an adjacent surface. However, there may be sites of irreversible tissue damage which heal following the organization of granulation tissue with scar formation. The healing process is discussed further as part of the outcome of chronic inflammation.

7.2 CHRONIC INFLAMMATION

Chronic inflammation may follow one or more episodes of acute inflammation

Table 7.3 Effects of interleukin-1 and tumour necrosis factors in inflammation

Endothelial effects
    Increased leucocyte adhesion molecules
    Increased prostanoid synthesis
    Increased platelet aggregation
    Anticoagulant
    Increased endothelial synthesis of IL-1

Acute phase response
    Fever
    Decreased appetite
    Increased synthesis of acute phase proteins
    Marrow stimulation to synthesize neutrophils
    Shock

Connective tissue cell effects
    Proliferation
    Increased collagen synthesis
    Increased collagenase synthesis
    Local prostanoid synthesis

Table 7.4 Probable *in vivo* mediators of inflammation

Effect	*Mediator*	*Source*
Vasodilatation	Prostanoids	Most tissue cells
Vascular permeability	Histamine	Mast cells
	5-Hydroxytryptamine	Platelets
	Complement products (C3a, C5a)	Liver via blood
	Kinins	Plasma
	Leukotriene	Leucocytes
Neutrophil chemotaxis	C5a	Plasma
	Leukotrienes	Leucocytes
Fever	Interleukin 1	Macrophages
	Tumour necrosis factors	Macrophages
	Prostanoids	Most cells
Pain	Prostanoids	Most cells
	Kinins	Plasma
Tissue damage	Free radicals	Neutrophils
	Lysosomal enzymes	Neutrophils and Macrophages

because resolution is interfered with, or the agent persists, or because of tissue damage after repeated acute episodes. But, most commonly it is, *ab initio*, a non-acute, low-grade reaction because the agent does not arouse the acute response. Sometimes there is prolonged exposure to non-degradable, but potentially toxic particulate substances, including foreign materials such as plastics and metals from implants, and naturally occurring substances such as silicates from rocks and biological materials such as wood splinters. Sometimes such material is ignored by the body, most often it initiates some type of non-immunological chronic inflammatory reaction (Figure 7.14). However, more frequently the agent is antigenic and presents a challenge to the immune system. This gives rise to a highly specific form of tissue reaction controlled by lymphocytes but involving numerous other cell types and is always in response to the presence, within the body, of molecules (either free or parts of cell surfaces) that are not normally present. This foreign material, or antigen, is the ultimate trigger to immune-mediated chronic inflammation. The typical stimulus to the immune system is a persistent infection by an organism that is only a weak stimulator of acute inflammation or which is facultatively intracellular, e.g. tubercule bacillus. Other stimuli are transplanted or implanted tissues, and normal molecules rendered antigenic. The latter process underpins autoimmunity and is of considerable importance in the understanding of joint disease.

7.2.1 THE HISTOLOGICAL FEATURES OF CHRONIC INFLAMMATION

Chronic inflammation is a prolonged response, taking a longer time to develop and with a longer duration than acute

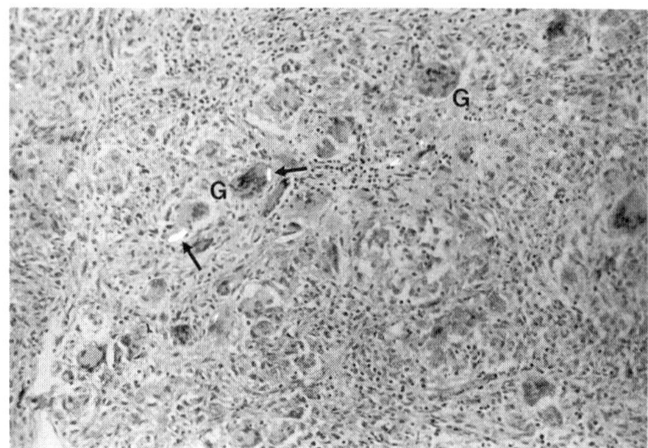

Figure 7.14 A giant cell (G) and macrophage response to immunologically inert particulate material (arrowed). (H and E viewed in polarized light.)

inflammation. The tissue is infiltrated by mononuclear cells, principally macrophages, lymphocytes and the effector cells of the lymphocyte lineage (activated lymphocytes and plasma cells). It is the peculiar functional attributes of these two cell types that is responsible for the nature and course of chronic inflammation. In addition there is destruction of normal host tissues associated with proliferation of fibroblasts, and in many instances small blood vessels. Although it was widely held that the lymphocyte was the major cell in initiating and controlling the processes of chronic inflammation, it is now clear that the mechanisms that underlie this host-tissue reaction require a close interaction between lymphocytes, macrophages and certain other tissue cells.

(a) Macrophages

Macrophages serve a variety of roles. They form from peripheral blood monocytes that have migrated into the tissue (Johnston, 1988). Cells of the monocyte–macrophage lineage develop into all the fixed tissue or resident macrophages (histiocytes) such as connective tissue histiocytes, alveolar macrophages, Kupffer cells of the liver, and microglia. These are the majority of macrophages and are important initiators of inflammation, both acute and chronic. In addition monocyte-derived macrophages can be recruited into sites of inflammation. Inflammation-associated macrophages are of two varieties: 'elicited' cells which respond to inert particulate and foreign material and immunologically 'activated' cells which participate in cell-mediated immunity and delayed hypersensitivity reactions (Gordon, 1986).

Macrophage migration is a key step in the development of chronic inflammation (Freemont, 1992). As in acute inflammation, endothelial cells are central to the initiation of the inflammatory response, for they also bear receptors to adhesion molecules present upon the circulating monocyte or lymphocyte. The production and expression of these molecules is up-regulated in the presence of a chronic inflammatory stimulus, enhancing the migration of the inflammatory cells into the tissue. Their entry is also promoted by factors such as C5a, fibrin, neutrophil cationic proteins, cytokines, platelet factors, collagen and fibronectin fragments.

Once within the tissue the monocyte is converted into a macrophage and activated (North, 1978). Macrophage activation in inflammation may be triggered by lymphokines, interferons, factors produced by activated lymphocytes and non-immune factors such as endotoxin. Once activated the monocyte differentiates along one of three cell lineages. Two of these cell types, the inflammatory macrophage and the multinucleated giant cell, are phagocytic and also produce a variety of degradative enzymes and lysosomal products, such as lysozyme and intracellular digestive enzyme, and oxygen and halide free radicals, with which phagocytosed particles are lysed. By and large phagocytosis is not a primary immunological phenomenon, thus these cells are 'elicited' and although activated are not immunologically active. That is not to say they do not play a part in immune responses, for phagocytosis of debris is essential if the macrophage is to act as an antigen presenting cell. Most commonly the cells are a secondary consequence of the immune-mediated inflammation rather than a primary effector mechanism. Why some macrophages should become multinucleated is not clear but it is known that certain intracellular organisms such as the tubercle bacillus and large non-cellular particles, particularly foreign material, may induce this process. The third product of macrophage differentiation is the epithelioid cell which is not phagocytic but functions as a secretory cell (Figure 7.15). It can manufacture neutral proteases, chemotactic factors, arachidonic acid metabolites, components of complement, coagulation

factors, growth factors, cytokines such as interleukin-1 and tumour necrosis factor and other factors such as the interferons and platelet deactivating factor and will vary the synthesis of these factors depending on environmental stimuli (Nathan, 1987).

It is the secretory products of these activated macrophages that, in part at least, induce the changes characteristic of chronic inflammation, including tissue destruction, by the release of proteases and free radicals into the tissue; neovascularization and fibroblast proliferation promoted by growth factors and nitric oxide synthesis; and the accumulation of connective tissue as the result of activating fibroblasts by substances such as interleukin-1 and tumour necrosis factor (Ross *et al.*, 1986; Gospodarowicz *et al.*, 1987; Sporn *et al.*, 1987).

(b) Lymphocytes

The lymphocyte is the main cell involved in the initiation and control of the chronic inflammatory response. There are two main types of lymphocytes. The T-lymphocyte (Sanders *et al.*, 1988) and the B-lymphocyte (MacLennan *et al.*, 1990). Both groups of cells are formed early in development from primitive bone marrow precursors. Each matures by passage through specific organs (in the

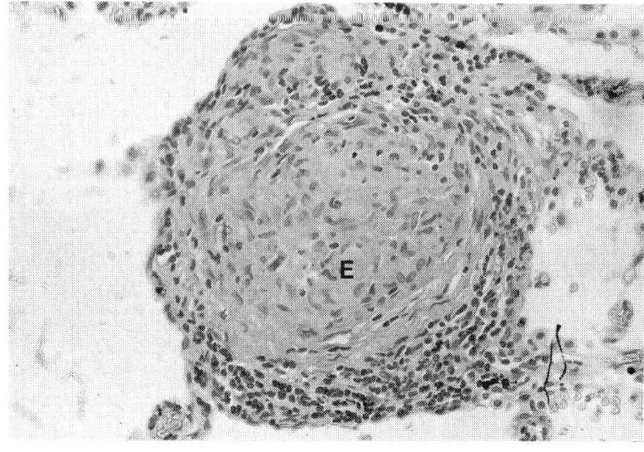

Figure 7.15 Epithelioid cells (E) within a granuloma.

case of human T-lymphocyte the thymus) into a non-specific B or T-lymphocyte. These cells encounter antigen and become activated. When activated the B-lymphocyte produces two cells, an effector cell, the plasma cell, which produces one of a group of toxic chemicals called antibodies (Burton, 1990), and a memory cell which is geared specifically to recognize the antigen that stimulated the original lymphocyte. There are three effector cells of the T-cell lineage. The cytotoxic T-cell, which will specifically destroy unwanted cells; the helper T-cell, which promotes chronic inflammatory reactions; and the suppressor T-cell which inhibits them. In addition, activation of T-cells also leads to formation of a memory cell. Although both types of lymphocyte can be stimulated non-specifically by substances like bacterial endotoxins, they are most commonly activated by contact with antigen.

The lymphocyte is confronted with the antigen either directly or more commonly by having it presented to it by cells, either specialized antigen-presenting cells or activated macrophages. These cells phagocytose, process and present antigen to lymphocytes.

Activated by antigen, either within the tissue, or following migration to one of a specific group of organs which include the lymph nodes, spleen and mucosal-associated lymphoid tissues, the lymphocyte division and maturation events lead to the production of many memory and effector cells. The effector cell of the B-cell lineage, the plasma cell, produces antibodies which bind to antigens, both free and cell bound. The principal consequence of antibody–antigen binding is the activation of the complement cascade through the classical pathway. If antigen is attached to a cell surface the end result of complement activation is cell lysis.

The secretion of antibodies may be at the site of inflammation or within an associated lymphoid organ, gaining access to the inflamed tissue from the circulation into which they are secreted.

This is known as humoral immunity. By contrast, the effector cells of the T-cell lineage have to be present within the tissue at the site of chronic inflammation and if not produced locally have to migrate from the lymphoid organs into the inflamed tissue. The activated T-helper and T-suppressor lymphocytes produce many lymphokines which are messenger and control compounds. Together with macrophage products they are the key to the complex interrelationships in chronic inflammation. The cytotoxic T-cell, as its name suggests, destroys cells. This it achieves by coming into contact with a cell expressing surface membrane antigen. In very general terms the cytotoxic T lymphocyte attacks host cells infested with intracellular organisms (notably viruses), neoplastic cells and cells bearing foreign histocompatibility antigens.

(c)   Autoimmunity

This exists when molecules, which the body has always recognized as being its own or 'self' molecules, come to be treated as foreign and initiate an inflammatory response. Autoimmunity may occur through a variety of mechanisms. For instance the antigen of a *Streptococcus* which has initiated an inflammatory response may be so similar in its molecular arrangement to that of a naturally occurring tissue molecule that, once primed, the lymphocytes may attack the latter. In the case of streptococcal-induced disease, these molecules are primarily in the endocardium, myocardium and pericardium and the autoimmune response that follows is manifest as rheumatic fever. In other circumstances tissue damage leads naturally occurring tissue molecules either to combine with other molecules or to fragment; when these come into contact with the immune system they are in a form which it has never 'seen' before. They are thus regarded as 'foreign' and initiate inflammation, an example is Dressler's syndrome which follows myocardial infarction. The mechanism underlying other autoimmune disorders is less well understood. Why it should be that in autoimmune gastritis antibodies are made against gastric parietal cells is not clear, nor is it known why, in rheumatoid arthritis, certain immunoglobulins become antigenic. Whatever the cause the misrecognition within, and destruction of, the tissue concerned is a major cause of disease. In both conventional immune responses and also in autoimmune responses, if the 'foreign' molecule is soluble and non-cell bound then it may bind to antigen to form complex molecules which will precipitate within tissues, either at the site of inflammation or, following a period circulating in the blood, in more distant organs, where they initiate an inflammatory response. This is almost certainly the mechanism by which diseases such as rheumatoid arthritis, systemic lupus erythematosus and polyarteritis nodosa come about.

(d) Granulomatous inflammation

This is a distinctive subtype of chronic inflammation (Gafaar and Turk, 1970). A granuloma is the basic cellular aggregation of this reaction; many more or less well-developed granulomas form the lesion. The least-structured lesions can generally be recognisable as granulomatous from their cellular composition. When well-organized, a granuloma has a near spherical structure (Figure 7.16) and a distinctive histological pattern. In the centre are cells of the macrophage lineage (Johnston, 1988): some or all of multinucleated cells, epithelioid cells and macrophages. These are surrounded by a mixture of B and T-lymphocytes. Beyond them is a zone of variable extent, predominating in plasma cells, which merge into contiguous granulomas. The centre of a granuloma may undergo necrosis.

Granulomatous inflammation is a non-specific reaction caused by many agents; for example, inorganic metals; dusts such as

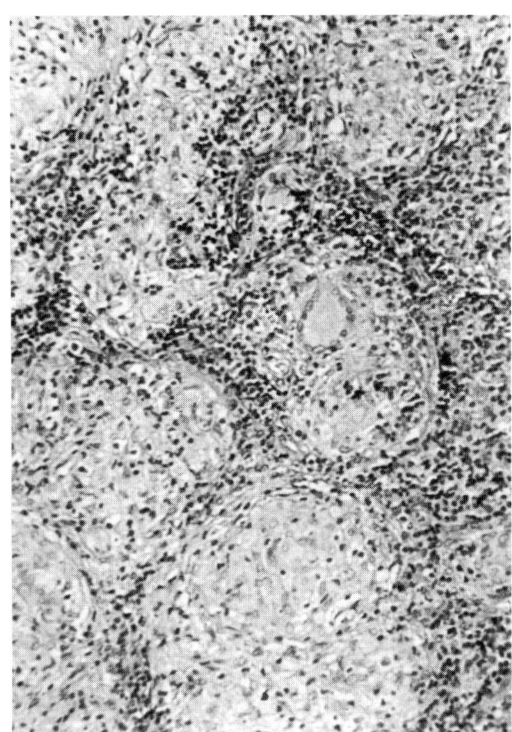

Figure 7.16 Granulomata of sarcoidosis within synovium.

silica; beryllium; introduced substances like plastics; certain types of bacteria, as in tuberculosis, leprosy, syphilis, cat-scratch disease; fungi such as cryptococcus, coccidioides and histoplasma. In addition there is a variety of disorders of unknown cause which includes sarcoidosis, primary biliary cirrhosis and Crohn's disease.

(e) Systemic effects

Like acute inflammation, chronic inflammation is associated with generalized features of illness which include fever, leucocytosis, alteration in blood chemistry and constitutional symptoms like weight loss and fatigue. These are related to the release from the inflamed sites of factors including the cytokines interleukin-1 and tumour necrosis factor, and prostanoids.

(f) Healing and repair

Tissue is never completely restored when a chronic inflammatory reaction abates, as can occur following acute inflammation, and is always marked by fibrosis and scarring. In cirrhosis of the liver, for example, hepatocytes may regenerate, but the overwhelming response may be to replace once-functioning tissue by fibrosis. Activated lymphocytes and macrophages induce fibrosis by producing two types of factor: one that stimulates division, migration and maturation of fibroblasts, and the other that stimulates growth and ingrowth of new vessels (neovascularization, or angiogenesis) (Rappoke *et al.*, 1988) which supply the fibroblasts with factors necessary for synthesizing collagen

(Figure 7.17) (Mantovini and Dejana, 1989). This combination of growing blood vessels and migrating, actively synthesizing fibroblasts, and granulation tissue, is initiated immediately chronic inflammation starts and is therefore a natural accompaniment of the process. Thus in chronic inflammation there may be seen, in varying amounts at any one site, cellular infiltration, tissue necrosis, and fibrous tissue formation and maturation.

7.2.2 SUMMARY

Inflammation is the body's response to tissue injury. This necessarily short description of the mechanisms involved can do little more than give a brief insight into these complex interactive processes. There are many excellent treatises on inflammation including some which form part of more general texts (Alberts *et al.*, 1989; Glynn *et al.*, 1989; McGee

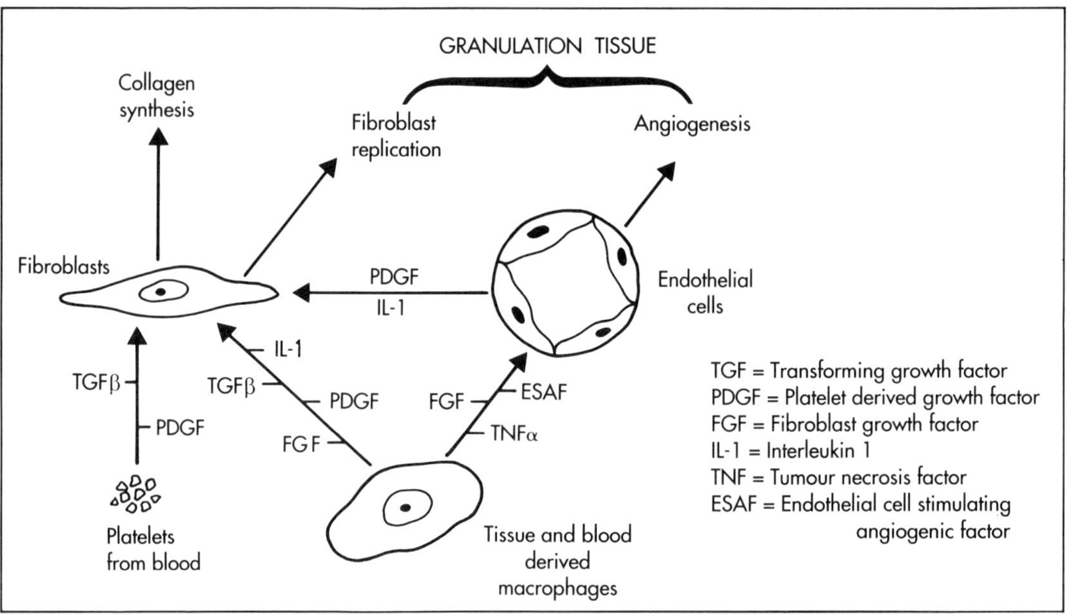

Figure 7.17 A diagrammatic representation of the cytokine-mediated interactions between inflammatory cells, fibroblasts and endothelial cells.

et al., 1992). It is important to appreciate the non-specificity of the inflammatory reactions vis-à-vis particular organisms, and that bacteriological culture is a source of valuable information for the histopathologist.

7.3   INFLAMMATION IN BONE

Over the past 100 years there has been a change in the way in which bone inflammation is perceived and possibly in the pattern of the disease. In the past there had been little understanding of aetiology or pathogenesis of inflammation. Suppuration, whose cause was not understood, but which had long been acknowledged as a complication of compound fractures and wounds generally, was regarded as a necessary stage of healing. From the Middle Ages, however, there were individuals who questioned this doctrine and felt it could and should be avoided. Through the 18th century clinical awareness increased and during the 19th century, together with the advent of the new science of pathology, there came an acquisition of knowledge that laid down the groundwork for the revolution in the understanding and treatment of inflammation of bone.

Through this knowledge, coupled with advances in antisepsis, and then asepsis and anaesthesia, great advances were made in the surgical management of bone inflammation. It became possible to draw a sharp line between neoplastic and inflammatory bone diseases, to distinguish infection from other types of inflammation and to segregate the bacterial diseases on the basis of their aetiology. At this time the major inflammatory disease of bone was recognized to be osteomyelitis caused predominantly by organisms leading to suppuration, or to granuloma formation.

As most of the inflammatory diseases of bone can be considered as either pyogenic or granulomatous osteomyelitis these subjects will be considered at length. It should not be forgotten, however, that osteomyelitis is not the only inflammatory disease of bone and these much rarer, but nonetheless interesting, disorders will also be discussed.

7.4   OSTEOMYELITIS

From the 1920s to the present day staphylococci and streptococci have remained the main pus-forming organisms causing osteomyelitis, and tuberculosis the most common cause of granulomatous inflammation. A number of other organisms (such as *Escherichia coli*, *Neisseria gonorrhoeae*, *Neisseria meningitidis* and *Haemophilus influenzae*) are also capable of leading to osteomyelitis (Table

Table 7.5 Organisms which can cause osteomyelitis

Organism	% of cases
Staphylococcus aureus	55
Streptococci	10
Haemophilus influenzae	4
Staphylococcus epidermidis	3
Streptococcus pneumoniae	2
Pseudomonas aeruginosa	2
Salmonella sp.	1
Enterobacter	1
Other identifiable organisms	2
No identifiable organism	20

7.5) and more are being recorded (Burkert and Watanakumakorn, 1991).

Such are the advances that have been made in the management of osteomyelitis that there has been a tendency to forget that even in 1930s the mortality from osteomyelitis was sometimes as high as 40% in the acute disease (White and Dennison, 1952) and a high proportion of cases developing chronic disease ended with the patient requiring amputation. The changes that have occurred since then have been many. Initially the availability of antibiotics, particularly penicillin and streptomycin, led to a dramatic reduction in the mortality of osteomyelitis and better control of chronic osteomyelitis. When these were coupled with public health measures which made tuberculosis a sporadic disease in the Western world the prospect of making osteomyelitis a rare condition seemed realistic. However, osteomyelitis is still far from rare. This is for two major reasons. First, such is the evolutionary ability of bacteria, because of their very high rate of division, that antibiotic-resistant forms have readily developed. Second, because of the changes that have occurred in orthopaedic management, notably fracture fixation and prosthetic joint replacement, there has been an increased possibility of infection being introduced at the time of surgery.

7.4.1 PYOGENIC OSTEOMYELITIS

Although it is probably realistic to say that all cases of pyogenic osteomyelitis are due to bacteria, in up to 20% of cases it is not possible to isolate an organism. This is almost certainly a reflection of our, as yet, incomplete understanding of microbiology. Infective organisms may gain access to the bone, or more accurately the bone marrow, via one of three routes.

1. Haematogenous: the organisms arrive in the bone from a distant origin, via the bloodstream. In these cases it necessarily follows that a primary focus of infection must be present elsewhere within the body (Winters and Cahen, 1960). The mechanism by which bacteria lodge within the bone is still uncertain. Thromboembolism was favoured for many years. Later the concepts of organisms being free or within cells was introduced and rheological factors were invoked to explain sites of deposition. Recently the potential role of cell adhesion molecules that might serve to adhere bacteria to one another and to the substratum have also been investigated as a possible source of lodgement of organisms within bone marrow (Rissing, 1990). Whatever the major cause or combination of causes, it is still generally believed that the anatomy of the vasculature, particularly of long bones, septic thromboembolism and its subsequent forward or retrograde propagation, are important in establishing the extent and position of pyogenic osteomyelitis.

The most common site for pyogenic osteomyelitis is within the diaphysis, but pus may also track into the epiphysis, disrupting the growth plate in children, and into the joint, particularly when the joint capsule is reflected onto the diaphysis (Alderson *et al.*, 1986)

It has long been held that mild trauma, perhaps by its effect on local blood flow, is a determinant of site, both within individual bones and between bones, the skeletal distribution reflecting the frequency of knocks and bruises in children. Ogden (1979) has suggested that the frequency at different sites is a reflection of the relative rates of growth and the associated blood flow.

2. Direct extension: here organisms spread to the bone marrow from an adjacent focus of infection.

3. Inoculation: organisms are introduced directly from outside. An obvious portal of entry is identifiable, usually an injury or site of surgery (Grogan *et al.*, 1986; Maderazo *et al.*, 1988).

Pyogenic osteomyelitis begins as a local response to bacteria at the point of lodgement. After deposition of the organisms by whatever route there is a latent period before the development of the inflammatory reaction. During this time bacteria multiply and spread, thus the few organisms which may have lodged within the marrow originally will have dramatically increased in number before the host defence system initiates an inflammatory response. Initially this is acute inflammation. There is hyperaemia, due to vascular dilatation, fluid exudation into the marrow, as a consequence of increased vascular permeability, and subsequent polymorph infiltration. The inflammation extends into the adjacent marrow and is associated with a sequence of important phenomena that characterize osteomyelitis:

1. The debris from the interaction between infection and inflammatory response leads to the local release of digestive enzymes and the formation of pus.
2. The presence of the pus and the exudate, both fluid and cellular, lead to an increase in the pressure within the enclosed environment of the bone.
3. The increased pressure together with the natural thrombogenic effect of the local tissue inflammation leads to the vascular supply and drainage of the bone becoming compromised with consequent bony infarction.

The two major macroscopic features of acute pyogenic osteomyelitis are, therefore, pus formation and bone necrosis (Gilmour, 1962). Tissue necrosis is an unusual sequel of acute inflammation in other tissues and the healing response in bone in acute pyogenic osteomyelitis is therefore rather different from that seen in other organs. In particular the presence of necrotic tissue leads to the persistence of organisms (Figure 7.18). Furthermore, within this avascular environment the organisms are not subject to ingress of antibiotics delivered systemically.

Histologically the stages of acute osteomyelitis are:

1. Organisms within the bone marrow.
2. An acute, polymorph-dominated, inflammatory response with pus formation.
3. Associated local bone infarction.
4. Granulation tissue formation at the periphery of the infarcted area.

Often the presence of necrotic tissue and residual bacteria inhibit healing or even progressive scarring. The granulation tissue is a

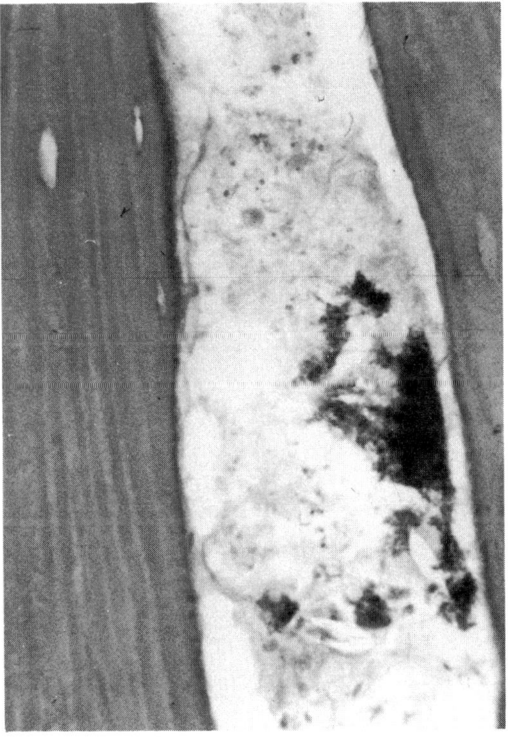

Figure 7.18 Bacteria within necrotic marrow and bone.

powerful stimulus to both osteoblasts and osteoclasts, but, due to a relative excess of osteoclasis possibly mediated through prostaglandin E (Plotquin *et al.*, 1991), the result is predominantly resorption. If the response is given time this zone of resorption will sever the connection between viable and necrotic bone, but often the infection spreads through the marrow cavity. The residual dead bone within the centre of the zone of infection remains intact and it is this dead bone that forms the sequestrum.

Pus not only tracks along the marrow cavity but through the Volkmann's canals in the cortex and thence into the surrounding soft tissues. In so doing it elevates the periosteum. This has two effects, the stripping of the periosteum and the vascular thrombosis that results from the inflammatory reaction deprives the outer cortex of its blood supply, which is not a part of the bone rendered avascular by raised intramedullary pressure. Through this mechanism necrosis of the whole local section of the original bone is completed. In addition elevation of the periosteum initiates a bone-forming response. This new viable periosteal bone, known as the involucrum, comes to surround the dead sequestrum and macerated specimens are seen to be perforated by holes through which pus extends from the medullary cavity into the surrounding tissue (Figure 7.19). This pus may ultimately point towards the surface skin and discharge at a sinus (Figures 7.20 and 7.21).

Not all cases of osteomyelitis have all the features described above, in particular the pattern varies with age. Trueta (1959) has speculated that the different patterns of bone infection and response are a function of the changing vasculature in developing bone. He describes three different types of acute haematogenous osteomyelitis.

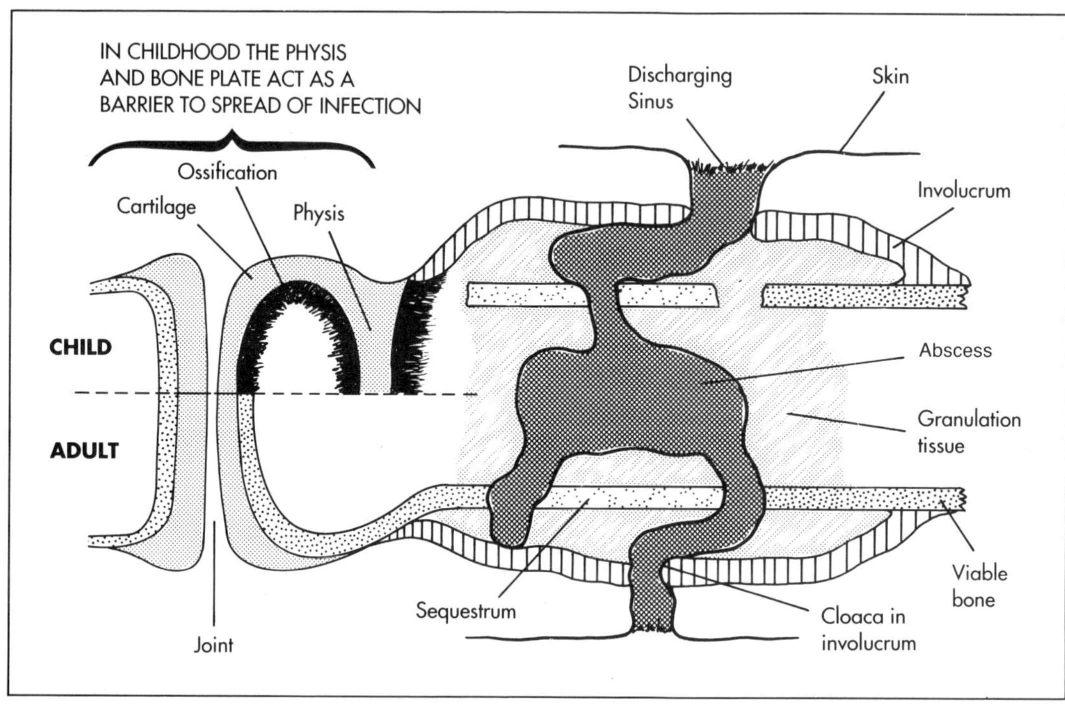

Figure 7.19 Diagram demonstrating the pathological features of osteomyelitis.

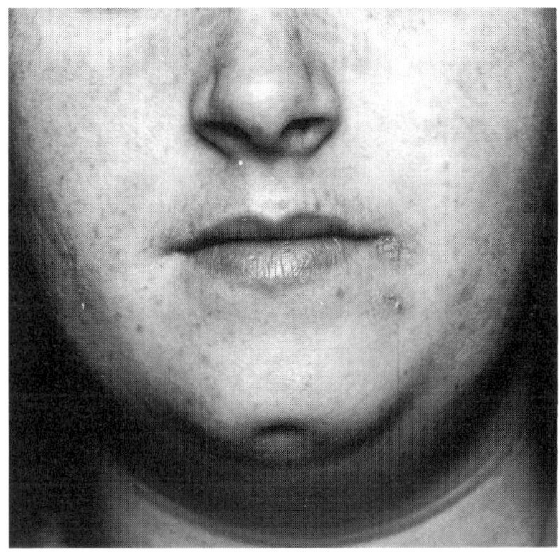

Figure 7.20 A discharging sinus on the chin of a woman with subacute osteomyelitis of the mandible.

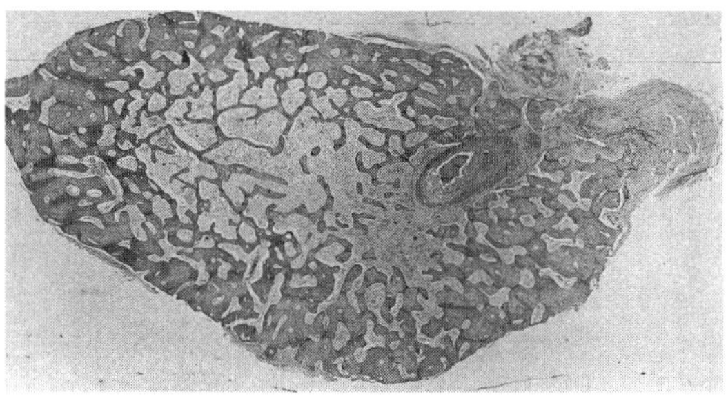

Figure 7.21 Transverse section of the fibula showing the changes of osteomyelitis including a cloaca.

Type 1: Infants up to one year. Until the epiphysis is established some vessels in the shaft extend into the epiphyseal cartilage to end in blood lakes, giving infection a route to the end of the bone and access to the joint. Even with extensive infection there can be deceptively little constitutional effect, contributing to the difficulty in making the diagnosis.

Type 2: Children to the age of epiphyseal fusion. This is the most common age group and pattern of acute haematogenous osteo-myelitis. The child is usually systemically ill and experiences fever and local pain. Most childhood infections start in the metaphysis; this is thought to be related to the metaphyseal venous sinuses, which are liable to thrombosis, and which can provide a nidus for bacterial growth. Once infection is established it spreads through the cortex and lifts the periosteum, which is weakly tethered to the shaft of a child's bone, giving rise to abscess and involucrum formation. There is, however, firm attachment of the periosteum at the level of the epiphyseal plate which prevents spread of infection into the joint. An exception occurs, where the capsular attachment, at least in part, is reflected onto the diaphyseal cortex. Several joints are so arranged (Ogden, 1979) with the hip and shoulder especially so. Because of the degree of localization and the healing powers of children childhood osteomyelitis is amongst the easiest to treat (Cole *et al.*, 1982).

Type 3: Adult. Acute haematogenous osteomyelitis is relatively rare in adults, being most common in the vertebrae. Once established, however, there is a rapid spread of the infection internally as there is no barrier to extension into the epiphysis and the joint. The periosteum is firmly adherent, and the cortex less easily penetrated than in the child, with the result that the cortex is resorbed internally. There is little periosteal reaction but a danger of fracture. The infection tracks to the exterior through the periosteum to form extraperiosteal abscesses and discharging sinuses, and on occasion, septic arthritis.

Although acute haematogenous osteomyelitis is rare in adults, osteomyelitis is not itself rare because of the incidence of surgically inoculated infection (McQuire, 1989).

Inevitably, because of the peculiar tissue reaction associated with acute osteomyelitis (Harris, 1960), and in particular the difficulty mobilizing a proper acute inflammatory response because of tissue necrosis, there is the possibility of incomplete resolution. In this way acute osteomyelitis may become subacute or chronic (Harris and Kirkaldy-Willis, 1965) (Figure 7.22).

(a) Subacute osteomyelitis

These are insidiously developing lesions of osteomyelitis, without constitutional symptoms, caused principally by *Staphylococcus aureus*. These started to come to notice particularly after the Second World War with an increasing incidence. Harris and Kirkcaldy-Willis (1965), among others, drew attention to this, aptly calling the lesions primary subacute pyogenic osteomyelitis. They drew attention to indolent development of lesions in both the appendicular and axial skeleton.

(i) *Appendicular lesions*

There were two radiographic appearances: cases with abscess formation (either Brodie's (small with abundant sclerosis) or large (metaphyseal accompanied by periosteal bone formation), and cases with dense sclerosis in which abscess was 'not usually demonstrable'. In addition they were impressed by the number of vertebral lesions developing in this indolent fashion.

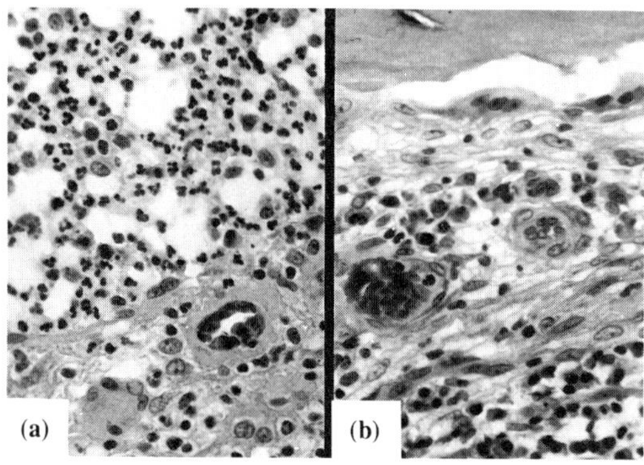

Figure 7.22 Inflammatory infiltrate of acute osteomyelitis (a) and chronic osteomyelitis (b).

(a) *Bone abscess*

Brodie, in 1872, described a small destructive metaphyseal lesion. Radiographically it may be up to several centimetres in size (Kozlowski, 1986), but is generally half that, with a limited bone reaction (Figure 7.23). The clinical history is of variable deep pain over months and years. Histologically there is a minute abscess with a dense fibrous capsule enclosed by actively remodelling reactive bone. Often the lesion is sterile; if organisms are present they are usually *Staph. aureus*. Much larger abscesses occur in the metaphysis, occupying most of the width of the diaphysis. Symptoms are referred to the locale, and are not generalized. Small abscesses also occur in the superficial diaphyseal cortex, just beneath the periosteum, which gives rise to local reactive bone. Their location makes eradication a simple procedure.

(b) *Bone scelerosis*

These lesions are generally referred to as sclerosing osteomyelitis: synonyms (primary) chronic sclerosing osteomyelitis (with and without the qualification 'Garre'). Although the topic has been raised here in connection with appendicular osteomyelitis, it is one of considerable concern in dentistry because of the involvement of the mandible (van Merkesteyn *et al.*, 1988), the lesion there goes by the same name, including the eponym. There is much confusion surrounding this term. Wood *et al.* (1988) studied Garre's original article of 1893 (57 pages in length) in which, without benefit of radiographs, bacteriology or tissue pathology (which were either not invented, developed or applied to clinical practice at the time), he described the clinical features of acute osteomyelitis. He labelled one form, characterized by thickening and 'rising' of the bone, as sclerosing non-purulent, even though, according to Wood *et al.* (1988), pus was

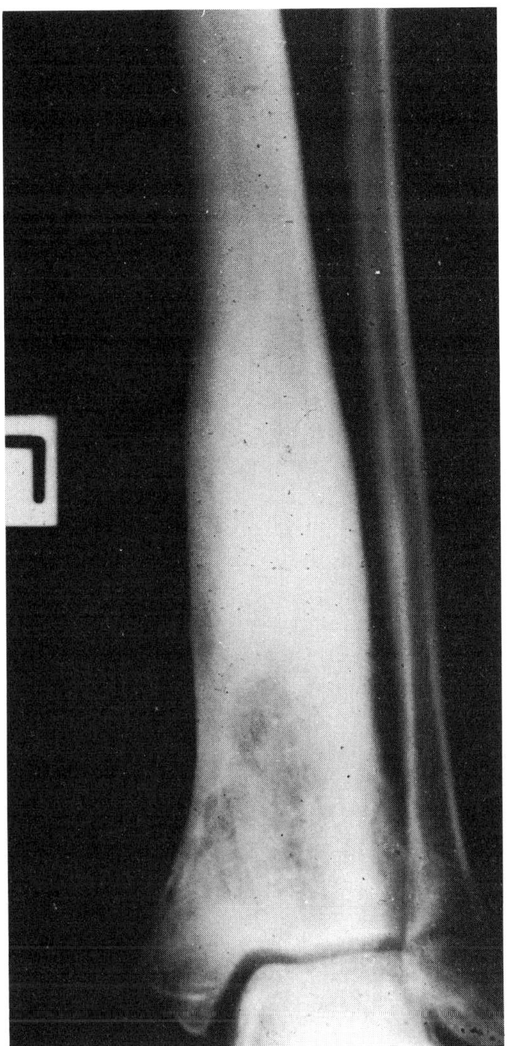

Figure 7.23 Clinical X-ray of a Brodie's abscess in the distal tibia.

attended a Stockholm hospital for the treatment of osteomyelitis, found eight who had chronic, non-fistulous, non-suppurative osteomyelitis dominated radiographically by severe sclerosis. Their ages were 6–30 years. Pain for an average of 7 months preceded consultation. Major long bones, sternum, clavicle and pelvis were the sites. A second lesion at a second site occurred in four after an interval of years. There was no growth from six lesions, and an anaerobic organism in two. Treatment (surgical and/or antibiotic) had little effect. Somewhat similar experience is quoted in dental journals. In 1934 Axhausen, on clinical and radiographic features, described the lesion in the mandible as pseudo-Pagetic. Hoppe (1964) described the marrow fibrosis and increased remodelling of the bone histologically, and the paucity of inflammatory foci.

Sclerotic lesions, particularly in the appendicular skeleton, give rise to concern about neoplasia, which may be difficult to put aside if biopsies do not include foci of inflammation (Lindenbaum and Alexander, 1984). Clavicular lesions, which sometimes are bilateral, may, in the adult, be confused with sternoclavicular hyperostosis (Kohler *et al.*, 1977; Kruger *et al.*, 1987). This is an uncommon, painful dense enlargement of the sternum, clavicles and upper ribs, which may also involve vertebral bodies; it is of unknown aetiology.

present in five of nine patients cited in this class. Moreover, two of these patients died within days of onset. After reviewing articles in the dental literature about 'Garre's sclerosing osteomyelitis' Wood *et al.* (1988) emphasize that all the statements of what Garre observed are apocryphal.

However, the condition to which it is applied is real enough. Collert and Isacson (1982), in a review of patients who had

(ii)   Axial lesions: Vertebral osteomyelitis

The term subacute osteomyelitis now includes vertebral disease, since it has the same insidious onset as other subacute forms and is without constitutional symptoms (Harris and Kirkcaldy-Willis, 1965). It involves the vertebral body. This is a pattern of disease that stands in striking contrast to the descriptions of vertebral osteomyelitis in the older literature (Kulowski, 1936; Griffiths and Jones, 1971) where vertebral osteomyelitis is recorded as an acute disease, mainly under the age of 30 years, taking the form seen in other parts of the skeleton, and with the same high morbidity and mortality. The parts of the neural arch were affected more often than the body; abscess formation was common, with tracking to a wide range of sites (skin, retropharynx, mediastinum, pleura, pericardium, abdominal cavity, retroperitoneum, pelvis, groin), as well as metastatic bone and joint involvement.

Histologically the subacute disease is pyogenic. Periosteal response is not striking, but the inflammation usually extends to adjacent soft tissues where it causes a soft tissue shadow on radiographs that can serve to distinguish it from neoplastic destruction of the bone. The infection may involve adjacent vertebrae, either *ab initio* or by spread. The intervening disc is at risk. It is more likely to be destroyed in pyogenic infection, but its preservation does not necessarily mean tuberculosis, where the disc often survives.

Because of the absence of constitutional effects, symptoms may be only mild chronic backache until the destruction causes vertebral collapse and the potential of cord compression and paraplegia.

(b)   Chronic pyogenic osteomyelitis

The eradication of infection from within bone has always been a difficult problem. Lack of success leads to chronic inflammation. Even at the present time there is a 15–30% incidence of this in patients with acute disease (Hayes *et al.*, 1990). In general terms, as the inflammatory response changes there is a progressive increase in the number of lymphocytes, macrophages and plasma cells. Cytokine synthesis by these cells stimulates bone cell activity leading to the bone's equivalent of the fibrotic reaction that typifies chronic inflammation. This is manifest as bone sclerosis around the lesion. The fibrosis itself is relatively poorly vascular, often incorporates necrotic bone fragments and appears to harbour the bacteria, which

are not easily reached by antibiotics, to which they may be resistant, nor by surgery short of amputation. The result is usually fistulation and chronic drainage of pus. There is a risk of generalized amyloidosis of the amyloid A variety, and a smaller risk of squamous carcinoma at the cloaca of a sinus, where epithelial hyperplasia is a feature.

(c)   Osteomyelitis of infancy

Acute osteomyelitis, usually with a bacteraemia and sometimes with a septicaemia, is occasionally seen in newborn or very young children (Green and Shannon, 1936; Blanche, 1952; Ogden, 1979). It was once considered to be a result of streptococcal infection, but increasingly the importance of staphylococci and *Escherichia coli* is being appreciated. Infection often starts within the first month after delivery and in the case of staphylococci and *E. coli* many bones may be involved. Despite the extent of the disease, not infrequently there is an absence of systemic symptoms which delays diagnosis. This can have disastrous consequences as in the small bones of very young children, in which the distinction between the diaphysis, metaphysis and epiphysis is relatively poor, a virulent organism can lead to involvement of the whole bone, shaft, epiphyses, periosteal tissues and adjacent joint (Ayre-Brook, 1960). Healing, if it occurs, is associated with the formation of distorted bones with large involucra and the danger of permanent inhibition of growth.

(d)   Diaphyseal osteomyelitis

Primary subacute diaphyseal osteomyelitis is a well-recognized but, relatively rare, entity. In one series 3% of cases of childhood haematogenous osteomyelitis showed this pattern (Hoffman *et al.*, 1990). The disease is of short duration and the radiographic appearances are of a linear periosteal reaction indistinguishable from round cell tumours of bone. The histological picture is that of a mixed acute and chronic inflammatory cell infiltrate and sometimes staphylococci can be cultured from the tissue. All patients heal completely within 6 months after treatment with flucloxacillin.

(e) Osteitis pubis

This is a name given to a variety of disorders that lead to inflammation within the bones adjacent to the symphysis pubis. It can occur following surgery to the lower urinary tract (Lavalle and Hamm, 1951) (particularly retropubic prostatectomy) and the female genital tract (Barnes and Malament, 1963). It is also seen in association with ankylosing spondylitis where it was originally believed to represent an extension of the enthesopathy. It is now recognized that patients with ankylosing spondylitis are prone to develop prostatitis (Freemont, 1988) and almost certainly the lesion seen in ankylosing spondylitis is of a similar nature to that associated with surgical manipulation of the lower urinary tract. Most often the affecting organisms are Gram negative bacilli, commonly of the genera *Proteus* and *Pseudomonas*. There is rarefaction of the bones within the pubic rami associated with surrounding bone sclerosis, a periosteal reaction and irregular destruction and new bone formation at the enthesis.

(f) Salmonella osteomyelitis

Bone infections following typhoid and paratyphoid have long been recognized (Murphy, 1916; Giaccia and Idriss, 1952). In Western countries they are now uncommon. Typically this type of osteomyelitis affects the vertebrae and ribs and may not be evident at the time of the initial illness, coming to light sometimes only many years later when pointed to by painful chronic abscesses (Saphra and Winter, 1957). Vertebral involvement is particularly interesting as it is believed to occur as a consequence of retrograde venous spread from the bowel. Salmonella infection is not nearly as destructive as other forms of pyogenic infection and repair and bony ankylosis may ensue. The most interesting association between Salmonella osteomyelitis and both sickle cell disease and trait is now well recognized (Hook *et al.*, 1957; Hook, 1961; Widen and Cardon, 1961; Kaye and Hook, 1963), although rare. Whether this characteristic linkage is a consequence of the other bony complications of sickle cell disease is not clear, but the association with the trait suggests not necessarily.

7.4.2 GRANULOMATOUS INFLAMMATION OF BONES

The general principles that govern the establishment of pyogenic infections also apply to those infections due to organisms which will stimulate a granulomatous inflammatory response. The organisms enter the bone marrow most commonly haematogenously, but can also infect the bone by extension or by inoculation. For the greater part tuberculosis is the cause, but a number of atypical acid-fast organisms, several fungi, brucella and syphilis are also causes.

(a) Tuberculous osteomyelitis

Before efforts to eradicate, or at least control, tuberculosis, tuberculous infection of bones and joints was one of the most common causes of admission to orthopaedic units. With the advent of antibiotic-resistant strains of *Mycobacterium tuberculosis*, and increasing numbers of patients with chronic debilitating disorders and those who, for one reason or another, are immunosuppressed, this situation may well recur.

Tuberculous osteomyelitis is always a consequence of haematogenous spread (Martini *et al.*, 1986) and there must therefore be a primary focus of infection elsewhere within the body. The most common site for a tuberculous infection that has arisen as a consequence of haematogenous spread is in or near a joint of a long bone (usually the hip or the knee) or within a vertebra. Most patients are below the age of 25 years and it is they who succumb most commonly to spinal or hip disease. It therefore follows that tuberculous osteomyelitis about the knee most commonly affects older individuals. Because of the association between bone and joint diseases, a pointless and unanswerable argument has been initiated as to whether this is primarily a bone or a joint infection.

Spinal tuberculosis affects the lower thoracic and lumbar vertebrae most commonly and spreads from vertebra to vertebra beneath the spinal ligaments and directly by erosion through the intervertebral disc (Lifeso *et al.*, 1985) (Figures 7.24 and 7.25). The destructive process leads to angulation (Pott's disease) and may cause compression of the spinal cord. In addition there is often bony ankylosis of the spine in end-stage disease. Tuberculous meningitis may occur and soft tissue extension into the psoas muscles and their sheaths is not uncommon. Tracking along the sheath leads to formation of a cold psoas abscess in the groin.

In tuberculous infection around the hip and knee both bone and joint tissues may be infected. There is often destruction of bone, cartilage and soft tissues with loss of the joint space on X-ray and joint instability.

Within bone tuberculous inflammation is very similar to that elsewhere. There is mixed giant cell and epithelioid granuloma formation with central caseous necrosis (Figure 7.26). Unfortunately, not infrequently the granulomatous quality of the inflammatory response is not readily apparent and may mimic subacute or chronic pyogenic osteomyelitis. The inflammation is more destructive and less invasive than pyogenic infection so that sequestrum formation is less prominent but the corollary that the reactive bone formation is less substantial is also true. Repair, if and when the infection is

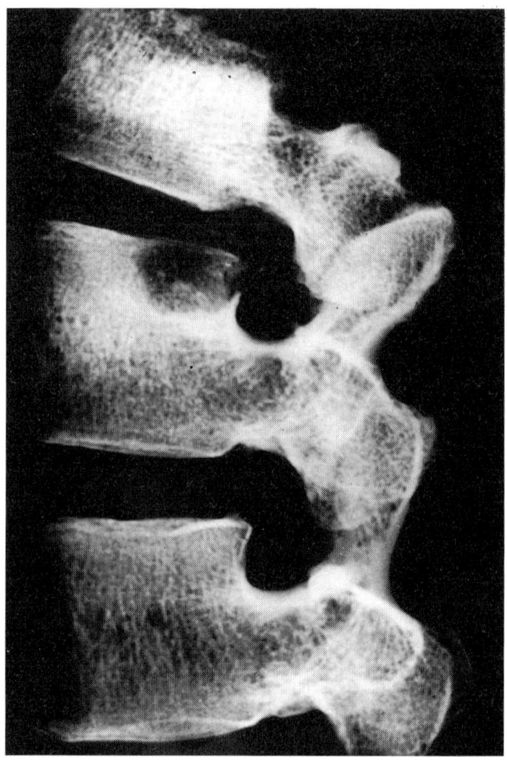

Figure 7.24 Radiograph of excised spine from a patient dying with destructive spinal tuberculous osteomyelitis.

overcome, is therefore less effective in tuberculous osteomyelitis than in pyogenic cases.

Since many organisms may cause a granulomatous reaction, diagnosis is dependent upon demonstration of the organisms in culture or tissue sections. In tissue sections diagnosis depends upon identifying the organism using conventional stains. These rely on the acid-fast properties of the saccharides in the bacterial cell wall. This staining is interfered with in nitric acid decalcified tissue, but not formic acid or EDTA decalcified tissue.

(b) Leprosy

Mycobacterial infections of bone are not restricted to tuberculosis. Atypical mycobacteria can cause osteomyelitis (Babulkar *et al.*,

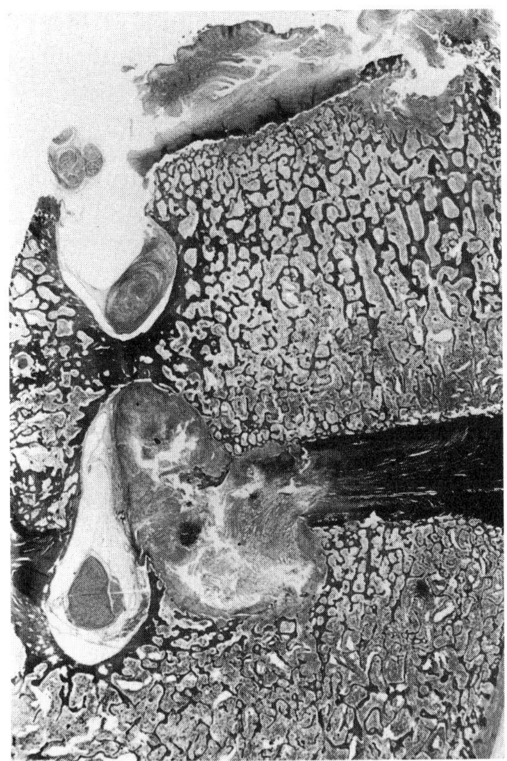

Figure 7.25 Histological section of the specimen in the radiograph in Figure 7.24.

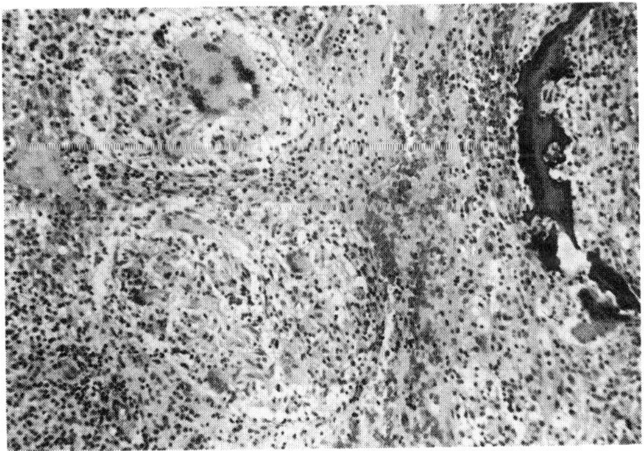

Figure 7.26 Tuberculous granuloma in bone.

1984), particularly in the immunosuppressed and *Mycobacterium leprae* may also affect bone as part of the general picture of leprosy (Fite, 1943). There are two principal forms of lepromatous involvement of bone – leprous osteitis and bone resorption associated with anaesthetic nerve lesions (Riordan, 1960).

In leprous osteitis, tuberculoid lesions – lepromata – develop in the bone marrow. Each consists of loosely formed collections of histiocytoid cells containing numerous bacilli. The lepromata which may be quite small and numerous, cause bone rarefaction and, because of their number and distribution, radiographically, infection often appears like tiny punched out holes throughout large areas of the bone.

Bone resorption secondary to local anaesthesia starts in the distal ends of digits. It is associated with increased osteoclasis. The cause of the osteoclasis is probably multifactorial but a significant component is the result of secondary infection.

(c) Granuloma inguinale

There are a very few cases of bone involvement with the organism *Calymmatobacterium granulomatosis* (Kalstone *et al.*, 1961). This venereally acquired organism usually causes skin and lymph node lesions consisting of aggregates of macrophages containing characteristic 'Donovan bodies', small cytoplasmic inclusions best recognized in Wright or Giemsa stained preparations. Such cells are typical of the bony lesions which most commonly affect the spine.

(d) Brucellosis

Most cases are caused by *Brucella melitensis*, but *Brucella abortus* and *Brucella suis* are also found. Brucellosis is transmissible from animal to human either through drinking infected milk, or through close contact with infected animals. Within the lymphoid system the disease is characterized by either epithelioid granulomata or by suppuration. Either form of inflammation may occur within bone (Kelly *et al.*, 1960), the predominant pattern in sternal or iliac crest marrow being granuloma formation whereas in the spine (vertebral brucellosis acounts for 75% of all cases), the pattern is that of suppuration, but with less necrosis and abscess formation and a greater degree of fibrosis and new bone formation than is normally associated with acute or subacute pyogenic osteomyelitis.

(e) Syphilis

Skeletal syphilis is now exceptionally rare in the West. In general terms both congenital and acquired syphilis are characterized by chronic inflammation, sometimes with associated granuloma formation and necrosis. There is bone destruction and repair (Walzman *et al.*, 1986). The exact nature of the lesion depends on whether the disease is periosteal or endochondral, and whether it proceeds to gumma formation.

The lesions of congenital syphilis are fully developed at birth. Spirochaetes are most commonly encountered within the area of active endochondral ossification and within the periosteum. The typical lesions are therefore a mixed epiphysitis and periostitis. Microscopically the epiphysitis affects the calcifying cartilage of the growth plate. Chronically inflamed, vascular granulation tissue infiltrates between and destroys the chondrocyte columns. This may lead to cessation of growth and even dislocation of the epiphyseal cartilage.

Periostitis causes stimulation of new bone formation at the periosteal region leading to a massive growth of periosteal new bone about the existing cortex.

In acquired syphilis the bone changes are usually seen first in early tertiary disease approximately 3–4 years after contracting the infection. The lesions are encountered most commonly in the tibia, bones of the nose and palate and in the skull. The lesions are, for the most part, similar to those of congenital disease, except that they do not occur in growing bones and may show the formation

of gummata. The disease may present as either a periostitis or as a form of osteomyelitis, although this is relatively rarer. If gummata form there is, in addition, bone necrosis with perforation of bone plates and collapse of bones. Secondary pyogenic osteomyelitis may develop.

(f) Yaws

Yaws is caused by the organism *Treponema pertenue*. In many respects the lesions of yaws are very similar to those of syphilis, but in bone the disease does not manifest itself as a periostitis as does syphilis, nor is epiphysitis a feature (Hackett, 1951). The lesions commonly present as small areas of rarefaction within the cortex which come to elicit a very active periosteal osteogenetic response. Histologically it is not possible to distinguish the lesions of syphilis and yaws.

Gummata form in flat bones but not long bones. Two characteristic lesions are described, a reactive exostosis of the mandible, called 'goundou' and massive necrosis of the nose, palate and nasopharynx ('gangosa').

(g) Fungal infections

Whenever granulomatous lesions are seen in bone, nowadays, fungal infection must be excluded (Figure 7.27). In some parts of the world pathogenic fungi such as *Blastomyces*, *Coccidioides*, *Paracoccidioides*, *Histoplasma* (Cockshott and Lucas, 1964), *Sporotrichosis* (Altner and Turner, 1970) and *Cryptococcus* may cause bone infection. Increasingly in Britain, a country not known for a high level of pathogenic fungal infections, fungi are causing granulomatous osteomyelitis. This is a reflection of the number of patients who are now immunosuppressed as a consequence of disease or its management.

In patients who are immunosuppressed any organism may cause disseminated disease, including bone involvement. Diagnosis

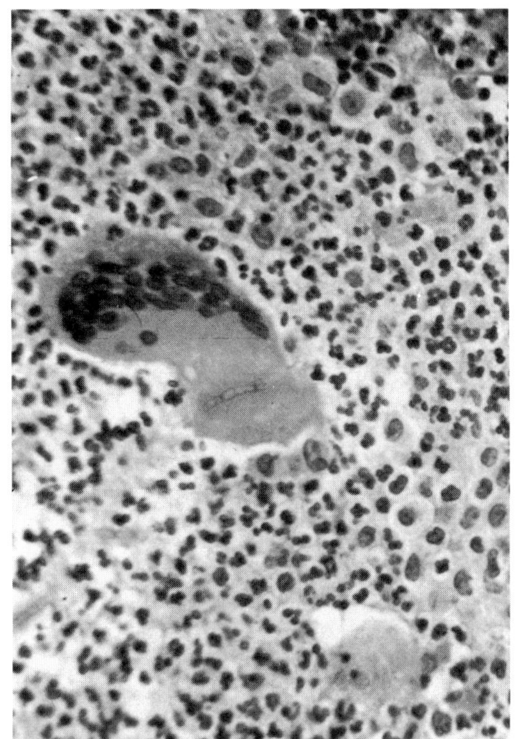

Figure 7.27 Fungal granuloma in bone.

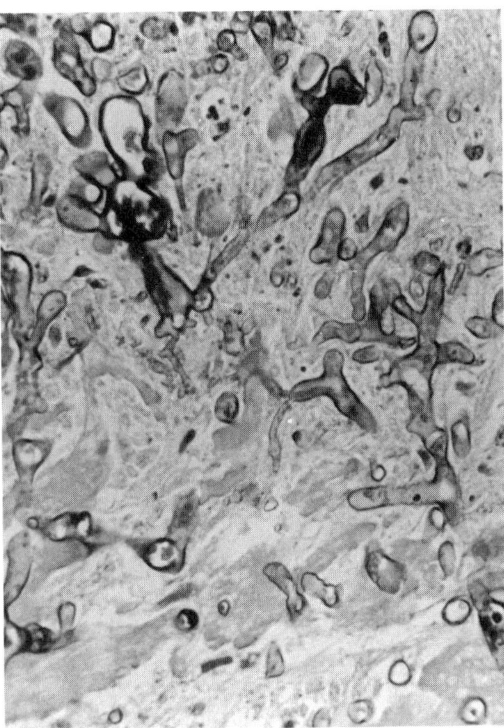

Figure 7.28 Fungal hyphae in the centre of the granuloma illustrated in Figure 7.27.

of this diverse group of infective organisms may well depend on biopsy. Periodic acid–Schiff (Figure 7.28) or a modified silver stain are important for making the diagnosis and lectin histochemistry may, when coupled with morphology, type the organism. Care with tissue handling is required as acid decalcification may so affect the structure of the complex saccharides that constitute the fungal wall as to render them unreactive with conventional stains and to give false results with panels of lectins.

The nature of the bony lesions caused by fungi is best illustrated by a brief description of three of the most common.

(i)   Coccidioidomycosis

Coccidioides immitis rarely progresses to a systemic disease. If it does, bone involvement may occasionally occur (Birsner and Smart, 1956). The infection specifically targets the small bones of the hand and feet, the vertebrae and ribs. The organism causes small lytic lesions in bone which persist after eradication of the infection, i.e. the lesions do not heal.

(ii)   Blastomycosis

Systemic infection with *Blastomyces dermatidis* is not infrequently associated with osteomyelitis (Witorsch and Utz, 1968). The favoured bones are spine, skull and small bones of the hand and feet. The infection is characterized by lytic lesions in bone, similar to those of *Coccidioides*.

(iii)   Cryptococcosis

About 10% of cryptococcal infections show skeletal involvement (Littman and Walter, 1968). The lesions, which are often multiple, are rounded radiolucencies (Kromminga *et al.*, 1990). Unlike all the other fungi the reaction is predominantly histiocytic and may be mistaken for a neoplasm. The histiocytes contain organisms which can be recognized by fungal stains (Abdul-Karim *et al.*, 1991).

7.5   OTHER TYPES OF INFLAMMATION WITHIN BONE

These disparate disorders are best considered under two headings, disorders associated with infective organisms (other than those already discussed) and non-infective forms of inflammation.

7.5.1   FORMS OF INFLAMMATION ASSOCIATED WITH INFECTIVE ORGANISMS

(a)   Parasitic infections

Only two parasites have been described in human bone. Much the more common is the tapeworm *Echinococcus.*

The larval form of the tapeworm *Echinococcus granulosus* (hydatid cyst) is a not uncommon finding within bones of individuals from areas in which the dog/sheep strain of the worm is particularly prevalent (e.g. Kenya, North Africa and the Middle East). The larval form of the worm enters the body through the bowel wall and either bypasses the liver or reseeds the circulation from hydatids in the liver. The organisms metastasize to the bone where they grow, not as the distinct cyst typical of hepatic hydatid disease, but by infiltrating the medullary spaces and vascular passageways (Howarth, 1945). The irregular 'cyst' that results contains little fluid and no scolices, instead being filled with a gelatinous material. The wall may consist of a dense capsule but there is little surrounding tissue reaction (Figure 7.29). With time expansion of the lesion leads to the development of an apparently multiloculated

cystic radiolucent space within the bone (Figure 7.30). This area, often towards the epiphyseal end of the bone, may be mistaken for a neoplasm, and may so weaken the bone that it leads to pathological fracture.

Much less common is involvement of bones by the larval forms of other tape worms. The pattern of involvement is similar to that seen in Echinococcal infestation.

(b)   Viral infections

A number of viruses have been described as causing inflammation within bone, some are better recorded than others and, with the increasing incidence of immunosuppressed patients, new types of viral infection of bone are still being described (Berman and Jensen, 1990). Of these some of the best recognized are the following:

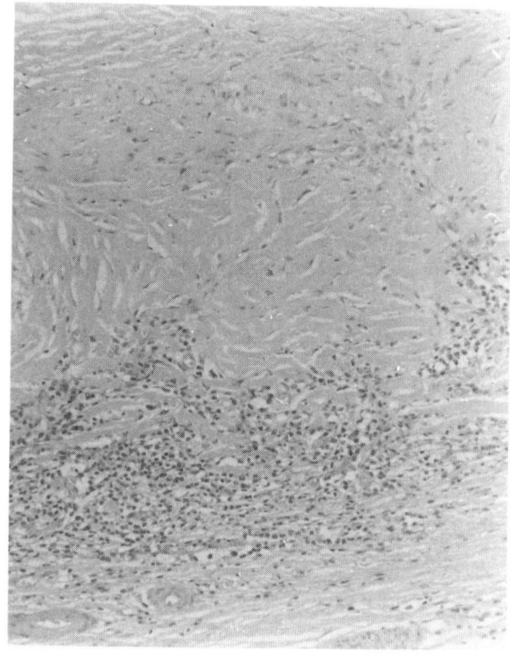

Figure 7.29 Male with hydatid disease. Wall of a cyst showing lamellar structure and a patchy inflammatory reaction.

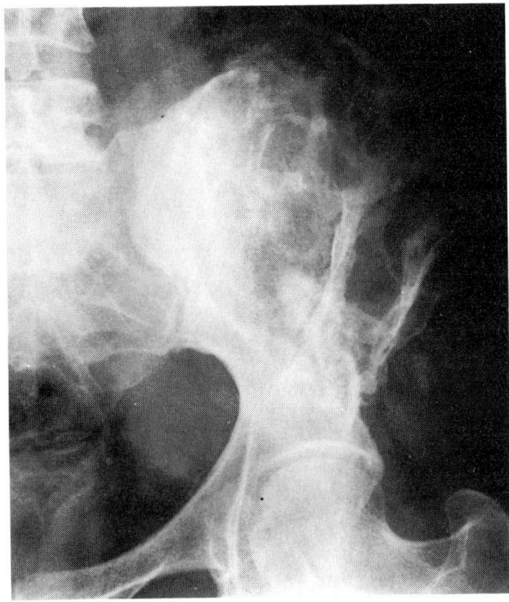

Figure 7.30 Male with hydatid disease. Radiograph of left ilium showing a large, multiloculated, osteolytic lesion expanding the wing of the ilium.

(i)   *Smallpox*

The finding of bony lesions in smallpox is an old observation. Thankfully, it is becoming increasingly rare and will soon be a thing of the past now that the infection has been eradicated. The bone lesion develops approximately two weeks after the initial infection (Davidson and Palmer, 1963). The bone is involved in a chronic inflammatory, non-suppurative osteomyelitis, predominantly in the area of the epiphysis. In children it leads to growth arrest and premature epiphyseal fusion. Sometimes it results in a periostitis with formation of an involucrum.

(ii)   *Vaccinia*

Vaccinial osteomyelitis has also been observed several weeks after inoculation (Elliott, 1959). There is a predilection for the upper extremities. Biopsy shows non-purulent chronic inflammation and marrow fibrosis. Viable vaccinia organisms have been cultivated from the lesions.

(iii)   *Rubella*

In cases of maternal rubella (German measles) the newborn infant has been reported as having irregular growth plates and a poorly defined trabecular pattern on X-ray. The histology of these lesions has not been described.

(c)   Paget's disease

Paget's disease (see Chapter 10 for detailed description) has been shown to have viral inclusions within osteoclasts. Recent immunohistochemical and *in situ* hybridization studies have shown the viral particles to be of the paramyxovirus group (Cartwright *et al.*, 1993). Although variously ascribed as measles or respiratory syncytial virus, the most recent data indicate that the virus is probably the canine distemper virus in the overwhelming majority of cases. Although it has not been possible yet to prove that the disease is caused by the virus the association with the virus and its distribution within the bone strongly support this conclusion.

(d)   SAPHO syndrome

SAPHO is an acronym for Synovitis, Acne, Pustulosis, Hyperostosis, Osteitis (Benhamou *et al.*, 1988). Palmoplantar pustulosis may be associated with peculiar bone and joint disorders. The initial descriptions localized these disorders to the anterior chest wall, but latterly more peripheral bones and joints have been associated with severe acne. Typically these patients present with pustulotic acne and sternoclavicular bone involvement. Other bones may be involved. The bone lesion combines a sterile active chronic inflammatory cell infiltrate with hyperostosis. Occasionally the bone resembles that seen in Paget's disease.

The aetiology is unknown although there are reports of the organism *Propionibacterium acnes* being isolated from the bone and there is a suggestion that there may be a genetic basis for the disorder (Kahn *et al.*, 1991). The most favoured explanation for SAPHO syndrome is that it represents a form of spondyloarthropathy with an enthesitis and inflammatory involvement of the adjacent marrow.

(e)   Lymphogranuloma venereum

Lymphogranuloma venereum is a venereal disease caused by the organism *Chlamydia trachomatis*. In lymph nodes the organism causes a macrophage response which develops into a characteristic 'stellate abscess' consisting of a central necrotic centre and peripheral palisaded macrophages. Very rare cases of osteomyelitis have been ascribed to this organism (Wright and Logan, 1939). The lesions in bone are histologically identical to those in lymph nodes.

(f)   Catch scratch disease

Catch scratch disease is believed to be caused by a chlamydial-like organism. The lesions are similar to those of lymphogranuloma venereum. Focal osteolysis, presumed to be caused by the infective lesions, is sometimes seen in association with this disease (Carithers *et al.*, 1969).

(g)   Actinomycosis

Although *Actinomyces israeli* rarely causes infection, when it does infect bone it tends to do so by direct extension (Young, 1960; Nathan *et al.*, 1962). As a commensal of the mouth, throat and respiratory passages it most commonly affects the bones of the jaw, ribs and vertebrae. The process is predominantly lytic. The lesions are often yellow on gross examination. The abscesses have a border of lipid-laden macrophages and contain colonies of branching bacilli in an amorphous matrix.

7.5.2   NON-INFECTIVE INFLAMMATION

(a)   Sarcoidosis

Sarcoidosis involves the bones in 25% of cases with systemic disease (James, 1974). The typical epithelioid granulomata with rare multinucleated giant cells and relatively few other inflammatory cells are frequently found on bone marrow biopsy in these cases. Less commonly the lesion causes circumscribed bone destruction often with an associated periosteal reaction. The destructive lesions have a particular tendency to involve phalangeal bones of the hands and feet.

(b)   Intraosseous inflammation associated with joint disease

Inflammatory joint disease is frequently associated with bone changes and in some of these inflammatory cells are seen within the marrow spaces. The archetypal inflammatory joint disease with bone involvement is rheumatoid disease. This disorder illustrates the wealth of lesions that can be found in bone marrow associated with local joint inflammation. There are three main types of lesion.

In severe active rheumatoid disease an inflammatory process, similar to that seen within the synovium, can also be found within the marrow immediately adjacent to the subchondral bone plate. The marrow contains macrophages and lymphocytes within a loose vascular granulation tissue.

Inflammation is also seen about rheumatoid pseudocysts, again in juxta-articular marrow. These lesions are not cysts at all but spaces filled by rheumatoid-type granulation tissue in continuity with the inflamed pannus through deficiencies within the articular surface or the juxta-articular cortex.

Finally lymphoplasmacytic aggregates are found diffusely within otherwise uninvolved bone marrow of patients with rheumatoid disease. They tend to be centrally placed within the marrow and have little effect on bone.

(c) Inflammation associated with marrow disease

Many disorders of the bone marrow are associated with inflammatory cells within the marrow spaces. This is particularly true of immune-mediated disorders, such as some types of aplastic anaemia in which the marrow contains an excess of lymphocytes and plasma cells, and certain types of chronic leukaemia in which the marrow infiltrate may mimic inflammation.

(d) Infantile cortical hyperostosis

This disorder was first described by Caffey and Silverman in 1945 (Pazzaglia *et al.*, 1985). It affects children between the ages of 2 and 6 months and is characterized by a peculiar self-limiting inflammatory osteoperiostitis found most commonly in the long bones of the limbs, mandible, clavicle, ribs and scapulae. The disease is associated with a systemic illness. It is suggested that there may be a viral aetiology (Pazzaglia *et al.*, 1985).

7.5.3 CONDITIONS MIMICKING OSTEOMYELITIS

In general terms inflammatory lesions give rise to bone destruction and adjacent new bone formation. Clinically and radiologically these changes may be confused with neoplastic lesions and histologically the same confusion can arise, particularly with small cell neoplasms, and certain leukaemias and lymphomas.

Radiologically and clinically osteomyelitis is also mimicked by bone tumour-like lesions of bone such as fibrous dysplasia and histologically disorders such as the storage disorder Gaucher's disease may be mistaken for inflammation (Hoffman *et al.*, 1990).

7.5.4 CHRONIC GRANULOMATOUS DISEASE AFFECTING THE SKELETON

Chronic granulomatous disease is the result of a heritable disorder of oxidative metabolism of neutrophils which prevents them from producing the oxidants that destroy bacteria. The usual test for the disease is nitroblue tetrazolium reduction by neutrophils. Infection usually begins in soft tissues or parenchymatous organs and skeletal involvement is secondary. Sponseller *et al.* (1991) reviewed the files of 42 children with the condition from the National Institutes of Health and the Johns Hopkins Hospital. Thirteen had bone involvement, in three of whom it was the first manifestation of the disease. The infection reaches bone either by direct spread, or haematogenously. Abscess formation follows, with both periosteal and endosteal bone reactions. The organisms are usually catalase positive, and include *Staphylococcus* species, *Serratia, Nocardia, Mycobacteria* and many fungi. Sponseller *et al.* (1991) suggest that many organisms produce peroxide which neutrophils can use to overcome them; but the catalase-positive organisms destroy peroxide. The inflammatory reaction is granulomatous, with a variable degree of granuloma formation. There are no special features for any particular organism; the bacterial organisms caused the same reaction. Antibiotics alone are not usually adequate treatment, and must be supplemented by surgical procedures.

REFERENCES

Abdul-Karim, F.W., Pathria, M.N., Heller, J.G.H. *et al.* (1991) Case report 664. *Cryptococcus neoformans* osteomyelitis. *Skeletal Radiol.*, **20**, 22–9.

Alberts, B., Bray, D., Lewis, J. *et al.* (1989) *Molecu-

lar Biology of the Cell, 2nd edn., Garland Publishing, New York.

Alderson, M., Speers, D., Emslie, K. *et al.* (1986) Acute haematogenous osteomyelitis and septic arthritis – a single disease. *J. Bone Joint Surg.*, **68B**, 268–74.

Altner, P.C. and Turner, R.R. (1970) Sporotrichosis of bones and joints; review of the literature and report of 6 cases. *Clin. Orthop.*, **68**, 138–48.

Axhausen, G. (1934) Uber Paget und PseudoPaget der Kiefer. *Dtsch. Kieferchir.* **1**, 4–27.

Ayre-Brook, A.L. (1960) Septic arthritis of the hip and osteomyelitis of the upper end of the femur in infants. *J. Bone Joint Surg.*, **42B**, 11–20.

Babulkar, S.S., Tayade, W.B. and Babulkar, S.K. (1984) Atypical spinal tuberculosis. *J. Bone Joint Surg.*, **66B**, 239–42.

Barnes, W.C. and Malament, M. (1963) Osteitis pubis. *Surg. Gynecol. Obstet.*, **117**, 277–84.

Benhamou, C.L., Chamot, A.M. and Kahn, M.-F. (1988) Synovitis-acne-pustulosis hyperostosis osteomyelitis syndrome (SAPHO). A new syndrome among the spondylarthropathies? *Clin. Exp. Immunol.*, **6**, 109–12.

Berman, S. and Jensen, J. (1990) Cytomegalovirus-induced osteomyelitis in a patient with the acquired immunodeficiency syndrome. *South. Med. J.* **83**, 1231–2.

Birsner, J.W. and Smart, S. (1956) Osseous coccidioidomycosis; a chronic form of dissemination. *Am. J. Roentgenol.*, **76**, 1052–60.

Blanche, D.W. (1952) Osteomyelitis of infants. *J. Bone Joint Surg.*, **34A**, 71–85.

Burkert, T. and Watanakumakorn, C. (1991) Group G streptococcus and septic arthritis and osteomyelitis. *J. Rhematol.*, **18**, 904–7.

Burton, D.R. (1990) Antibody: the flexible adaptor molecule. *Trends Biochem. Sci.*, **15**, 64–9.

Caffey, J. and Silverman, W.A. (1945) Infantile cortical hyperostoses: preliminary report on a new syndrome. *Am. J. Roentgenol.*, **54**, 1–16.

Carithers, H.A., Carithers, C.M. and Edwards, R.O. (1969) Cat scratch disease: its natural history. *J. Am. Med. Assoc.*, **207**, 312–8.

Cartwright, E.J., Gordon, M.T., Freemont, A.J. *et al.* (1993) Paramyxovirus and Paget's disease. *J. Med. Virol.* **40**, 133–41.

Cockshott, W.P. and Lucas, A.O. (1964) Radiological findings in *Histoplasma duboisii* infections. *Br. J. Radiol.*, **37**, 653–60.

Cole, W.G., Dalziel, R.E. and Leitl, S. (1982) Treatment of acute osteomyelitis in childhood. *J. Bone Joint Surg.*, **64B**, 218–23.

Collert, S. and Isacson, J. (1982) Chronic sclerosing osteomyelitis (Garre) *Clin. Orthop,* **164**, 136–40.

Davidson, J.C. and Palmer, D.E.S. (1963) Osteomyelitis variolosa. *J. Bone Joint Surg.*, **45B**, 687–93.

Edelman, G.M. (1986) Cell adhesion molecules. *Science*, **219**, 450–7.

Elliott, W.D. (1959) Vaccinial osteomyelitis. *Lancet*, **ii**, 1053–5.

Felsberg, G.J., Gore, R.L., Schweitzer, M.E. *et al.* (1990) Sclerosing osteomyelitis of Garre (sclerosing periostitis ossificans). *Oral Surg. Oral Med. Oral Pathol.*, **70**, 117–20.

Fite, G.L. (1943) Leprosy from the histologic point of view. *Arch. Pathol.*, **35**, 611–23.

Freemont, A.J. (1988) Pathology of ankylosing spondylitis. in *New Clinical Approaches – Rheumatology – Ankylosing Spondylitis* (eds D.C. Calabro and W. Carson Dick), MTP Press, Lancaster, pp. 1–22.

Freemont, A.J. (1992) High endothelial venules. *Adv. Rheumatol. Inflamm.*, **28**, 129–36.

Gaafar, S.M. and Turk, J.L. (1970) Granuloma formation in lymph nodes. *J. Pathol.*, **100**, 9–20.

Giaccia, L. and Idriss, H. (1952) Osteomyelitis due to *Salmonella* infection. *J. Paediatr.*, **41**, 72–8.

Gilmour, W.N. (1962) Acute haematogenous osteomyelitis. *J. Bone Joint Surg.*, **44B**, 841–53.

Glynn, L.E., Houck, J.C. and Weissman, G. (1989) *The Handbook of Inflammation.* Vols. 1–5. Elsevier, Amsterdam.

Goldberg, D.G. and Arbesfeld, D. (1991) Squamous cell carcinoma arising in a site of chronic osteomyelitis. Treatment with Mohs micrographic surgery. *J. Dermatol. Surg. Oncol.*, **17**, 788–90.

Gordon, S. (1986) Biology of the macrophage. *J. Cell Sci.*, **4 suppl.**, 267–8.

Gospodarowicz, D., Neufeld, G. and Schweigerer, L. (1987) Fibroblast growth factor: structural and biological properties. *J. Cell Physiol.*, **5 suppl.**, 15–26.

Green, W.T. and Shannon, J.G. (1936) Osteomyelitis of infants; a disease different from osteomyelitis of older children. *Arch. Surg.*, **32**, 462–93.

Griffiths, H.E.D. and Jones, D.M. (1971) Pyogenic infection of the spine; a review of 28 cases. *J. Bone Joint Surg.*, **53B**, 383–91.

Grogan, T.J., Dorey, F., Rollins, J. *et al.* (1986) Deep sepsis following knee arthroplasty. *J. Bone Joint Surg.*, **68A**, 226–34.

Hackett, C.J. (1951) *Bone lesions of Yaws in Uganda.* Blackwells, Oxford.

Harris, N.H. (1960) Some problems in the diagnosis and treatment of acute osteomyelitis. *J. Bone Joint Surg.*, **42B**, 535–41.

Harris, N.H. and Kirkaldy-Willis, W.H. (1965) Primary subacute osteomyelitis. *J. Bone Joint Surg.*, **47B**, 526–32.

Hayes, C.S., Heinrich, S.D., Craver, R. *et al.* (1990) Subacute osteomyelitis. *Orthopaedics*, **13**, 363–6.

Henson, P.M. and Johnston, R.B. (1987) Tissue injury in inflammation. Oxidants, proteinases and cationic proteins. *J. Clin. Invest.*, **79**, 669–74.

Herron, G.S., Werb, Z., Dwyer, K. *et al.* (1986) Secretion of metalloproteinases by stimulated capillary endothelial cells. I and II. *J. Biol. Chem.*, **261**, 2810–18.

Hoffman, E.B., de Beer, J.D., Keys, G. *et al.* (1990) Diaphyseal primary subacute osteomyelitis in children. *J. Paediatr Orthop.*, **10**, 250–4.

Hook, E.W. (1961) Salmonellosis; certain factors influencing the interaction of *Salmonella* and the human host. *N. Y. Acad. Med. Bull.*, **37**, 499–512.

Hook, E.W., Campbell, C.G., Weens, H.S. *et al.* (1957) Salmonella osteomyelitis in patients with sickle cell anaemia. *N. Engl. J. Med.*, **257**, 403–7.

Hoppe, W. (1964) Zur Pathogenese der Osteomyelitis Sicca Mandibulae (Pseudo-Paget). *Fortsehr. Kiefer-n. Geschtechir.*, **9**, 162–50.

Howarth, M.B. (1945) Echinococcus of bone. *J. Bone Joint Surg.*, **27**, 401–12.

Hynes, R.O. (1987) Integrins: a family of cell surface receptors. *Cell*, **48**, 549–54.

James, D.G. (1974) The many faces of sarcoidosis. *J. Irish Med. Assoc.*, **67**, 329–36.

Johnston, R.B. (1988) Monocytes and macrophages. *N. Engl. J. Med.*, **318**, 747–52.

Kahn, M.-F., Bouvier, M., Palazzo, E. *et al.* (1991) Sternoclavicular pustulotic osteitis (SAPHO). 20 year interval between skin and bone lesions. *J. Rheumatol.*, **18**, 1104–8.

Kalstone, B.M., Howell, J.A. and Cline, F.X. (1961) Granuloma inguinale with haematogenous dissemination to the spine. *J. Am. Med. Assoc.*, **176**, 152–6.

Kaye, D. and Hook, E.W. (1963) The influence of haemolysis on susceptibility to Salmonella infection; additional observations. *J. Immunol.*, **91**, 517–27.

Kelly, P.G., Martin, W.J., Schirger, A. *et al.*, (1960) Brucellosis of the bones and joints. Experience with 36 patients. *J. Am. Med. Assoc.*, **174**, 347–53.

Kohler, H., Uehlinger, E., Kutzner, J. *et al.* (1977) Sternoclavicular hyperostosis: painful swelling of the sternum, clavicles and upper ribs. **Ann. Intern. Med.**, **87**, 192–4.

Kozlowski, K. (1986) Brodie's abscess in the first decade. *Paediatr. Radiol.*, **10**, 73–7.

Kromminga, R., Staib, F., Thalmann, U. *et al.* (1990) Osteomyelitis due to *Cryptococcus neoformans* in advanced age. *Mycoses*, **33**, 157–66.

Kruger, G.D., Rock, M.G. and Munro, T.G. (1987) Condensing osteitis of the clavicle. *J. Bone Joint Surg.*, **69A**, 550–7.

Kulowski, J. (1936) Pyogenic osteomyelitis of the spine; an analysis and discussion of 102 cases. *J. Bone Joint Surg.*, **18**, 343–64.

Lavalle, L.L. and Hamm, F.C. (1951) Osteitis pubis; its aetiology and pathology. *J. Urol.*, **66**, 418–23.

Lifeso, R.M., Weaver, P. and Harder, E. (1985) Tuberculous spondylitis in adults. *J. Bone Joint Surg.*, **67A**, 1405–13.

Lindenbaum, S. and Alexander, H. (1984) Infections simulating bone tumours: a review of subacute osteomyelitis *Clin. Orthop.*, **184**, 193–203.

Littman, M.L. and Walter, J.E. (1968) Cryptococcosis: current status. *Am. J. Med.*, **45**, 922–32.

Lowman, M.A., Rees, P.H., Beynon, R.C. *et al.* (1988) Human mast cell heterogeneity: histamine release from mast cells dispersed from skin, lung, adenoids, tonsils and intestinal mucosa in response to IgE dependent and non-immunologic stimuli. *J. Allergy Clin. Immunol.*, **81**, 590–7.

MacLennan, I.C.N., Liu, Y.-J., Oldfield, J. *et al.* (1990) The evolution of B-cell clones. *Curr. Top. Microbiol. Immunol.*, **159**, 38–63.

Maderazo, E.G., Judson, S. and Pasternak, H. (1988) Late infections of total joint prostheses. *Clin. Orthop.*, **229**, 131–42.

Malich, H.D. and Gallin, G.I. (1988) Neutrophils in human disease. **37**, 687–94.

Mantovani, A. and Dejana, E. (1989) Cytokines as communications signals between leukocytes and endothelial cells. *Immunol. Today*, **10**, 371–5.

Martini, M., Adjrad, A. and Boudjemaa, A. (1986) Tuberculous osteomyelitis. *Int. Orthop.*, **10**, 201–7.

McGee, J.O'D., Isaacson, P.G. and Wright, N.A. (1992) *Oxford Textbook of Pathology*, Vol. I. Oxford University Press, Oxford.

McGuire, M.H. (1989) Pathogenesis of adult osteomyelitis. *Orthop. Rev.*, **18**, 564–70.

Murphy, J.B. (1916) Bone and joint disease in relation to typhoid fever. *Surg. Gynecol. Obstet.*, **23**, 119–43.

Nathan, C. (1987) Secretory products of macrophages. *J. Clin. Invest.*, **79**, 319–26.

Nathan, M.H., Radman, W.P. and Barton, H.L. (1962) Osseous actinomycosis of the head and neck. *Am. J. Roentgenol.*, **87**, 1048–53.

North, R.J. (1978) Opinions: the concept of the activated macrophage. *J. Immunol.*, **121**, 806–9.

O'Flaherty, J.T. (1982) Lipid mediators of inflammation and allergy. *Lab. Invest.*, **47**, 314–29.

Ogden, J.A. (1979) Paediatric osteomyelitis and septic arthritis: The pathology of neonatal disease. *Yale J. Biol. Med.*, **52**, 423–8.

Pazzaglia, U.E., Byers, P.D., Beluffi, G. *et al.* (1985) Pathology of infantile cortical hyperostosis (Caffey's Disease): report of a case. *J. Bone Joint Surg.*, **67A**, 1417–26.

Plotquin, D., Dekel, S., Katz, S. *et al.* (1991) Prostaglandin release by normal and osteomyelitic human bones. *Prostaglandins Leukotrienes Essent. Fatty Acids*, **43**, 13–15.

Rappolee, D.A., Mark, D., Banda, M.J. *et al.* (1988) Wound macrophages express TGF-β and other growth factors in-vivo: analysis by mRNA phenotyping. *Science*, **241**, 708–12.

Riordan, D.C. (1960) The hand in leprosy. Part II. Orthopaedic aspects of leprosy. *J. Bone Joint Surg.*, **42A**, 683–92.

Rissing, J.P. (1990) Animal models of osteomyelitis. Knowledge, hypothesis and speculation. *Infect. Dis. Clin. North Am.*, **4**, 377–90.

Ross, R., Raines, E.W. and Bowen-Pope, D.F. (1986) The biology of platelet-derived growth factor. *Cell*, **46**, 155–69.

Ryan, G. and Majno, G. (1977) Acute inflammation; a review. *Am. J. Pathol.*, **86**, 185–93.

Sanders, M.E., Makgoba, M.W. and Shaw, S. (1988) Human naive and memory T-cells: reinterpretation of helper–inducer and suppressor–inducer subsets. *Immunol. Today*, **9**, 195–9.

Saphra, I. and Winter, J.W. (1957) Clinical manifestations of Salmonellosis in man; an evaluation of 7779 human infections identified at the New York Salmonella Center. *N. Engl. J. Med.*, **256**, 1128–34.

Sponseller, P.D., Malech, H.L., McCarthy, E.F. *et al.* (1991) Skeletal involvement in children who have chronic granulomatous disease. *J. Bone Joint Surg.*, **73A**, 37–51.

Sporn, M.B., Roberts, A.B., Wakefield, L.M. *et al.* (1987) Some recent advances in the chemistry and biology of transforming growth factor-beta. *J. Cell Biol.*, **105**, 1039–45.

Trueta, J. (1959) The three types of acute haematogenous osteomyelitis: a clinical and vascular study. *J. Bone Joint Surg.*, **41B**, 671–80.

Van Merkesteyn, J.P., Root, R.H., Bras, J. *et al.* (1988) Diffuse sclerosing osteomyelitis of the mandible: clinical radiographic and histologic findings in 27 patients. *J. Oral Maxillofac. Surg.*, **46**, 825–9.

Walzman, M., Wade, A.A.H., Drake, S.M. *et al.* (1986) Rest pain and leg ulceration due to syphilitic osteomyelitis of the tibia. *Br. Med. J.*, **293**, 804–5.

White, M. and Dennison, W.M. (1952) Acute haematogenous osteitis in childhood. *J. Bone Joint Surg.*, **34B**, 608–23.

Widen, A.L. and Cardon, L. (1961) *Salmonella typhimurium* osteomyelitis with sickle cell haemoglobin c disease: a review and case report. *Ann. Intern. Med.*, **54**, 510–21.

Winters, J.L. and Cahen, I. (1960) Acute haematogenous osteomyelitis; A review of 66 cases. *J. Bone Joint Surg.*, **42A**, 691–704.

Witorsch, P. and Utz, J.P. (1968) North American blastomycosis; A study of 40 patients. *Medicine*, **47**, 169–200.

Wood, R.E., Grotepass, F., Schmidt, S. *et al.* (1988) Periostitis ossificans versus Garre's osteomyelitis. Part I. What did Garre really say? *Oral Surg, Oral Med. Oral Pathol.*, **65**, 773–7.

Wright, L.T. and Logan, M. (1939) Osseous changes associated with lymphogranuloma venereum. *Arch. Surg.*, **39**, 108–21.

Young, W.B. (1960) Actinomycosis with involvement of the vertebral column; Case report and review of the literature. *Clin. Radiol.*, **11**, 175–82.

ARTHRITIS 8

Anthony J. Freemont

8.1 JOINT INFLAMMATION

Joints enable bones to move relative to one another. In the simplest joints, such as the symphysis pubis, which permit only limited movement, the bone ends are separated by a band of fibrous tissue which tethers the bone ends together and yet gives a degree of flexibility. As the functional demands of the joint increase so too does the complexity of the joint structure up to the most highly sophisticated synovial joints, such as the knee.

Any joint may show inflammatory changes but, as might be predicted, the nature and effects of the inflammation vary with the structure of the joint because many of the characteristics of inflammation are dependent upon blood flow, endothelial cells, and substances brought to the tissue by the blood. Inflammation is essentially a tissue reaction dependent upon the presence of a blood supply. It necessarily follows that an avascular structure such as cartilage cannot be a primary site of inflammation, but vascular structures can, and of those the most susceptible are synovium and the insertions of capsule and ligament into bone (the entheses). The story of inflammation within joints is therefore centred about the vascularized tissues, but also encompasses the effects of inflammation on other tissues such as cartilage and synovial fluid. The two major groups of inflammatory joint diseases (the arthritides) are therefore the synovitides and the inflammatory enthesopathies. These two groups of disorders are typified by rheuma-toid disease and ankylosing spondylitis respectively.

8.1.1 THE NATURE OF INFLAMMATION WITHIN JOINTS

The arthritides are of two types: primary inflammatory disorders, which encompasses a group of diseases which, as yet, have no clearly defined cause, and secondary inflammatory disorders which do. Both the primary and secondary arthritides have acute and chronic variants, but as a broad general view the primary inflammatory disorders tend to be chronic and the secondary, acute.

Another way in which to consider the inflammatory arthropathies is on the basis of the nature of the inflammatory response elicited in each. Tables 8.1 and 8.2 both list the main inflammatory arthropathies and classify them.

Acute and chronic inflammatory reactions in joints are in most respects the same as those occurring in any site but are modified locally by the variable nature of the matrix. In order to understand the influence of the matrix on inflammation it is necessary to examine the nature and effects of inflammation on the various tissues that make up joints.

Diarthrodial (or synovial) joints have four major components: cartilage, synovial fluid, synovium and capsule (together with its thickenings, the ligaments). Non-synovial joints have different components but inflammatory lesions in these are usually very

Table 8.1 Inflammatory arthropathies

Primary inflammatory arthropathies
    Connective tissue diseases
        Rheumatoid disease
        Juvenile chronic arthritis
        Systemic lupus erythematosus
        Polyarteritis nodosa
        Behçet's disease
        Polymyalgia rheumatica
        Systemic sclerosis
    Seronegative spondylarthropathies: infection associated (reactive, postinfective, postvaccinial, rheumatic fever)
        Ankylosing spondylitis
        Psoriatic arthritis
        Inflammatory bowel disease

Secondary inflammatory arthropathies
    Infective
        Bacterial
        Viral
        Fungal
    Crystal-induced arthritis
        Monosodium urate
        Calcium pyrophosphate
        Hydroxyapatite

Table 8.2 Inflammatory arthropathies: classification

Diagnosis	Organism in joint	Antigen in joint	Circulating antibody
Crystal arthritis	−	−	−
Infective arthritis	+	+	+
Reactive arthritis	−	+	+
Rheumatoid disease	−	−	+

similar to those within the equivalent component of the synovial joint. For instance the intervertebral disc has end-plate cartilage very similar to articular cartilage, a nucleus pulposus which in consistency and structure is midway between articular cartilage and synovial fluid, and an annulus fibrosus which is directly analogous to a capsule; and fibrous joints could, for practical purposes, be considered as joints made up of capsule and ligament only.

The detailed structure of these components is discussed elsewhere but may be summarized as follows.

(a) Articular cartilage

Articular cartilage forms a hard cap to the bone end. It has three major components, cells (chondrocytes), type II collagen and proteoglycans, which together account for its physical properties. Type II collagen is a fibrillar protein with the main orientation of the fibrils such that, in practical terms, the fibres form arcades arising from, and anchoring the cartilage to, the underlying bone. The spaces between the collagen fibres are filled by proteoglycans which are strongly hydrophilic. This hydrophilic property causes the cartilage to swell, an expansion resisted by the collagen fibrils. These two opposing forces eventually reach an equilibrium. Providing this balance is retained the cartilage behaves normally; the disturbance of this equilibrium, either through altered chondrocyte synthesis of matrix or by matrix damage at the molecular level by endogenously or exogenously produced degradative enzymes, will result in abnormal cartilage function.

At its interface with bone the cartilage is calcified. It has been suggested that chondrocytes in this region are nonviable, but *in situ* hybridization studies have shown that this is not the case (Marles *et al.*, 1991). The mineral in this zone is hydroxyapatite.

(b)   Synovium

Synovium consists of a vascular, innervated connective tissue, usually fibrous tissue or fat, covered by an incomplete synoviocyte layer. There are two main types of synoviocyte, the macrophage-derived phagocytic type A cells remove debris from the joint and the type B cells, which are modified 'fibroblasts', synthesize components of synovial fluid, notably hyaluronans.

(c)   Capsule

The capsule is an enclosing layer of dense fibrous connective tissue that surrounds the joint and gives it stability. It is attached to both bones, but unlike the fibrous joint described above the capsule of the synovial joint attaches to the cortex of the bone shaft some little distance from the articular surfaces. The area where the capsule inserts into bone is known as the enthesis. In places the capsule is thickened to form ligaments which give added strength at sites of extreme load. This structure is not restricted to synovial joints but is found around other joints such as the intervertebral disc, and is effectively the sole component of fibrous joints.

(d)   Synovial fluid

Synovial fluid is best regarded as a semi-liquid, avascular, hypocellular, connective tissue. It consists of a transudate of serum from synovial vessels supplemented with hyaluronans synthesized by synoviocytes. Normal synovial fluid is a clear pale yellow, viscid substance. When acetic acid is added the hyaluronans and proteins form a white flocculant precipitate, the mucin clot.

There is a tendency to regard the joint as being multicompartmental; however, close examination shows that there are no distinct boundary layers within the joint (Figure 8.1). There is an incomplete layer of cells on the surface of synovium (Figure 8.2). Although each has an individual basement membrane they do not fuse to form a complete layer. There are even fewer cells on the surface of cartilage (Figure 8.3) and, again, no limiting membrane. There is therefore, potentially, free flow of molecules from synovium to synovial fluid and from synovial fluid into cartilage.

Although one might predict that free movement of molecules would mean that the pattern of inflammation within the different parts of the joint would be the same, and occur simultaneously, this is not the case. This apparent anomaly is almost certainly a function of the anatomy and physicochemical composition of the individual zones of the joint.

1.   Anatomy: that synovium is the most vascular of the components and contains innate inflammatory cells (mast cells and macrophage-derived synoviocytes), means that, of the different regions of the joint, it is in a privileged position from the point of view of inflammation.
2.   Physical structure: dense connective tissue matrices such as cartilage and capsular fibrous tissue can physically inhibit entry of cells. As cellular cytokines are essential to inflammation, denying cells access to the tissue significantly alters

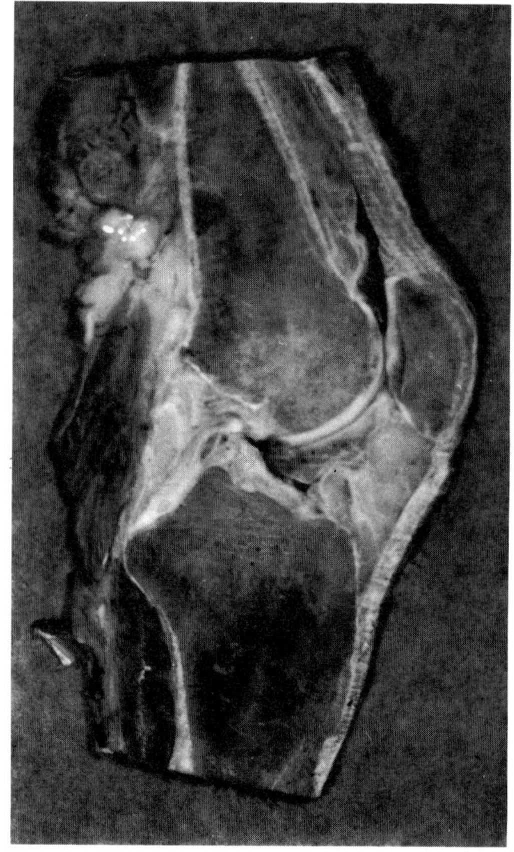

Figure 8.1 Sagittal section through the knee showing the major components of the joint.

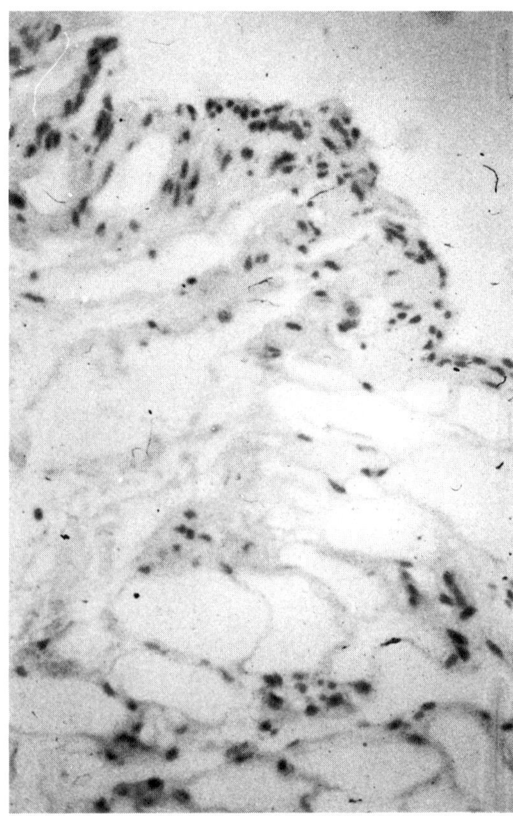

Figure 8.2 Normal synovium showing the incomplete surface layer of synoviocytes. (H and E ×70)

the inflammatory response.

3. Chemical structure: the molecular structure of individual components can impede entry of exogenous molecules. This is best demonstrated by cartilage which, with its strong negative charge, repels all other strongly negatively charged molecules.

As a consequence of this variation the inflammatory response in different areas of the joint, and its effect on the function of the joint, varies dramatically.

8.1.2 SYNOVIAL INFLAMMATION

The synovium is the main site within diarthrodial joints in which inflammation is initiated. The highly vascular tissue is the portal through which inflammatory cells gain access to the joint. The synovium is advantageously positioned to permit this to occur. It has an innate complement of fixed inflammatory cells – mast cells, macrophages, nerve cells and endothelial cells – and is therefore subject to inflammatory stimuli and capable of initiating inflammatory responses.

There are three aspects to cellular inflammation within synovium.

1. In all types of joint disease, but particularly the inflammatory arthropathies, there is recruitment of synoviocytes leading to a thickening of the synoviocyte layer from a single incomplete layer

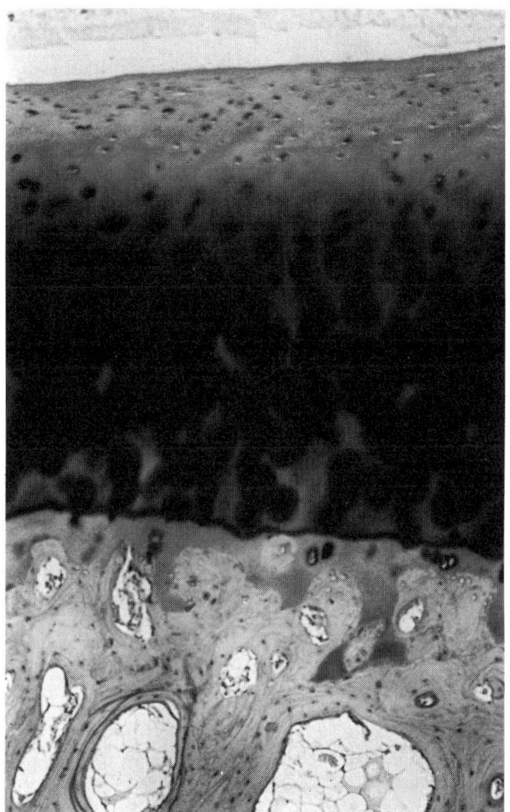

Figure 8.3 Normal cartilage. Note the absence of a surface layer of cells. (H and E ×40)

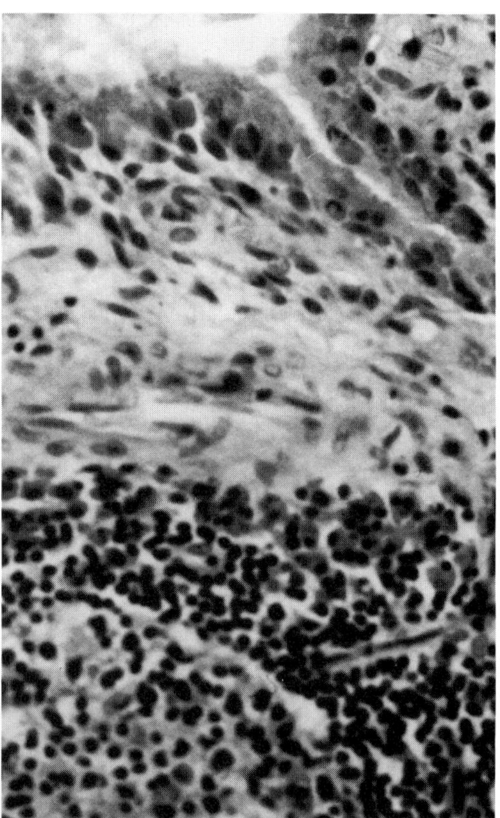

Figure 8.4 Rheumatoid synovium showing subintimal chronic inflammation with germinal centre formation and synoviocyte hypertrophy and hyperplasia. (H and E ×100)

to a multilayer of hypertrophied cells (Figure 8.4) (Henderson *et al.*, 1988). These are always active cells, capable of phagocytosis and cytokine synthesis. Often in inflammatory arthropathies it is not possible to recognize a synoviocyte layer because of heavy fibrin deposition on the synovial surface (Figure 8.5) (Gardner, 1972). The apparent loss of synoviocytes does not represent destruction of the cells but is a reflection of the fact that the interface between synovium and synovial fluid is a preferred site of cell accumulation. Fibrin deposition disturbs the physical and chemical nature of the interface and the synoviocytes migrate away from this, now alien, environment.

2. There is an influx of inflammatory cells into the synovium. Synovial inflammation, like all inflammation, is associated with changes in vascular function. There is one specific vascular change that occurs in most sites of chronic inflammation that was first described in synovium. This is the formation of high endothelial venules, vessels lined by distinct endothelial cells which specifically promote lymphocyte entry into the tissue through the synthesis of a unique range of molecules (Freemont, 1987). These vessels are seen normally only in lymphoid organs.

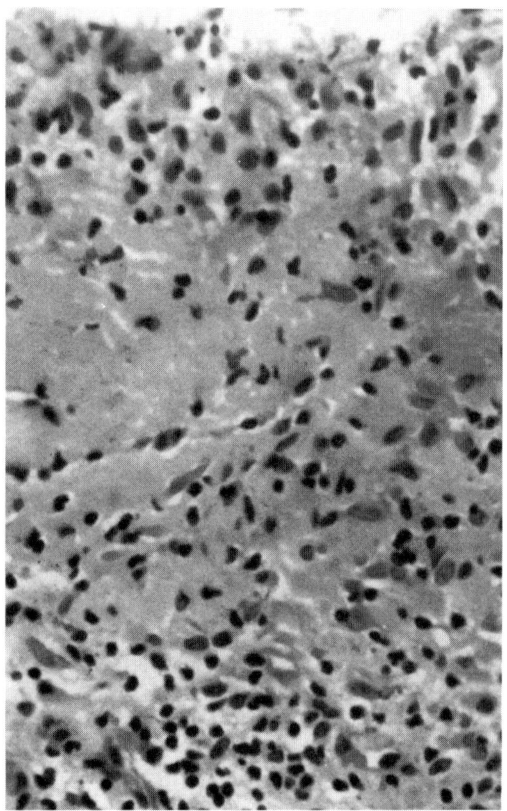

Figure 8.5 Surface fibrin. There is no synoviocyte layer. (H and E × 100)

in a significant minority the infiltrate consists predominantly of lymphocytes.

In addition to these major inflammatory events a number of associated phenomena also occur to and within the synovium that are worthy of note.

1. The synovium in certain inflammatory disorders contains numerous antigen presenting cells (Henderson and Edwards, 1987) and the overall pattern of chronic inflammation can come to resemble the structure of a lymph node.
2. The synovium is a site of sequestration of debris within the joint. Thus if there is damage to the articular surface, fragments of bone and cartilage can be identified either within the synoviocyte layer, or more commonly within the layer of supporting connective tissue immediately beneath the synoviocytes, sometimes called the subintima (Figure 8.6). This debris can cause inflammation itself by initiating a macrophage response. Nowadays with the increasing use of joint replacement surgery, extraneous debris can also be found within the joint, including polyethylene (the most commonly employed plastic for artificial articular surfaces), methylmethacrylate (a plastic resin used to cement the artificial components of the joint into place), metal (from the metal supports and articular surfaces of the prostheses), silicone (from small joint prostheses) and dacron and carbon fibre (used to manufacture artificial internal ligaments for joints such as the knee).

3. There is transmigration of inflammatory cells through synovium into the synovial fluid. Although in acute inflammation both the synovium and synovial fluid contain polymorphs, in chronic inflammatory synovitides the synovial infiltrate is predominantly lymphocytes and plasma cells but the synovial fluid contains mainly polymorphs in the majority of cases. This is the most obvious example of how the inflammatory response differs in different parts of the joint. The mechanism is not known, nor is it clear why in certain types of chronic arthritis (e.g. rheumatoid disease) the majority of synovial fluid specimens are predominantly polymorph rich whereas

(a) Synovial biopsy in diagnosis

Unfortunately for the histopathologist the pattern of synovial inflammation is rarely specific.

Aggregates of crystals within the subintima may give a clue to the origin of the arthropathy. Unfortunately crystals of mono-

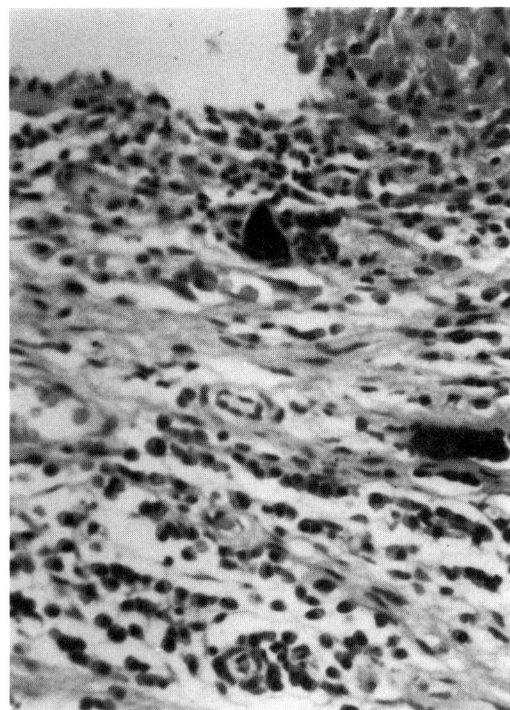

Figure 8.6 Joint debris within the synovium. (H and E ×80)

Figure 8.7 Aggregates of urate crystals within the synovium. (H and E ×70)

sodium urate are very soluble in water and are removed during tissue processing (unless the tissue has been fixed in ethanol). Fortunately the protein that surrounds the crystals remains and, in fixed tissue, the needle-like spaces left by the crystals are clearly seen, surrounded by the stained protein (Figure 8.7). Calcium pyrophosphate crystals are not as soluble in water but are dissolved by acid. Conventional stains (such as H and E) often have an acid base. To ensure the crystals remain in the tissue it is best to stain the sections with an alkaline stain, such as alkaline toluidine blue. Although the crystals do not stain they can be visualized because of their birefringence in polarized light (Figure 8.8). In H and E sections the presence of sites of accumulation of calcium pyrophosphate crystals can be recognized, even if the crystals have been removed, because the glyco-

proteins with which they aggregate are a blue–mauve colour.

Very rarely one might encounter synovial rheumatoid nodules typical of seropositive rheumatoid disease. It is safe to suggest that if an inflamed synovium contains bone or cartilage fragments there is a good chance that the patient has rheumatoid disease, which is the most common of the erosive arthritides (see below). It has also been shown that having more than 10% of the synovial plasma cells react positively for mu heavy chain, immunohistochemically, is specific for rheumatoid disease (Freemont and Rutley, 1986).

With these exceptions there are few specific histological features. However, some patterns of synovial cellular infiltrate are more suggestive of certain types of arthritis.

1. A predominantly polymorph infiltrate is typical of acute inflammatory disorders such as septic arthritis and crystal-induced disease. If there is tissue necrosis, septic arthritis is more likely.
2. Granulomatous inflammation is typical of tuberculosis, sarcoidosis and atypical mycobacterial infections, although the latter do not necessarily present with granulomata.
3. A chronic synovitis with a moderately heavy, diffuse polymorph infiltrate (5–10% of the inflammatory cells) in the subintima and synoviocyte layer is most commonly seen in disorders such as Reiter's and Behçet's disease.
4. A low-grade, predominantly lympho-plasmacytic infiltrate associated with extensive fibrosis in the subintima is the characteristic pattern of synovial involvement in systemic sclerosis.
5. Vasculitis sometimes can be seen in rheumatoid disease, systemic lupus erythematosus and polyarteritis nodosa.

8.1.3 CARTILAGE IN INFLAMMATION

The cartilage is not a primary site of inflammation. However, it is frequently involved in the inflammatory process. The main effects of inflammation are mediated through adjacent synovium and synovial fluid and by chondrocytes and exogenous inflammatory cells.

Chondrocytes not only synthesize the individual components of cartilage but also have the potential to synthesize matrix-digesting enzymes. This process is known as chondrocytic chondrolysis. Chondrocytic chondrolysis can be stimulated by inflammatory mediators such as IL-1 and mast cell products which can also induce changes in the normal synthesis of collagen. These inflammatory mediators are secreted into the synovial fluid from synovial cells (Wood *et al.*, 1985), and then enter cartilage by simple diffusion. As the weakened cartilage breaks down, the surface becomes roughened, exposing fibrillar matrix molecules to synovial fluid. These exposed molecules become sites of adherence for immunologically active molecules (Cooke *et al.*, 1980) which may

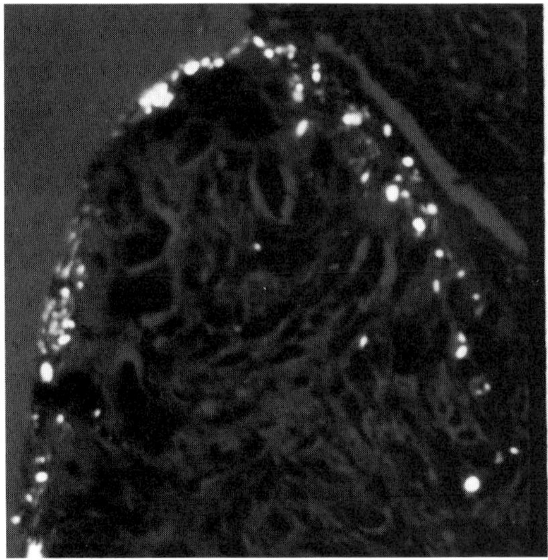
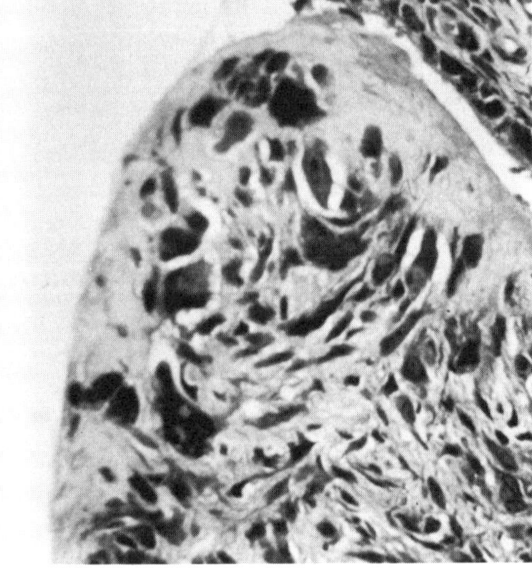

Figure 8.8 Calcium pyrophosphate crystals in the synovium. Polarizing microscopy on alkaline toluidine blue section (×100), alkaline toluidine blue (×100)

promote further immune-mediated tissue damage.

Direct cartilage damage occurs in severe acute inflammation usually with synovial fluid polymorph counts in excess of 50 000 cells/mm^3. These cells release lysosomal enzymes into the fluid which digest cartilage matrix, and lead to chondrocyte death. The cartilage is invaded by polymorphs and rapidly disintegrates due to enzymic digestion. This is most common in articular sepsis and can lead to complete loss of articular cartilage in as little as 24 hours.

Normal joints are lined throughout with synovium except over the cartilaginous articular surfaces. This state is probably maintained through two mechanisms: (a) loading of the surface of the articular cartilage and (b) the production by chondrocytes of substances that inhibit synovial growth. In rheumatoid disease this inhibition is lost and the inflamed synovium starts growing over the surface of the cartilage (Figure 8.9) (Shepherd, 1983). As it does so, cells, including polymorphs, macrophages, mast cells and endothelial cells, produce substances that degrade cartilage directly or stimulate

chondrocytic chondrolysis (Dodge and Poole, 1989). These same cells can produce cytokines which, where synovial tissues are reflected onto the periarticular bone, initiate osteoclastic bone resorption. This mechanism accounts for the erosions typical of rheumatoid disease.

8.1.4 SYNOVIAL FLUID IN INFLAMMATORY JOINT DISEASE

There have been a number of recent studies that have shown the significance of microscopic changes within the synovial fluid in the understanding of the mechanisms of joint disease and the diagnosis of arthritis (Revell, 1982; Freemont and Denton, 1985). This is a reflection of the diversity of cytological changes seen in this medium due to the different inflammatory processes that underlie the various clinical arthritic syndromes (Freemont and Denton, 1991).

In inflammatory arthritides the number of blood-derived nucleated inflammatory cells exceeds 1000/mm^3. In most inflammatory arthropathies the synovial fluid is characterized by a predominance of polymorphs, but

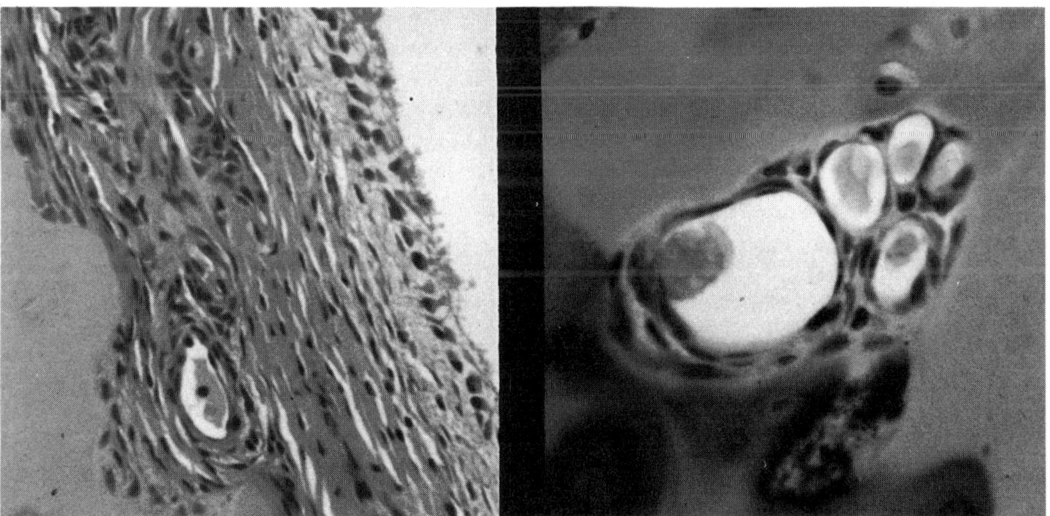

Figure 8.9 Pannus growing over and eroding cartilage. (H and E ×70)

other general patterns exist. In addition the presence of specific single cells have diagnostic significance.

8.1.5 THE GENERAL SYNOVIAL FLUID FEATURES OF THE PRIMARY INFLAMMATORY ARTHROPATHIES

In inflammatory arthropathies the fluid is typically pale yellow and translucent. There is poor mucin clot formation because the structure of the hyaluronans, either through degradation by digestive enzymes or because of atypical synthesis through the effects of inflammation on the function of type B synoviocytes, is altered (Cohen *et al.*, 1975). As a consequence the fluid is often of low viscosity.

Macroscopic particles consisting of small aggregates of fibrin and joint debris, are seen in most inflammatory synovial fluids.

Crystals are found in the crystal arthropathies but are rare in the primary inflammatory arthropathies. If present they are usually either an incidental finding, for instance it is not uncommon to find crystals of calcium pyrophosphate in an elderly patient who, in addition to the inflammatory disorder, has chondrocalcinosis in the aspirated joint; or evidence of articular surface damage, manifest by crystals of hydroxyapatite released from the bone or calcified cartilage either by direct inflammatory damage to the joint or as part of secondary osteoarthritis.

With a few notable exceptions the overall cytological pattern of synovial fluids in the inflammatory arthropathies falls into one of two groups:

1. Non-specific inflammatory: a pattern in which polymorphs predominate.
2. Seronegative: this pattern has a predominance of either macrophages or lymphocytes, or both, but always polymorphs account for less than 40% of the nucleated cells.

The first pattern is characteristic of all inflammatory arthropathies (hence its name) and is seen in approximately 80% of all aspirates. The second is rarely seen in rheumatoid disease but is encountered in a proportion of all other forms of arthritis. Both patterns may have more specific features superimposed upon them, and it is the recognition of these features that is the key to the use of synovial fluid cytoanalysis diagnostically. The different types of cell that are found in synovial fluid are discussed at length in several recent publications (Freemont and Denton, 1985, 1991; Freemont *et al.*, 1991) but there are a few that require mention here because of their significance.

(a) Mast cells

Mast cells are found in many arthropathies. The highest numbers (>1% of all nucleated cells) are seen in the seronegative spondylarthropathies (see below) and following joint trauma.

(b) Cytophagocytic mononuclear cells (CPM)

CPM are large mononuclear cells which contain phagocytosed neutrophils. The neutrophils are always apoptotic. The formation of CPM has become better understood in recent years.

The polymorph is a small 'time bomb' full of destructive substances. Once within synovial fluid there is a danger that the polymorphs might die and release their potent lysosomal products. Fortunately a mechanism exists for clearing them from the joint. First they undergo apoptosis, a process of cell death characterized by a burst of metabolic activity in the cell, a change in polymorph surface receptors and the active breakdown of DNA (Savill *et al.*, 1989). In this state the polymorph is unable to degranulate or respond to external stimuli. The apoptotic state lasts 24 h and is followed by autolysis and release of lysosomal enzymes. In the apoptotic state the neutrophil is particularly susceptible to phagocytosis by activated macrophages to form CPM (Figure 8.10). The whole process can be regarded as a way of neutralizing and then removing unwanted polymorphs from the synovial fluid and synovium. CPM are particularly prominent in the seronegative spondylarthropathies and juvenile chronic arthritis whereas apoptosis in the absence of CPM formation is virtually specific to rheumatoid disease. It is not clear why phagocytosis of apoptotic polymorphs is impaired in rheumatoid disease but this failure and subsequent release of lysosomal enzymes may well account for some of the tissue destruction in this disorder.

(c) Lymphocytes

The lymphocytes in various arthropathies have been characterized immunohistochemically. In rheumatoid disease, they are predominantly T lymphocytes with a CD4:CD8 ratio of 4:3, which compares with a peripheral blood ratio of 10:1. Moreover

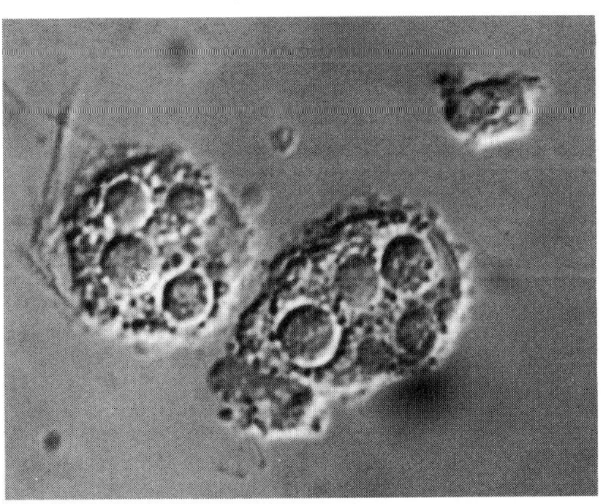

Figure 8.10 Cytophagocytic macrophages: the included apoptotic nuclear inclusions are clearly seen. (Unstained, Nomarski optics ✕500)

there is an increased expression of class II histocompatibility antigen by cells in rheumatoid fluid – a possible reflection of the numbers of activated CD8-positive cells.

(d) Ragocytes

Ragocytes were first described in rheumatoid disease. They are cells containing one or more distinct granules when viewed using phase contrast microscopy. The granules are believed to be phagocytosed immune complexes. These cells are found in greatest numbers in rheumatoid disease and septic arthritis.

(e) Reider cells

These cells bear a striking resemblance to the Reider cells seen in blood preparations; hence their name. Their most characteristic feature is the morphology of the nucleus: it is multi-lobed, the lobes usually showing symmetry about a pale, attenuated central region. Cells with this morphology may be either T lymphocytes or macrophages.

The peculiar nuclear morphology of Reider cells is a function of changed cytoskeletal and nuclear membrane function. This type of cellular dysfunction is typical of cells in rheumatoid synovial fluid.

8.1.6 CAPSULE IN INFLAMMATION

The capsule is not itself a common site of inflammation, but the insertion of capsule and certain ligaments into bone (the enthesis) is. The inflammatory lesion that occurs at this site is the enthesopathy (Ball, 1971). Inflammation, usually characterized by a lymphocytic infiltrate, leads to erosion at the insertion of the capsule or ligament into bone with local destruction of the bone and ligament (Figure 8.11). The inflammation is of remitting and relapsing type. When the inflammation dies down there is a reactive response in the connective tissues with formation of new bone and fibrous tissue. The reactive bone tends to be exuberant and not only fills the deficit in the bone, but also part of that in the ligament resulting in calcification in the capsule or ligament at the junction with bone (Figure 8.12). As the inflammation comes and goes this process cycles and gradually the whole ligament, particularly short ones such as the annulus fibrosus, may calcify completely, rendering the joint fixed or ankylosed (Figure 8.13).

The capsule of a joint may also be involved in an inflammatory process initiated elsewhere. For instance in rheumatoid

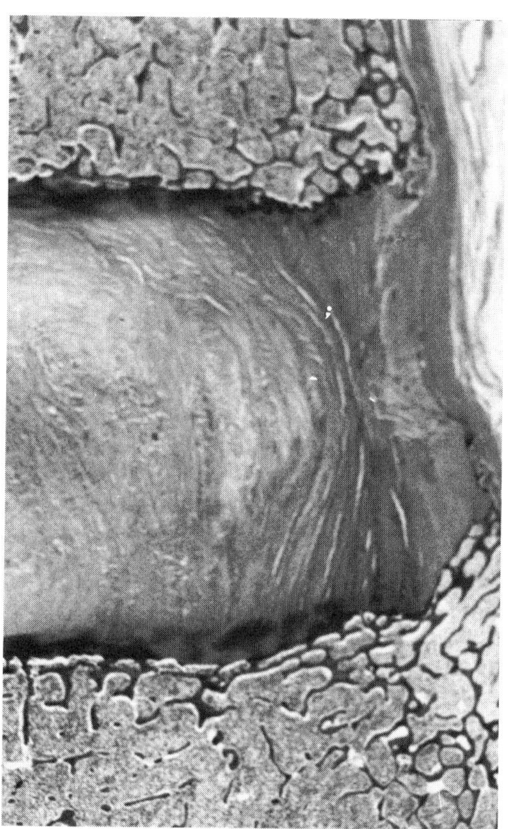

Figure 8.12 Ossification extending into the fibres of the annulus fibrosus. (H and E ×30)

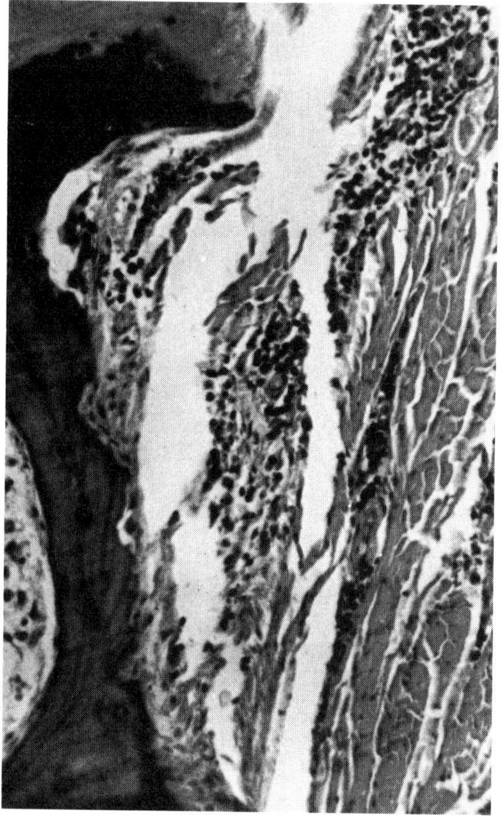

Figure 8.11 Erosion of the vertebral rim at the insertion of the annulus fibrosus in an acute erosive lesion of ankylosing spondylitis. (H and E ×100)

disease inflammation in the synovium tracks to the capsule and extends into it initiating, as it goes, inflammatory responses including angiogenesis. Both inflammation and angiogenesis lead to activation of collagenases locally within the capsule causing degradation of matrix, which weakens the tissue. Because of its structural role, damage to the capsule of this type increases joint instability (Gardner, 1972).

These general principles cover the overwhelming majority of situations in which inflammation occurs within a joint. In the rest of this chapter specific inflammatory arthropathies will be discussed in more detail.

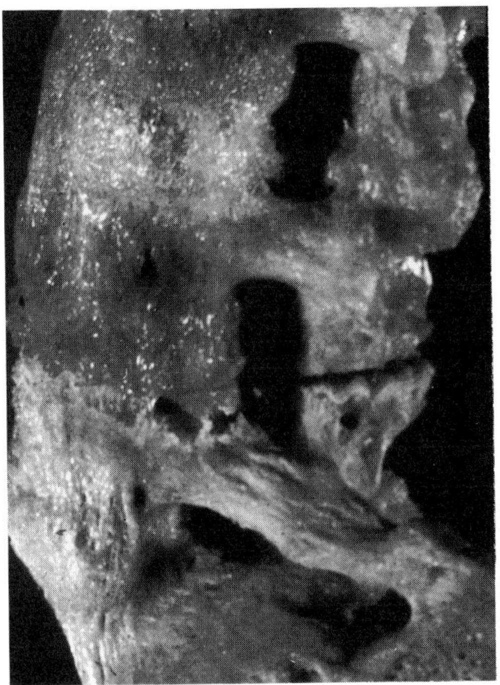

Figure 8.13 An ankylosed spine in ankylosing spondylitis.

8.2 SECONDARY INFLAMMATORY ARTHROPATHIES

8.2.1 INFECTIVE ARTHRITIS

An infectious agent may cause arthritis by one of two mechanisms.

1. The microorganism may gain access to the joint either from the blood or following a penetrating injury. The infecting agent then replicates within the synovium and synovial fluid and can be retrieved from either.

2. A microorganism may cause an acute or chronic arthritis without the intact organism being present within the joint. In this type of arthritis joint disease is associated with infection anywhere within the body, other than the involved joint; this may include another joint. The synovium and synovial fluid are sterile. Sometimes pro-

tein fragments of the organism (epitopes) can be identified immunochemically within the joint. It is now recognized that these epitopes are usually present within the joint bound to specific anti-epitope antibodies in the form of large molecular aggregates called immune complexes. These disorders represent a group of joint diseases known as reactive, infection-associated or postinfective arthropathies. They are discussed in more detail under the seronegative spondylarthropathies.

(a) True infective arthropathies

The infective agents may be bacteria, viruses or fungi. Most infectious agents enter the joint from the bloodstream. The synovial membrane is extremely vascular and it is believed that as a result the joint is capable of trapping circulating foreign particles including organisms. The infectious agents replicate in the synovium and synovial fluid. Here they are phagocytosed by synoviocytes and inflammatory cells. During phagocytosis, proteolytic enzymes are released from the phagocytes, causing further inflammation and tissue degradation. The nature and extent of the inflammation varies with the type of organism, but in all infections synoviocyte hyperplasia, progressive inflammation and granulation tissue formation will ensue. If the infection is untreated, cartilage erosion, destruction of the joint and fibrous or bony ankylosis may result.

The rapidity and final extent of joint tissue destruction depends on a number of factors, notably the nature of the organism and the degree of the cellular response. The greatest tissue destruction is seen in patients with acute pyogenic arthritis. In this type of arthritis the joint frequently contains more than 50 000 polymorphs/mm^3. Release of proteolytic enzymes from so many cells can cause rapid and complete cartilage destruction, if untreated.

Other bacteria, such as *Neisseria gonorrhoea*, which induce a lower grade polymorph response, cause less tissue destruction. Most viruses do not generally cause irreversible joint damage.

Host defence mechanisms also influence the development of infectious arthritis. If the host is immunocompromised by chronic illness or medication, the risk of septic arthritis is increased. This is particularly well illustrated in rheumatoid disease in which changes in innate immunity and the effects of drugs used in treatment make the patients more prone to infection. Severe joint damage such as occurs in neuropathic joints, articular trauma and surgery may also predispose to infection.

In any type of infectious arthritis the diagnosis is definitive only if the infectious agent is recovered from the synovial fluid or synovium. Synovial fluid analysis must always include microbiological investigation but microscopic analysis of suitably stained cytospin preparations has a high diagnostic yield in bacterial and fungal infections (87%) and although the organism is rarely seen, cytological features strongly suggestive of a viral arthritis are described which can assist in diagnosis.

(b) Specific forms of infective arthritis

(i) Non-gonococcal bacterial arthritis

Staphylococcus aureus, several *Streptococcus* species, and various Gram-negative bacilli are common causes of non-gonococcal bacterial arthritis in adults (Goldenberg and Cohen, 1976; Rosenthal *et al.*, 1980). In neonates, *Haemophilus influenzae* is one of the most common organisms infecting the joint (Ward and Atcheson, 1977). The most common source of bacteria in infected joints is an extra-articular infection. The causal agent is therefore the same at both sites.

Non-gonococcal bacterial arthritis generally affects a single joint, most commonly the weight-bearing joints and especially the knee. Most patients are usually either very young or very old. It is especially important to be aware that bacterial infection may be superimposed on debilitating illness such as rheumatoid disease so as not to mistake infective arthritis for a flare of the underlying joint disease thereby delaying diagnosis and appropriate therapy.

(ii) Gonococcal arthritis

Disseminated gonococcal infection generally occurs in young, healthy, sexually active patients. It has been estimated that it will occur in approximately 0.1–0.5% of patients who develop gonorrhoea (McCord *et al.*, 1977; Eisenstein and Masi, 1982). Women are more likely to develop the infection than men. Patterns of arthritis include migratory polyarthralgia, tenosynovitis, and polyarthritis. A purulent type of joint effusion is present in 30–50% of patients but organisms can be recovered in less than 50% of these. The synovium shows an acute inflammatory cell infiltrate. In most other patients scant transient sterile joint effusions or tenosynovitis of reactive type is the only articular manifestation of the disease.

(iii) Tuberculous arthritis

The frequency of tuberculosis of bones and joints has decreased over the past half century paralleling the decline in pulmonary tuberculosis. Tuberculous arthritis is relatively rare compared to other forms of extrapulmonary tuberculosis occurring in less than 1% of all patients with proven tuberculosis (Berney *et al.*, 1972; Wallace and Cohen, 1976). Tuberculous arthritis occurs at all ages. The most common sites are the intervertebral discs and large weight-bearing joints such as hips and knees. Predisposing factors such as local trauma, alcoholism, drug addiction, intra-articular corticosteroid injections or systemic illness are found in a large proportion of patients. Only a small number have overt miliary tuberculosis and less than half have a history of tuberculosis or radiological evidence of inactive disease. However, almost all have a positive tuberculin skin test. A negative skin reaction therefore militates strongly against the diagnosis of tuberculous arthritis. The synovium often shows a granulomatous infiltrate but sometimes the granulomata are hard to find.

The synovial fluid is usually of the non-specific pattern. Organisms may be retrieved from either site.

(iv) Fungal arthritis

Worldwide a significant proportion of chronic granulomatous arthritis is due to mycotic infection (Greenman *et al.*, 1975). Joint infection may result from systemic fungal infection or from penetrating cutaneous inoculation by plant material.

In Britain most patients developing fungal arthritis have some impairment of host defence mechanisms. Untreated fungal arthritis usually follows a chronic indolent course with progressive destruction of bone and joints (Bayer and Guze, 1978). Radiologically the disease cannot be distinguished from other forms of granulomatous arthritis.

Histologically the synovium contains a granulomatous infiltrate but because of immunosuppression the pattern of synovial fluid response is often unusual.

It may be difficult to identify fungi. Hyphal forms predominate in the synovium and yeast forms in the fluid. In all suspected cases a concentrated cytocentrifuge preparation of synovial fluid can be stained with an appropriate fluorescein-labelled lectin, which improves detection of fungal elements.

(v) Syphilitic arthritis

Congenital and acquired syphilitic infections are uncommon causes of joint disease (Gray and Philp, 1963; Reginato *et al.*, 1979). An effusion is frequently restricted to a single joint and may mimic a pyogenic infection. As most patients with inflamed joints have secondary syphilis, serological tests for syphilis are strongly positive. In tertiary syphilis a granulomatous arthritis is not uncommon. In both groups the synovial fluid contains a low-grade lymphocyte-rich inflammatory cell infiltrate.

(vi) Viral arthritis

Viral arthritis is of two types. The more common is a reactive type of disorder associated with a viral infection elsewhere in the body (Hyer and Gottleib, 1978). This is discussed with the seronegative spondylarthropathies. The second is also associated with extra-articular viral infection but the arthritis is due to colonization of the synovium by virus.

Direct infection is always associated with viraemia and tends to be a mono- or asymmetrical oligoarthropathy. It typically affects young people in winter months and is usually associated with upper respiratory tract infections, influenza and rubella (Alpert *et al.*, 1971; Thompson *et al.*, 1973).

The reactive pattern is more common and tends to be of sudden onset and a symmetrical polyarthropathy. This is particularly common in patients with viral meningitis and hepatitis and following inoculation with live attenuated viruses.

(vii) Lyme disease

Lyme disease is named after the Connecticut town where it was first recognized (Kay *et al.*, 1988). It is a systemic inflammatory disorder recognized clinically by the skin lesion erythema chronicum migrans. The disease is caused by a spirochaete which can be identified in synovium and rarely in synovial fluid.

Articular symptoms of migratory polyarthritis and longer episodes of inflammation in large joints such as the knee occur in

50% of patients. The synovium and synovial fluid findings are similar to rheumatoid disease.

8.2.2 CRYSTAL-INDUCED ARTHROPATHIES

The three most common crystals encountered in synovial fluid are those of monosodium urate, calcium pyrophosphate dihydrate and a salt of calcium and phosphorus which by X-ray diffraction approximates most closely to hydroxyapatite. Other crystals, such as calcium oxalate, have also been described.

A very great deal has been written about the identification and significance of crystals, and there are a number of excellent texts which go further and deeper into the subject than is possible here (McCarty, 1974; Dieppe *et al.*, 1979; Dieppe and Calvert, 1983). There are also numerous excellent dissertations on polarizing microscopy which is the technique employed most frequently to demonstrate and identify crystals (Peterson and Kuhn, 1965; Gatter, 1974; Gordon *et al.*, 1989). Such discussions, although interesting and of academic importance, are of limited practical value. Much more important is a series of simple rules, which if applied, will permit most crystals to be identified readily.

To identify crystals and understand their significance it is essential to note: crystal size and shape; the degree of birefringence and its sign; and the cellular tissue reaction.

1. Crystal shape: crystals are commonly needle-shaped (e.g. monosodium urate), elongated rhomboids (e.g. calcium pyrophosphate), large rhomboidal plates (e.g. cholesterol), fine amorphous granules (e.g. hydroxyapatite), pyramidal polygons (e.g. calcium oxalate), and dumb-bell shaped (e.g. calcium oxalate), but many other possible forms exist. As a general rule any one type of crystal tends to have a predictable structure, but unfortunately this is not always the case.

2. Birefringence: in addition to its shape a crystal can be identified by its birefringence. For this some sort of polarizing attachment is required on the diagnostic microscope, preferably one in which a first order red compensator can be interposed between the polarizer and the analyser. Polarization makes crystals much more easily detectable. The compensator is important in differentiating between different types of crystal, particularly those of monosodium urate and calcium pyrophosphate dihydrate. A correctly orientated compensator gives a red background to the polarized image on which crystals appear either yellow or blue. Elongated crystals with their axes in one direction will appear yellow when viewed in polarized light with the compensator in place, and those whose long axis is at right angles to that of the yellow crystals will be blue. This is true of all suitable crystals. Round crystals and crystalloids (notably liquid crystals, starch granules and urate and hydroxyapatite beach balls) will be segmentally yellow and blue.

    The value of the compensator comes in the identification of crystals. The direction in which the molecular lattice of the crystal refracts light relative to its long axis determines if the crystal is described as being positively or negatively birefringent. Although strictly inaccurate, crystals that have a positive sign and are birefringent are colloquially said to be positively birefringent, and those with a negative sign, negatively birefringent. If two crystals, one positively birefringent (e.g. calcium pyrophosphate) and the other negatively birefringent (e.g. monosodium urate) are orientated with their long axes parallel to one another in the same microscope field, then one would appear blue and the other yellow.

Using these criteria the common crystals have the following characteristics:

- Monosodium urate: needle shaped, strongly negatively birefringent crystals (Figure 8.14). These crystals are water soluble. They either aggregate as collections in tissue, called tophi, or are free in synovial fluid as single crystals.
- Calcium pyrophosphate dihydrate: these crystals are usually more rhomboidal than the needle-shaped crystals of monosodium urate (Figure 8.15). They are positively birefringent, and soluble in weak acids (including acid dye solutions). One of the peculiar properties of crystals of calcium pyrophosphate is that the crystal structure can sometimes be built up with the long axis of the crystal running in the 'wrong direction', so that it appears to be negatively birefringent. Rarely, L-shaped crystals may form in which the two arms of the crystal are the same colour when viewed in polarized light with an interposed quarter wave plate.
- Hydroxyapatite: crystals of hydroxyapatite do not have a crystal structure that allows them to exhibit birefringence. With the condenser diaphragm partially closed, and using the highest powers of the optical microscope, these crystals appear as fine granules within synovial fluid. They are much more clearly demonstrated by

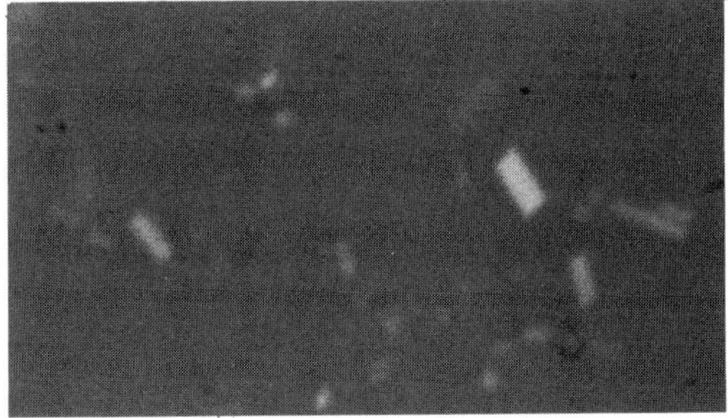

Figure 8.15 Crystals of calcium pyrophosphate viewed between crossed polarizers with an interposed quarter wave plate. (×1000)

Nomarski phase optics which tend to accentuate granular structures (Figure 8.16). Like all salts of calcium and phosphorus, these crystals will react with alizarin red S to form an alizarin–calcium complex which is both birefringent and red. The crystals will stain black with von Kossa's stain.

Occasionally in destructive periarthritis crystals of hydroxyapatite form spherical aggregates known as spherulites.

Hydroxyapatite within joints is usually derived from calcified cartilage or subchondral bone. Its presence within the synovial fluid and synovium indicates

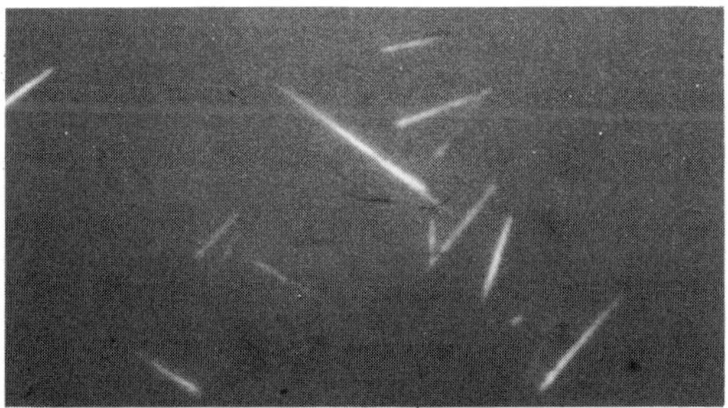

Figure 8.14 Crystals of monosodium urate viewed between crossed polarizers with an interposed quarter wave plate. (×1000)

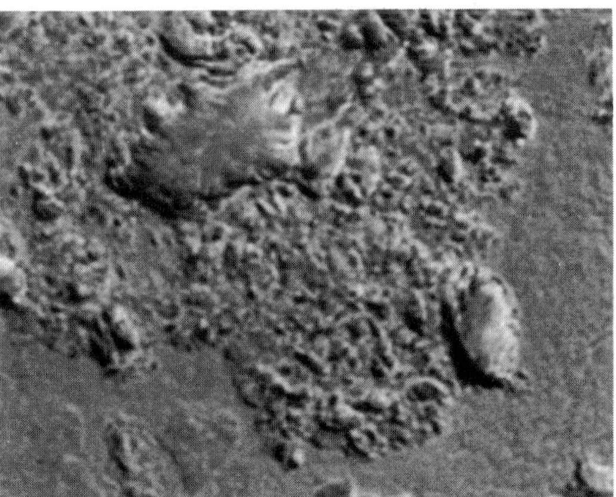

Figure 8.16 Crystals of hydroxyapatite. Nomarski phase optics. (×1500)

destruction of articular cartilage with exposure and wear of deeper, calcified structures. In inflammatory arthropathies hydroxyapatite is seen most commonly in rheumatoid disease and occasionally in psoriatic arthritis and ankylosing spondylitis.

- Lipid: lipid of many different sortes (cholesterol, trigylcerides, phospholipid, neutral fats) – either free or as part of lipoproteins – have been described within synovial fluid but not synovium. In smears of fresh synovial fluid lipids appear as spherical or elongated crystals, fatty acids and triglycerides, flat rectangular plates (cholesterol) and amorphous aggregates (depot steroids). They also exhibit differential solubility in hydrocarbon solvents.

Intra-articular lipids may be derived from blood or from fatty tissues adjacent to or within the joint (Freemont and Denton, 1988). Blood-derived lipids are evidence of recent and/or old intra-articular haemorrhage. Cholesterol is found in any blind-ended sac, and is evidence of long-standing arthropathy. Crystals of free fatty acid (Figure 8.17) are found within fat globules in the synovial fluid of patients immediately following intra-articular trauma. Globules of lipid are an almost universal finding in the traumatic arthropathies.

(a)   Crystal-induced disease

There are three main crystals of pathogenic significance – monosodium urate, calcium pyrophosphate dihydrate and hydroxyapatite. The first two are associated with an acute inflammatory arthritis and a chronic destructive arthropathy the last with a destructive periarthritis. Monosodium urate crystals cause the acute inflammatory arthritis gout, but also a destructive arthropathy secondary to tophus formation in the synovium and periarticular structures (Dieppe and Calvert, 1983). Calcium pyrophosphate

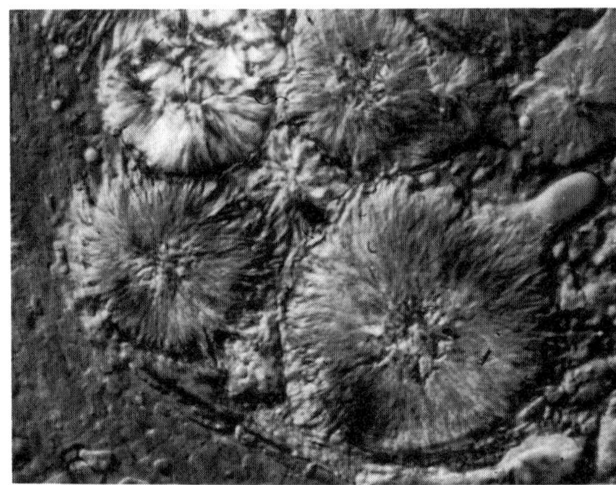

Figure 8.17 Lipid crystals in lipid droplets. (Nomarski phase ×1000)

crystals cause an acute arthritis similar to gout and a destructive arthropathy similar to osteoarthritis. Hydroxyapatite causes an inflammatory periarthritis which may progress to a destructive arthritis.

(i)   Gout

Gout is one of the oldest recorded forms of arthritis and is characterized by recurrent episodes of acute inflammation due to the release of microcrystals of monosodium urate into the joint cavity. The disease represents a complication of prolonged hyperuricaemia although it is occasionally found in patients with a normal serum urate (Boss and Seegmiller, 1979). Uric acid is a breakdown product of nucleic acid metabolism and the crystals are relatively insoluble in body fluids. Higher concentrations, such as seen in hyperuricaemia, are the result of formation of a supersaturated solution. Supersaturation can be reversed leading to a tendency for crystal deposition into the synovium, synovial fluid, cartilage and other body tissues.

The serum urate concentration is continuously varying and throughout the population represents the result of a multifactorial inheritance modified by numerous other factors including diet, body weight, haemoglobin concentration, social class and life style. Investigation has shown that 5% of adults may have hyperuricaemia.

Uric acid is formed by oxidation of purines which may orignate exogenously or endogenously. About two-thirds of the daily production of uric acid is excreted in the urine and most of the rest via the gastrointestinal tract. In most cases hyperuricaemia is the result of either an increase in uric acid production or decreased renal excretion. Hyperuricaemia may be primary, secondary or idiopathic. Primary hyperuricaemia includes X-linked enzyme defects such as congenital hypoxanthine-guanine phosphoribosyltransferase (an enzyme important in purine metabolism) deficiency and polygenic, otherwise undefined, molecular defects which lead to overproduction or underexcretion of monosodium urate. Secondary hyperuricaemia refers to cases that develop in the course of another disease or as a consequence of drug treatment. Increased uric acid production occurs in diseases with increased nucleic acid turnover and include myelo- and lymphoproliferative disorders and haemolytic anaemias as well as other haematological diseases. Decreased renal excretion can occur in renal insufficiency, treatment with most diuretic agents, lead intoxication and various types of organic poisoning. Idiopathic hyperuricaemia refers to cases where a raised serum urate is found in the absence of gout and with no other association. Gout is characterized by recurrent episodes of acute joint inflammation. Gout is a disease chiefly of middle-aged and elderly men and postmenopausal women, with the peak incidence in the fourth and fifth decades. It is the most common form of inflammatory arthritis in men over 40 years of age.

Most episodes of gout are monarticular and tend to affect the lower limbs, especially the first metatarsophalangeal joint. Initially attacks occur at intervals of months or years but may become more frequent with the passage of time when other joints become involved.

The acute attacks are believed to be due to acute precipitation of crystals within the synovial fluid. The crystals become coated with plasma proteins, including immunoglobulin, and are then phagocytosed by polymorphs. The immunoglobulin coating may improve phagocytosis through polymorph recognition of the Fc fragments. It has been postulated that following phagolysosome formation the surface proteins are removed, unmasking the crystals' ability to disrupt cell membranes. Thus ingestion of urate crystals is followed by rapid polymorph degranulation and disintegration with release of powerful intracellular digestive enzymes into the joint. Macrophages recruited in response to the crystals will phagocytose crystals and as a result will produce eicosanoids directly and collagenases indirectly which contribute to the joint damage.

Progression of the disease leads to the development of permanent swelling and joint deformity as the result of deposition of aggregates of urate crystals within articular and pararticular structures. These aggregates are known as tophi and may occur at a distance from joints in organs such as the skin and kidneys.

Para-articular cysts and bursae may also be involved in gout. Olecranon bursitis develops with notable frequency in patients with gout.

The synovium contains an acute inflammatory infiltrate, and the synovial fluid contains negatively birefringent crystals and a high cell count with a preponderance of polymorphs.

(ii)   Calcium pyrophosphate deposition disease

The crystals deposited within the joint in this group of conditions are crystals of calcium pyrophosphate dihydrate (CPPD).

There are essentially three conditions associated with CPPD crystals within the joint –

chondrocalcinosis; acute pseudogout and a destructive arthropathy very similar to osteoarthritis (McCarty, 1979).

The term chondrocalcinosis is often used to describe the radiological appearance of calcified cartilage (either hyaline or fibrocartilage), although CPPD can be deposited in synovium and in periarticular sites such as capsule, tendon, etc. This condition is often symptomless (Zitan and Sitaj, 1963). It is very common particularly in the elderly and it is not surprising therefore that crystals of CPPD are seen in synovial fluid specimens from joints affected by other disorders both inflammatory and non-inflammatory.

Acute pseudogout is the term given to an acute inflammatory arthropathy, which is, as its name might suggest, clinically similar to gout (McCarty *et al.*, 1962). Unlike gout the disease tends to affect the knees most commonly. Provocation of attacks by surgery or severe intercurrent illness occurs in gout and pseudogout.

Nearly 50% of all patients with CPPD deposition disease experience a progressive destruction of multiple large joints. The knees are the most frequently affected, followed in order of frequency by the wrists, hips, shoulders and ankles. Although there is some overlap with primary generalized (nodal) osteoarthritis the absence of small joint involvement or Heberden's node formation allows the two to be distinguished.

(iii) Hydroxyapatite crystal disease

Hydroxyapatite is the normal form of calcium phosphate salt within the bone and sites of physiological and pathological calcification elsewhere within the body.

Hydroxyapatite crystals are causally implicated in syndromes of periarticular calcium deposition including the calcific periarthritis around the shoulder that leads to frozen shoulder, and acute and chronic erosive arthropathies (Alwan *et al.*, 1989), including disorders such as Milwaukee shoulder (Hal-

verson *et al.*, 1981). Diseases associated with hydroxyapatite deposition arthritis include scleroderma, hyperparathyroidism, neurological disorders, tumoral calcinosis and dermatomyositis. Hydroxyapatite deposition is also seen in patients receiving haemodialysis and chronic ambulatory peritoneal dialysis (CAPD). In addition crystals are frequently seen in osteoarthritic joints and joints of patients with erosive inflammatory joint disease such as rheumatoid disease.

Individual hydroxyapatite crystals are so small that they can only be visualized clearly with the electron microscope. They are generally rod shaped with a diameter of approximately 1 µm. Crystals frequently aggregate in the joint fluid to form microspherulites between 10 and 50 µm in diameter. They can be seen by phase microscopy in synovial fluid, and in synovium following von Kossa stain.

8.3 PRIMARY INFLAMMATORY ARTHROPATHIES

8.3.1 RHEUMATOID ARTHRITIS

Rheumatoid arthritis, or more correctly rheumatoid disease, is the most common of the primary inflammatory arthropathies.

Rheumatoid disease is a symmetrical polyarthropathy predominantly of the small joints of the hands, feet and neck. It affects women more often than men and the age of onset varies from 16 to 71 (Short *et al.*, 1957). Radiologically erosive changes are seen within affected joints.

The majority of patients with this disease have specific antibodies within their blood and synovial fluid which are known as rheumatoid factors (Torrigiani and Roitt, 1967). Both within the blood and within the synovial fluid, rheumatoid factors bind to other host immunoglobulins (acting as antigens), to form immune complexes.

Patients with significant titres of rheumatoid factor in their serum are said to be seropositive. The diagnosis of rheumatoid disease is not based entirely on this finding but rather on the presence of specific permutations of a group of clinical and laboratory features defined by the American Rheumatism Association (The Rheumatoid Arthritis Subcommittee of the ARA, 1988). Rheumatoid factor is only one of the diagnostic criteria. As only a proportion of the total criteria need be present in an individual patient to make the diagnosis of rheumatoid disease it follows that there are patients who have an acceptable number of clinical characteristics for the diagnosis of rheumatoid disease to be made, but who do not have detectable rheumatoid factor. These patients are said to have seronegative rheumatoid disease. Patients with seronegative rheumatoid disease may acquire rheumatoid factor (seroconvert) and it is also recognized that seropositive patients may become seronegative. The disease tends to persist as a chronic arthritis with remission and exacerbations. The joint destruction caused by the inflammatory process predisposes to the development of osteoarthritis.

In addition to the joint symptoms and signs, patients with rheumatoid disease may develop extra-articular abnormalities (Hollingsworth, 1968), that include vasculitis, polyserositis, fibrosing alveolitis, tenosynovitis, bursitis, muscle wasting, scleritis, rheumatoid nodules (which are areas of collagen necrosis surrounded by macrophages found most commonly in the subcutaneous tissue over pressure points, but may also be found in the lung, heart, sclera and other organs) (Figure 8.18), neuropathies, lymphadenopathy (which may mimic a lymphoma), splenomegaly (Felty's syndrome is hypersplenism associated with rheumatoid disease), anaemia, osteoporosis (most commonly juxta-articular) and amyloidosis.

Infective arthritis is more common in patients with rheumatoid disease than in

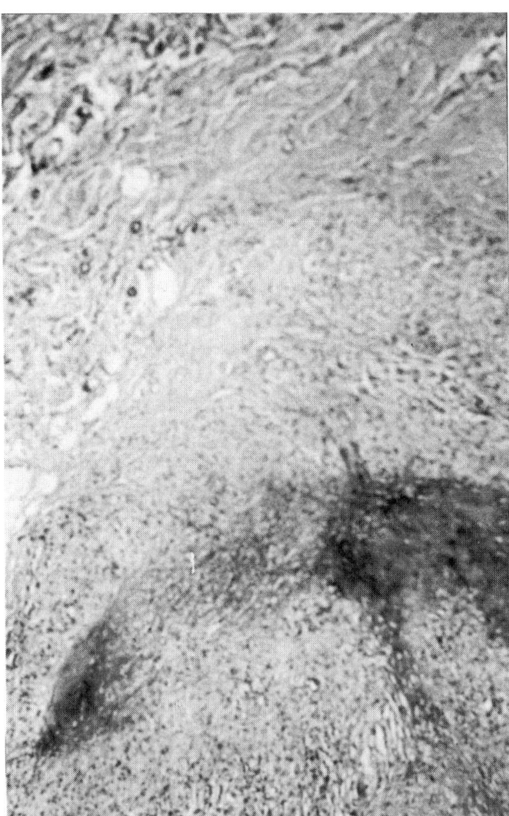

Figure 8.18 Section of a rheumatoid nodule. (H and E ×50)

the general population, both for reasons of constitution and drug therapy. Any specimen from a patient with rheumatoid disease taking immunosuppressive agents should be regarded as potentially infected. This has implications for laboratory staff and patient management. The degree of inflammation may be less than in a non-immunosuppressed patient and specific stains for organisms should be undertaken.

Non-immunosuppressed rheumatoid patients are also at a higher risk than the general population of developing intra-articular infection. A careful search for infective organisms is therefore indicated in all rheumatoid patients in whom there is a clinical suspicion of infection.

(a) Secondary osteoarthritis

Destructive inflammatory arthropathies predispose to the development of secondary osteoarthritis. If this develops and the inflammatory arthritis disappears (burnt-out rheumatoid disease) the joint has only features of osteoarthritis. All intermediate states exist.

(b) Crystals and rheumatoid disease

Hydroxyapatite from the damaged articular surface is a common finding in rheumatoid disease, as is the presence of crystals of calcium pyrophosphate dihydrate in elderly patients with relatively quiescent disease. It is said that gout and rheumatoid disease do not co-exist. Although not entirely true it is an exceptionally rare occurrence.

(c) Periarticular cysts and bursae

There is a tendency in rheumatoid disease for the development of periarticular cysts and bursae. These may become lined by a structure identical to rheumatoid synovium and contain rheumatoid 'synovial fluid'. With disease chronicity these cysts tend to become distended with thick, turbid fluid heavily laden with crystals of cholesterol and cholesterol ester (Freemont, 1992).

(d) Pathology of rheumatoid disease

The synovium in rheumatoid disease is thickened and thrown into finger-like processes, or villi (Figure 8.19). The surface is covered either by fibrin or multilayered hypertrophied synoviocytes. The cause of the synovial thickening varies with the activity of the disease (Figure 8.20). Oedema and inflammatory cells typify the active disease, whereas fibrosis is more common as the disease burns itself out.

As described earlier the synovium grows over and destroys cartilage and the inflam-

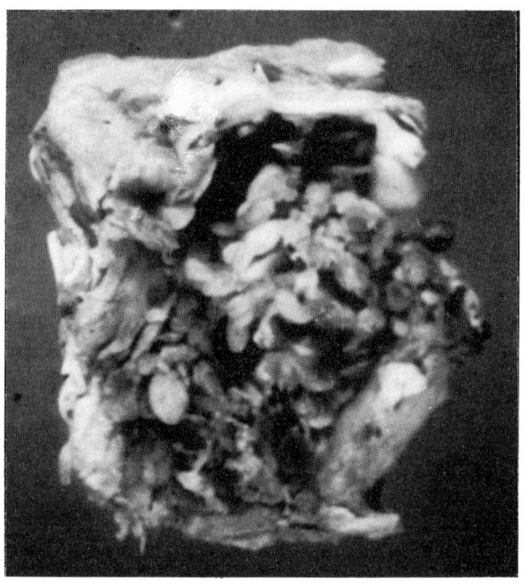

Figure 8.19 Macroscopic view of villous rheumatoid synovium.

mation within the synovium may initiate capsule and bone damage (Figure 8.21). The synovium may contain fragments of cartilage and bone.

Because there seems to be a fault in cytophagocytosis apoptotic polymorphs are found in the synovial fluid but no CPM. Failure to clear polymorphs may explain part at least of the joint destruction. Peculiar cell forms also typify rheumatoid synovial fluid, as a consequence of altered cytoskeleton and cellular membrane function. In addition, in seropositive rheumatoid disease synovial fluid ragocytes are common.

8.3.2 SERONEGATIVE SPONDYLARTHROPATHIES

This is an interesting group of clinically related inflammatory oligo- and polyarthropathies. Moll *et al.* (1986) have listed the disorders now included in, and the criteria for membership of, the seronegative spondylarthropathies.

The disorders are:

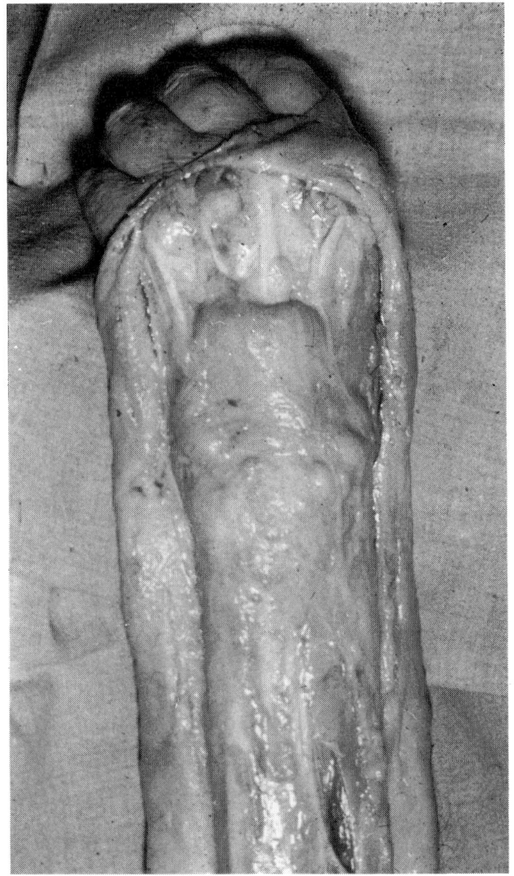

Figure 8.20 Thickened extensor tenosynovium in a patient with rheumatoid disease.

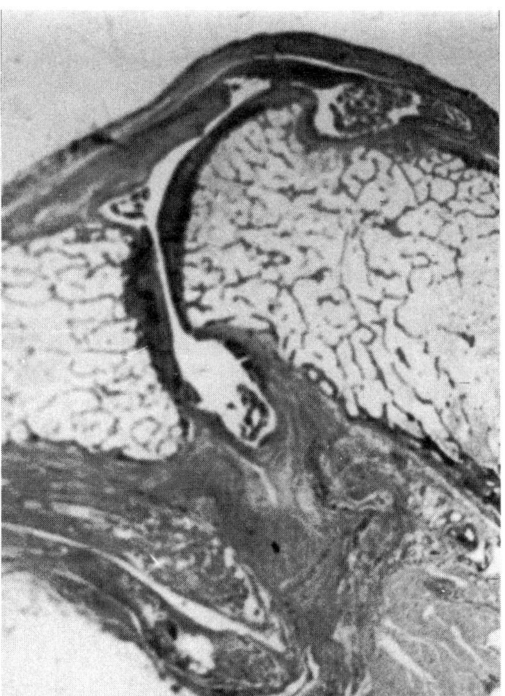

Figure 8.21 Section through a subluxed interphalangeal joint in a patient with rheumatoid disease. Damage to the capsule has resulted in joint laxity. (Masson's trichrome ×1)

- Uncomplicated ankylosing spondylitis
- Psoriatic arthritis
- Reiter's disease
- Ulcerative colitis
- Crohn's disease
- Whipple's disease
- Reactive and post-infective arthritis

The criteria for a disorder to be included in this group are:

1. Absence of rheumatoid factor in the serum – hence the name 'seronegative'.
2. Absence of subcutaneous ('rheumatoid') nodules – these nodules have an almost invariable association with seropositiv-

ity and are pathognomonic of rheumatoid disease. This criterion strengthens the point that these diseases are distinct from rheumatoid disease.
3. Inflammatory peripheral arthropathy (may be asymmetrical) – the increase in synovial fluid in these joints is often sufficient to allow aspiration.
4. Radiological sacroilitis with or without radiological erosion and/or new bone formation at the margins of vertebral bodies – all these disorders are characterized by an inflammatory enthesopathy at sites of ligamentous insertions into bone, most particularly the insertions of the ligaments around intervertebral discs and the sacro-iliac joints. It is this feature that gives the group the name 'spondylarthritis'.

5. Evidence of clinical overlap between members of the group – the clinical syndromes of each of the disorders in the group share characteristics with one or more of the others. Sometimes the patient presents with a set of symptoms and signs that do not conform to a single syndrome but have features of two or more. This degree of overlap is not uncommon in the seronegative spondylarthropathies.

6. Tendency to familial aggregation – the disorders in this group have a familial tendency and some families contain related individuals who have different disorders in the group.

7. Significant association with HLA-B27 antigen – there is a genetic predisposition to develop this group of disorders that corresponds to having the HLA-B27 allotype. In addition, an environmental element, usually inflammation of a body surface, is needed to trigger the disorder. There are also an increasing number of reports suggesting that local trauma could precipitate the arthritis in susceptible individuals.

Two types of joint disease occur in the seronegative spondylarthropathies, an inflammatory enthesopathy and a peripheral inflammatory arthritis.

The enthesopathy is as described earlier with inflammatory bone destruction followed by exuberant bone repair and ossification within the fibres of the annulus fibrosis, forming a lesion referred to as a syndesmophyte. Finally, the annulus ossifies completely and the joint, now immobilized, is resorbed and replaced by bone. There is then a danger of fracture (Figure 8.22).

The synovium in the peripheral arthropathy is similar to rheumatoid disease but the inflammation is much less, and there is little if any associated cartilage, bone and capsular destruction.

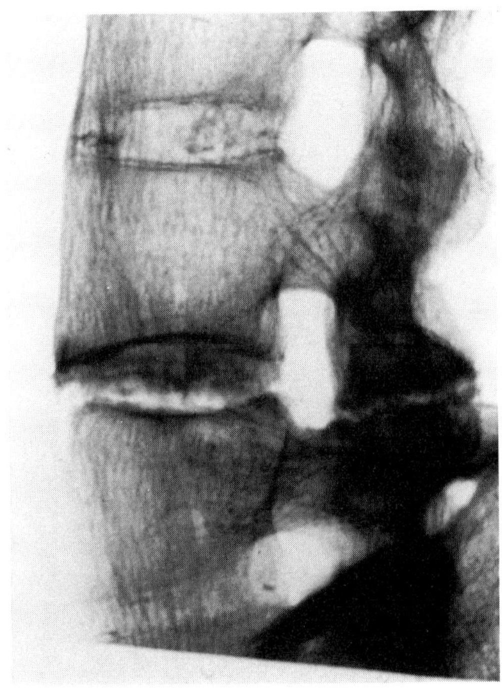

Figure 8.22 Radiograph showing fracture through an ankylosed intervertebral joint.

The synovial fluid typically contains CPM and mast cells.

(a) Ankylosing spondylitis

Ankylosing spondylitis is a disorder characterized by inflammation at entheses. The enthesopathy of ankylosing spondylitis is most common within the axial skeleton, although it can occur at other ligamentary and capsular insertions (Freemont, 1988). A third of patients develop a peripheral arthropathy.

(b) Reactive arthritis

Reactive arthritis is a form of inflammatory oligo- or polyarthropathy that follows an infection, usually in the genitourinary or gastrointestinal tracts (Ford, 1986). Until recently, no organism or antigen had been identified within the joint. However, a sub-group of patients with reactive arthritis associated with genitourinary tract infection, so-called sexually acquired reactive arthritis or SARA (Wordsworth *et al.*, 1990), have now been shown to have chlamydial antigen within the synovial fluid, but not chlamydial DNA, suggesting that this reactive arthritis is due to microbial antigens, presumably in the form of immune complexes, rather than whole intra-articular organisms. These findings open the way towards demonstrating the reactive arthritides, as a group, to be due to immune complex deposition in which the antigenic component of the complex is an epitope of an infective organism.

(c)   Reiter's disease

Reiter's disease can be considered as a form of reactive arthritis in which the patient also has conjunctivitis and urethritis (Keat, 1986). The disease usually follows a bout of non-gonococcal urethritis. Men are more commonly affected with the peak age of onset between 20 and 40. The disorder is an asymmetrical polyarthropathy particularly affecting the joints of the lower limb.

(d)   Psoriatic arthritis

Psoriasis is a skin disorder of variable severity. Some patients have only barely noticeable scaly patches within the hairline or over the elbows and knees as the outward manifestation of this disease. About 10% of patients with psoriasis develop peripheral arthritis most commonly in the finger joint (Baker *et al.*, 1963).

There are various clinical patterns to the arthritis, and some lead to swelling of joints sufficiently large to enable synovial fluid to be aspirated. An arthropathy of this type can occur independently of the degree of skin involvement, thus the first manifestation of psoriasis may be the arthropathy, and only subsequent careful examination of the patient unmasks the presence of skin disease. Because of the prognostic and management implications the possibility that joint disease might precede clinically overt skin diseases emphasizes the importance of the early recognition of psoriatic arthritis and, in particular, of distinguishing it from other types of inflammatory arthropathy.

Very similar remarks could be made for the peripheral arthropathy of ankylosing spondylitis and inflammatory bowel disease, as in both of these disorders, arthritis may precede the onset of the typical clinical syndrome.

(e)   Inflammatory bowel disease

It has long been recognized that patients with Crohn's disease, ulcerative colitis and Whipples's disease have an associated arthropathy (Haslock and Wright, 1973). This is identical to the other seronegative spondylarthropathies.

(f)   Post-infectious arthritis

In addition to the recognized seronegative spondylarthropathies the microscopic features of this group of disorders are also found following infections such as meningococcal meningitis, hepatitis (A and B), upper respiratory tract infections and, in patients with rheumatoid disease, viral pneumonia. It may also follow vaccination, particularly with rubella vaccine.

(g)   Poncet's disease (tuberculous rheumatism)

Poncet's disease is a polyarthritis associated with visceral tuberculosis, in which there is no evidence of bacteriological involvement of the joints themselves (Isaacs and Sturrock, 1974). In Poncet's disease the synovial fluid and synovium is indistinguishable from that of the seronegative spondylarthropathies and post-viral infections.

8.3.3 JUVENILE ARTHRITIS

Joint disease is not rare in childhood. There is, however, a specific group of inflammatory arthritides beginning in childhood labelled variously as 'juvenile chronic arthritis', 'juvenile rheumatoid arthritis' or 'juvenile arthritis'. The multiplicity of terminology reflects a lack of consensus among clinicians internationally, rather than significant differences in the pattern of disease (Wood, 1978). It is perhaps best to classify chronic inflammatory arthropathies in childhood into three groups (i) juvenile chronic arthritis, (ii) juvenile onset rheumatoid disease and (iii) others. The one unifying factor in these disease groups is that they begin before the child's sixteenth birthday.

(i) *Juvenile chronic arthritis*

Juvenile chronic arthritis is characterized by chronic synovial inflammation of unknown cause. It is a relatively common chronic childhood disease and the most common of the three groups in the preferred classification (80–85% of cases) (Holt, 1990).

In general the disease may begin at any age during childhood and girls are more often affected than boys. There are, however, specific subgroups and these have rather more restricted age and sex associations. Affected joints are swollen, stiff, limited in movement and tender. Juvenile chronic arthritis is subclassified on the basis of the number of joints involved and the presence or absence of systemic features, particularly fever and a rash, during the first six months after onset. The three subgroups of juvenile chronic arthritis are systemic, polyarticular and pauciarticular.

Systemic type of juvenile chronic arthritis
Systemic onset disease accounts for approximately 20% of cases. In this subgroup the sex ratio is approximately one. The disease can start at any age in childhood. Clinical charac-teristics include high intermittent fever, rash, polyserositis, lymphadenopathy, hepatomegaly, splenomegaly, leucocytosis and anaemia.

Arthritis is often only a minor part of the syndrome, affects few or many joints and tends to be of variable severity. Less than a quarter of the patients progress to chronic arthritis.

Polyarticular disease Polyarticular (five or more joints involved) onset disease, without the systemic features of the systemic type occurs in approximately 60% of children with juvenile chronic arthritis. There is a female preponderance and the disease most commonly starts before the age of 5 years. It causes a symmetrical polyarthritis affecting larger limb joints more commonly than the small joints of the hands. Approximately 20% progress to a chronic debilitating arthritis.

Pauciarticular juvenile chronic arthritis Pauciarticular onset juvenile chronic arthritis accounts for 20% of cases of juvenile chronic arthritis. Such children have arthritis affecting only a few joints (four or less) within the first 6 months of onset of symptoms.

Several subgroups of pauciarticular juvenile chronic arthritis are described. One subgroup is characterized by early childhood onset (i.e. <6 years of age) and female preponderance. These patients often have positive titres of antinuclear antibodies, but are rheumatoid factor negative. Usually the disease involves the knees, ankles and elbows, the hips are spared and sacroilitis is not seen. Up to 50% of these patients develop iridocyclitis.

A second subgroup of patients with pauciarticular disease is characterized by older age of onset and strong male preponderance. These patients are generally negative for rheumatoid factor and antinuclear antibodies but more than half have the HLA-B27 phenotype and often a family history of spondylarthropathy. Arthritis affects predominantly the joints of the lower limb. Because of the difficulty of diagnosing sacroilitis in developing sacro-iliac joints it is not possible to say if this is a variant of typical ankylosing spondylitis, but many patients have an enthesopathy and a variable proportion will develop the features of ankylosing spondylitis in early adulthood.

The synovial pathology is that of a nonspecific chronic synovitis. The synovial fluid resembles a seronegative spondylarthropathy.

(ii) Juvenile onset rheumatoid disease

In Britain this disease is widely regarded as an entity separate from juvenile chronic arthritis. It affects, predominantly, girls more than 14 years old. It is a syndrome identical in every way to adult rheumatoid disease.

In the USA, juvenile chronic arthritis and juvenile onset rheumatoid disease are considered together as juvenile rheumatoid arthritis. This classification has the same three subdivisions as juvenile chronic arthritis, but juvenile onset rheumatoid arthritis is incorporated into the polyarticular group, sometimes as a seropositive (high serum titres of rheumatoid factor) variant.

The original term for the most dramatic cases of chronic arthritis in childhood was Still's disease named after G. F. Still who described the condition in 1897. All the systemic type patients and some from the other two subgroups of juvenile chronic arthritis would have been included under this diagnosis.

(iii) Other arthropathies

A number of conditions that cause musculoskeletal disease in children may mimic juvenile chronic arthritis. These include other autoimmume diseases, joint infections, para-articular primary and secondary malignancies, inherited and congenital disorders of bone and cartilage, trauma and avascular bone necrosis.

Two diseases require special note – juvenile ankylosing spondylitis and juvenile systemic lupus erythematosus.

Juvenile ankylosing spondylitis Ankylosing spondylitis developing in childhood may pose diagnostic difficulties. In many children the disease starts in peripheral joints, mimicking pauciarticular juvenile chronic arthritis. Often there is no evidence of sacroilitis for weeks, months or, rarely, years after the onset of peripheral joint symptoms. Even if symptomatic it is often difficult to confirm radiologically because of continuing growth of the joint. The patients are usually male, older than 8 years and may have a family history of spondylitis. The diagnosis is made by identifying new bone formation in the outer fibres of the annuli fibrosi of the intervertebral discs radiologically.

Juvenile systemic lupus erythematosus Systemic lupus erythematosus in childhood, as in adult life, is a multisystem disease with diverse and varied manifestations associated with the presence, in patients' serum, of antibodies to double-stranded DNA. The most common presentation in childhood is with fever, arthralgia, arthritis and rash. The joint disease may be migratory or symmetrical but is rarely deforming. About three quarters of children have laboratory evidence of renal disease at the time of presentation.

The synovium and synovial fluid are no different from those of their adult counterparts.

8.3.4 SYSTEMIC LUPUS ERYTHEMATOSUS

Systemic lupus erythematosus (SLE) is a complex, serious, multisystem, autoimmune disorder with an appreciable mortality at 5 years (approximately 25%) (Ropes, 1976). It affects women far more commonly than men and has its peak age of onset between 20 and 40 years. Immune complex deposition on vascular and epidermal basement membranes is a feature of the disease. Arthritis is only one of its manifestations but occurs in 90% of patients and may precede the onset of other systemic features by many years. The arthritis is polyarticular and symmetrical, affecting the finger joints, wrists, knees, ankles and shoulders. Unfortunately for the pathologist the arthritis is rarely biopsied and the joints seldom aspirated.

The synovial inflammation has no specific features but it may be associated with aggregates of smudged nuclei. These artefacts, although common, are not diagnostic, but afford a small pointer that sometimes impresses if correct.

The synovial fluid is often of a seronegative type with large numbers of LE cells. Unfortunately these are even less specific when found in synovial fluid than in blood.

8.3.5 LYMPHOCYTIC ARTHRITIS

In 1980 Utsinger *et al.* described an acute relapsing oligoarthropathy of young adult women which did not appear to conform to any known arthritic syndrome. The disorder is characterized by a high proportion of lymphocytes (>90%) within the synovial fluid. Of these >95% are T lymphocytes. Each episode is of short duration, rarely lasting more than a month or so and the intervals between the bouts of acute painful inflammatory joint disease may be as much as 10 years. All the patients are seronegative for rheumatoid factor.

The nature of the disease in unknown. It appears to be self-limiting.

8.3.6 POLYARTERITIS NODOSA

This is an uncommon multisystem disorder characterized by vasculitis, predominantly of arteries (Travers *et al.*, 1979). The disease may present at any age and affects men more commonly than women. Approximately three-quarters present with generalized joint pain and one quarter have an arthritis at some stage during the disease. In addition the disease affects the kidneys (renal failure or the nephrotic syndrome), peripheral nerves (peripheral neuropathy), heart (myocardial infarction and heart failure), lung disease (bronchitis or pneumonia) and skin (necrosis, nodules).

Polyarteritis nodosa carries a poor prognosis even on treatment.

8.3.7 POLYMYALGIA RHEUMATICA

This is a relatively common syndrome characterized by pain and stiffness around the shoulder and pelvic girdle (Chuang *et al.*, 1982). The importance of the disease is that it is associated with giant cell arteritis, which in the elderly most commonly affects the arteries of the head (temporal arteritis) and may cause severe pain and blindness.

Women are affected more often than men. The onset of polymyalgia rheumatica is typically after the age of 60 years.

Joints are always affected, most commonly sternoclavicular, acromioclavicular, shoulder, cervical spine, hips and knees, and effusion is common. There is mild synovial inflammation only.

8.3.8 SYSTEMIC SCLEROSIS

This is the systemic variant of a group of disorders characterized by dermal fibrosis and known collectively as scleroderma (Rodnan and Medsger, 1968). There are two main variants of systemic sclerosis, progressive systemic sclerosis (PSS), in which the bowel, kidney, arteries, heart and lung may become involved in the disease process, and the CREST syndrome (Calcinosis, Raynaud's phenomenon, Oesophageal disease, Sclerodactyly and Telangiectasia) in which the only systemic involvement is of arteries and the oesophagus. In addition to the systemic features already mentioned, an arthropathy is seen in most cases and often manifests itself early in the disease. Systemic sclerosis is more common in women, has a peak age of onset in the fourth decade and affects the joints of the fingers most commonly.

In systemic sclerosis the synovium is fibrotic and the synovial fluid has a low inflammatory cell count (1000–4000 cells/mm^3) and a predominance of macrophages.

8.3.9 BEHÇETS DISEASE

This is a rare disorder of unknown aetiology characterized by the triad of oral ulceration, iritis and genital ulceration (Shimizu *et al.*, 1979). Men are affected more commonly than women and the peak incidence is in the third and fourth decades. Arthritis occurs in half of all cases and is polyarticular with the knee being the most commonly involved joint. The synovial pathology is notable for the number of polymorphs in the synoviocyte layer and superficial subintima.

8.3.10 SJOGREN'S SYNDROME

Sjögren's syndrome is a rare disorder characterized by diminished lacrimal and salivary gland secretion (sicca complex). The original syndrome consisted of a triad of dry eyes, dry mouth and rheumatoid disease but it is now accepted that other 'connective tissue diseases' such as systemic lupus erythematosus and systemic sclerosis can replace rheumatoid disease in the triad and indeed that the sicca complex can exist as a primary pathological entity (Primary Sjögren's syndrome) (Mason *et al.*, 1973). The lack of exocrine gland secretions in Sjögren's syndrome is due to destruction of glandular acini by a chronic inflammatory cell infiltrate which in rare cases may progress to lymphoid malignancy.

The disease affects women predominantly and the mean age at diagnosis is 50 years.

Arthritis occurs in a high proportion of patients, usually as part of the associated connective tissue disease, but also in the primary form of the disease.

The synovium and synovial fluid findings are non-specific.

8.3.11 MIXED CONNECTIVE TISSUE DISEASE

It is not uncommon for patients to present with a 'connective tissue disease' that does not conform exactly to a defined syndrome. Sometimes the syndrome is incomplete, but equally the patient's presentation may incorporate features considered specific for more than one syndrome (Sharp *et al.*, 1972). Although there is some controversy as to how mixed connective tissue disease should be classified it can, for simplicity's sake, be regarded as one of these overlap syndromes, with features of systemic lupus erythematosus, systemic sclerosis and an inflammatory condition of muscle known as polymyositis. It is much less common than systemic lupus erythematosus, affects women much more commonly than men, and occurs most commonly in young adults.

It must be reiterated that most of these primary inflammatory arthropathies cannot be distinguished on synovial biopsy or synovial fluid analysis other than in the ways specified above. Even then it is rare that a certain diagnosis can be made.

REFERENCES

Alpert, E., Isselbacher, K.J. and Schur, P.H. (1971) The pathogenesis of arthritis associated with viral hepatitis. *N. Engl. J. Med.*, **285**, 185–9.

Alwan, W.H., Dieppe, P.A., Elson, C.J. *et al.* (1989) Hydroxyapatite and urate crystal induced cytokine release by macrophages. *Ann. Rheum. Dis.*, **48**, 476–82.

Baker, H., Golding, D.N. and Thompson, M. (1963) Psoriasis and arthritis. *Ann. Intern. Med.*, **58**, 909–25.

Ball, J. (1971) Enthesopathy of rheumatoid and

ankylosing spondylitis. *Ann. Rheum. Dis.*, **30**, 213–23.

Bayer, A.S. and Guze, L.B. (1978) Fungal arthritis. *Semin. Arthritis Rheum.*, **8**, 142–50.

Berney, S., Goldstein, M. and Bishko, F. (1972) Clinical and diagnostic features of tuberculous arthritis. *Am. J. Med.*, **53**, 36–42.

Boss, G.R. and Seegmiller, J.E. (1979) Hyperuricaemia and gout: classification, complications and management. *N. Engl. J. Med.*, **300**, 1459–68.

Chuang, T.Y., Hunder, G.G., Ilstrup, D.M. *et al.* (1982) Polymyalgia rheumatica: a ten year epidemiologic and clinical study. *Ann. Intern Med.*, **97**, 672–80.

Cohen, A.S., Brandt, K.D. and Krey, P.R. (1975) In *Laboratory Diagnostic Procedures in the Rheumatic Diseases* 2nd edn (ed. A.S. Cohen). Little Brown, Boston.

Cook, T.D.V., Bennett, E.L. and Ohno, O. (1980) The deposition of immunoglobulins and complement components in osteoarthritic cartilage. *Int. Orthop.*, **4**, 211–7.

Dieppe, P.A. and Calvert, P. (1983) *Crystals and Joint Disease*. Chapman & Hall, London.

Dieppe, P.A., Crocker, P.R., Corke, C.F. *et al.* (1979) Synovial fluid crystals. *Q. J. Med.*, **192**, 533–53.

Dodge, G.R. and Poole, A.R. (1989) Immunohistochemical detection and immunochemical analysis of type II collagen degradation in human normal, rheumatoid and osteoarthritic articular cartilage and explants of bovine articular cartilage cultured with interleukin 1. *J. Clin. Invest.*, **83**, 647–61.

Eisenstein, B.J. and Masi, A.T. (1982) Disseminated gonococcal infection and gonococcal arthritis. *Semin. Arthritis Rheum.*, **10**, 155–72.

Ford, D.K. (1986) Reactive arthritis: a viewpoint rather than a review. *Clin. Rheum. Dis.*, **12**, 389–400.

Freemont, A.J. (1987) Molecules controlling lymphocyte-endothelial interactions in lymph nodes are produced in vessels of inflamed synovium. *Ann. Rheum. Dis.*, **46**, 924–8.

Freemont, A.J. (1988) The pathology of ankylosing spondylitis. In *New Clinical Applications – Rheumatology – Ankylosing spondylitis* (eds D.C. Calabro and W. Carson Dick), MTP Press, Lancaster, pp. 1–22.

Freemont, A.J. (1992) Clinical conundrum – what is the significance of synovial fluid lipid crystals in a patient with an isolated monoarthritis? *Br. J. Rheumatol.*, **31**, 183.

Freemont, A.J. and Denton, J. (1985) The disease distribution of synovial fluid mast cells and cytophagocytic mononuclear cells in inflammatory arthritis. *Ann. Rheum. Dis.*, **44**, 312–5.

Freemont, A.J. and Denton, J. (1991) *Atlas of Synovial Fluid Cytopathology*. Kluwer Academic Publishers, Dordrecht, The Netherlands.

Freemont, A.J. and Rutley, C. (1986) The distribution of immunoglobulin heavy chains in diseased synovia. *J. Clin. Pathol.*, **39**, 731–5.

Freemont, A.J., Denton, J., Chuck, A. *et al.* (1991) Diagnostic value of synovial fluid microscopy: a reassessment and a rationalisation. *Ann. Rheum. Dis.*, **50**, 101–7.

Gardner, D.L. (1972) *Pathology of Rheumatoid Arthritis*. Edward Arnold, London.

Gatter, R.A. (1974) The compensated polarized light microscope in clinical rheumatology. *Arthritis Rheum.*, **17**, 253–5.

Goldenberg, D.L. and Cohen, A.S. (1976) Acute infectious arthritis: a review of patients with non-gonococcal joint infections. *Am. J. Med.*, **60**, 369–76.

Gordon, C., Swan, A. and Dieppe, P.A. (1989) Detection of crystals in synovial fluid by light microscopy: Sensitivity and reliability. *Ann. Rheum. Dis.*, **48**, 737–42.

Gray, M. and Philp, T. (1963) Syphilitic arthritis: diagnostic problems with special reference to congenital syphilis. *Ann. Rheum. Dis.*, **22**, 19–25.

Greenman, R., Becker, J., Campbell, R. *et al.* (1975) Coccidioidal arthritis of the knee. *Arch. Intern. Med.*, **135**, 526–30.

Halverson, P.B., Cheung, H.S., McCarty, D.J. *et al.* (1981) 'Milwaukee shoulder' – association of microspheroids containing hydroxyapatite crystals, active collagenase, and neutral protease with rotator cuff defects. II. Synovial fluid studies. *Arthritis Rheum.*, **24**, 474–83.

Haslock, I. and Wright, V. (1973) The arthritis associated with intestinal disease. *Bull. Rheum. Dis.*, **24**, 750–4.

Henderson, B. and Edwards, J.C.W. (1987) *The Synovial Lining in Health and Disease*. Chapman & Hall, London.

Henderson, B., Revell, P.A. and Edwards, J.C.W. (1988) Synovial lining cell hyperplasia in rheumatoid arthritis; dogma and fact. *Ann. Rheum. Dis.*, **47**, 348–9.

Hollingsworth, J.W. (1968) *Local and Systemic Complications of Rheumatoid Arthritis*. W. Saunders, Philadelphia.

Holt, P.J.L. (1990) The classification of juvenile chronic arthritis. *Clin. Exp. Rheumatol.*, **8**, 331–3.

Hyer, F.H. and Gottleib, N.L. (1978) Rheumatic disorders associated with viral infections. *Semin. Arthritis Rheum.*, **8**, 17–31.

Isaacs, A.J. and Sturrock, R.D. (1974) Poncet's disease – Fact or fiction? *Tubercle*, **55**, 125–42.

Kay, J., Eichenfield, A.H., Athreya, B.H. *et al.* (1988) Synovial fluid eosinophilia in Lyme disease. *Arthritis Rheum.*, **31**, 1384–9.

Keat, A. (1986) Reiter's syndrome and reactive arthritis. *Reports on Rheumatic Diseases.* Series 2. The Arthritis and Rheumatism Council, London.

Marles, P.J., Hoyland, J.A., Parkinson, R. *et al.* (1991) Demonstration of variation in chondrocyte activity in different zones of articular cartilage – an assessment of the value of in-situ hybridisation. *Int. J. Exp. Pathol.*, **72**, 171–82.

Mason, A.M., Gumpel, J.M. and Golding, P.L. (1995) Sjögren's syndrome: a clinical review. *Semin. Arthritis Rheum.*, **2**, 301–31.

McCarty, D.J. (1974) Crystal deposition joint disease. *Ann. Rev. Med.*, **25**, 279–88.

McCarty, D.J. (1979) Calcium pyrophosphate crystal deposition disease: pseudogout, articular chondrocalcinosis. *Arthritis and Allied Conditions* (ed. D.J. McCarty), Lea and Febiger, Philadelphia, pp. 1276–99.

McCarty, D.J., Kohn, N.N. and Faires, J.S. (1962) The significance of calcium phosphate crystals in the synovial fluid of arthritic patients: the 'pseudogout syndrome'. *Ann. Intern. Med.*, **56**, 711–37.

McCord, W.C., Nies, K.M. and Louie, J.S. (1977) Acute venereal arthritis. *Arch. Intern. Med.*, **137**, 858–63.

Moll, J.M.H., Haslock, I. and Wright, V. (1986) Seronegative spondarthritides. In *Copeman's Textbook of the Rheumatic Diseases.* Churchill Livingstone, Edinburgh.

Peterson, B.J. and Kuhn, R.J. (1965) Optical characterisation of crystals in tissue. Cystine and calcium oxalate monohydrate. *Am. J. Clin. Pathol.*, **43**, 401–8.

Reginato, A.J., Schumacher, H.R., Jimenez, S. *et al.* (1979) Synovitis in secondary syphilis. Clinical, light, and electron microscopic studies. *Arthritis Rheum.*, **22**, 170–6.

Revell, P.A. (1982) The value of synovial fluid analysis. *Curr. Top. Pathol.*, **71**, 1–24.

Rodnan, G.P. and Medsger, T.A. (1968) The rheumatic manifestations of progressive systemic sclerosis (scleroderma). *Clin. Orthop.*, **57**, 81–93.

Ropes, M.W. (1976) *Systemic Lupus Erythematosus.* Harvard University Press, Cambridge.

Rosenthal, J., Bole, G. and Robinson, W.B. (1980) Acute non-gonococcal infectious arthritis. *Arthritis Rheum.*, **23**, 889–97.

Savill, J.S., Wyllie, A.H., Henson, J.E. *et al.* (1989) Macrophage phagocytosis of aging neutrophils in inflammation. *J. Clin. Invest.*, **83**, 865–75.

Sharp, G.C., Irwin, W.S., Tan, E.M. *et al.* (1972) Mixed connective tissue disease – an apparently distinct rheumatic disease syndrome associated with a specific antibody to an extractable nuclear antigen. *Am. J. Med.*, **52**, 148–59.

Shepherd, H. (1983) An update of mechanisms of cartilage destruction in rheumatoid arthritis. *Aust. N. Z. J. Med.*, **13**, 195–200.

Shimizu, T., Ehrlich, G.E., Inaba, G. *et al.* (1979) Behçet's disease (Behçet's syndrome). *Semin. Arthritis Rheum.*, **8**, 223–60.

Short, C.L., Bauer, W. and Reynolds, W.S. (1957) *Rheumatoid Arthritis.* Harvard University Press, Cambridge, MA.

The Rheumatoid Arthritis Criteria Subcommittee of the Diagnostic and Therapeutic Criteria Committee of the American Rheumatism Association (18 authors). (1988) The American Rheumatism Association 1987 revised criteria for the classification of rheumatoid arthritis. *Arthritis Rheum.*, **31**, 315–24.

Thompson, G.R., Weiss, J.J., Shillis, J.L. *et al.* (1973) Intermittent arthritis following rubella vaccination. *Am. J. Dis. Child.*, **125**, 526–30.

Torrigiani, G. and Roitt, I.M. (1967) Antiglobulin factors in sera from patients with rheumatoid arthritis and normal subjects. *Ann. Rheum. Dis.*, **26**, 334–40.

Travers, R.L., Allison, D.J., Brettle, R.P. *et al.* (1979) Polyarteritis nodosa: a clinical and angiographic analysis of 17 cases. *Semin. Arthritis Rheum.*, **8**, 184–99.

Utsinger, P.D., Hicks, J.T. and McLaughlin, G.E. (1980) Chronic lymphocytic arthritis [abstract]. *Arthritis Rheum.*, **23**, 758.

Wallace, R. and Cohen, A.S. (1976) Tuberculous arthritis. *Am. J. Med.*, **61**, 277–9.

Ward, J.R. and Atcheson, S.G. (1977) Infectious arthritis. *Med. Clin. North Am.*, **61**, 313–24.

Wood, D.D., Ihrie, E.J. and Hammerman, D. (1985) Release of interleukin-1 from human synovial tissue in vitro. *Arthritis Rheum.*, **28**, 853–62.

Wood, P.H.N. (1978) Nomenclature and classification of arthritis in children. In *The Care of Rheumatic Chidren* (ed. E. Munthe), EULAR Publishers, Basel.

Wordsworth, B.P., Hughes, R.A., Allan, I. *et al.*, (1990) Chlamydial DNA is absent from the joints of patients with sexually acquired reactive arthritis. *Br. J. Rheumatol.*, **29**, 208–10.

Zitan, D. and Sitaj, S. (1963) Articular chondrocalcinosis. *Ann. Rheumat. Dis.*, **22**, 142–70.

8.4   NON-INFLAMMATORY ARTHROPATHIES

By far the most common of the diseases of joints are the non-inflammatory arthropathies; it is said that every person over the age of 20 has one or more joints affected.

The non-inflammatory arthropathies can be divided into three major groups.

1.   Osteoarthritis
2.   Traumatic arthritis
3.   Others

As for the inflammatory arthropathies, it is best to consider the pathology of the non-inflammatory arthropathies in synovial and non-synovial joints separately, although there are some generalizations that apply to both.

8.4.1   OSTEOARTHRITIS

Osteoarthritis (OA) is the name given to a very common disorder of synovial joints which probably represents the final common pathology of a variety of pathogenic mechanisms which lead to joint failure (Doyle, 1986). The peak onset is at 50 years of age and the joints most commonly involved are the knees and small joints of the hands.

A similar disorder affecting the intervertebral discs, and known as spondylosis, will be discussed later.

The joint derangement in osteoarthritis is progressive but the course of the disorder is often punctuated by episodes of acute pain and swelling (Kellgren, 1961). Sequential radiological features of the disease include gradual loss of joint space (narrowing of the gap between the bones on the two sides of the joint); formation of cysts beneath the articulating surfaces; progressive subarticular bone sclerosis (an increase in the amount of bone at the bone ends adjacent to the affected joint); and formation of bony buttresses (osteophytes) at the periphery of the joint (Lawrence *et al.*, 1966) (Figure 8.23).

The essential pathological features of osteoarthritis match the radiological changes and are: cartilage damage, culminating in loss of cartilage and exposure of subchondral bone; formation of thin-roofed cysts within subarticular marrow, often connected to the joint cavity by narrow channels, and the development of bony outgrowths at the margin of the joint which together with wear to the exposed subchondral bone distort the shape of the articular surface.

Cartilage damage is irregularly progressive, starting with a loss of matrix and forma-

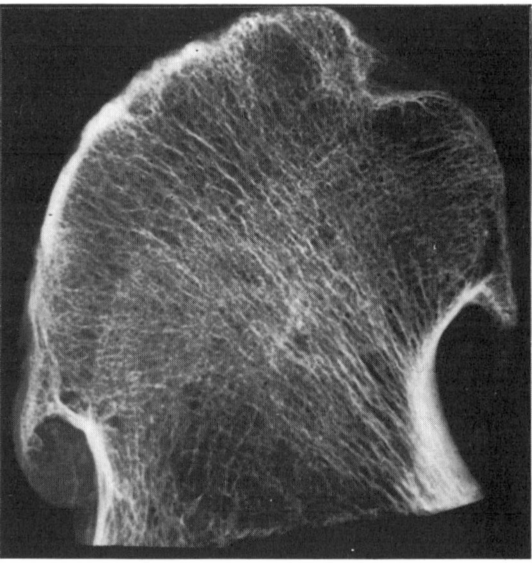

Figure 8.23 A slab radiograph of an osteoarthritic femoral head.

tion of numerous vertical fissures ('fibrillation') in the surface layers. The fissures propagate downwards towards the subchondral bone. The cartilage between the fissures takes on a characteristic crimped pattern superficially (Figure 8.24) and the chondrocytes proliferate to form clusters (Figure 8.25). Eventually, in load-bearing areas, as the fissures extend down to the underlying bone the cartilage is lost and the underlying bone exposed. This process occurs at the two opposing surfaces of the joint and thus bone comes to articulate on bone. As the two bone surfaces rub over one another, they become smooth – a process know as eburnation. During this course of events crimped cartilage, cartilage containing chondrocyte clusters, and wear debris from bone (predominantly hydroxyapatite crystals) are shed into the synovial fluid (Ball, 1986).

As the cartilage is lost the joint becomes less stable. This is compensated for, in part, by very active formation of new bone by enchondral ossification of growing cartilage, mainly at the edges of the articular cartilage,

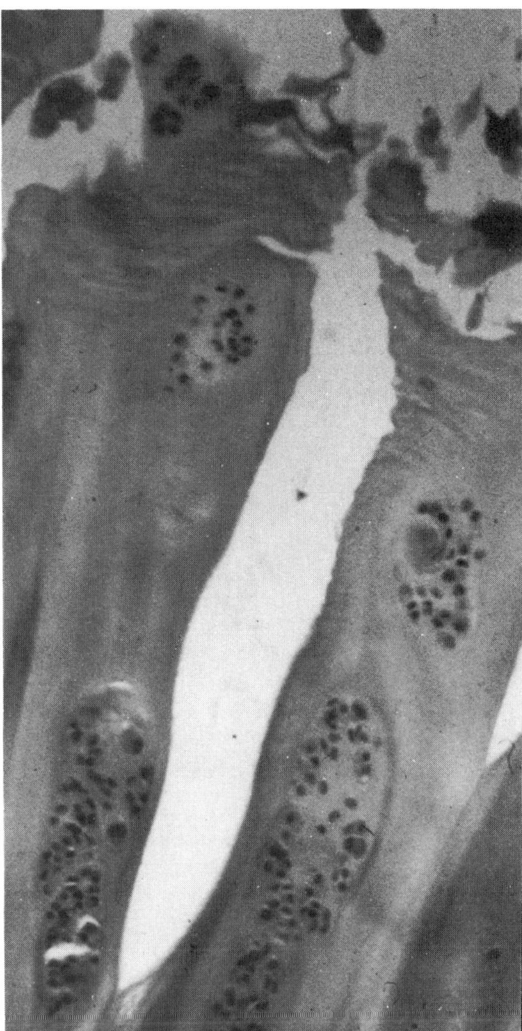

Figure 8.25 Deep cartilage clefts with clusters of chondrocytes in the adjacent cartilage. (H and E ×80)

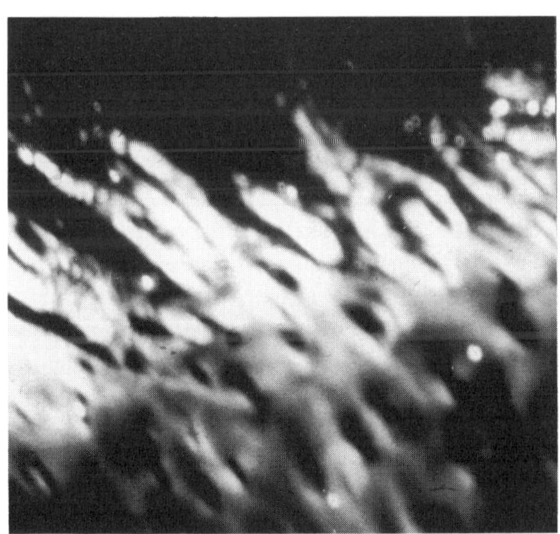

Figure 8.24 Polarizing photomicrograph of early osteoarthritis showing crimped superficial cartilage. (H and E ×20)

sometimes from metaplastic periosteal cartilage (Figure 8.26).

The synovium is thrown into finger-like folds or villi which may become fibrotic. There is an increase in the number of synoviocytes in the synovial membrane (Figure 8.27), and usually none or very few inflammatory cells are found within the synovium. These are, for the most part, lymphocytes

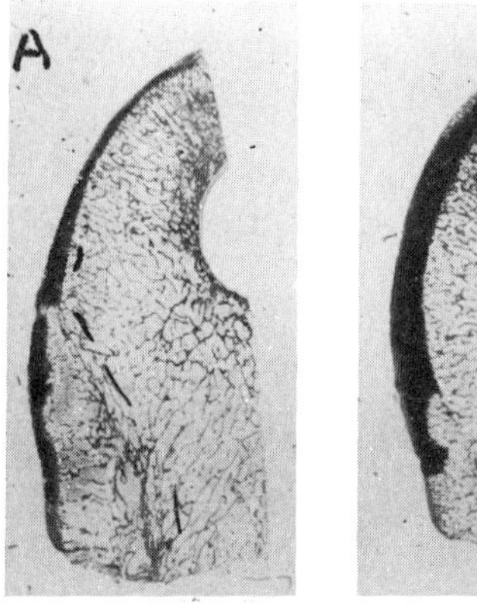

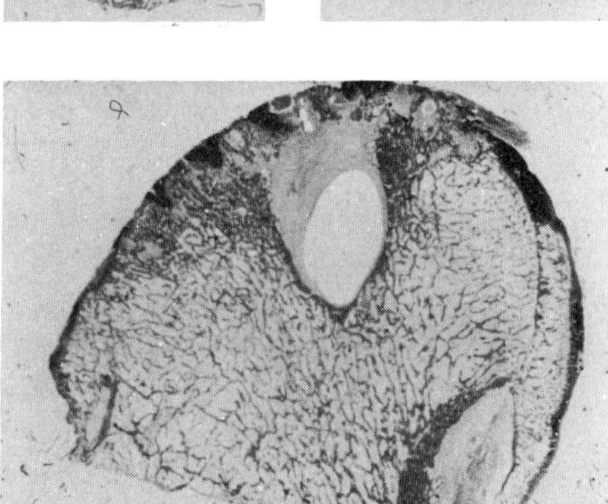

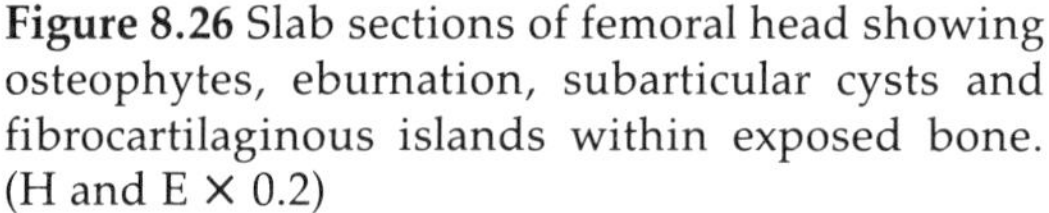

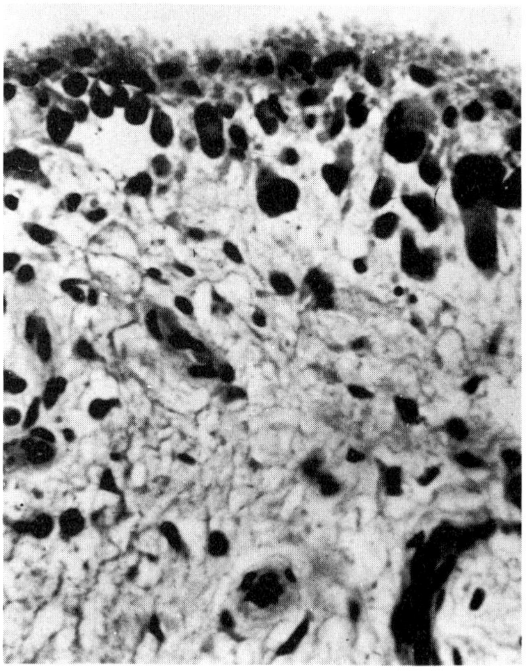
Figure 8.27 The synovium in osteoarthritis with no inflammation, synoviocyte hyperplasia and multinucleate synoviocytes. (H and E ×150)

Figure 8.26 Slab sections of femoral head showing osteophytes, eburnation, subarticular cysts and fibrocartilaginous islands within exposed bone. (H and E × 0.2)

(Figure 8.28). Occasionally, bone debris enters the synovium and elicits a macrophage response (Figure 8.29).

It is unusual for the early events of this sequence to be observed in human joints except at post-mortem (Byers *et al.*, 1970) (Figure 8.30). Most material removed from the joints of patients with osteoarthritis comes to the pathologist at the time of joint replacement surgery. By this time the disease has reached an end stage with the full gamut of histological characteristics, including eburnation, osteophyte formation, the development of subarticular cysts (Figure 8.31) and synovial fibrosis. Occasionally, particularly in multicompartmental joints like the knee, osteoarthritis is sufficiently severe in one compartment to warrant replacement of the whole joint. Material derived from other compartments may then show lesser changes of the disease and, the changes then seen are presumed to represent an earlier stage of the disease. Occasionally, particularly in private practice, the synovium of osteoarthritic joints is biopsied earlier in the course of the disease. From these two sources and animal models of the disease it is possible to piece together the story of the joint changes that occur in osteoarthritis. Although briefly described above, the presumed sequential changes seen in the cartilage are worthy of more detailed consideration as they give an insight, at the morphological level, into the molecular events that must be occurring.

It is believed that the following sequence of events typifies the progressive cartilage loss in osteoarthritis.

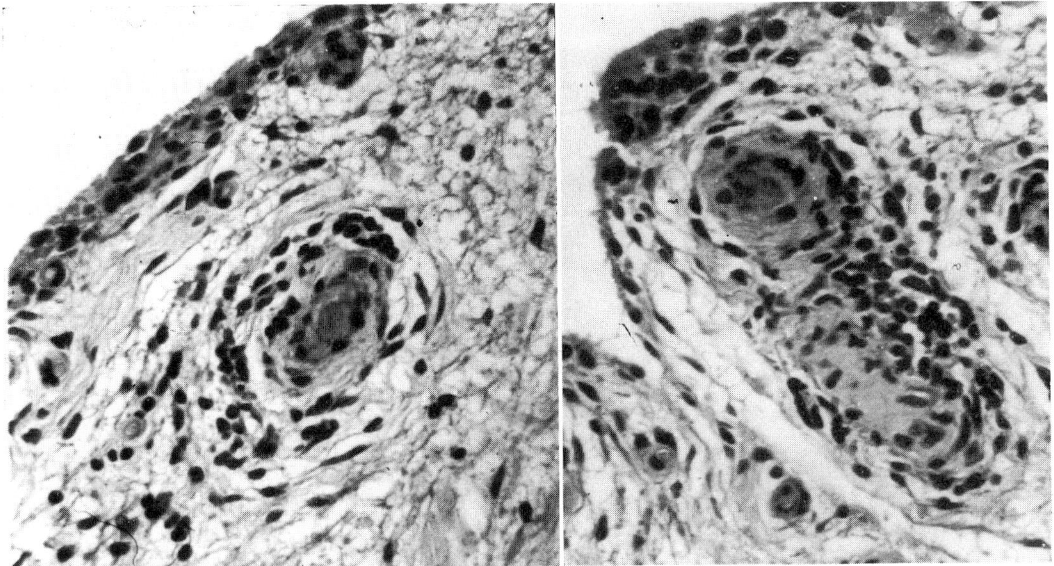

Figure 8.28 Osteoarthritic synovium showing the frequently encountered perivascular lymphocyte aggregates. (H and E ×150)

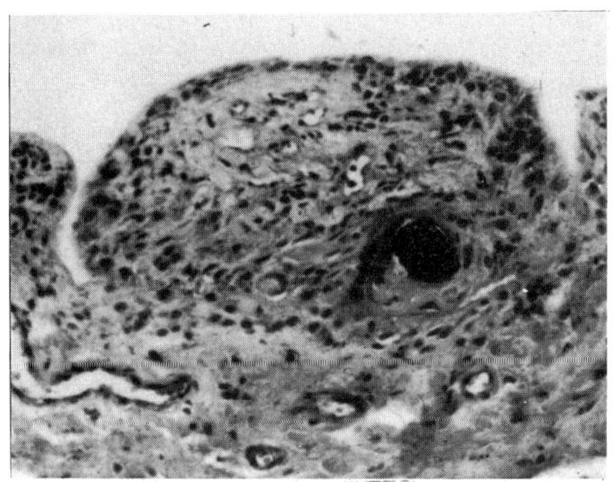

Figure 8.29 Osteoarthritic synovium with included hydroxyapatite nodule (H and E, von Kossa ×50)

1. Loss of metachromasia adjacent to chondrocytes in the superficial layers of the cartilage.
2. Fibrillation of the superficial cartilage. The term fibrillation describes a process in which the superficial cartilage layer breaks up to give a velvet quality to the articular surface. Microscopically the cartilage surface consists of tiny irregular protrusions consisting of strands of chondroid material separated by fine fissures (Figure 8.30b). Under the polarizing microscope the strands appear crimped, as if the tension on a fibril had been suddenly released.
3. Extension of the superficial fissures deeper into the cartilage, until they finally reach the underlying bone.
4. Proliferation of chondrocytes adjacent to the fissures. These chondrocytes form circumscribed collections of up to 50 cells by division.
5. Loss of the fibrillated cartilage and eburnation of bone.

In molecular terms it would seem that chondrocyte dysfunction is the initial abnormality. The glycosaminoglycans that are normally synthesized by local chondrocytes would appear either to be formed abnormally or not to be formed at all. Glycosaminoglycans are avid for water, and it is this

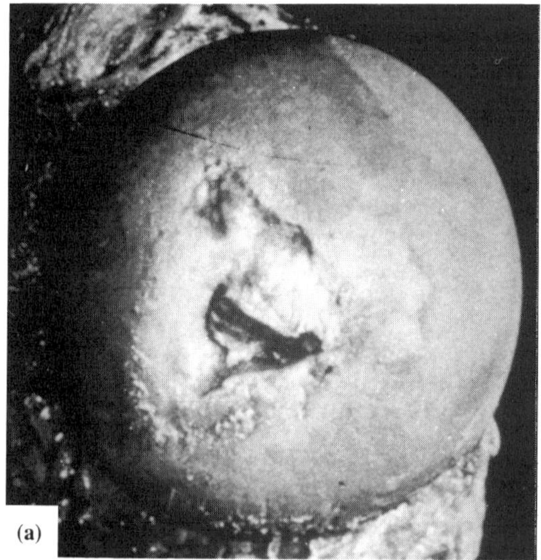

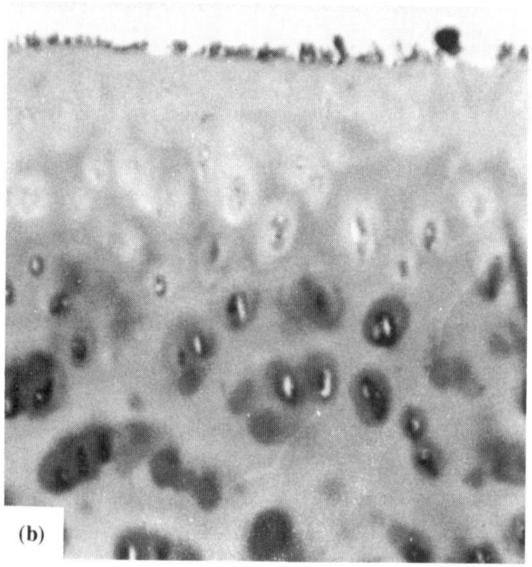

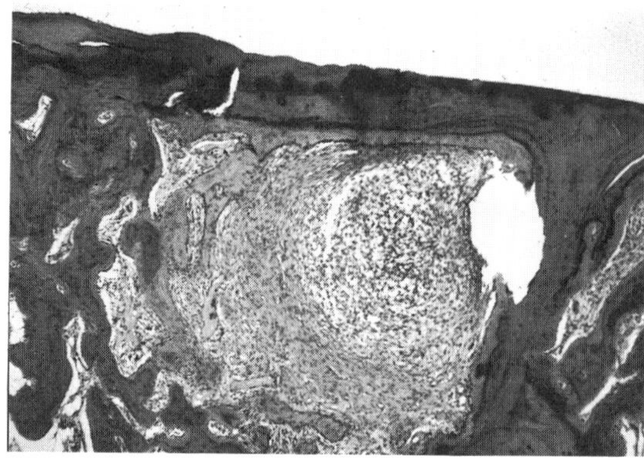

Figure 8.31 A subarticular cyst beneath an eburnated bone surface. (H and E ×50)

Figure 8.30 Female 68 years. (a) Femoral head obtained at autopsy. There are perifoveal osteophytes and lesions of limited progression in the cartilage around the fovea and inferiorly. On the skyline of the anterosuperior surface there is an area which was of velvety texture. This represents the progressive lesion of osteoarthritis (Byers *et al.*, 1970, 1976). Histological section of this area (b) showed very fine surface fibrillation. The contralateral hip had advanced osteoarthritis in the comparable area. Reproduced with permission from the *Annals of Rheumatic Diseases*.

hydrophilic property that hydrates and expands the cartilage matrix – an expansion opposed by the tension within the type II collagen fibres – that gives cartilage its resilience. Absent or abnormal synthesis of glycosaminoglycans, therefore, leads to a decrease in the internal expansive forces within the cartilage, reducing its resilience and making it vulnerable to load. Under load this partially expanded cartilage starts to wear superficially and the shearing forces acting across the surface cause the type II collagen fibres, running parallel to the surface, to rupture. The tension in these ruptured fibres is released and it is they that appear as the crimped superficial strands.

It is presumed that the proliferation of chondrocytes is part of the attempted repair response within the cartilage. Whether this is true or not is immaterial as, if repair is attempted, it invariably fails. The exact reason for this is uncertain but the proliferating chondrocytes do not function normally. Although these cells accumulate sulphate from their environment they do not synthesize the normal complement of glycosaminoglycans.

Under load the fissures in the now weakened cartilage proliferate along the lines of the major orientation of the type II collagen fibres, (i.e. towards the underlying bone). Once the matrix has been fully breached the cartilage is rapidly worn away exposing bone. A similar process occurs on both sides of the joint and, as a consequence, bone articulates on bone. The exposed bone becomes very smooth. The exposed and worn bone is also very vulnerable, and in areas undergoes infarction, and may fracture under load particularly where it overlies cysts. Repair responses to these events lead to focal areas of cartilage and fibrous tissue within the bone.

Although cartilage damage and loss is a major feature of osteoarthritis it is only one of the two changes in connective tissue matrix that occur in this disorder. The other is new bone formation. New bone forms at the periphery of the joint, from cartilage growth (as described above), to form large buttresses called osteophytes. Excessive new bone is also a characteristic of the subarticular region of the joint in response to the loss of cartilage, and arises by osteoblastic apposition to the existing structures.

It is not entirely clear what the stimulus to new bone formation is in these sites. There is an increasing body of evidence that points towards osteophyte formation being due to a regression of the phenotype of mid-zone chondrocytes in the cartilage at the edge of the articulating surface towards that seen normally in fetal development. The mid-zone chondrocytes suddenly start to express type X collagen gene (Hoyland *et al.*, 1991). This, through an unknown mechanism, leads to calcification within the mid-zone of the cartilage and ingrowth of capillaries. These two phenomena together stimulate ossification in the mid-zone of the cartilage. As the disease progresses this zone of new bone formation extends centrally. Once initiated progressive new bone formation within the cartilage separates the two layers of cartilage, one of which comes to lie on the surface of

the osteophyte and the other appears to be buried deep within the bone in the line of the original articular surface. The process of osteophyte formation is, therefore, a form of active endochondral ossification occurring from two directions at once.

By contrast the subarticular bone sclerosis forms only in part through this mechanism. Residual articular cartilage expresses type X collagen basally and endochondral ossification occurs at this site. The rest of the bone forms *de novo* under the action of cytokines. Cytokines were first recognized as mediators of inflammatory processes. It is now recognized that certain cytokines such as IL-6 are involved physiologically in the control of cellular activity. The source and stimulus to cytokine synthesis in the subarticular bone in osteoarthritis remains a mystery but there is now little doubt that it represents the key stimulus to new bone formation at the interface between marrow and subarticular bone.

The pathogenesis of subchondral bone cysts is controversial. One school of thought proposes that, as a consequence of the high intra-articular pressures achieved during some activities, such as rising from a chair, synovial fluid is forced through defects in the eburnated bone into the underlying bone marrow. Unlike cartilage, bone is naturally permeated by narrow channels, either in the form of Haversian systems or the canaliculi linking osteocyte lacunae and these make convenient routes for synovial fluid under pressure to be forced through the bone. Once in the marrow the synovial fluid elicits a connective tissue reaction which walls off the fluid into a rounded cyst surrounded by a rim of sclerotic bone. Histologically, the edge of the cyst consists of fibrous tissue and woven new bone. The alternative view is that reactive marrow fibrosis undergoes mucoid degeneration, the fluid accumulating to form a cyst with fibrotic walls, in a process identical to the formation of soft tissue ganglia. If fluid accumulation continues, expansion occurs by initiating osteoclastic resorption. Some cysts communicate with the joint surface and discharge into the joint cavity (Byers *et al.*, 1976).

It is not known why osteoarthritis is initiated. Over the past four decades there has been an increasing impetus to investigate the causes of osteoarthritis, which has led to research by many in the fields of bioengineering, biophysics, biochemistry and tissue biology, down to the molecular level. The result is a very large body of knowledge on every aspect of articular cartilage and joint function (Sokoloff, 1969, 1978, 1980; Moskowitz *et al.*, 1992). Despite many hypotheses, the aetiopathogenesis of osteoarthritis still remains elusive. The recent growth in knowledge of control factors is adding to understanding of how stimulus and response are linked. There is an increasing body of evidence derived from a variety of sources which suggests that much of the stimulus to changed chondrocyte activity is chemically mediated through the synovium. Two substances have been implicated as initiators of osteoarthritis – mast cell products and cytokines produced by synoviocytes. Mast cells and synoviocytes are innate components of the synovial membrane. In early osteoarthritis there is an increase in the number and size of the synoviocytes and the number of mast cells, a significant proportion of which are degranulated. Both cells seem to be activated in osteoarthritis. The investigation of the mediators of the early stages of osteoarthritis is in its earliest stages and remains, still, a matter of considerable investigation.

(a) Risk factors in the development of osteoarthritis

As mentioned above OA is not so much a disease as a common group of clinical radiological and pathological characteristics that together form a distinct entity. It is well recognized from clinical and epidemiological studies that a variety of conditions may predispose to the development of OA. These can be placed into ten major groups (Solomon, 1976).

1. Abnormal articulation – this is usually the result of an anatomical aberration which leads to loads passing through the joint at mechanically inefficient angles. Sometimes it is caused by excessive joint movement as a result of increased laxity of the ligaments and other structures which stabilize the joint (hypermobility syndrome).

2. Structural disorders arising in childhood – these are abnormalities either of blood supply (e.g. idiopathic aseptic bone necrosis), or of postnatal development (e.g. slipped upper femoral epiphysis).

3. Trauma and mechanical disorders – these include meniscal injuries (and surgical menisectomy), intra-articular fracture and recurrent dislocation of the joint.

4. Neuropathic joints – in diabetes, syphilis and syringomyelia (cystic change and neuronal loss in the upper spinal cord), nerve damage or dysfunction leads to a failure of pain sensation. The joints are not protected from misuse by pain and progressive joint damage ensues.

5. Drugs – it has been suggested that patients taking non-steroidal anti-inflammatory drugs to control symptoms arising from joint disease may progress to end-stage osteoarthritis more rapidly than patients not taking these drugs. A mechanism similar to that of neuropathic joints is proposed.

6. Crystal deposition diseases – gout, calcium pyrophosphate deposition disease and calcific periarthritis can all stimulate damage to the articular surfaces which may progress to osteoarthritis. This is usually by altering the structure of cartilage through crystal deposition within the chondroid matrix, or by stimulated

release of polymorph lysosomal enzymes in acute flares of crystal-induced arthritis.

7. Avascular bone necrosis (see below).
8. Ochronosis (see below).
9. Primary, generalized or nodular osteoarthritis (see below)
10. Following inflammatory damage to cartilage – this is most commonly seen in patients with rheumatoid arthritis but may follow sepsis and other types of primary inflammatory arthropathy.

In mechanistic terms these groups of disorders have certain similarities. Points 1, 2 and 3 are disorders leading directly to abnormal load distribution through the articular surfaces. Points 4 and 5 prevent adequate protection of the joint by removing pain sensation, thus increasing the risk of traumatic injury to the various components of the joint. Points 6–10 lead to abnormalities of the articular cartilage either through genetic aberrations of cartilage or cell-mediated cartilage damage. In general terms, however, the risk factors can be summarized as any factor that damages cartilage; abnormal load, chemical alterations in the matrix and inflammatory damage.

(b)   Generalized osteoarthritis

One of the most common types of osteoarthritis is a genetically determined oligo- or polyarthropathy which presents predominantly in middle age. It is characterized by the development of osteophytic bony swellings over the distal interphalangeal joints of the fingers. These are known as Heberden's nodes (Kellgren and Moore, 1952). Large joints are also involved and the distribution may be asymmetrical. This disease therefore differs from the other types of osteoarthritis in that it is not restricted to single, large, weight-bearing joints. This together with a family history, which typically occurs in this

disorder, indicates a genetic origin (Kellgren *et al.*, 1963).

The histological appearances are, however, almost identical except that frequently there is a generalized loss of cartilage rather than the more commonly seen focal loss, and sometimes relatively little osteophyte formation.

(i)   *'Inflammatory' osteoarthritis*

Much has been made in the literature of the presence of inflammatory cells within the synovium of patients with the unmistakeable clinical syndrome of osteoarthritis. Such inflammatory infiltrates are rarely heavy, and consist predominantly of perivascular aggregates of lymphocytes deep in the synovial subintima. Examination of synovial biopsies from joints with long-standing established osteoarthritis shows lymphocytic infiltrates to be a common finding in the subintima. The synovial fluid always has less than 1000 cells/mm^3, but lymphocytes often predominate.

The significance of these findings is still unclear. Whether patients with these changes have a true 'inflammatory osteoarthritis' or osteoarthritis secondary to an as yet undefined primary inflammatory arthropathy will only be determined when our ability to recognize and classify inflammatory arthropathies becomes more refined (Ehrlich, 1972; Utsinger and Fite, 1982).

(ii)   *'Osteoarthritis' of non-synovial joint*

Certain non-synovial joints are also susceptible to osteoarthritis, or at least a disorder which in many respects mimics osteoarthritis. This is particularly common in intervertebral discs and is known as spondylosis. In this condition, changes in the structure of the nucleus pulposus of the intervertebral disc, either following trauma (Weber, 1983) or the age-related alterations in the chemical composition of the nucleus pulposus (Pritzker, 1977) which lead to a reduction in the intervertebral distance, cause instability in the spine (Kirkaldy-Willis *et al.*, 1978). The annulus fibrosus does not contract in the same way as the nucleus pulposus and movement of the unstable spine places abnormal load upon the annulus. Traumatic lesions known as rim lesions form at the insertion of the annulus into the edge of the vertebral body (Hilton *et al.*, 1980). These amount to vascular deficiencies from which new blood vessels grow into the normally avascular intervertebral disc. Trauma to the insertion of the outer fibres of the annulus also stimulates production of the new buttressing bone at the edge of the vertebral bodies (Figure 8.32). Sometimes, if they grow posteriorly the vertebral osteophytes compress the nerve root and vessels within the intervertebral root canal (Figure 8.33) giving rise either to back pain or sciatica, if in the lumbar spine, or neck pain and finger paraesthesia, if in the cervical spine.

These lesions are rarely biopsied; much more commonly traumatized intervertebral disc is removed at discectomy. The only clue to the pathologist that this may be associated with a vertebral rim lesion or an osteophyte is the presence of blood vessels within this otherwise avascular structure.

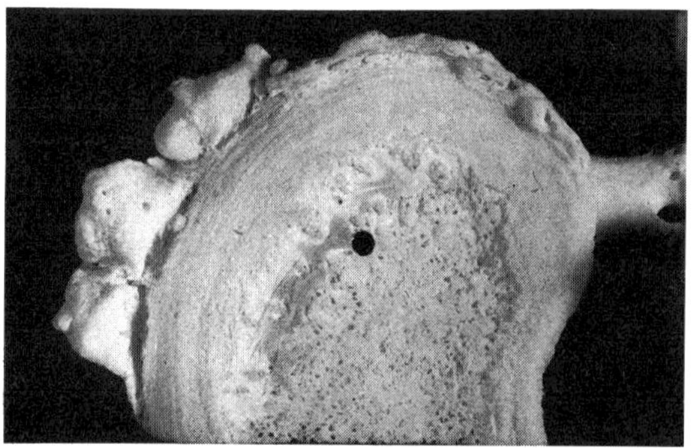

Figure 8.32 A macerated specimen showing osteophytes of the vertebral body. (×0.25)

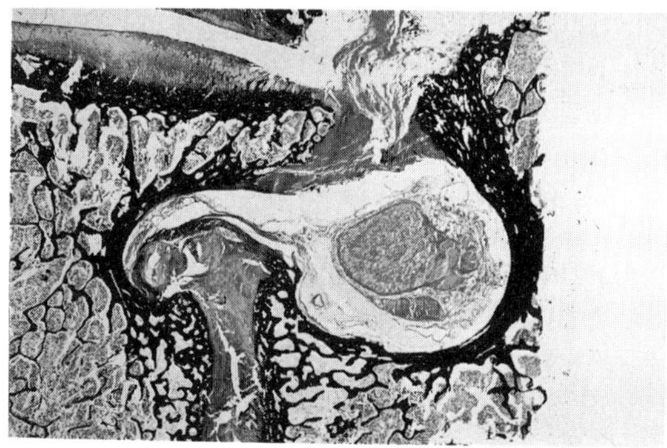

Figure 8.33 A posterolateral osteophyte projecting into the intervertebral root canal. (EVG ×1)

8.4.2 TRAUMATIC ARTHRITIS

Both synovial and non-synovial joints are, because of their complexity and function, highly susceptible to injury. The effects of trauma will vary depending upon:

1. The force of the injury.
2. The direction of the injurious force acting on the joint.
3. Whether the injury is a single occurrence or repetitive.
4. The type of joint.

Trauma to joints may therefore vary from relatively mild with ligamentous or capsular injury, to severe with damage to cartilage or underlying bone.

Forces acting in different directions on the joint may have different effects on articular structures. For instance loading in compression may lead, in a synovial joint, to disruption of articular cartilage and in a vertebral joint to fracture of the end plate. By contrast, twisting injury, such as occurs to footballers, knee joints, or to the intervertebral discs in people lifting with a poor action, lead to disruption of the capsule and intra- or peri-articular ligaments.

(a) Traumatic arthritis in synovial joints

Synovial joints exhibit two common patterns of joint disease following acute trauma –

haemarthrosis and non-haemorrhagic acute effusion.

Intra-articular haemorrhage is a common finding following trauma, and is always associated with significant internal disruption of the joint. In complex joints, such as the knee, this could be one or more of a multitude of abnormalities from meniscal tears and ligament injury to intra-articular fracture.

The synovium is always oedematous and if there has been previous injury there may be synoviocyte hyperplasia and iron deposition within the synovium. The synovial fluid is invariably blood stained or frankly haemorrhagic and may contain fragments of the injured structure, be it cartilage, ligament or meniscus. The cell count is below 1000 cells/ mm^3. The nucleated cells are predominantly macrophages, lymphocytes and synoviocytes, some of which may be multinucleate.

It is rare to encounter an acute traumatic effusion that contains no blood but in minor twisting injuries, particularly of the knee, this may occur. The extent of internal injuries is invariably less than in haemarthroses and so the synovial fluid contains neither blood nor fragments of articular structures. The synovium is oedematous and may show a minor increase in synoviocytes. The basic cell complement of the synovial fluid is very similar to that of osteoarthritis, but, in addition, it invariably contains mast cells, which may account for up to 5% of all nucleated cells (Malone *et al.*, 1986).

(b)   Recurrent trauma

In synovial joints the most common form of repetitive trauma occurs in patients with a permanent abnormality of the internal anatomy of the joint (an internal derangement). Rarely in an internal derangement is the joint loaded without causing at least minor tissue injury. Examples include meniscal tears and capsular laxity.

The synovium in patients with long-standing episodic trauma is villous. There is synoviocyte hypertrophy but little hyperplasia. The subintima is highly vascular and shows an increase in the number of mast cells. It may be fibrotic. Mast cells and synoviocytes are also increased in the synovial fluid. The total nucleated cell count may be up to 1000 cells/mm^3. The cell population is, in general terms, similar to that of non-haemorrhagic acute traumatic effusions but lymphocytes may be the most numerous cells.

Even in these long-standing effusions fragments of damaged intra-articular structure can be identified including cartilage, synovium (which may be normal or fibrotic), meniscal fibrocartilage (Royle *et al.*, 1992), bone marrow, bone, adipose tissue or ligament, depending upon the type of joint and the extent of trauma (Freemont and Denton, 1988). An interesting finding of uncertain cause is that traumatized synovial joint fluids feel greasy and microscopic examination reveals them to contain lipid droplets (Gregg *et al.*, 1978), some of which contain needle-shaped lipid crystals. It is believed that these come either from intra-articular fat-pads or exposed bone marrow.

(c)   Penetrating injury

Penetrating injuries, particularly of the knee, are not uncommon. The penetrating object is usually sharp (e.g. glass, nail or plant thorn) and almost invariably carries with it other foreign material. Usually the result of a penetrating injury is local swelling and inflammation for a few days which settles spontaneously. Occasionally, there is persistent inflammation (usually in response to the introduced foreign material) or delayed inflammation in the affected joint.

A rare condition – plant thorn synovitis – has been described (Sugerman, 1977). In this childhood disorder an inflammatory polyarthropathy develops in response to introduction of plant material into a single joint. It can be treated by removing the plant thorn. It has also been reported that trauma can initiate an episode of seronegative spondylarthropathy (Olivieri *et al.*, 1989).

(d) Trauma to non-synovial joints

Repetitive injury is also encountered in non-synovial joints. Indeed, the most common site for repetitive injury is in the intervertebral joints. Although intra-articular haemorrhage in the intervertebral disc is very rare, severe trauma to the intervertebral joint may cause fracture of end plate bone and cartilage (Hilton *et al.*, 1976) (Figure 8.34). The pathology of traumatic joint disease in non-synovial joints is centred about trauma to the insertions of fibrous components of the joint into bone. This is effectively a traumatic enthesopathy and the pathology is described above. Local tissue damage, neovascularization and attempted repair are the hallmarks of this lesion, and indeed, this general pattern also typifies trauma at all entheses, and interfaces between bone and fibrous tissue of fibrous joints.

8.4.3 OTHER DISORDERS

Although osteoarthritis, acute traumatic arthropathies and internal derangements account for the majority of non-inflammatory arthropathies, there are very many other diseases which can give rise to a non-inflammatory type of disorder. Most will lead, ultimately, to the development of osteoarthritis but some have characteristic features in the pre-osteoarthritic phase of the disease. It is implicit in this statement that a patient with one of these disorders may have synovial fluid and articular findings characteristic of the primary disorder, typical of osteoarthritis or a hybrid pattern, depending on the local stage of the disease. This has to be taken into account when interpreting the findings.

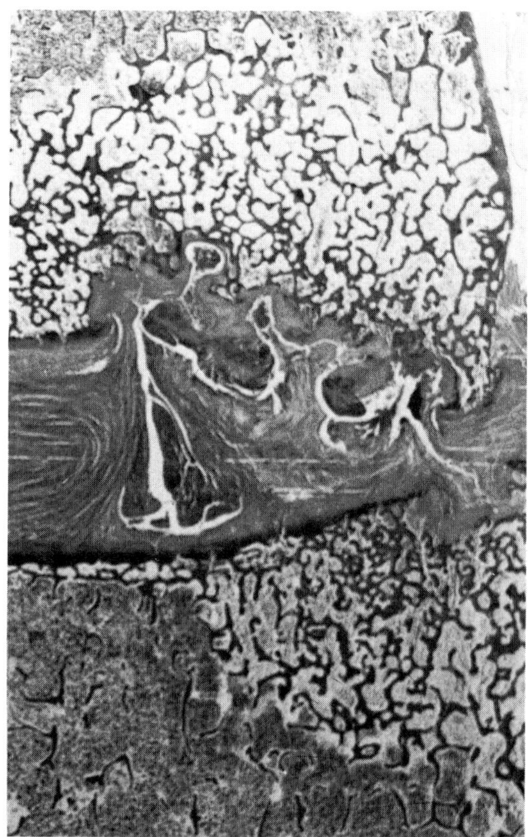

Figure 8.34 Post-traumatic fracture of the vertebral end plate. (H and E ×1)

(a) Amyloidosis

Amyloidosis is a generalized disorder characterized by the deposition of abnormal proteins in many organs in the body, amongst these being synovium and cartilage (Franklin, 1975). The principal characteristic of the protein is that, instead of the usual helical arrangement of the amino acid chains, it has a beta-pleated sheet configuration. Proteins with a beta-pleated sheet configuration are less easily degraded and less soluble than those with the conventional helical pattern. Thus, they accumulate in the body and are deposited within the tissues. Many proteins can take on this structure but it is a particular property of immunoglobulin, acute phase proteins, β_2-microglobulin (Freemont, 1986) and prealbumin. These proteins increase in the serum in a variety of neoplastic, inflammatory and other disorders. Because of the particular types of protein that preferentially form amyloids, amyloidosis is seen, most frequently, in conditions such as multiple myeloma, where the major protein in the amyloid is immunoglobulin; chronic inflammatory diseases, such as rheumatoid arthritis, bronchiectasis and ulcerative colitis, where the protein is amyloid A protein (derived from serum protein A, an acute phase reactant); and chronic haemodialysis where the protein is β_2-microglobulin (which accumulates because it cannot be dialysed out of the blood using conventional cellophane dialysis membranes). In addition to the major protein, almost all forms of amyloid contain the same minor protein, known as protein P. Amyloid can be recognized by the use of non-specific histochemical stains, such as Congo red, or specifically by immunohistochemical techniques against the protein of the amyloid or protein P.

Patients with amyloid in their joints (amyloid arthropathy) tend to develop a polyarticular disorder of the small joints of the hands, wrists, shoulders and knees, which, on X-ray, is associated with joint erosions. Therefore, it may be confused with rheumatoid disease clinically.

The synovial fluid has non-inflammatory features and may contain fragments of amyloid material.

(b) Acromegaly

Acromegaly is a disease of the pituitary gland which results in the over-production of growth hormone with the enlargement of bones, joints and other internal organs. Half the patients develop an arthropathy (Bluestone *et al.*, 1971), most commonly of the fingers, spine and knees. Histologically, weight-bearing cartilage develops undercut deficiencies as a result of focal cartilage

necrosis and subsequent dispersal (Figure 8.35). These may fill with fibrocartilage. The cartilage adjacent to these areas may become hypertrophic and the chondrocytes hyperplastic. Progression to osteoarthritis is usual.

(c) Ochronosis

Ochronosis is a rare hereditary disease in which deficiency of the enzyme homogentisic acid oxidase leads to the accumulation of the pigment polymeric homogentisic acid in tissues. The pigment binds to cartilage collagen (Figure 8.36) and decreases its resilience. As a result, the cartilage becomes brittle and fragments under load. The onset of the arthropathy is in the fourth and third decades and progresses relentlessly towards osteoarthritis (Schumacher and Holdsmith, 1977). The knees, shoulders and hips are the joints most commonly involved. The cartilage contains deposits of dark-brown ochronotic pigment, most commonly within the mid and basal zones. The cartilage surface tends to be fragmented and fragments of the dark cartilage are seen within the synovial fluid and the synovium (Figure 8.37). So much pigment can be deposited that the inside of the joint can appear black and the synovial fluid is said to resemble black pepper particles in suspension.

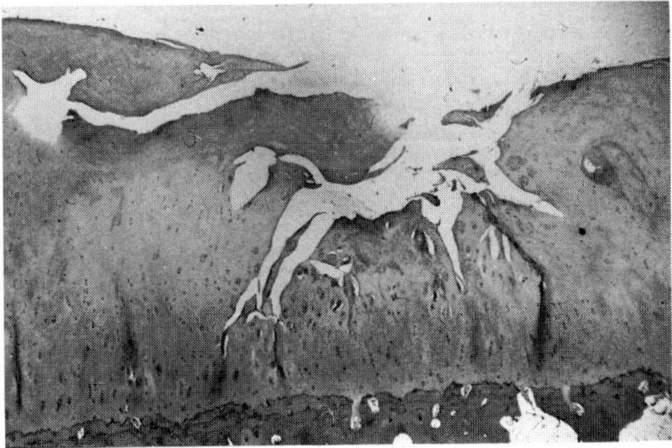

Figure 8.35 Undermining of the cartilage in acromegaly. (H and E ×2)

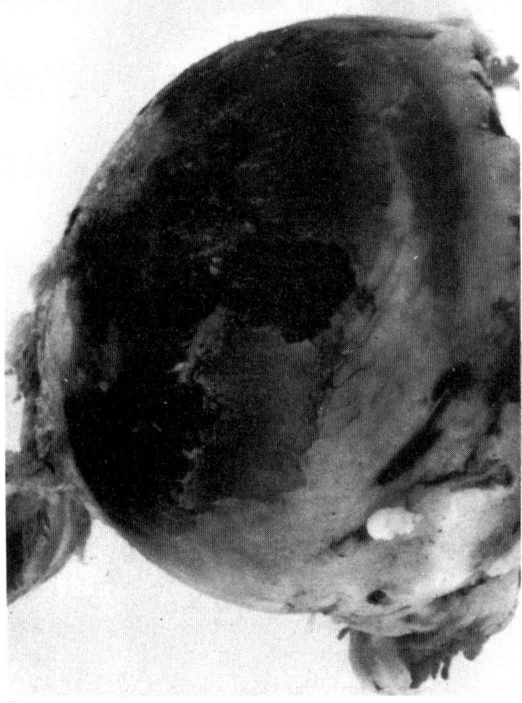

Figure 8.36 The femoral head from a patient with ochronosis. (×0.25)

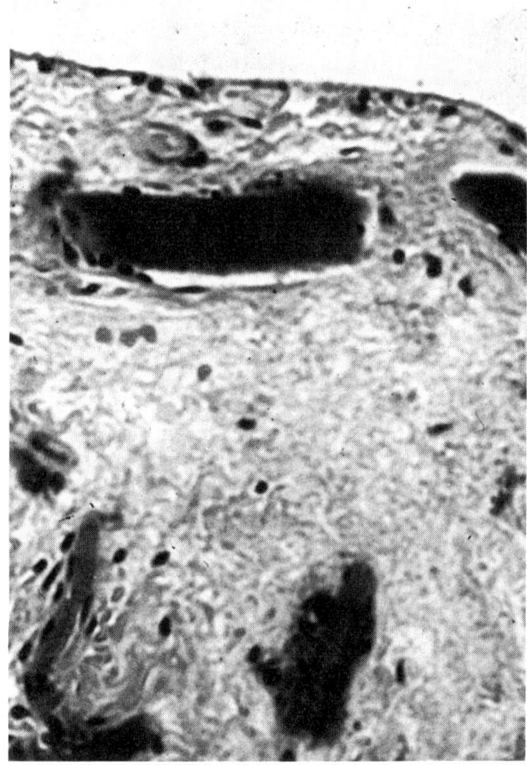

Figure 8.37 Ochronotic cartilage deposited in the synovium. (H and E ×50)

(d) Avascular bone necrosis (see also Chapter 9)

Avascular bone necrosis typically occurs at bone ends as subarticular wedge-shaped areas of bone and bone marrow necrosis. The overlying articular cartilage, which is nourished by the synovial fluid, remains viable. The dead bone becomes separated from the viable bone by a zone of fibrous tissue. Ultimately, dead bone with attached live overlying cartilage may detach from the articular surface and form a loose body within the joint space (Jones, 1978).

Trauma is implicated in some cases of aseptic bone necrosis (Green, 1966), as are disorders that interfere with bone blood flow, including sickle cell disease, vasculitis, rapid decompression ('the bends') and steroid therapy. The knee and hip are the most commonly involved joints.

The loose bodies are characteristic in that they consist, for the most part, of viable cartilage with an attached fragment of necrotic bone. The synovium, in addition to showing synoviocyte hyperplasia, contains fragments of dead bone, some of which are only tiny particles of hydroxyapatite. These are best demonstrated using von Kossa's stain for calcium. Sometimes these tiny particles elicit a marked macrophage response.

The synovial fluid is haemorrhagic and contains fragments of cartilage and large numbers of hydroxyapatite crystals.

(e) Hypertrophic pulmonary osteoarthropathy (see also Chapter 9)

This is a syndrome characterized by digital clubbing, periostitis, synovitis and thickening of skin. It is associated with a variety of non-musculoskeletal system disorders, notably malignant tumours of the bronchus (Dixon, 1963), stomach and oesophagus, but also, more rarely, benign tumours, pulmonary suppuration and cirrhosis and cyanotic congenital heart disease. Because of its association with bronchial carcinoma, hypertrophic osteoarthropathy is predominantly a disease of middle age and affects men more than women. It may precede other manifestations of the neoplasm by many months.

The macroscopic, microscopic and cytological features of the joint and synovial fluid are simply those of a non-inflammatory arthropathy.

(f)   Overt and imminent failure of joint prosthesis

Joint replacement surgery is being performed increasingly frequently, usually for irreversible damage to articular surfaces. In addition synthetic prostheses are being used regularly for repair of ligaments, particularly within the knee.

Replacement joints are of two types. The articular surfaces of large joints are usually replaced with prostheses consisting of high- or ultrahigh-density polyethylene on a supporting framework of cobalt or chromium doped steel. Smaller joints, such as the interphalangeal joints of the fingers, are replaced by hinged silastic prostheses. Prostheses are usually held in place using a bone cement of polymerized methylmethacrylate.

Ligament protheses may consist of any one of many polymers or composites. Dacron and carbon fibre are among the most common to be used.

Both the synovium and the synovial fluid contain fragments of prosthetic material during prosthesis failure (Evans and Mears, 1981). These vary from tiny black particles of metal to larger fragments of plastic (Figure 8.38) or other synthetic polymers; the synovium usually contains large quantities of

this debris much of which is birefringent. In addition this material will cause a foreign body type giant cell reaction which often dominates the histological picture.

(g)   Synovial chondromatosis and 'Snowstorm knee' (see also Chapter 13)

'Snowstorm knee' is one of the extreme manifestations of synovial chondromatosis, a disorder characterized by small nodules of cartilage within the synovium and synovial fluid. It has been suggested that these form as a result of chondroid metaplasia within the connective

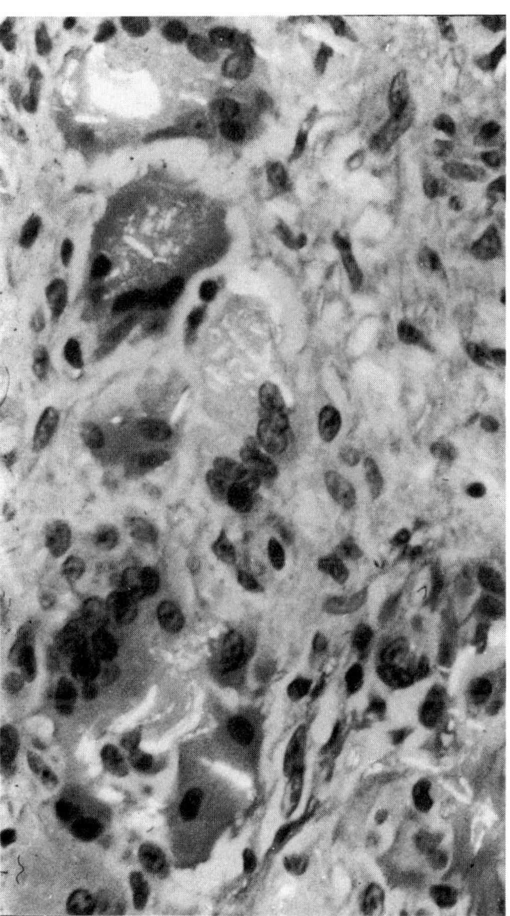

Figure 8.38 Giant cell reaction to prosthesis debris within synovium. (H and E ×100)

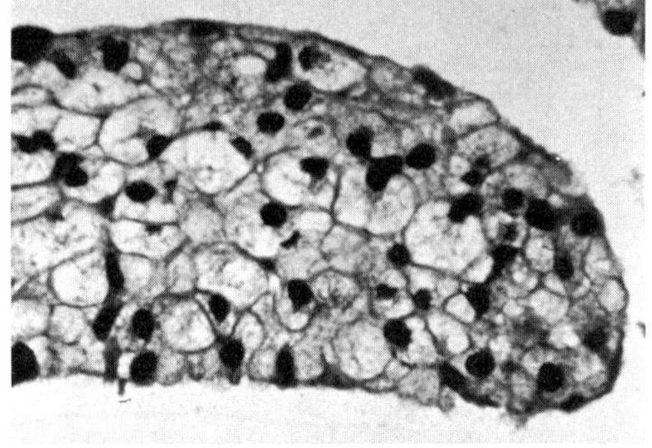

Figure 8.39 Lipid-laden macrophages within synovial villi in a patient with congenital type II hyperlipidaemia. (H and E ×100)

tissues of the synovium. Much more probable is that the nodules grow from chondrocytes or small clusters of chondrocytes shed from the surface of the articular cartilage (Kaye *et al.*, 1989). Early in the disease, the synovial fluid contains chondroid nodules and, in snowstorm knee, may be numerous, when the total volume of the nodules may exceed that of the articular cartilage by 10–20-fold. Arthroscopy in patients with snowstorm knee shows a soft, flaky surface to the cartilage and so many chondroid nodules in the fluid that the appearance has been likened to being in a blizzard (hence the name). The nodules in all forms of synovial chondromatosis consist of cartilage, but may have a central core of bone.

(h) Multicentric reticulohistiocytosis

Multicentric reticulohistiocytosis is a rare disease of unknown aetiology and pathogenesis which presents clinically with a polyarthropathy, mucocutaneous nodular itchy eruptions and constitutional symptoms. In approximately 25% of patients the disorder is associated with an underlying malignancy, and in many of the others the arthritis becomes severely destructive and unresponsive to treatment.

The synovial fluid is most unusual in this disease. It is usually bloodstained. The nucleated cell count is less than 1000 cells/

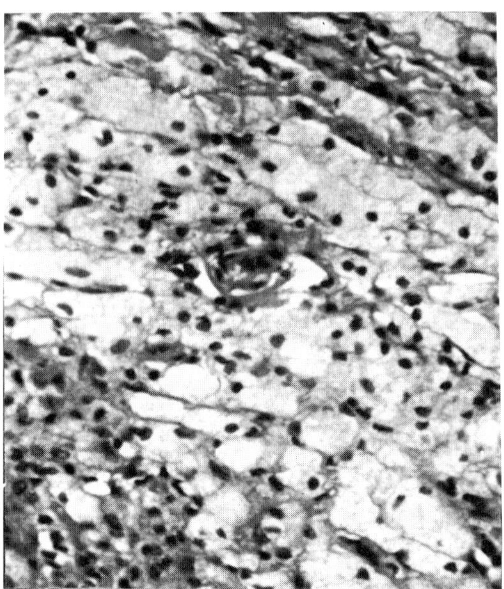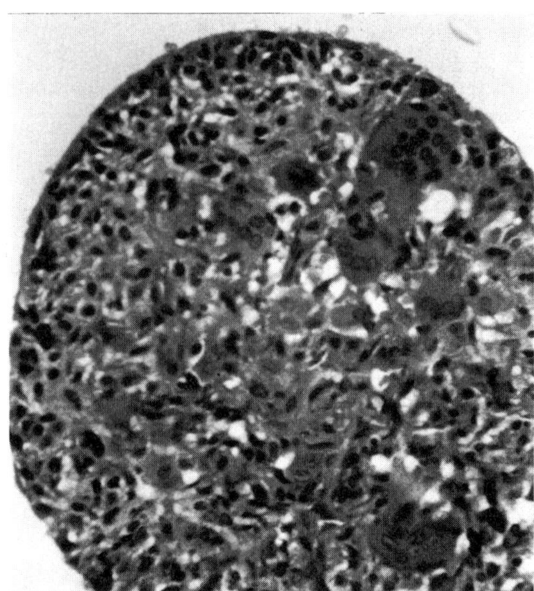

Figure 8.40 Giant cells, lipophages and iron-laden macrophages in the synovium in pigmented villonodular synovitis. (H and E ×100)

mm^3, and the predominant cells are macrophages and lymphocytes. Unusually the majority of the lymphocytes are of the B cell lineage. Immunoblasts account for about 10% of all cells. An unusual cell type called a megalocyte (Freemont *et al.*, 1983) is found in small numbers in the synovial fluid. Megalocytes are very large mononuclear macrophages, up to 70 μm in diameter, in cytocentrifuge preparations. The synovium contains clusters of similar cells. The megalocytes contain PAS-positive granules and stain immunohistochemically for lysozyme and α_1-antitrypsin.

The importance of making the diagnosis of multicentric reticulohistiocytosis is that the joint disease may predate the symptoms of malignancy by several years, although more typically, it is by only weeks or months. Investigation for occult neoplasia should be undertaken immediately.

(i) Hyperlipidaemia

Hyperlipidaemia is sometimes associated with joint swelling. Synovial biopsy is characterized by aggregates of lipid-laden macrophages (Figure 8.39).

(j) Pigmented villonodular synovitis

Pigmented villonodular synovitis is a joint disease characterized by nodular aggregates of macrophages in the synovium. Some of the macrophages contain lipid and others large quantities of iron (Figure 8.40). Multinucleate forms are common. The cause of pigmented villonodular synovitis is not known.

Clinically the disorder is associated with recurrent haemarthroses and joint destruction.

(k) The arthropathy of bleeding diatheses

Haemarthroses secondary to bleeding diatheses such as haemophilia are associated with a persistent or progressive arthropathy. In its early stages haemophilic arthropathy is char-

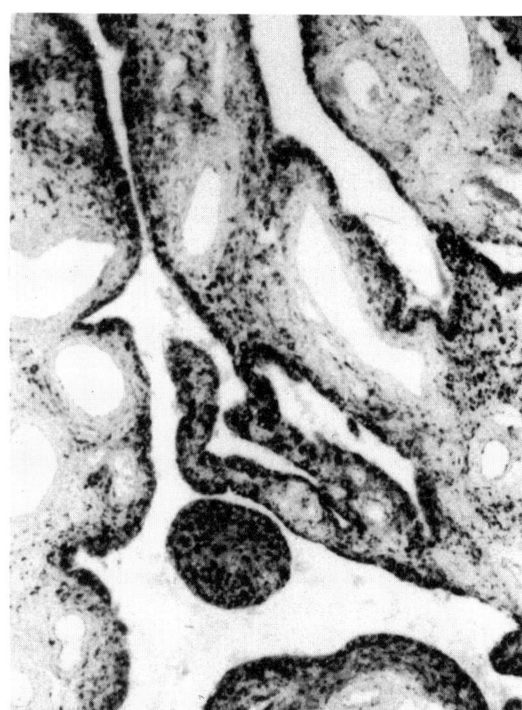

Figure 8.41 Iron deposition within the synovium of a haemophiliac. (H and E ×50)

acterized by recurrent joint swelling interposed with episodes of recovery. Iron is deposited in the synovium (Figure 8.41) and comes to be associated with a predominantly lymphocytic infiltrate in the synovium. With time the synovium and perisynovial tissues become fibrosed leading to fixed deformities and there is erosion of the articular surfaces. Untreated the disorder progresses towards gross destruction of the articular surfaces associated with marked joint deformity and contractures.

Unfortunately many haemophiliacs have become infected with hepatitis B and HI viruses and great care must be taken when handling synovial fluid from these patients.

REFERENCES

Ball, J. (1986) Aetiology and pathology of osteoarthrosis, In *Copeman's Textbook of the Rheumatic Diseases*. Churchill Livingstone, Edinburgh.

Bluestone, R., Bywaters, E.G.L., Hartog, M. *et al.* (1971) Acromegalic arthropathy. *Ann. Rheum. Dis.*, **30**, 243–58.

Byers, P.D., Contepomi, C.A. and Farkas, T.A. (1970) A post mortem study of the hip joint. I. Including the prevalence of the features of the right side. *Ann. Rheum. Dis.*, **29**, 15–31.

Byers, P.D., Contepomi, C.A. and Farkas, T.A. (1976) A post mortem study of the hip joint. II. Histological basis for limited and progressive cartilage alterations. *Ann. Rheum. Dis.*, **35**, 114–21.

Dixon, A.St J. (1963) Unusual effects of bronchial carcinoma and other lung tumours. *Thorax*, **18**, 197–204.

Doyle, D. (1986) Clinical aspects of osteoarthrosis, In *Copeman's Textbook of the Rheumatic Diseases.* Churchill Livingstone, Edinburgh.

Ehrlich, G.E. (1972) Inflammatory osteoarthritis. *J. Chron. Dis.*, **25**, 635–43.

Evans, C.H. and Mears, D.C. (1981) The wear particles of synovial fluid: their ferrographic analysis and pathophysiological significance. *Bull. Prosthesis Res.*, **10**, 13–26.

Franklin, E.C. (1975) Amyloidosis. *Bull. Rheum. Dis.*, **26**, 832–7.

Freemont, A.J. (1986) Amyloid arthropathy in patients with chronic renal failure. *Ann. Rheum. Dis.*, **45**, 349

Freemont, A.J. and Denton, J. (1988) Synovial fluid findings early in traumatic arthritis. *J. Rheumatol.*, **15**, 881–2.

Freemont, A.J., Jones, C.J.P. and Denton, J. (1983) The synovium and synovial fluid in multicentric reticulohistiocytosis – a light microscopic, electron microscopic and cytochemical analysis of one case. *J. Clin. Pathol.*, **36**, 860–6.

Green, J.P. (1966) Osteochondritis dissecans of the knee. *J. Bone Joint Surg.*, **48B**, 82–91.

Gregg, J.R., Nixon, J.E. and DiStefano, V. (1978) Neutral fat globules in traumatised knees. *Clin. Orthop.*, **132**, 220–4.

Hilton, R.C., Ball, J. and Benn, R.T. (1976) Vertebral endplate lesions (Schmorl's nodes) in the dorsolumbar spine. *Ann. Rheum. Dis.*, **35**, 127–38.

Hilton, R.C., Ball, J. and Benn, R.T. (1980) Annular tears in the dorsolumbar spine. *Ann. Rheum. Dis.*, **39**, 533–40.

Hoyland, J.A., Thomas, J.T., Donn, R. (1991) Distribution of type X collagen in normal and osteoarthritic human cartilage. *Bone Miner.*, **15**, 151–64.

Jones, J.P. (1978) Osteonecrosis. *Clin. Orthop.*, **130**, 2–4.

Kaye, P., Freemont, A.J. and Davies, D.R.A. (1989) The aetiology of multiple loose bodies: Snowstorm knee. *J. Bone Joint Surg.*, **71B**, 501–4.

Kellgren, J.H. (1961) Osteoarthrosis in patients and populations. *Br. Med. J.*, **2**, 1–6.

Kellgren, J.H., Lawrence, J.S. and Bier, F. (1963) Genetic factors in generalised osteoarthrosis. *Ann. Rheum. Dis.*, **22**, 237–55.

Kellgren, J.H. and Moore, R. (1952) Generalised osteoarthritis and Heberden's nodes. *Br. Med. J.*, **1**, 181–7.

Kirkaldy-Willis, W.H., Wedge, J.H., Yong-Hing, K. *et al.*, (1978) Pathology and pathogenesis of lumbar spondylosis and stenosis. *Spine*, **3**, 319–31.

Lawrence, J., Bremner, B.M. and Bier, F. (1966) Osteoarthrosis. *Ann. Rheum. Dis.*, **25**, 1–24.

Malone, D.G., Irani, A.M., Schwartz, L.B. *et al.* (1986) Mast cell numbers and histamine levels in synovial fluids from patients with diverse arthritides. *Arthritis Rheum.*, **29**, 956–63.

Moskowitz, R.W., Howell, D.S., Goldberg, V.M. *et al.* (1992) *Osteoarthritis. Diagnosis and Medical/ Surgical Management.* WB Saunders Harcourt Brace Jovanovich, Philadelphia.

Olivieri, I., Gemignani, G., Christou, C. *et al.* (1989) Trauma and seronegative spondyloarthropathy: report of 2 more cases of peripheral arthritis precipitated by physical injury. *Ann. Rheum. Dis.*, **48**, 520–1.

Pritzker, K.P.H. (1977) Aging and degeneration in the lumbar intervertebral disc. *Orthop. Clin. North Am.*, **8**, 65–72.

Royle, S.G., Noble, J., Parkinson, R.W. *et al.* (1992) The diagnostic potential of synovial fluid effusion in meniscal pathology. *Arthroscopy*, **8**, 254–7.

Schumacher, H.R. and Holdsmith, D.E. (1977) Ochronotic arthropathy. I. Clinicopathologic studies. *Semin. Arthritis Rheum.* **6**, 207–46.

Sokoloff, L. (1969) *The Biology of Degenerative Joint Disease.* University of Chicago Press, Chicago.

Sokoloff, L. (1978) *The Joints and Synovial Fluid.* Vol. 1. Academic Press, New York.

Sokoloff, L. (1980) *The Joints and Synovial Fluid.* Vol. 2. Academic Press, New York.

Solomon, L. (1976) Patterns of osteoarthritis of the hips. *J. Bone Joint Surg.*, **55B**, 176–83.

Sugerman, M. (1977) Plant thorn synovitis. *Arthritis Rheum.*, **20**, 1125–9.

Utsinger, P.D. and Fite, F.L. (1982) Immunologic evidence for inflammation in osteoarthritis. *Arthritis Rheum.*, **25**, 44–51.

Weber, H. (1983) Lumbar disc herniation. A controlled prospective study with ten years of observation. *Spine*, **8**, 131–8.

CIRCULATORY DISORDERS 9

Paul D. Byers

This chapter will discuss injury as a consequence of deprivation of blood supply to bone.

Necrosis of bone as an organ, i.e. the bone plus its contained tissues, is nearly always the result of impairment of blood supply. Necrotic bone *per se* retains the strength of live bone, but, in the absence of viable marrow, has no capacity to remodel or repair. Unless and until associated events or responses are manifested and recognized the fact of necrosis will not be evident. In the case of fracture, one knows *a priori* that there is bone necrosis, and its extent can be predicted from the nature of the fracture; but the necrosis need not be clinically or radiologically evident. However, this may alter as the result of the reaction in the surrounding viable tissue. The necrotic bone will not participate in the regional acceleratory phenomenon (RAP), and the contrast will stand out on a radiograph. This may, of course, be obscured by the callus response. But should vascular impairment come about non-traumatically, inciting little or no RAP, the necrosis would not be detected until such time as associated events or responses drew attention.

In peripheral vascular occlusive disease, apart from the involvement of bone in gangrenous tissue, the bones higher in the limb may also show changes. These may simply be the effects of disuse osteoporosis in slowly developing occlusive disease or of the regional acceleratory phenomenon (see Chapter 20) in embolic or thrombotic cases. There may also be death of osteocytes due to interruption of the blood supply (in older patients allowance must be made for the natural loss of osteocytes with age, particularly in interstitial cortical bone), or even infarction of marrow or cortex (Jaffe, 1972). In the latter instance, if there has been time for a collateral circulation to develop, remodelling of the necrotic tissue can occur. Such changes are of little consequence and the fate of the limb will be determined by the condition of soft tissues.

It is more localized impairment of circulation that gives rise to problems. Epiphyseal infarction eventually leads to organ failure: of the epiphysis, and possibly, subsequently of the joint. Marrow infarction is much less prone to give trouble. In general the pathology of the necrotic lesion is understood, but the events leading to the infarction are, with exceptions, obscure. The exceptions are fracture and traumatic dislocation of the hip. This group are frequently called avascular necrosis, in recognition of the known pathogensis. The others are usually designated idiopathic osteonecrosis.

The classification of the entities under consideration is shown in Table 9.1.

Something of the history of bone necrosis is helpful in getting to grips with the subject. The following resume is drawn from McCarthy *et al.* (1982), Zinn (1971), McCallum *et al.* (1966) and Burrows (1959). Bone necrosis was a subject of interest in the 18th century, largely in the context of inflammation. The discovery of bacteria in abscesses by Pasteur in 1860 opened the way to recognizing bone necrosis in the absence of inflammation; however, the term aseptic necrosis was not

Table 9.1 Classification of entities related to circulatory disorders (from Catto, 1976)

Intracapsular fracture of the femoral neck
Traumatic dislocation (of the hip)
Dysbarism
Idiopathic – no associated conditions
Idiopathic – in association with
  Alcoholism
  Hyperuricaemia and gout
  Collagen disorders, especially SLE
  Obesity
  Drugs – steroids and NSAIDs*
Sickle cell disease
Pancreatic disease
Gaucher's disease
Perthes' disease
Other eponymous conditions
  Kohler – tarsal navicular
  Freiberg – metatarsal head
  Kienbock – lunate
  Osgood–Schlatter – tibial tubercle
  Sindig–Larsen – patella, lower pole
  Sever – calcaneal hypophysis
  Calve – vertebral body epiphysis
  Scheuerman – vertebral ring epiphysis
Osteochondritis dissecans (Konig's disease)

* The conditions for which the drugs are administered are not thought to be contributory unless listed separately.

used until 1907, by Axhausen.

In 1888 Konig published the conclusions of his interest in joint loose bodies, which he thought resulted from a low-grade tissue reaction. Necrosis, a common feature of these, led to their inclusion in bone necrosis. Axhausen's interest in the subject came through the study of bone grafts. The fate of the graft, did it live or die, was investigated in the exploration of their use in bone tumour surgery during the 19th century, and was answered in 1893 by Barth. Influenced by Cohnheim's concept of embolization and anaemic infarction, Axhausen applied it in the study of bone lesions, with particular interest in the causation of arthritis deformans (osteoarthritis). At this time X-rays had become available and in the period 1908-1910 Kohler, Legg, Perthes, Calve and Kienboch described entities affecting epiphyses, followed by Freiberg in 1914. In 1923 Axhausen demonstrated necrosis in their pathology. He and Schmorl, independently in 1924, and Freund in 1926 described the pathology of idiopathic necrosis of the femoral head (McCarthy, 1982). Phemister, influenced by Axhausen, studied bone necrosis, emphasizing the correlation of radiographs and histology in 1920, in a variety of conditions affecting the femoral head and other sites. In 1939 with colleagues he described aseptic necrosis in caisson disease and of undetermined aetiology. Chandler, an associate of Phemister, had published three years earlier a study of femoral head necrosis without apparent cause, in effect idiopathic osteonecrosis. From about this time interest in necrosis of bone became more widespread, the number of conditions in which it was recognized grew, and special interest groups emerged.

Burrows (1959), writing editorially in the *Journal of Bone and Joint Surgery*, pointed out that osteochondritis deformans juvenilis was a term of convenience used by Perthes to make a distinction from arthritis deformans juvenilis. Without a pathological basis, it came to be used for any puzzling appearance in any centre of ossification. With the recognition of necrosis and fragmentation in Perthes' disease, and similar observations in Freiberg and Kienbock lesions, some of which macroscopically resembled lesions of osteochondritis dissecans, and with the assertion by Fairbank that osteochondritis dissecans was a fracture, and, further, with the view of Smillie that Freiberg's was a stress fracture there was a strong feeling for these to be related. But, as it was possible to argue about fracture preceding the necrosis or vice versa, uncertainty was rife. In 1971 there was still a place for the re-affirmation of the traumatic nature of osteochondritis dissecans (Aichroth, 1971a, b), including Freiberg's disease.

Uncertainty over the cause, apart from trauma, of bone necrosis in many cases, particularly of the femoral head, but with quite definite associated conditions in a high proportion, has led to the singling out of idiopathic disease of the femoral head as of special interest. Zinn (1971) gives a brief historical résumé of idiopathic osteonecrosis, starting from and including Konig's osteochondritis dissecans. He emphasizes the small number of cases reported up until the 1960s when Mankin and Brower found only 24 cases in the English literature. Welfling, in publications starting in 1951, was responsible for stimulating the interest of French physicians. In 1963 Volle wrote about the cases in the French literature, which, together with his 52, amounted to 199. It is now recognized that the condition is not uncommon, with cases appearing from the second decade onwards, with a peak incidence around the fifth decade, and males exceeding females by between 2 and 4:1.

The incidence of bone necrosis is difficult to establish in many instances. Some idea of prevalence following fracture is given by Sevitt (1981) (Chapter 6). The populations exposed to dysbaric osteonecrosis offer better opportunity for assessment. The incidence varies according to the conditions causing it: it is low among aviators and up to 50% in Japanese shellfish divers. In 1966 it was reported by the MRC Decompression Sickness Panel (McCallum *et al.*, 1966) that of 241 tunnel workers employed between 1955 and 1963, who were symptom free, 19% had lesions. The distribution of lesions in

Table 9.2 Distribution of lesions found in tunnellers and divers (Davidson, 1976)

	Tunnellers	*Divers*
Juxta-articular		
Humerus	35	15
Femur	11	8
Metaphyseal		
Humerus		
Proximal	11	24
Femur		
Proximal	3	15
Distal	30	34
Tibia		
Proximal	10	4

tunnellers and shellfish divers is shown in Table 9.2 (Davidson, 1976).

Arlot *et al.* (1983) reported 77 cases of idiopathic necrosis from Lyon, seen over eight years, all with normal kidneys. The mean ages were: male, 49 +/– 10, range 24–73 years; female 64 +/– 9, range 49–91 years. Of these 15 were on long-term steroid therapy, 33 were alcoholics, and 27 were normal. In 22 both femoral heads were affected. In addition ten femoral condyles, five humeral heads and ten feet were involved.

Excepting the eponymous conditions (section 9.3), the sites affected by the various categories are mainly the following:

- Metaphyseal/diaphyseal segment (medullary infarcts)
    Commonest sites: lower femur and upper tibia, humerus
- Epiphyseal/juxta-articular region
    Head of femur
    Head of humerus
    Femoral condyles
    Talus
    Carpal scaphoid
    Capitate and capitulum of the humerus

The basic pathology of the lesions, regardless of aetiology but given the starting point of established necrosis, is regarded as essentially similar. For epiphyseal sites the paradigm is the femoral head. The pathology as modified in Gaucher's, pancreatic and sickle cell disease, and Perthes' and the other eponymous conditions are discussed in separate sections.

9.1 THE PATHOLOGY OF BONE INFARCTION

The pathological descriptions of bone infarction begin from the point of established osteonecrosis. The events leading up to the necrosis have not been found to influence the events which follow.

9.1.1 MEDULLARY INFARCTS (FIGURE 9.1)

These are most often seen in dysbarism and haemoglobinopathies, but they are also seen as idiopathic events. Catto (1976) fully describes the lesion. If only marrow is affected there will not be an alteration of bone density and the lesion will not be visualized on X-ray, unless, at a later stage, dystrophic mineralization occurs or contiguous bone undergoes appositional reaction. It is unusual for such lesions to be discovered, let alone examined pathologically at an early stage so there is little detail about the reparative process. Seen at a late stage residual marrow is dry, opaque, possibly patchily calcified, and enclosed by a fibrous membrane, which also may contain mineral. Neighbouring trabeculae are thick-

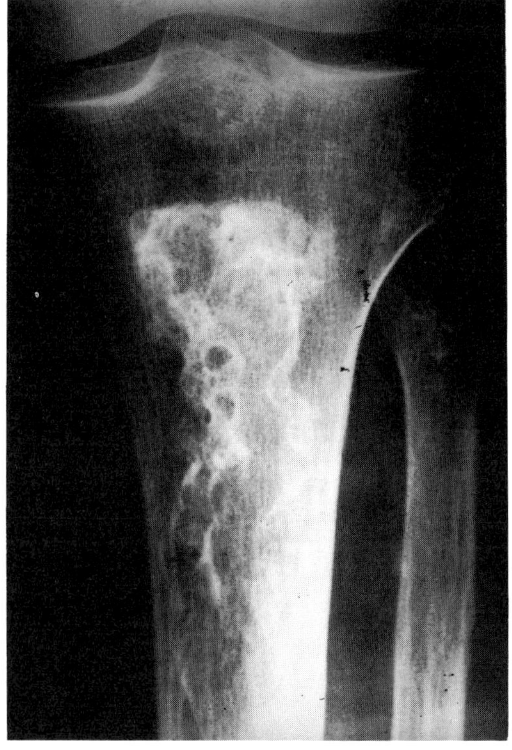

Figure 9.1 Medullary infarct in the proximal tibial metaphysis. The affected area, outlined by linear densities, is of variable density.

ened by appositional bone, and if the endosteal bone has been involved it too may be thickened. Mineral deposition and bone apposition will make the lesion detectable by radiograph, which may come about as an incidental finding.

A small but uncertain proportion of metaphyseal infarcts are associated with the

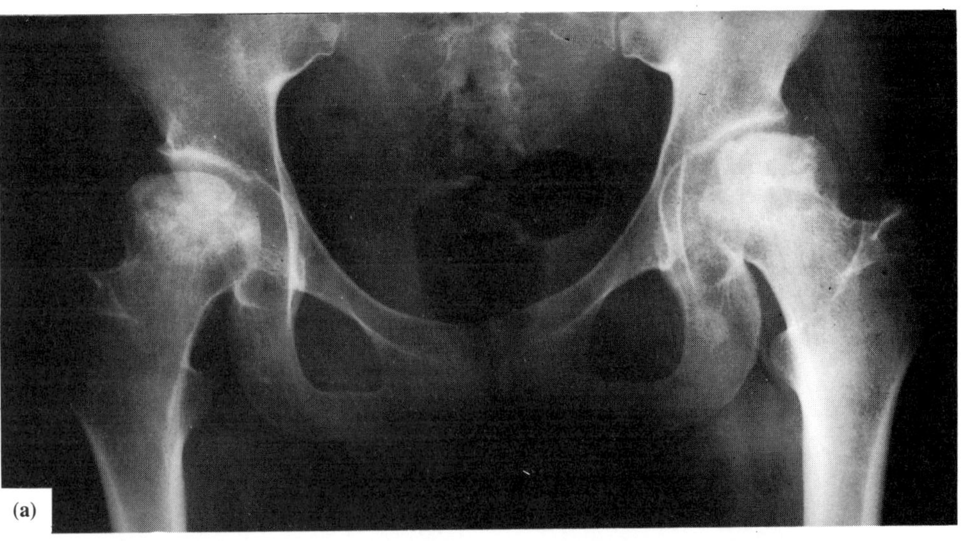

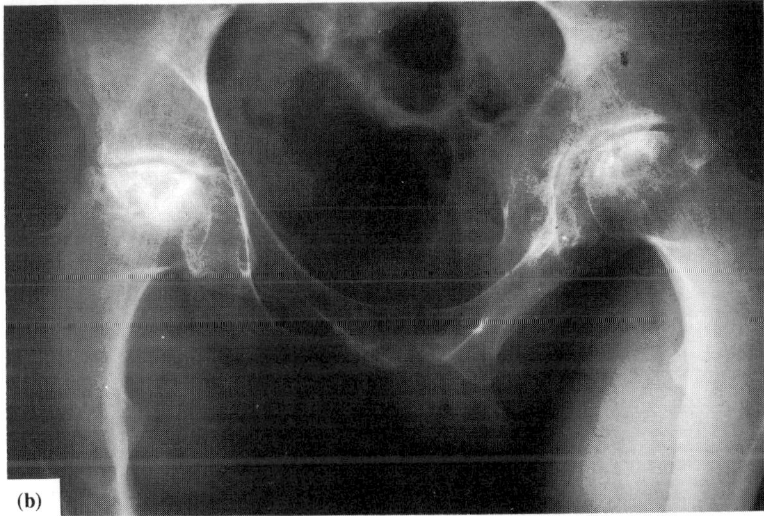

Figure 9.2 Avascular necrosis of femoral head, bilateral. (a) Avascular necrosis affects both femoral heads. The superior segment is denser than the remainder of the head. In the right hip this is marked by a band of decreased density, the site of reparative granulation tissue penetrating the infarct and leading to bone resorption. This is bordered by a dense zone due to reactive bone apposition in the viable boundary. These developments are not yet apparent in the left hip. (b) Some weeks later both femoral heads have collapsed: the infarcted tissue can no longer support the loads on the subchondral bone and cartilage and they subside.

development of sarcoma, presumably arising out of the reactive tissue. There is nothing about the neoplasm itself to distinguish it from those without such an antecedent history The reasons for suspecting the possibility may arise from an occupational history, radiographic findings, or features of infarction in histological material. The last may be difficult to attribute to a cause – antecedent infarction or following tumour invasion. Usually these are spindle celled tumours such as malignant fibrous histiocytoma (Galli *et al.*, 1978).

Sickle cell dactylitis is a special example of medullary infarct and is described below in connection with that condition.

9.1.2 EPIPHYSEAL INFARCTION

This also induces a reparative reaction (Figures 9.2–9.5). It is difficult to know the extent to which it may be successful; this will be considered again below. The usual sequence of events has been extensively studied and has been described as three stages (Catto, 1976):

1. Before the onset of structural failure and collapse.
2. Structural failure followed by collapse.
3. Development of secondary osteoarthritis.

Glimcher and Kenzora (1979a,b,c) adopt a similar division. First, macroscopically the

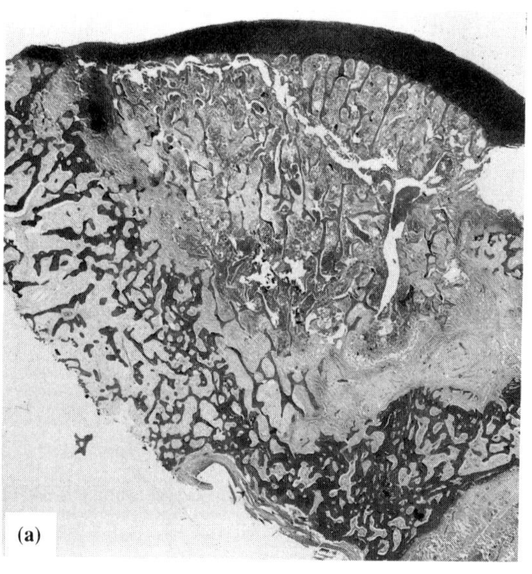

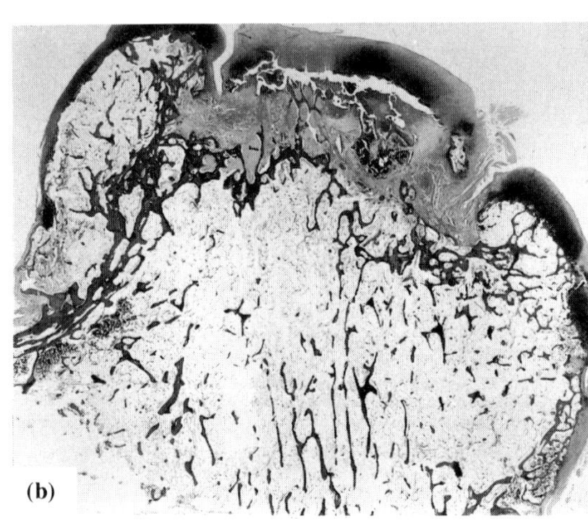

Figure 9.3 Avascular necrosis of humeral heads. (a) Histological section of humeral head (fragmentation artefact on right) resected prior to collapse. Normal cartilage overlies the triangular infarct which is bounded on its deep surface by a band of fibrous tissue containing only a few remnants of bone. Beyond this is a zone of viable dense bone: the thickness of the trabeculae here can be compared with the trabeculae in the infarct which, unaltered, represent the bone density in the head prior to the infarction. On the left at the point where the granulation tissue reaches and brings about the resorption of the subchondral bone plate, a point of weakness is created from which a subchondral fracture extends through the upper levels of the infarct. This fracture is detectable radiologically and is a diagnostic sign of infarction. Disintegration of necrotic bone is evident in the depths of the infarct. (b) Histological section of humeral head after collapse. The infarct has the same zoning and subchondral fracture. The infarcted bone has largely disintegrated, the articular cartilage has fractured at the extremities of the infarct, and is held in place by contact with the reparative tissue; if this gives way a flap or loose body will result.

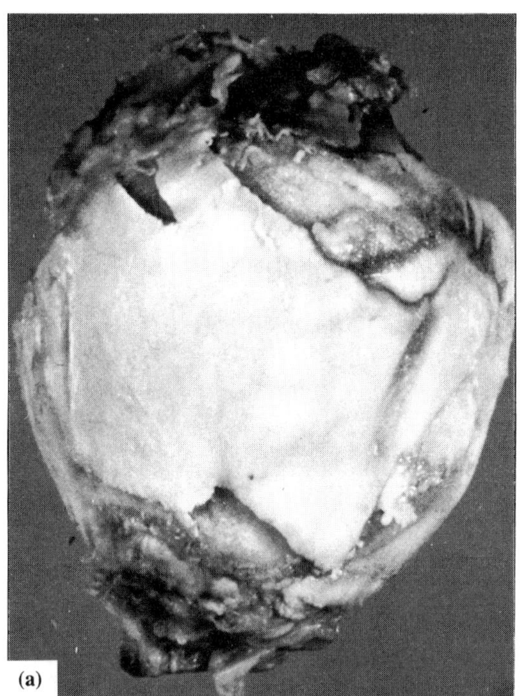

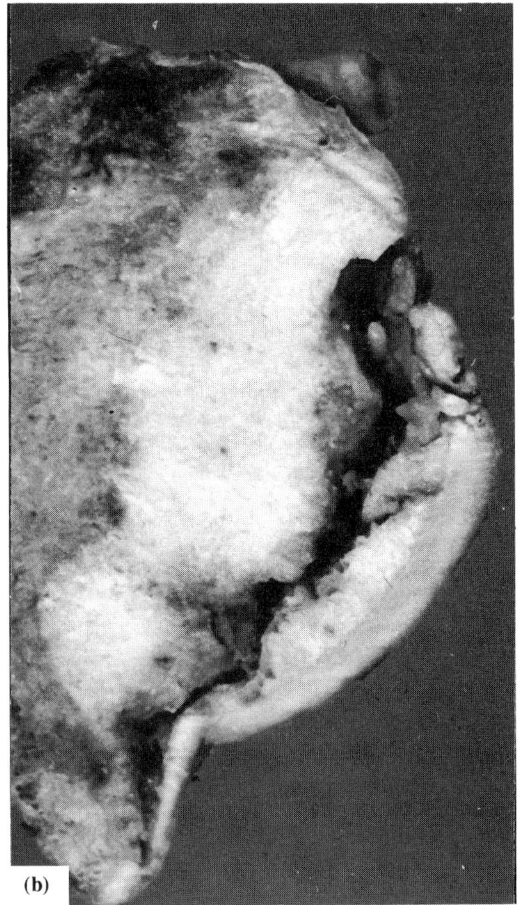

Figure 9.4 Avascular necrosis of humeral head. (a) A view of the articular surface which has a circular defect where it has folded and fractured with collapse of its support. (b) The cut surface of the specimen. The zoning seen in Figure 9.3 is discernible here. The articular cartilage, only partially attached, is now a flap.

cut surface of the infarct is yellow in colour, and dry. Depending on the progress of repair it will be abruptly demarcated from the adjacent viable tissue or there will be a zone of demarcation red or greyish in colour, depending on the proportion of vascular and fibrous proliferation, and possibly a band of denser bone. Repair starts in the viable tissue at the margin of the infarct, and consists of fibrovascular proliferation (granulation tissue) in the marrow and apposition of bone to trabecular surfaces. The latter will be on both viable and necrotic trabeculae at the margin, but will involve only dead bone as the granulation tissue penetrates the infarct. This local increase in bone volume becomes detectable in radiographs. The penetration of the granulation tissue is usually limited to some millimetres. The osteoblastic activity, following behind, also comes to a halt. The interface between repair and necrosis is gradually maturing fibrovascular tissue in which osteoclasts become active. Over time within the reparative tissue there may appear chondroid tissue. The articular cartilage is unaffected by these developments, as it receives its nutrition from the synovial fluid. However the calcified cartilage and the subchondral plate are necrotic.

Second, there can be an interval of months to years before collapse occurs. Two planes of weakness, where fracture occurs, have been recognized: the subchondral trabecular bone, and the reparative zone between

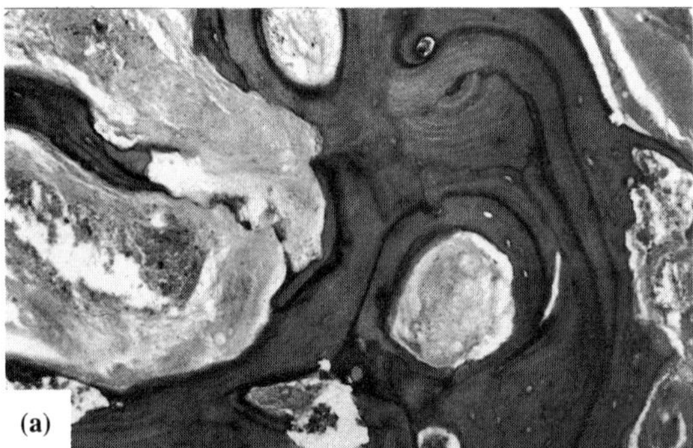

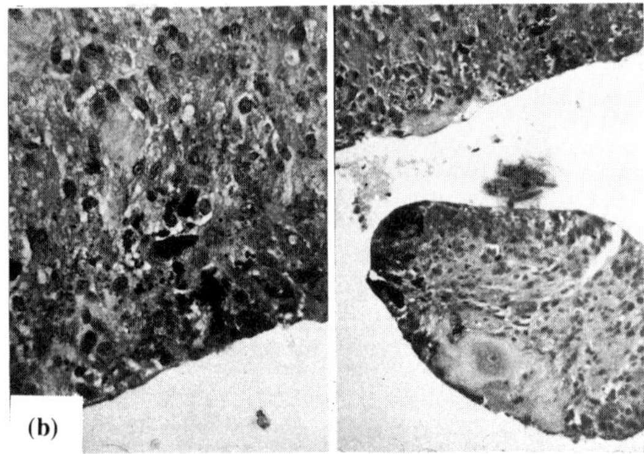

Figure 9.5 Avascular necrosis. (a) The zone of reactive bone. The linear cement lines indicate successive waves of apposition. The small area of mosaic pattern, and the several resorption cavities and small osteoid seams are signs of active turnover: but this has been in the past, for all this tissue is necrotic, indicating that a second episode of infarction has occurred. (b) Synovium, von Kossa stain. As the infarcted bone disintegrates it is able to escape into the joint space through the chondral fracture from where it is picked up by the synovium.

necrotic and viable tissue. The basis for the latter is the osteoclastic resorption and weakening of trabeculae. There has been uncertainty about the reason for the former. Glimcher and Kenzora (1979c) maintain from their studies that extension of the reaction to the subchondral region leads to a band of resorption of the subchondral plate lying along the perimeter of the necrotic zone; this alters the mechanics of the bone support system, leading to the propagation of fracture. It has been their experience that in the femoral head the plane of the propagated fracture differs as between necrosis following subcapital fracture and an idiopathic event. In the former they observed fracture through both planes, but only through the subchondral plane in idiopathic cases. They note Catto's experience, in some cases of post-fracture necrosis, of finding only the subchondral fracture. The subchondral fracture appears in radiographs as a crescent overlying the femoral head (the 'crescent sign' of osteonecrosis). Abrasion between the surfaces erodes the bone and leads the cartilage to sink in. The effect on the articular cartilage is that at least it must buckle at the margin between normal and necrotic bone; but it may also crack along this line, creating a flap of cartilage (Figures 9.3 and 9.4).

This same end point is reached if the bone at the deep surface of the infarct fractures. The cartilage loses its support, folds at the margins of the infarct, and eventually separates along the plane between subchondral plate and bone, splits at the fold and becomes a flap.

In either case abrasive movement of the flap creates bone detritus which escapes into the synovial space to be picked up by the synoviocytes where it induces a reaction. The presence in synovium of fragmented bone is certain indication of bone exposure within the joint; disintegrating infarct or Charcot joint are usually responsible.

Thirdly, if the situation is allowed to persist the flap will progressively disintegrate, possibly separating to become a loose body, exposing the infarcted bone which wears and fragments in its turn. When the viable bone is reached it will react, producing more bone to create an eburnated surface. The long-term result is usually a small flattened head with few osteophytes.

These are descriptions of large zones of infarction. Lesser zones can be more successfully handled by the reparative phenomena, with revascularization and stable repair, as seems to happen in many examples of osteochondritis dissecans (section 6.3.4)

9.2 AVASCULAR NECROSIS IN OSTEOARTHRITIS

As indicated above and in Chapter 8, osteoarthritis can develop following osteonecrosis, particularly in the femoral head. But, in addition, it is quite possible to demonstrate avascular necrosis in a small proportion of femoral heads resected in the treatment of osteoarthritis where there is no reason to invoke a preceding osteonecrosis (Figure 9.6). Necrotic bone is sometimes only

evident in histological sections, and is observed in bone that has been isolated by extensive fibrovascular proliferation, somewhat similar to a sequestrum. In other cases the infarct is larger, and macroscopically evident on the exposed bone of the articular surface as a yellowish-white area. Sawing through this reveals extension of the discoloured region into the substance of the head. It is rare for these to exceed 2 cm in size; absence of a substantial reactive zone around them, and the preserved contour of the articular surface, speak in favour of their having developed late in the disease.

9.3 THE AETIOPATHOGENESIS OF BONE INFARCTS

The spontaneous explanation for bone necrosis is deprivation of blood. The failure to establish the mechanism for this in idiopathic osteonecrosis has led Kenzora and Glimcher (1985) to postulate cumulative cell stress as the cause. The argument turns on the many associated conditions, the effect of corticosteroids on cell metabolism, on

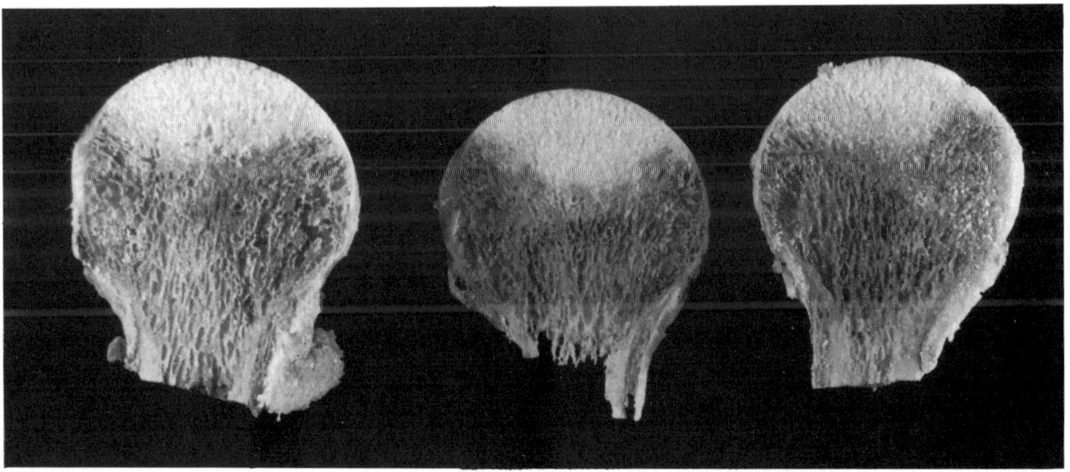

Figure 9.6 Femoral head resected in the treatment of osteoarthritis. The disease was not based on a preceding osteonecrosis. The intact specimen showed extensive loss of cartilage and eburnation of bone, the central portion of which was yellow. The cut surfaces show an exceptionally large infarct outlined by a zone of reactive tissue.

other risk factors upsetting cell metabolism, and on the concept of accumulating multifactorial damage to cells leading to the death of cells in bone as an organ. The experimental work of Matsui *et al.* (1992) seems relevant. The hypothesis does not as yet account for the localization of the disease.

The cause of the disruption of the supply to segments of bone is obvious in fractures and traumatic dislocations of the hip (Sevitt, 1981). But in other situations the circumstances may be less clear. Physiologically, bone is a rigid container filled with fluid under pressure through which pass compressible vessels containing pressurized fluid. This offers several ways in which flow can be impaired: intravascular obstruction to inflow or outflow by emboli, thrombi or disease of the vessels; disruption or compression of the vessels inside or outside the bone by local pathological events; compression of the vessels within the bone by altered pressure relationships. During infiltration of the marrow by inflammatory, neoplastic, histiocytic (Michael and Dorfman, 1976) or fibrous tissue with associated marrow infarction and sequestrum formation, the blood vessels are, or are assumed to be, destroyed or compressed. Microvascular obstruction of blood flow is usually considered to occur in sickle cell disease (Nachamie and Dorfman, 1974), but this has been questioned (Francis, 1991). In dysbarism it is assumed that gas bubbles cause the obstruction, although unequivocal evidence for this is wanting (Davidson, 1976). The difficulties are greater in the idiopathic cases where pathophysiological mechanisms are even more obscure, especially in those patients who are in good health. The problem with this last group is particularly taxing and of some interest to bone pathologists.

The increased incidence, and growing clinical problem has led to a number of reviews (Kenzora, 1985; Ono, 1992), in addition to a growing literature. Over the years a variety of hypotheses to explain the aetio-

pathogenesis of idiopathic osteonecrosis, particularly with reference to that of the femoral head, have been explored without a definitive conclusion. The mechanisms which have been considered are as follows.

1. Primary obstructive lesions of the intraosseous vasculature (Saito *et al.*, 1988, 1992; Atsumi *et al.*, 1989; Ohzono *et al.*, 1992). These have been microangiographic studies, some coupled with histology. They show intracapital obstruction of one or more of the arteries supplying the head, and, in some, arterial pathology, as well as extensive arterial proliferation. But aetiopathogenesis remains obscure. Ohzono *et al.* (1992) see a link with the mechanical obstructive mechanism suggested by Fergusson (1985).
2. Intravascular coagulation (Jones, 1992).
3. Raised intramedullary pressure (Wang *et al.*, 1975, 1977; Ficat, 1985; Hungerford and Lennox, 1985).
4. Fat embolism (Jones, 1985, 1989) as a result of a disturbance of fat metabolism.
5. Stress patterns in the head leading to arterial compression (Fergusson, 1985) or to accumulating microdamage affecting, in turn, the intracapital vasculature (Frost, 1960, 1964; Lagier, 1971; Freeman *et al.*, 1974).

Kenzora and Glimcher (1985) have proposed that multifactorial elements in the pathogenesis lead to cumulative stress on cells and their final necrosis. Their hypothesis does not state what determines the sites at which this occurs.

Although none of these has found general favour, and aetiology and pathogenesis remain obscure, for the bone fancier the hypothesis of microtrauma is the most intriguing, even though it now seems to command little attention.

It is not proposed to discuss the mechanics that cause the damage. Various observations of microdamage to bone have been made

(Frost, 1960, 1964, 1973, 1986; Lagier, 1971; Todd *et al.*, 1972; Freeman *et al.*, 1974; Fazzalini *et al.*, 1987; Benaissa *et al.*, 1989). The damage is either clefts and splits without discontinuity, or complete fractures of individual trabeculae. The former have been demonstrated by Frost (1960) by bulk staining of bone in fuchsin before sectioning. The latter have been shown in macerated bones at low magnification and histologically.

The hypothesis is that microdamage caused by repetitively applied forces accumulates more rapidly than it can be repaired, by remodelling in the case of incomplete lesions, or by fracture callus in complete lesions. In reading the literature it is not always clear as to what exact consequences authors are envisaging. However, two outcomes seem to be anticipated.

1. In due time the progressively weakening bone gives way and fractures, as a result of which necrosis ensues. (This is the thesis of Frost.)
2. The reactive tissue engendered by the microdamage impedes the blood flow to part of the head which undergoes necrosis. Lagier (1971) suggests this possibility. Further changes follow this.

Glimcher and Kenzora (1979c) have assembled a catalogue of evidence to counter these hypotheses, based on their own experience and that of others. Their thesis is similar to that of Catto (1976). The premise from which they start is that the first evidence of fracture is in the subchondral region, where a crescent of subchondral bone of the superior surface separates from the underlying cancellous bone. They pose the question, does osteonecrosis precede the crescent fracture (see pathology) through dead bone, or is the fracture first and the osteonecrosis follows. In answering this they emphasize that a fracture at this site is not going to cause necrosis of the deeper tissue, which argues for necrosis before fracture. They also state that osteopenia, a usual antecedent to fracture in femoral heads, is not a feature of

idiopathic osteonecrosis, even in patients with renal transplants. They add that if osteopenia and microfracture were the underlying cause, a much higher incidence of idiopathic osteonecrosis should be seen in patients with primary or secondary osteopenia than in patients of similar age without osteopenia. Additionally, they quote both Catto's (1976) and Jones' (1971) observations that superior segments of femoral heads at an early stage were necrotic, the repair response was underway, there was no evidence of a subchondral fracture, nor any change in the trabecular architecture.

Several of the foregoing statements are open to argument. First, the question of underlying osteoporosis. The morphometric analysis of iliac crests in idiopathic osteonecrosis in renal transplantation by Nielsen *et al.* (1977) and Charon *et al.* (1982), and in non-renal cases by Arlot *et al.* (1983) (see above) established the presence of reduced bone volume in all the cases and of reduced osteoblastic activity. The age range of the cases seen by Arlot *et al.* (1983) extended well into old age. Furthermore, Freeman *et al.* (1974) quantitated the number of trabecular fractures in 10 post-fracture femoral heads, and in the femoral necks and heads of 15 cadavers ranging in age from 20 to 90 years, and assessed the bone density of the specimens. The specimens were macerated, dried, weighed, their volume determined, and then divided into 3–5 mm slices and the number and distribution of fracture calluses counted (Figure 6.11). Some fractures were present in all, except for one of three 20-year olds. As bone density fell the number of fractures rose; the critical point for a steep rise was 0.5 g/ml. They concluded that:

1. Occasional fatigue fracture is physiological.
2. There is a critical bone density at which the number of fractures rises steeply.
3. Gross fracture of the femoral neck is a terminal event of progressive trabecular failure due to fatigue, not impact.

The controls in a study by Fazzalini *et al.*

(1987) provide corroboration of the association of falling trabecular density and increasing trabecular fractures (Freeman *et al.*, 1974).

These rebuttals do not touch upon the absence of trabecular alteration or of fracture in the early cases of Catto (1976) and Jones (1971), nor upon the observation by Glimcher and Kenzora (1979b) that there was no sign of microfracture at the interface of viable and necrotic bone as predicted by the microdamage hypothesis. These are observations which seriously weaken the microdamage hypothesis. Nevertheless, the weight of the rebuttals warrants a close appraisal of femoral heads in the earliest stages of idiopathic osteonecrosis by maceration and morphometric techniques. More detail about the distribution of fractures in the head and neck (e.g. Benaissa *et al.*, 1989), combined with morphometric analysis should also lead to further understanding.

There is a group of lesions affecting epiphyses or epiphysoid bones (small bones with a single centre of ossification which grow from the cartilage end plate as in epiphyses) whose name suggests inflammation of bone and cartilage – osteochondritis, osteochondrosis, epiphysitis – but in which neither cartilage nor inflammation play a part. Jaffe (1972), in a discussion of these lesions, quotes Burrows' (1959) reference to them as 'the most eponymous of affections'. Following that lead they are so listed in Table 9.3 with their site and the currently held views on pathogenesis.

It seems desirable to mention here other conditions affecting epiphyses in which necrosis may occur so as to consider, in one place, a sometimes confusing group of lesions. To do so necessitates confronting the term osteochondritis dissecans, which might be translated as dissecting osteochondral disorder, and to include slipping capital femoral epiphysis, and physeal fractures.

In most of these, it is generally agreed that both trauma and avascular necrosis play a part, but there is not always agreement as to cause and effect. The exceptions are Calvé's disease and Scheuerman disease. Calvé described vertebral collapse (vertebra plana); Compere and Coventry (Burrows, 1959) recorded eosinophil granuloma as one cause, since when vertebra plana due to eosinophil granuloma has become Calvé's disease. In Scheuerman disease, the nucleus pulposus is forced through a weak point of the vertebral end plate.

Kohler's disease affects children between 3 and 7 years, predominantly boys (4:1), and gives rise to flattening and increased density of the bone. Over a period of 2 to 3 years the bone recovers its normal appearance. A few biopsies have shown necrosis and bone fragmentation. The sequence of events is readily explained by avascular necrosis followed by healing. (Something similar is seen in milder cases of Perthes' disease.)

Kienboeck's disease affects mainly the right wrist of males aged 20–40 years, which

Table 9.3 Eponymous conditions

	Site	*Pathogenesis*
Kohler	Tarsal navicular	Necrosis
Kienboeck	Lunate	Fracture, necrosis
Freiberg	Metatarsal head	Fracture, necrosis
Osgood–Schlatter	Tibial tubercle	Avulsion
Sindig–Larsen	Patella, lower pole	Avulsion
Sever	Calcaneal apophysis	Avulsion
Calvé	Vertebral body epiphysis	Eosinophil granuloma
Scheuerman	Vertebral ring epiphysis	Intrusion of disc

inclines one to regard it as traumatic. Symptoms are not severe at first, leading to a long interval before excision of the flattened, irregularly dense bone. This reveals necrosis and fracture without repair, findings which give precedence to either fracture/necrosis or necrosis/fracture. Other carpal bones can be similarly affected: scaphoid involvement is Preiser's disease.

Freiberg's disease can arguably be considered as an osteochondritis dissecans (try as one will the term osteochondritis is not to be avoided).

Osgood–Schlatter, Sindig–Larsen and Sever (and other) avulsion lesions lead to necrosis of the avulsed bone fragment. At one time it was argued that this represented an underlying cause and led to use of the term osteochondritis in connection with them. Active adolescents are affected; limitation of activity seems adequate treatment, but requires months to be effective. Complete loss of continuity between ligament and bone does not occur, but only a fragment of bone and cartilage is torn from the apophyseal surface; and sometimes there is laceration of the apophyseal cartilage plate (Jaffe 1972, and references, therein).

Calvé's disease is a manifestation of eosinophil granuloma.

Scheuerman's disease affects one or several vertebral bodies, usually of the thoracic region, but less frequently of lumbar or cervical level, in adolescents. There is generally some pain associated. The result is anterior wedging leading to accentuation of the thoracic curve, or diminution of the lumbar or cervical curves. Ischaemic necrosis of the secondary ossification centre (the ringlike epiphysis) was thought to be the cause. It is now believed to result from the herniation of nucleus pulposus through weak points in the cartilaginous end plate, with subsequent tracking anteriorly to isolate the ring epiphysis; the material may eventually end up beneath the anterior ligament to cause pressure atrophy of the vertebral surface (Jaffe, 1972).

Osteochondritis dissecans is a condition in which there is partial or complete separation of a segment of articular cartilage and subchondral bone from the joint surface. The lesion has been recognized since the studies by Konig, published in 1888. Many of the separated fragments are necrotic, leading to its inclusion in the category of avascular necrosis, although debate has been waged over trauma vs necrosis as the primary event (Nagura, 1960). At the present time the weight of opinion favours trauma on the basis of epidemiological and experimental evidence (Aichroth, 1971a, b). The condition is further discussed and illustrated in Chapter 6.

Slipping of the femoral capital epiphysis is discussed in section 6.3.3.

An additional potential cause of epiphyseal avascular necrosis in the child is physeal fracture (section 6.3.3). Dale and Harris (1958) and Salter and Harris (1963) correlated animal and clinical studies of this condition. The blood vessels supplying most epiphyses enter through the periosteum at the sides. In a few, notably the femoral head, articular cartilage overlaps the physeal plate and the nutrient vessels must enter through the cartilage. In the event of a physeal fracture the latter arrangement exposes the vessels to damage and puts the epiphysis at risk of necrosis. Since the epiphyseal vessels supply the reserve zone of the physis, its growth is also at risk.

9.4 GAUCHER'S DISEASE AND AVASCULAR NECROSIS

In this heritable metabolic disorder in which cerebrosides accumulate in histiocytic cells of the reticuloendothelial system, principally the spleen, liver and marrow, the bone is affected and may undergo infarction. The disease is severe and may be fatal in infancy, due to involvement of the central nervous system (Goldblatt *et al.*, 1978). Non-neuropathic cases are manifest later in childhood, or at any time into adult life, depending on the severity. The disease, in its mild expression, can be compatible with survival into old age. Orthopaedic aspects of the disease have been presented by Amstutz and Carey (1966), Goldblatt *et al.* (1978), Bell *et al.* (1986) and Katz *et al.* (1987). The problems are the result of marrow infiltration by Gaucher cells, and are an expression of the age and extent of the involvement. Clinically the bone involvement may result in attacks of severe bone pain with constitutional symptoms. The differentiation between osteomyelitis and a 'Gaucher crisis' is an important and difficult decision in which bone scans (Katz *et al.*, 1991) and MRI (Horev *et al.*, 1991) seem to have a place.

Substantial marrow involvement at an early age may cause expansion of the metaphyseal cortex with endosteal resorption. In the femur this is responsible for the Ehrlenmyer-flask shape demonstrated by imaging. In some the cellular accumulation gives rise in metaphyses to small focal loss of trabeculae, either by pressure atrophy or by infarction (of Gaucher cells and bone) with subsequent resorption and fibrosis, causing focal osteolytic foci in radiographs. Cortices may be porotic as the result of enlarged Haversian canals associated with the presence of Gaucher cells. More substantial medullary infarction can occur, which can lead to scarring and bone resorption. These reductions in bone volume weaken the bone, which may be accentuated by disuse, putting the patient at risk of pathological fracture and vertebral collapse.

Epiphyseal infarction occurs, mainly in the femoral head. In children it resembles Perthes' disease, and may show degrees of restoration over time; in adults degrees of collapse occur; in each case ensuing joint deformity leads ultimately to osteoarthritis. Cases with humeral head infarction have been reported (James, 1952; Rourke and Heslin, 1965).

The marrow of an affected bone is greyish, in which necrotic areas stand out as paler areas, and firmer if there has been fibrosis. The Gaucher cells are large, polyhedral or elongated, with a grainy, stranded cytoplasm that is lightly eosinophilic in conventional haematoxylin and eosin sections. Bone volume may be reduced. The Gaucher cells seem to crowd out the vascular tree and zones of necrosis may be found. Fibrous replacement of these takes place to produce densely collagenized foci. Enclosed trabeculae tend to become necrotic. Larger areas of necrosis assume the character of medullary or epiphyseal infarcts (see above).

There is a substantial literature on the imaging of Gaucher disease, but there are not many pathological studies (see Cushing and Stout, 1926; Melamed and Chester, 1938; Battaglia and Chiandussi, 1965; Jaffe, 1972; Catto, 1976).

9.5 PANCREATIC DISEASE AND AVASCULAR NECROSIS

For a century and more there have been studies of the distribution and pathogenesis of pancreatic fat necrosis (Gerle *et al.*, 1965). It follows acute and chronic pancreatitis and sometimes acinar pancreatic carcinoma (Jackson *et al.*, 1952; Virship and Slivinski, 1973; Radin *et al.*, 1986). Most patients are adults, often alcoholic, but drug-induced pancreatitis has been known (Baron *et al.*, 1984). In addition children are affected following post-traumatic pancreatitis (Allen and Jinkins, 1978).

Adipose tissue of the abdominal and thoracic cavities is primarily involved but in a proportion of cases subcutaneous, synovial and marrow fat is affected. These cases usually present with abdominal symptoms, with the skin, articular and bone lesions as secondary problems. However, in some cases these lesions are primary in the presentation, as a syndrome of subcutaneous nodules and polyarthritis (Simkin *et al.*, 1983; Wilson *et al.*, 1983; Baron *et al.*, 1984), or as pain and disability in one or more large joints, leading to discovery of pancreatitis or occasionally carcinoma (Radin *et al.*, 1986).

The skin nodules are usually small red and painful, and regress over some weeks; larger ones may liquefy and discharge. They consist of necrotic fat in the form of 'ghost cells' surrounded by a zone of inflammatory cells (lymphocytes and some polymorphs).

Both small and large joints may be affected in a variety of combinations. The pathogenesis is periarticular and synovial fat necrosis, giving rise to painful swollen joints which subside over some weeks (Smukler *et al.*, 1979). Free fatty acids are a prominent constituent of the synovial fluid. The synovial fat necrosis conforms with the pattern in the skin nodules (Wilson *et al.*, 1983; Simkin *et al.*, 1983).

Originally the bone lesions were regarded as being in the long bones, mainly femur and tibia. But latterly the involvement of small bones of hands and feet, wrists and ankles has been recognized (Lucas and Owen, 1962; Immelman *et al.*, 1964; Slovis *et al.*, 1975). These are painful, and may add to the joint symptoms. Consequently, they are seen in radiographs fairly early in their course, as foci of osteolysis affecting cortex and cancellous bone. There is often a periosteal reaction, particularly in children. Similar lesions appear in long tubular bones of arms and legs; and vertebral involvement has been reported in one case (Allen and Jinkins, 1978). Sometimes only the periosteal reaction is seen. These lesions generally resolve over some months without sequelae. However, cases with collapse requiring surgical intervention have been recorded (Allen and Jinkins, 1978; Baron *et al.*, 1984). Descriptions of the pathology come from the resected fragmented material, in which necrotic fat and bone trabeculae, fibrous tissue and inflammatory cells were seen.

In addition to the foregoing there are lesions which fit with descriptions of the intramedullary and epiphyseal dysbaric infarcts (Jackson *et al.*, 1952; Immelman *et al.*, 1964; Jaffe, 1972). These are silent, and appear in radiographs only after they have acquired a deposit of mineral. But with the advent of MRI they can be detected much earlier by imaging (Haller *et al.*, 1989). They have been observed mainly in the long bones of adults. Similarly, the epiphyseal lesions are found in the heads of femora and humeri. Here they too can give rise to collapse and secondary osteoarthritis. In the short term the anatomical findings are foci of fat necrosis with surrounding reaction in keeping with the time scale. Long term, a lesion resembles avascular necrosis of the medulla or epiphysis; in the latter instance if the site is a femoral head, collapse is likely. The necrotic adipose tissue takes up calcium, is surrounded by reactive fibroblastic tissue, and appositional, and possibly membranous, bone response.

The pathogenesis of the bone lesions has been attributed to circulating lipolytic enzymes or fat embolism. Perry (1947) demonstrated experimentally that the lipolytic enzymes spread in the abdomen and thorax by lymphatics. The more distant lesions must be the result of vascular transport following introduction into the circulation via the thoracic duct. But, dispute about pathogenesis continues (Potts, 1975; Simkin *et al.*, 1983; Wilson *et al.*, 1983; Jones, 1985).

The original and early descriptions of the lesions were pathological. Scarpelli (1956) reported the largest number of cases. In 67 autopsies of pancreatitis there were seven with necrosis in the single marrow sample taken (site not specified); these were all cases with widespread abdomino-thoracic necroses. But pathological descriptions of bone lesions are few compared with clinical and radiological reports. There is place for histopathological descriptions of the more acute healing lesions.

9.6 SICKLE CELL DISEASE AND AVASCULAR NECROSIS

The traditional view of the pathogenesis of avascular necrosis in sickle cell disease is microvascular obstruction by sickled cells, with thrombosis as a secondary phenomenon. This view is questioned by Francis (1991), who proposes that major vascular thrombosis is the pathogenesis. Nevertheless, the composition of the haemoglobin correlates with the severity of the disease (Powers, 1990). The question is still open.

Each of an individual's two haemoglobin genes forms its own type. As many as 17 haemoglobins are known, which are labelled alphabetically; only A is the normal adult type, and S is the sickling type. Genetic inheritance leads to a variety of hetero- and homozygous combinations. Heterozygotes formed with A are carriers and generally disease free. Homozygotes of abnormal types are usually anaemic. Abnormal heterozygotes may be anaemic (Middlemiss and Raper, 1966).

The globin component of haemoglobin consists of two paired polypeptide chains, alpha and beta. In haemoglobin S, beta-peptide chains have valine substituted for glutamic acid at position 6. When de-oxygenated, this produces a ring structure which locks with an alpha-peptide chain of another molecule; a sequence of such events produces rows of interlocked molecules. As the proportion of the haemoglobin arranged in this way increases, the cell assumes an elongated shape, and becomes progressively more rigid. If oxygen tension improves the sickling is reversed (Diggs, 1967). As mentioned above, conventional opinion is that there is a danger that the rigid sickled cells arrest at restriction points in capillary beds, further reducing oxygen tension and setting up a cycle which results in vascular occlusion. The likelihood of this occurring is determined by the genetic structure: homozygous or heterozygous for S; and if the latter, whether the allele is normal or another abnormal haemoglobin, such as thalassaemia.

The thalassaemia gene fails to produce beta-polypeptide chains. In the homozygous state the disease is very serious (major), usually resulting in death in infancy; heterozyogous individuals, even with A, are severely anaemic; and with S they are exposed to sickling.

The geographical distribution, both natural and as affected by migration (and the slave trade), of haemoglobin variants determines regional patterns of associated disease. The natural distribution (Middlemiss and Raper, 1966) of those associated with avascular necrosis is:

S: Tropical Africa; Mediterranean, Middle East; South India
C: West Africa
Thal: mainly Mediterranean; less commonly Middle East, India, Myanmar, Thailand, Indonesia, China; rarely Britain

There are five haemoglobinopathies known to be associated with avascular necrosis of bone (femoral head) (Chung and Ralston, 1969): SS, CS, S Thal, AS, SF (Thal = thalassaemia; F = fetal). These abnormalities have effects throughout the body, and death usually results from these, from infancy onwards, depending on the severity of the haemoglobinopathy. The marrow hyperplasia causes osteoporosis through increased resorption: the space between trabeculae is widened; the cortices are thinned and the osteonal canals enlarged; if the condition is sufficiently severe from early on there may be metaphyseal widening (Jaffe, 1972). These changes are notable in the skull (which may acquire a spicular periosteal reaction), mandible, ribs and vertebrae (which may collapse), and iliae. The condition of the marrow makes the bones susceptible to osteomyelitis, particularly by *Salmonella* organisms. In some severely affected children there is interference with physeal growth, attributed to blocking of vessels by marrow hyperplasia; some believe the cupped vertebral end plates are due to interference with growth of the central region.

The course of the disease is episodic, with exacerbations (crises) between intervals of relative well being (Diggs, 1965). In crises there are frequently attacks of abdominal and bone pain. The latter is commonly attributed to marrow infarction, but in a biopsy investigation only three out of seven cases were demonstrated to have infarcts (Charache and Page, 1967). An important and difficult differential diagnosis is osteomyelitis (generally *Salmonella*), to which bone scintigraphy and MRI may contribute. In children from 6 months to 2 years of age the tubular bones of hands and feet are affected (the unaffected fetal haemoglobin is gone by 6 months, and susceptible haemopoietic marrow has gone by 2 years). Necrosis involves the marrow and the inner portion of the cortex supplied by medullary vessels (Weinberg and Currarino, 1972; Catto, 1976). The overlying soft tissues soon become oedematous, but bone changes do not appear radiologically before 10–14 days when there is a substantial periosteal reaction. In the ensuing months this is gradually remodelled to increase the diameter of the bone. The episode interferes with growth in length; if the hands are asymmetrically involved inequality of finger length will result (Middlemiss and Raper, 1966).

In adults medullary infarction occurs mainly in the major long bones. This may not give rise to radiological signs if the cortex is not involved since there is little bone available to react. Such infarcts will be surrounded by fibrous tissue and may in time undergo some mineral deposition. If, however, the cortex becomes necrotic, through involvement of its medullary supply there will be periosteal and endosteal reaction, leading to concentric rings of bone (Diggs, 1967). The radiological pattern of 'a bone within a bone' is thought to result from successive infarcts and healing

reactions, although the pathogenesis is far from clear (Catto, 1976).

Epiphyseal infarcts involve the femoral head more than that of the humerus; the knee, talus or elbow are sometimes affected. In children a Perthes'-like condition results. In adults the developments are as in other causes of epiphyseal infarction. However, Sherman (1959) described a case where, although the load-bearing cartilage of the femoral head was detached, the epiphyseal bone was not necrotic. Between the two surfaces there was granulation and fibrous tissue containing necrotic bone fragments. There are abundant descriptions of the imaging features of these conditions; but pathological observations are comparatively few, and sometimes at odds with the former.

9.7 LEGG–CALVE–PERTHES' DISEASE

This condition is due to avascular necrosis of the femoral capital epiphysis before closure of the physis. Treatment is aimed at preservation of the affected joint and there is no basis for surgical intervention, so that, apart from a few core biopsies, knowledge of the pathology has come from postmortem studies. The condition is not fatal, so the opportunities for this have arisen because of co-existing disease. Much of the available material (11 cases) was reviewed by Catteral *et al.* (1982a). Unanswered questions remain and opportunities to study additional material should not be missed.

It is a non-genetic, developmental disease of unknown aetiology; undersized, disadvantaged children are at greatest risk (Wynne-Davies, 1980). Details of age range and incidence are given in Table 9.4.

The condition manifests itself as a painful irritable hip. The natural history has been studied by many; the conclusions of Catteral (1971) are widely used. He proposed four categories of disease based on radiological findings at the initial examination and fur-

Table 9.4 Perthes' disease: some epidemiological data (Kemp, 1983)

Sex	Ratio	Age range (years)	Age maximum incidence	Bilateral Incidence
Male	4	1–14	5	9.61/3000
Female	1	1–10	4	0.41/11 800

ther progress. Pathological studies (Catterall *et al.*, 1982a, b) support his thesis that the size and number of ischaemic episodes determine the course of the disease. Small, single episodes give rise to small infarcts which heal; larger, and second or third episodes, cause more extensive infarction, a longer reparative period and a risk of collapse of the epiphysis and permanent deformity (Catterall, 1971).

No studies have established the cause of the vascular occlusion (Catterall, 1981). Animal experiments have not reproduced the disease, leading to the conclusion that constitutional factors as well as local ones must play a part.

Devas (1975) concluded from his clinical observations that it seemed more likely that stress fracture of the femoral head was responsible for the necrosis. He reasoned this to be the case in both adults and children, and postulated that this is the basis of Perthes' disease. His argument turned largely on the similar distribution of stress fractures in the child and the elderly, and the absence from conventional classification of a condition in children comparable to stress fracture of the femoral head.

The material reported on by Catteral *et al.* (1982a, b) included two unaffected hips and five normal controls. From this it was established that the articular cartilage of unaffected hips was thicker than normal controls, with less active ossification and sporadic calcification within its substance. The physis of these femurs was thinner than normal with irregularity of the cell columns and of the primary spongiosa. The affected femoral

heads (Figures 9.7 and 9.8) also had thick articular cartilage. This was pronounced at the periphery, where the cartilage continued to grow and ossify causing broadening of the head, which is associated with a broadening of the neck. The head enlargement leads to a remodelling deformity of the acetabulum, which nevertheless ceases adequately to contain the femoral head, with pressure of the rim of the acetabulum adding to the deformity of the head (Figure 9.7).

Given optimum circumstances the infarcted zone is invaded by granulation tissue; accompanying osteoclasts resorb the necrotic bone, and the fibrous tissue undergoes metaplasia to chondroid tissue which ossifies and restores the integrity of the head. Trabecular bone peripheral to this is strengthened by apposition, the new bone demarcated by cement lines. Should some of these marginal trabeculae be necrotic then the core of the buttressed bone will be free of osteocytes. The basis for the conclusion that several episodes of infarction occur is the finding in some cases of successive layers of appositional bone of which one or more are also necrotic.

During the course of the disease there tends to be overgrowth of the articular cartilage and enlargement of the head. This in turn can have an effect on the moulding of the acetabulum as it adapts to the head (Catteral *et al.*, 1982b).

Abnormality of the femoral neck occurs in this condition (Robichon *et al.*, 1974). The neck widens as the result of growth and ossification of (articular) cartilage extending down over the neck beyond the limits of the

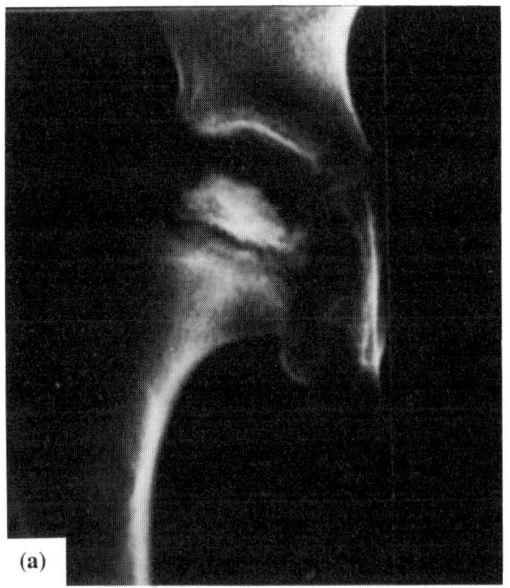

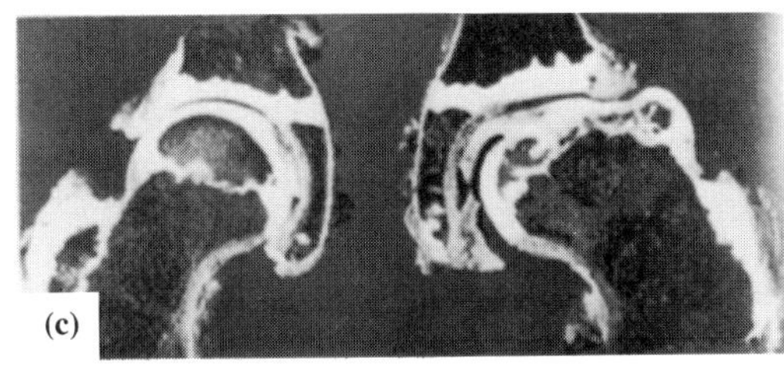

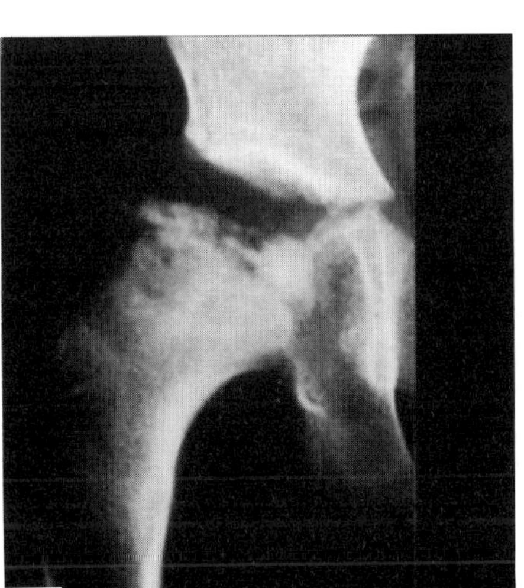

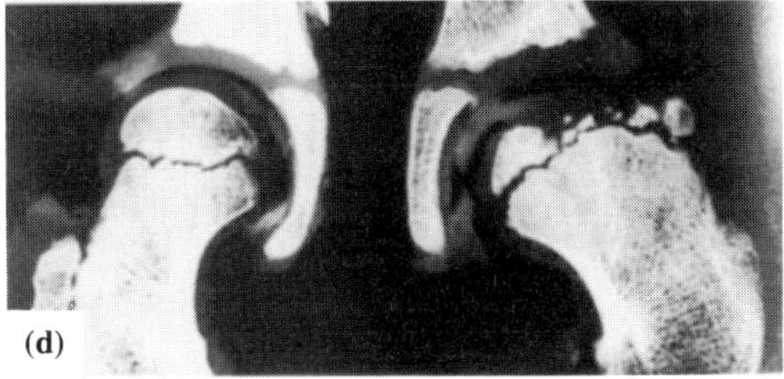

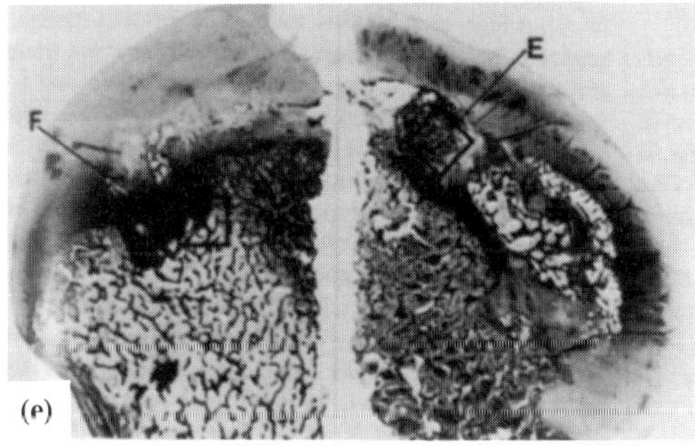

Figure 9.7 Perthes' disease. Male age 8 years. Presented because of hip disease and was then discovered to have leukaemia, from which he died. The hip was untreated. Both hips were obtained at autopsy. (a) Initial radiograph with dense region in the mid-region of the epiphysis. (b) One year later the density has largely been resorbed; the medial and lateral elements have grown. The neck is broad. (c) Cut surface of both hips. The affected epiphysis has collapsed; the acetabulum has adapted to it, but the head is too large and hinges on the labrum which has indented the head. There is widening of the neck; articular cartilage extends down it. (d) Fine detail radiograph shows most of these changes. (e) Histological sections of anterior and posterior slabs (i.e. the plane at right angles to c/d): at E fragmented necrotic bone; on its right a pale zone of granulation tissue; at this interface the necrotic tissue is being resorbed; on its right side the granulation tissue is differentiating to form a dark band of fibrocartilage, the right hand surface of which is ossifying; further to the right again a large region of viable cancellous bone which is being augmented by growth and ossification of the articular cartilage. At F the physis is disorganized, failing to ossify and forming a mass which can be responsible for a radiological defect. (Reproduced with permission from Catterall *et al.*, 1982b.)

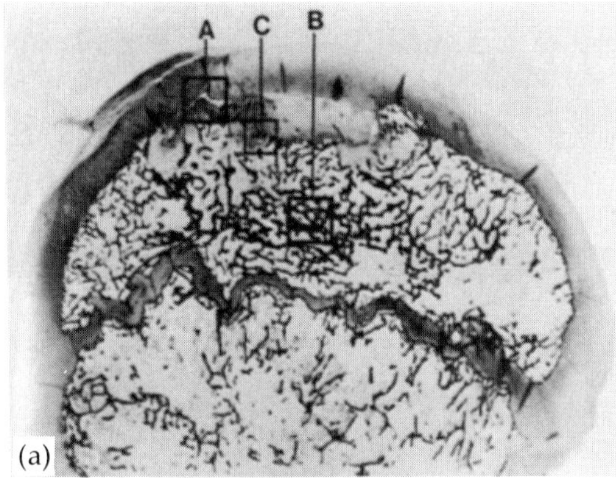

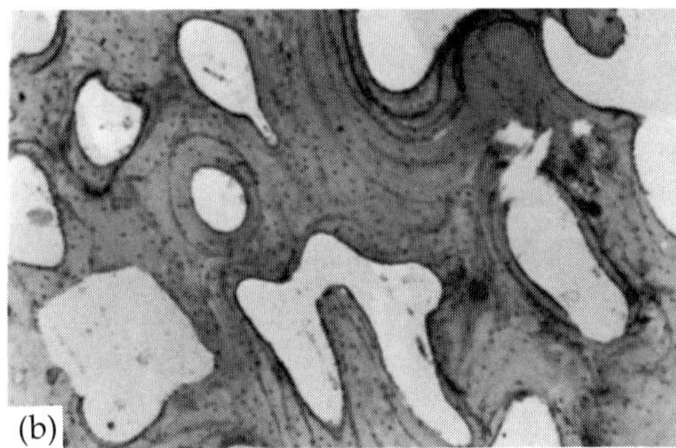

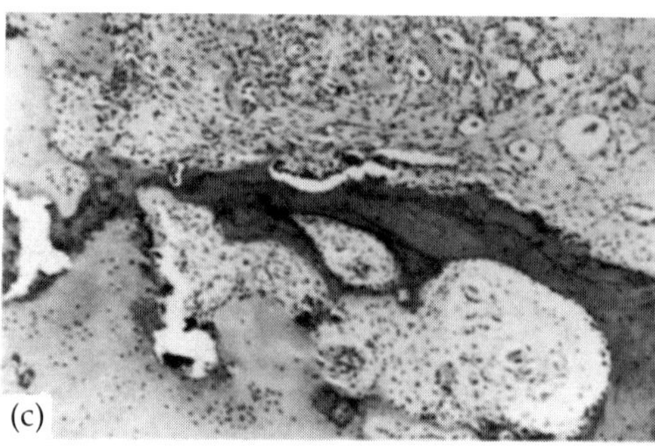

Figure 9.8 Perthes' disease. Male 12 years. Died of renal failure. Perthes' recognized at 10 years of age; 6 months weight relieving caliper. (a) Coronal section of femoral head. It is enlarged, slightly flattened, with a widened neck covered by cartilage. In the centre, beneath the cartilage, a pale zone of fibrovascular and fibrocartilaginous tissues engaged in replacement and repair (area C). To their left a subchondral fracture (area A). The dense bone here and at area B have many appositional cement (arrest) lines (b), and show some remodelling (c). (Reproduced with permission from Catterall *et al.*, 1982b.)

physis. In addition there are sometimes extensions or remnants of cartilage in the metaphysis resulting from disorganization of the physis (Catterall *et al.*, 1982b).

Circumstances are not always optimal, and the infarction may collapse before repair and restoration can be completed with a resultant flat head (coxa plana). Repair of the infarct and bone remodelling continue without correcting the deformity, which leads to risk of osteoarthritis in early adult life.

9.8 HYPERTROPHIC PULMONARY OSTEOARTHROPATHY

Clubbing of the digits was recorded in ancient Egypt, but the association with changes in bones and joints was recognized only in the 1890s (Altman, 1989). Because it was found to occur secondarily to pulmonary disease the term hypertrophic pulmonary osteoarthropathy was introduced. But, subsequently its presence secondary to other intrathoracic disease (e.g. congenital heart disease (Pineda *et al.*, 1985), neoplasia) and intra-abdominal infective and neoplastic conditions, led to the more general 'hypertrophic osteoarthropathy'. When cases without associated disease, but with the same features including thickening of the skin, were recognized, the qualifying terms primary and secondary were introduced. The primary disorder was also named pachydermoperiostitis (Anderson and Jayson, 1992). Some thyroid disease is occasionally accompanied by clubbing and periosteal bone formation, which is termed thyroid acropachy.

The features of the syndrome are:

- Clubbing of fingers and toes
- Periosteal bone formation on tubular bones ('periostitis')
- Arthritis or arthralgia
- Hypertrophic skin changes (uncommon in secondary forms)
- Seborrhoea with hyperhidrosis (uncommon in secondary forms)

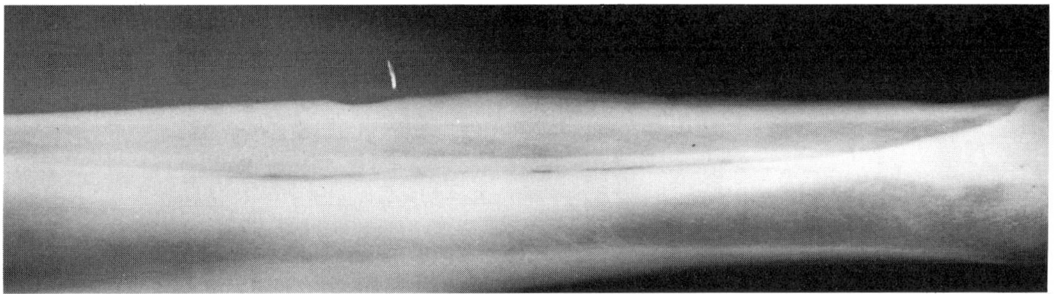

Figure 9.9 Dense periosteal bone formation in hypertrophic pulmonary osteoarthropathy.

Table 9.5

Measurement	Patient	Controls
Trabecular bone volume (%)	16.1	23.1 (4.5)
Trabecular osteoid (%)	20.0	23.1 (5.4)
Trabecular resorption surface (%)	5.0	3.6 (1.7)
Osteoclasts (mm ^{2})	0.467	0.045 (0.001–0.196)
Apposition rate (per/day)		
Trabecular	0.44	0.70
Cortical	1.17	(0.12)

The secondary disease occurs over a wide age range (Altman, 1989). Martinez-Lavin *et al.* (1988), in a review of 132 primary cases, found a bimodal age distribution with peaks at 1 year and at 15 years. There was a 9:1 male preponderance. The skin abnormalities were varied, and joint effusions uncommon. They favoured a genetically controlled growth factor as the pathogenesis.

Radiographs show symmetrical, periosteal new bone on distal diaphyseal/metaphyseal regions of long bones (Figure 9.9): particularly the forearm and legs, metacarpals and metatarsals. The phalanges are less affected. There is increased radioactive uptake at affected sites. Advanced imaging techniques can also demonstrate soft tissue changes (Pineda, 1992: Pineda *et al.*, 1990).

Gall *et al.* (1951) have described the pathology. The dermis and subcutaneous tissues are oedematous, with some increase in round cell infiltration, fibroblastic prolifera-

tion and collagen production. The periosteum is oedematous, infiltrated by small numbers of round cells, and produces immature bone. There appears to be associated remodelling of bone, with loss of endosteal and trabecular bone. The synovium, capsule and periarticular tissues were also oedematous and lightly infiltrated by round cells. A more detailed study of the skin changes, including TEM, has been reported by Matucci-Cerinic *et al.* (1989). Cooper *et al.* (1992) examined a labelled iliac crest biopsy from one severely affected primary case; the results, compared with 10 age and sex matched controls are given in Table 9.5.

The increased resorption and decreased formation on trabecular surfaces is in keeping with the trabecular osteoporosis. The increased cortical formation rate suggested to the authors that there were 'differential functional changes affecting these two envelopes'.

Hypertrophic pulmonary osteoarthropathy was attributed to a disorder of circulation following Mendlowitz and Leslie's (1941) observation that increased blood flow could cause it in dogs and was present in human cases (Mendlowitz, 1942). A neurogenic theory has also been examined (Martinez-Lavin, 1987).

REFERENCES

Aichroth, P.M. (1971a) Osteochondritis dissecans of the knee. A clinical survey. *J. Bone Joint Surg.*, **53B**, 440–7.

Aichroth, P.M. (1971b) Osteochondral fractures and their relationship to osteochondritis dissecans of the knee. An experimental study in animals. *J. Bone Joint Surg.*, **53B**, 448–54.

Allen, B.L. and Jinkins, W.J. (1978) Vertebral osteonecrosis associated with pancreatitis in a child. *J. Bone Joint Surg.*, **60A**, 985–7.

Altman, R.D. (1989) Hypertrophic pulmonary osteoarthropathy. In *Arthritis and Allied conditions*, 11th edn. (ed. D.J. McCarty) Lea and Febiger, Philadelphia, pp. 1360–7.

Amstutz, H.C. and Carey, E.J. (1966) Skeletal manifestations and treatment of Gaucher's disease. Review of 20 cases. *J. Bone Joint Surg.*, **48A**, 670–701.

Arlot, M.E., Bonjean, M., Chavassieux, P.M. *et al.* (1983) Bone histology in adults with aseptic necrosis. Histomorphometric evaluation of iliac biopsies in 77 patients. *J. Bone Joint Surg.*, **65A**, 1319–27.

Atsumi, T., Kuroki, Y. and Yamamoto, K. (1989) A microangiographic study of idiopathic osteonecrosis of the femoral head. *Clin. Orthop.*, **246**, 186–94.

Baron, M., Paltiel, H. and Lander, P. (1984) Aseptic necrosis of the talus and calcaneal insufficiency fractures in a patient with pancreatitis, subcutaneous fat necrosis and arthritis. *Arthritis Rheum.*, **27**, 309–13.

Battaglia, L. and Chiandussi, D. (1965) Manifestazioni osse della lipoidosi cerebrosidica di Gaucher. *Chir. Organi. Mov.*, **54**, 151–60.

Bell, R.S., Mankin, H.J. and Doppelt, S.H. (1986) Osteomyelitis in Gaucher disease. *J. Bone Joint Surg.*, **68A**, 1380–8.

Benaissa, R., Uhthoff, H.K. and Mercier, P. (1989) Repair of trabecular fractures. Cadaver studies of the upper femur. *Acta Orthop. Scand.*, **60**, 585–9.

Burrows, H.J. (1957) Slipped upper femoral epiphysis. Characteristics of 100 cases. *J. Bone Joint Surg.*, **39B**, 641–58

Burrows, H.J. (1959) Osteochondritis juvenilis. *J. Bone Joint Surg.*, **41B**, 455–6.

Catterall, A. (1971) The natural history of Perthes' disease. *J. Bone Joint Surg.*, **53B**, 37–53.

Catterall, A. (1981) Legg–Calvé–Perthes syndrome. *Clin. Orthop.*, **158**, 41–52.

Catterall, A., Pringle, J., Byers, P.D. *et al.* (1982a) A review of the morphology of Perthes' disease. *J. Bone Joint Surg.*, **64B**, 269–75.

Catterall, A., Pringle, J., Byers, P.D. *et al.* (1982b) Perthes' disease: is the epiphyseal infarction complete? *J. Bone Joint Surg.*, **64B**, 276–81.

Catto, M. (1976) Pathology of aseptic bone necrosis. In *Aseptic Necrosis of Bone* (ed. J.K. Davidson), Elsevier, Amsterdam, pp. 3–100.

Catto, M. (1982) Pathology of aseptic necrosis. In *Postgraduate Textbook of Clinical Orthopaedics* (ed. N.H. Harris), John Wright, Bristol, pp. 417–42.

Charache, S. and Page, D.L. (1967) Infarction of bone marrow in the sickle cell disorders. *Intern. Med.*, **67**, 1195–200.

Charon, S., Bavery, E., Malik, M.E. *et al.* (1982) Osteonecrose de la transplantation renale. *Lyon Med.*, **247**, 339–47.

Chung, S.M.K. and Ralston, E.L. (1969) Necrosis of the femoral head associated with sickle cell anaemia and its genetic variants. *J. Bone Joint Surg.*, **51A**, 33–58.

Cooper, R.G., Freemont, A.J., Riley, M. *et al.* (1992) Bone abnormalities and severe arthritis in pachydermoperiostitis. *Ann. Rheum. Dis.*, **51**, 416–19.

Cushing, E.H. and Stout AP. (1926) Gaucher's disease with report of a case showing bone disintegration and joint involvement. *Arch. Surg.*, **12**, 539–60.

Dale, G.S. and Harris, R.W. (1958) Prognosis of epiphyseal separation. *J. Bone Joint Surg.*, **40B**, 1116–22.

Davidson, J.K. (1976) Dysbaric osteonecrosis. In *Aseptic Necrosis of Bone* (ed. J.K. Davidson), Elsevier, Amsterdam, pp. 147–212.

Devas, M. (1975) *Stress Fractures*. Churchill Livingstone, Edinburgh.

Diggs, L.W. (1965) Sickle cell crises. *Am. J. Clin. Pathol.*, **44**, 1–19.

Diggs, L.W. (1967) Bone and joint lesions in sickle cell disease. *Clin. Orthop.*, **52**, 119–43.

Fazzalini, N.L., Vernon-Roberts, B. and Darracott, J. (1987) Osteoarthritis of the hip. Possible protective and causative roles of trabecular microfractures in the head of the femur. *Clin. Orthop.*, **216**, 224–33.

Fergusson, A.B. (1985) Segmental vascular changes in the femoral head in children and adults. *Clin. Orthop.*, **200**, 291–8.

Ficat, P. (1985) Idiopathic necrosis of the femoral head; early diagnosis and treatment. *J. Bone Joint Surg.*, **67B**, 3–9.

Francis, R.B. (1991) Large vessel occlusion in sickle cell disease: pathogenesis, clinical consequences and therapeutic implications. *Med. Hypotheses*, **35**, 88–95.

Freeman, M.A.R., Todd, R.C. and Pirie, C.J. (1974) The role of fatigue in the pathogenesis of femoral neck fractures. *J. Bone Joint Surg.*, **56B**, 698–702.

Frost, H.M. (1960) Presence of microscopic cracks in vivo in bone. *Henry Ford Hosp. Med. Bull.*, **8**, 25–35.

Frost, H.M. (1964) The etiopathogenesis of aseptic necrosis of the femoral head. In *Proceedings of the Conference on Aseptic Necrosis of the Femoral Head*. St Louis, Missouri, pp. 393–413.

Frost, H.M. (1973) *Orthopaedic Biomechanics*. Charles C. Thomas, Springfield, IL.

Frost, H.M. (1986) Intermediary organisation of the skeleton. CRC Press, Boca Raton, FL, Vol I, p. 300, Vol II, pp. 219–20.

Gall, E.A., Bennett, G.A. and Bauer, W. (1951) Generalised hypertrophic pulmonary osteoarthropathy. *Am. J. Pathol.*, **27**, 349–81.

Galli, S.J., Weintraub, H.P. and Proppe, K.H. (1978) Malignant fibrous histiocytoma and pleomorphic sarcoma in association with medullary bone infarcts. *Cancer*, **41**, 607–19.

Gerle, R.D., Walker, L.A., Achroid, J.L. *et al.* (1965) Osseous changes in chronic pancreatitis. *Radiology*, **85**, 330–7.

Glimcher, M.J. and Kenzora, J.E. (1979a) The biology of osteonecrosis of the femoral head and its clinical implications: I. Tissue biology. *Clin. Orthop.*, **138**, 284–309.

Glimcher, M.J. and Kenzora, J.E. (1979b) The biology of osteonecrosis of the femoral head and its clinical implications: II. The pathological changes in the femoral head as an organ and in the hip joint. *Clin. Orthop.*, **139**, 283–312.

Glimcher, M.J. and Kenzora, J.E. (1979c) The biology of osteonecrosis of the femoral head and its clinical implications: III. Discussion of the aetiology and genesis of the pathological sequelae. *Clin. Orthop.*, **140**, 273–312.

Goldblatt, J., Sucks, S. and Beighton, P. (1978) The orthopaedic aspects of Gaucher's disease. *Clin. Orthop.*, **137**, 208–14.

Hall, J.E. (1957) The results of treatment of slipped upper femoral epiphysis. *J. Bone Joint Surg.*, **39B**, 655–73.

Haller, J.O., Greenway, B., Resnick, D. *et al.* (1989) Intraosseous fat necrosis associated with acute pancreatitis: MR imaging. *Radiology*, **173**, 193–5.

Horev, G., Kornreich, L., Hadar, H. *et al.* (1991) Haemorrhage associated with 'bone crisis' in Gaucher's disease identified by magnetic resonance imaging. *Skeletal Radiol.*, **20**, 479–82.

Hungerford, D.B. and Lennox, D.W. (1985) The importance of increased intraosseous pressure in the development of osteonecrosis of the femoral head: implications for treatment. *Orthop. Clin. North Am.*, **16**, 635–54.

Immelman, E.J., Bank, S., Krige, H. *et al.* (1964) Roentgenologic and clinical features of medullary fat necrosis in bones in acute and chronic pancreatitis *Am. J. Med.*, **36**, 96–105.

Jackson, S.H., Savidge, R.S., Stein, L. *et al.*, (1952) Carcinoma of the pancreas associated with fat necrosis. *Lancet*, ii, 962–7.

Jaffe, H.L. (1972) Certain disorders of individual epiphyses, apophyses, and epiphysioid bones. In *Metabolic, Degenerative, and Inflammatory Diseases of Bones and Joints* (ed. H.L. Jaffe), Lea and Febiger, Philadelphia, Chapter 19, pp. 565–631.

James, N.E. (1952) Gaucher's disease. Report of a case. *J. Bone Joint Surg.*, **34B**, 464–5.

Jones, J.P. (1971) Alcoholism, hypercortisonism, fat embolism and osseous necrosis. In *Idiopathic Ischaemic Necrosis of the Femoral Head in Adults* (ed. W.M. Zinn), Georg Thieme Publishers, Stuttgart, pp. 112–32.

Jones, J.P. (1985) Fat embolism and osteonecrosis. *Orthop. Clin. North Am.*, **16**, 595–633.

Jones, J.P. (1989) Osteonecrosis. In *Arthritis and Allied Conditions* (ed. D.J. McCarty), Lea and Febiger, Philadelphia, pp. 1356–73.

Jones, J.P. (1992) Intravascular coagulation and osteonecrosis. *Clin. Orthop.*, **277**, 41–53.

Katz, K., Cohen, I.J., Ziv, N. *et al.* (1987) Fractures in children who have Gaucher disease. *J. Bone Joint Surg.*, **69A**, 1361–70.

Katz, K., Mechlis-Frish, S., Cohen, I.J. *et al.* (1991) Bone scans in the diagnosis of bone crisis in patients who have Gaucher disease. *J. Bone Joint Surg.*, **73A**, 513–7.

Kemp, H.B.S. (1983) Perthes' disease. In *Postgraduate Textbook of Clinical Orthopaedics* (ed. N.H. Harris), John Wright, Bristol, pp. 110–9.

Kenzora, J.E. (ed.) (1985) Symposium on Idiopathic osteonecrosis. *Orthop. Clin. North Am.*, **16** (4).

Kenzora, J.E. and Glimcher, M.J. (1985) The pathogenesis of idiopathic osteonecrosis: the ubiquitous crescent sign. *Orthop. Clin. North Am.*, **16** (4), 681–96.

Lagier, R. (1971) Idiopathic aseptic necrosis of the femoral head. An anatomo-pathological concept. In *Idiopathic Ischaemic Necrosis of the Femoral Head in Adults* (ed. W.M. Zinn), Georg Thieme Publishers, Stuttgart, pp. 49–67.

Lucas, P.F. and Owen, T.K. (1962) Subcutaneous fat necrosis, polyarthritis and pancreatic disease. *Gut*, **3**, 146–8.

Martinez-Lavin, M. (1987) Digital clubbing and hypertrophic pulmonary osteoarthropathy: a unifying hypothesis. *J. Rheumatol.*, **14**, 6–8.

Martinez-Lavin, M., Pineda, C., Valdez, T. *et al.* (1988) Primary hypertrophic osteoarthropathy. *Semin. Arthritis Rheum.*, **17**, 156–62.

Matsui, M., Saito, S., Ohzono, K. *et al.* (1992) Experimental steroid-induced osteonecrosis in adult rabbits with hypersensitivity vasculitis. *Clin. Orthop.*, **277**, 61–72.

Matucci-Cerinic, M., Cinti, S., Morroni, M. *et al.* (1989) Pachydermoperiostitis (primary hypertrophic osteoarthropathy): report of a case with evidence of endothelial and connective tissue involvement. *Ann. Rheum. Dis.*, **48**, 240–6.

McCallum, R.I., Walder, D.N., Barnes R. *et al.* (1966) Bone lesions in compressed air workers. *J. Bone Joint Surg.*, **48B**, 207–35.

McCarthy, E. (1982) Aseptic necrosis of bone: an historic perspective. *Clin. Orthop.*, **168**, 216–21.

Melamed, S. and Chester, W. (1938) Osseous form of Gaucher's disease. *Arch. Intern. Med.*, **61**, 798–807.

Mendlowitz, M. (1942) Clubbing and hypertrophic osteoarthropathy. *Medicine*, **21**, 269–306.

Mendlowitz, M. and Leslie, (1942) Experimental simulation in dog of cyanosis and hypertrophic osteoarthropathy which are associated with congenital heart disease. *Am. Heart J.*, **24** 141–52.

Michael, R.H. and Dorfman, H.D. (1976) Malignant fibrous histiocytoma associated with bone infarcts. Report of a case. *Clin. Orthop.*, **118**, 180–3.

Middlemiss, J.H. and Raper, A.B. (1966) Skeletal changes in the haemoglobinopathies. *J. Bone Joint Surg.*, **48A**, 693–702.

Nachamie, B.A. and Dorfman, H.D. (1974) Ischaemic necrosis of bone in sickle cell trait. *J. Mt Sinai Hosp.*, **41**, 527–36.

Nagura, S. (1960) The so-called osteochondritis of Konig. *Clin. Orthop.*, **18**, 100–22.

Nielsen, H.E., Melsen, F. and Christensen, M.S. (1977) Aseptic necrosis following renal transplantation. Clinical and biochemical aspects, and bone morphometry. *Acta Med. Scand.*, **208**, 127–32.

Ohzono, K., Takaoka, K., Saito, S. *et al.* (1992) Intraosseous arterial architecture in nontraumatic avascular necrosis of the femoral head. Microangiographic and histologic study. *Clin. Orthop.*, **277**, 79–88.

Ono, K. (ed.) (1992) Symposium on recent advances in avascular necrosis. *Clin. Orthop.*, **277**, 2–138.

Perry, T.T. (1947) Role of lymphatics in the transmission of lipase in disseminated pancreatic fat necrosis. *Arch. Pathol.*, **43**, 456–65.

Pineda, C. (1992) Diagnostic imaging in hypertrophic osteoarthropathy. *Clin. Exp. Rheumatol.*, **10**, **suppl 7**, 27–33.

Pineda, C., Guerra, J., Weisman, M.H. *et al.* (1985) The skeletal manifestations of digital clubbing: a study of patients with congenital heart disease and hypertrophic pulmonary osteoarthropathy. *Semin. Arthritis Rheum.*, **14**, 263–73.

Pineda, C., Fonseca, C. and Martinez-Lavin, M. (1990) The spectrum of soft tissue and skeletal abnormalities of hypertrophic osteoarthropathy. *J. Rheumatol.*, **17**, 626–32.

Potts, D.E., Man, F.M. and Iseman, M.D. (1975) Syndrome of pancreatic disease, subcutaneous fat necrosis and polyserositis. *Am. J. Med.*, **58**, 417–23.

Powers, D.R. (1990) Sickle cell anaemia and major organ failure. *Hemoglobin*, **14**, 573–98.

Radin, D., Colletti, P., Forrester, D. *et al.* (1986) Pancreatic acinar cell carcinoma with subcutaneous and intraosseous fat necrosis. *Radiology*, **158**, 67–8.

Robichon, J., Desjardin, J.P., Koch, M. *et al.* (1974) The femoral neck in Legg–Perthes' disease. *J. Bone Joint Surg.*, **56B**, 62–8.

Rourke, J.A. and Heslin, D.J. (1965) Gaucher's disease. Roentgenological changes over 20 years interval. *Am. J. Roentgenol.*, **94**, 621–30.

Saito, S., Ohzono, K. and Ono, K. (1988) Minimal osteonecrosis as a segmental infarct within the femoral head. *Clin. Orthop.*, **231**, 35–50.

Saito, S., Ohzono. K. and Ono, K. (1992) Early arteriopathy and postulated pathogenesis of osteonecrosis of the femoral head. *Clin. Orthop.*, **277**, 98–110.

Salter, R.B. and Harris, R.W. (1963) Injuries involving the epiphyseal plate. *J. Bone Joint Surg.*, **45A**, 587–622.

Scarpelli, D.G. (1956) Fat necrosis of bone marrow in acute pancreatitis. *Am. J. Pathol.*, **32**, 1077–87.

Sevitt, S. (1981) *Bone Repair and Fracture Healing in Man.* Churchill Livingstone, Edinburgh, pp. 203 ff for incidence and assessment of necrosis of femoral head.

Sherman, M.S. (1959) Pathogenesis of disintegration of the hip in sickle cell anaemia. *South Med. J.*, **52**, 632–7.

Simkin, P.A., Brunzell, P., Wisner, D. *et al.* (1983) Free fatty acids in the pancreatic arthritis syndrome. *Arthritis Rheum.*, **26**, 127–32.

Slovis, T.L., Borden, W.E., Haller, J.O. *et al.* (1975) Pancreatitis and the battered child syndrome: report of 2 cases. *Am. J. Roentgenol.*, **125**, 456–61.

Smukler, N.M., Schumaker, H.R., Pascual, E. *et al.* (1979) Synovial fat necrosis associated with pancreatitis. *Arthritis Rheum.*, **22**, 547–53.

Todd, R.C., Freeman, M.A.R. and Pirie, C.J. (1972) Isolated trabecular fatigue fractures in the femoral head. *J. Bone Joint Surg.*, **54B**, 723–8.

Virship, A.M. and Slivinski, A.J. (1973) Polyarthritis and subcutaneous nodules associated with carcinoma of the pancreas. *Arthritis Rheum.*, **16**, 388–92.

Wang, G.J., Guterman, I.A., Vinh, T.N. *et al.* (1975) Modification of fatty accumulation in the osteocyte in steroid treated rabbits using lipid clearing agents. In *Bone Circulation* (eds J. Arlet and B. Maxieres), Springer, Berlin, p. 399.

Wang, G.J., Sweet, D.E., Reger, S.I. *et al.* (1977) Fat-cell changes as a mechanism of avascular necrosis of the femoral head in cortisone treated rabbits. *J. Bone Joint Surg.*, **59A**, 729–35.

Weinberg, A.G. and Currarino, G. (1972) Sickle cell dactylitis. Histopathological observations. *Am. J. Clin. Pathol.*, **58**, 518–23.

Wilson, H.A., Askan, A.D., Neiderhiser, D.H. *et al.* (1983) Pancreatitis with arthropathy and subcutaneous fat necrosis. *Arthritis Rheum.*, **26**, 121–6.

Wynne-Davies, R. (1980) Some aetiological features of Perthes' disease. *Clin. Orthop.*, **150**, 12–15.

Zinn, W.M. (1971) Introduction. In *Idiopathic Ischaemic Necrosis of the Femoral Head in Adults* (ed. W.M. Zinn), Georg Thieme, Stuttgart, pp. 1–8.

Colin G. Woods

10.1 GENERAL INTRODUCTION

This chapter will consider the pathology of disorders of the skeleton resulting from disturbances of the ordered processes of bone formation and resorption whch are required to achieve normal growth, modelling, remodelling and turnover of bone, which processes are described in detail in Chapter 19.

The conditions which come, by common usage, under this heading include osteoporosis, rickets and osteomalacia, hyperparathyroid bone disease, Paget's disease of bone and fibrogenesis imperfecta ossium. Some of these diseases are the consequence of metabolic abnormalities producing changes in extracellular fluid and have a logical place in this category of bone disease whereas others appear to be internal derangements of bone 'metabolism' which are not the result of any known change in the general metabolic state. Other metabolic disorders having an effect on skeletal development and not customarily included in the category 'metabolic bone disease' are described in other chapters.

When describing the histological appearances associated with any pathological condition of the skeleton the cause of the observed abnormalities is often assumed to be due entirely to the disease process. It must be remembered that the skeleton is required for and responsive to the mechanics of locomotion and that some of the histological features of a pathological state may be the response to a change in the mechanical efficiency of the bone which has been brought about by the primary disease process, in short a form of bone reaction.

Histopathological examination of metabolic bone disease requires the selection of the appropriate section preparation and employment of histomorphometric techniques. These matters, being common to all the disorders, are considered in the last two sections of the chapter. The sections devoted to specific disorders describe the clinical, radiological, biochemical and histological features in general terms. Details of histological section preparation and staining are provided in Chapter 21.

10.2 OSTEOPOROSIS

10.2.1 INTRODUCTION

Osteoporosis is the commonest generalized disorder of the skeleton. In developed countries it occurs mainly in middle-aged and elderly people in whom it may cause severe disability. The condition is defined as that in which there is a reduced mass of bone, with a normal ratio of mineralized matrix to osteoid (Sissons, 1955), and excepting severe forms of osteogenesis imperfecta, the matrix is of normal mature lamellar type. The name derives from the porosity of macerated specimens, since the reduced bone volume increases the size of the marrow spaces.

Examination of bone samples from patients and cadavers of either sex by several observers has shown that there is a decrease in bone mass in the majority of people from the fifth decade onwards, a change which, in general, begins at an earlier age in women, commencing after the menopause, or oophorectomy in the premenopausal. These observations have led to the suggestion that 'osteopenia' should be used to describe asymptomatic 'physiological' bone loss, and the term 'osteoporosis' be used either when the bone mass is below the 95 percentile of the mean for the age and sex of the patient or is thought to be the cause of symptoms. Although this distinction may be of value to clinicians the histologist cannot determine in most cases whether the degree of abnormality seen in the section is causing, or likely to cause, symptoms. In this chapter only the term 'osteoporosis' will be used, to include both types of bone loss.

10.2.2 CLINICAL PRESENTATION

The consequence of loss of bone is mechanical failure. Virtually the only presentations of the disease are pain, which is thought to be caused by microfractures, loss of height because of collapse of vertebral bodies and overt fractures. However, there is not a close correlation between calculated bone mass and mechanical failure, the unmeasurable

Table 10.1 Types of osteoporosis

Generalized
   Idiopathic or uncertain aetiology
      Age-related (senile, idiopathic, physiological)
      Postmenopausal
      Idiopathic juvenile
      Osteoporosis in young adults
      Pregnancy related
   Cause identifiable
      Hypogonadism, oophorectomy
      Thyrotoxicosis
      Hypercorticosteroidism (adrenal tumour or iatrogenic)
      Hypopituitarism
      Vitamin C deficiency
      Immobilization
      Liver disease (biliary cirrhosis)
      Marrow infiltration (mycloma, mctastascs, leukaemia)
      Mastocytosis and prolonged heparin administration
   Chromosomal and genetic
      Turner's syndrome
      Down's syndrome
      Osteogenesis imperfecta
      Homocystinuria
   Associated with other metabolic bone diseases
      Hyperparathyroidism
      Osteomalacia
      Fibrogenesis imperfecta ossium
Localized
   Immobilization
   Acute joint inflammation especially rheumatoid arthritis
   Paget's disease, notably in the skull vault
   Transient osteoporosis
   Sudek's atrophy

variable being the load applied to the bone which precipitates the break.

10.2.3 CLASSIFICATION OF TYPES AND CAUSES

A classified list of types and causes of osteoporosis is set out in Table 10.1. In many cases there is no clear link between a primary disease and bone loss and these are properly classified as 'idiopathic'. When osteoporosis occurs as a predictable feature of a condition listed in Table 10.1, a bone biopsy will seldom be required to establish a diagnosis of osteoporosis, and in the event, is rarely obtained during the early stages of bone loss. As a consequence, there is a limited amount of histological information about the cellular activity which leads to loss of bone mass, such information coming from the planned examination of series of patients or experimental studies.

10.2.4 PATHOGENESIS

The constant removal and deposition of bone which occurs in life must, at least for a few decades after growth has ceased, be in balance if the skeletal mass is to be maintained. The influences, as currently known, which bear on that balance are dealt with in greater detail in Chapter 19. Suffice to say here that we do not fully understand the mechanisms by which those influences achieve their effects nor the relative importance of each in the normal adult. Our understanding of the pathogenesis of

osteoporosis is consequently limited. What can be said is that the change from normal to osteoporotic is the result of a preponderance of bone resorption over deposition. Within that outline one can imagine five possible changes in the relationship between rates of formation and removal of bone which will result in net loss (Table 10.2). The advantage in knowing which of the possible combinations is responsible is that it might lead to preventative or therapeutic measures against symptomatic osteoporosis. Examination of histological sections can make a contribution to identification of proximate cause and may disclose the presence of abnormalities additional to the osteoporosis but there are limitations on the information available in one biopsy.

10.2.5 RADIOLOGY

Radiographic changes resulting from osteoporosis include those which could be anticipated from the presenting signs and symptoms indicated above (Figures 10.1 and 10.2). They may not be specific; multiple pathological fractures occur in osteomalacia. Techniques for the detection of asymptomatic bone loss have included analyses of standard radiographs of specified parts of the skeleton (lateral view of lumbar spine, femoral neck, mid-diaphysis of femur, metacarpals) and more recently the use of photon absorptiometry to estimate the density of the distal forearm and the use of computed axial tomography (Genant *et al.*, 1989).

Table 10.2 Changes in cellular activity resulting in osteoporosis

Osteoclastic activity	*Osteoblastic activity*
Normal	Decreased
Decreased	Decreased
Increased	Increased
Increased	Normal
Increased	Decreased

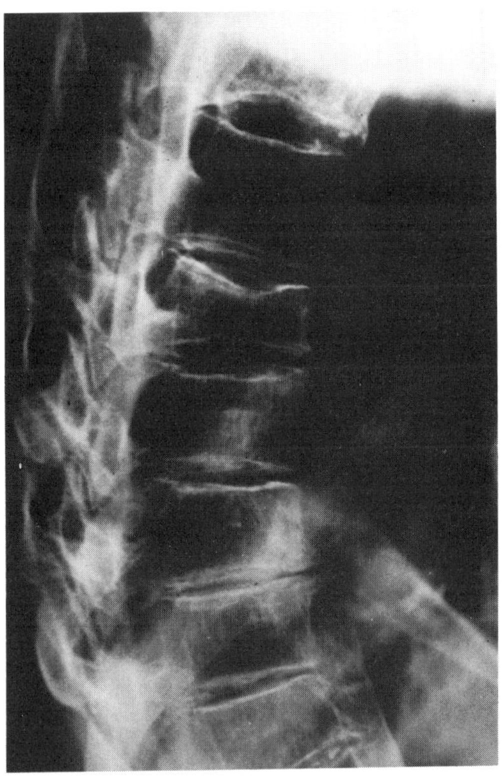

Figure 10.1 Osteoporosis. Radiograph of lateral spine. Collapsed vertebra.

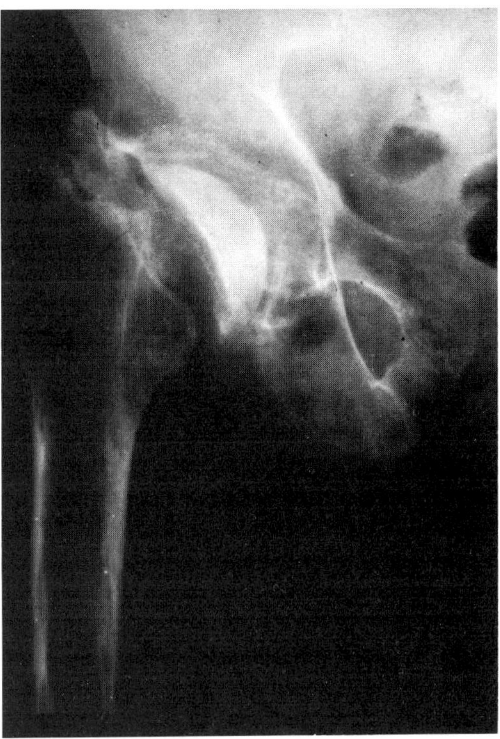

Figure 10.2 Osteoporosis. Radiograph of femur. Generalized osteoporosis following steroid therapy. The femoral cortex is thinned and there is a pathological fracture of the femoral neck.

10.2.6   BIOCHEMISTRY

The biochemical indicators of bone disease (plasma calcium, phosphorus, alkaline phosphatase, 25-hydroxy and 1,25-dihydroxy vitamin D metabolites and urinary calcium and hydroxyproline) are not consistently abnormal in age-related osteoporosis. Plasma calcium may be elevated and urinary output of calcium increased following acute total immobilization. Some of the diseases causing osteoporosis will have symptoms, signs, radiographic changes and biochemical abnormalities arising from the primary condition.

This background information must be known to the pathologist.

10.2.7   HISTOLOGY

As previously stated, bone biopsy is seldom required to establish a diagnosis of osteoporosis, and is more likely to be undertaken if the clinician wishes to exclude the presence of some other disease of or in the bone. Bone biopsy may be used by a clinician as part of the investigation of the effect of treatment of osteoporotic patients. Histomorphometric analysis (section 10.8) may then be required. What follows is a suggested procedure for the systematic examination of a bone section which will serve no matter for what reason the biopsy was taken.

There are observations whereby a prediction as to whether the bone is likely to be osteoporotic or not can be made even before mensuration begins. Bone loss occurs in both cortical and cancellous tissue and if both types are included in the section, comment should be made about each separately. In respect of cortical bone the dimensions of Haversian canals is the vital clue, enlargement being the indicator of bone loss and relatively easy to recognize (Figure 10.3). In cancellous bone, loss from trabeculae may affect all or only some of them and it is necessary to estimate both the width of normal trabeculae and the amount of marrow between them. So far as width is concerned, it is useful to compare the transverse diameter of the struts of bone with the diameter of fat-cells in the marrow; in young adult bone they are approximately equal (Figures 10.4 and 10.5). Some thinned trabeculae appear as isolated round structures rather than inter-connected struts. Estimation of the amount of marrow between trabeculae relies on counting the number of trabeculae in a standard microscopic field; lower magnification objectives cover a larger area of section and are the most useful. Histomor-

phometry may encompass measurement of trabecular width and spacing, but it is only necessary to determine that the area of cancellous bone tissue is below normal to make the basic diagnosis of osteoporosis.

Different patterns of bone loss have been described. In age-related loss from the cortex the Haversian canals in the inner (endosteal) part enlarge first and continue to enlarge until the residual bone merges with the adjacent cancellous bone (cancellization); this process leads to the radiographic appearance of thinning of the cortex of tubular bones and a widening of the medullary cavity. When bone loss occurs more quickly than it does in 'physiological' osteoporosis it may do so in an apparently random distribution within the cortex. Removal of bone from trabeculae

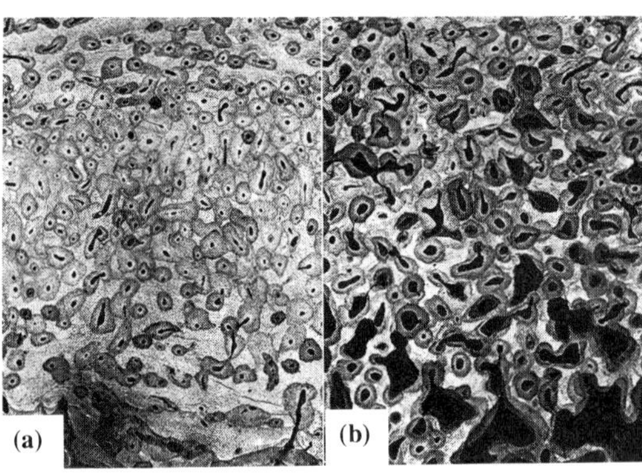

Figure 10.3 Osteoporosis. Microradiographs of transverse sections of femur diaphysis. (a) 17-year-old male showing normal bone density. (b) 77-year-old female with enlarged osteonal canals, particularly of the inner portion where the cortex has undergone some cancellization

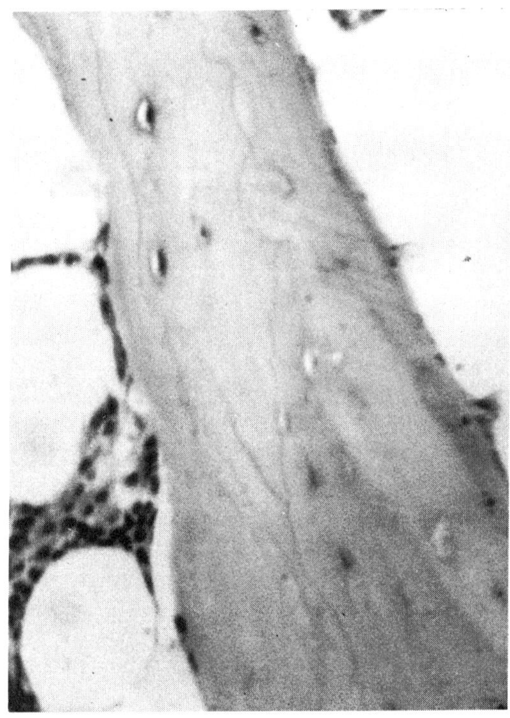

Figure 10.4 Trabeculae of normal width, note relative diameters of fat cells in marrow. Decalcified, paraffin embedded section.

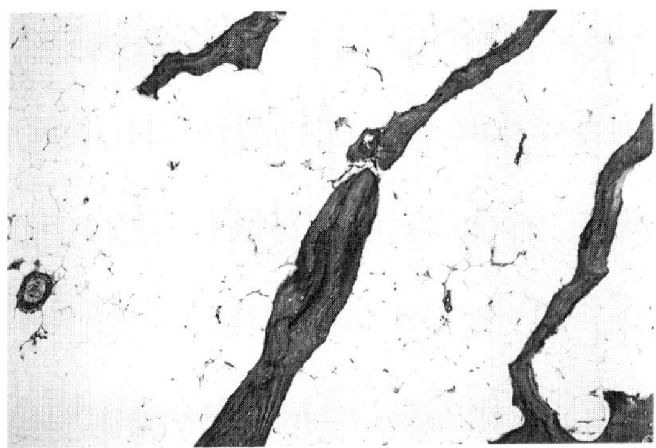

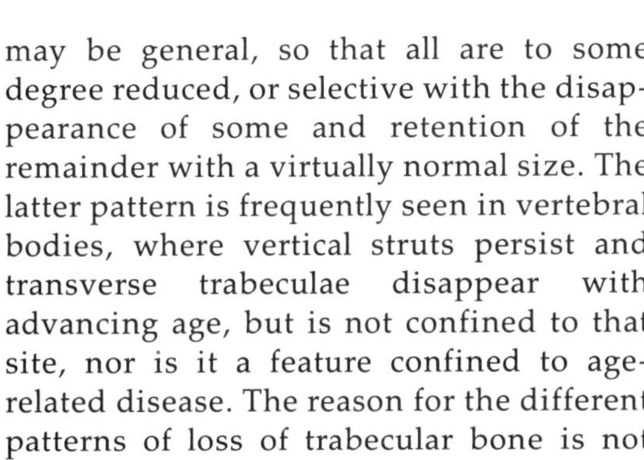

Figure 10.5 Osteoporosis. Cancellous bone showing narrowed trabeculae and an ovoid, detached trabecular remnant. Decalcified, paraffin embedded section.

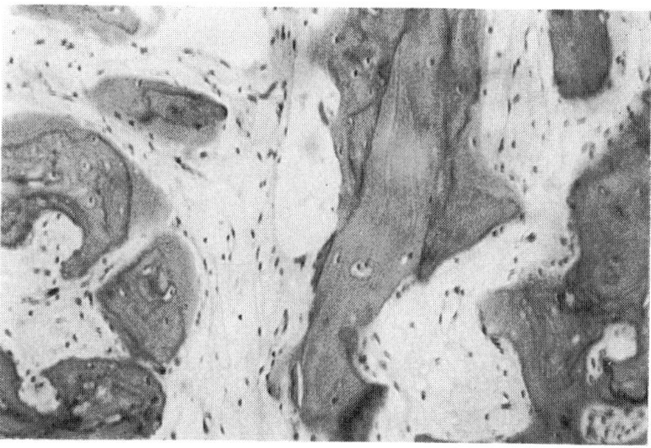

Figure 10.6 Reactive, woven, bone formation following fracture of osteoporotic femoral neck. Woven bone is attached to pre-existing trabeculae and is also deposited in the marrow. Decalcified, paraffin embedded section.

may be general, so that all are to some degree reduced, or selective with the disappearance of some and retention of the remainder with a virtually normal size. The latter pattern is frequently seen in vertebral bodies, where vertical struts persist and transverse trabeculae disappear with advancing age, but is not confined to that site, nor is it a feature confined to age-related disease. The reason for the different patterns of loss of trabecular bone is not known.

In the majority of biopsies of osteoporotic bone seen by the author the only type of original bone tissue present has been of mature lamellar type. However, immature (woven) bone persists in the skeleton in some types of osteogenesis imperfecta (see Chapter 5); and repair of microfractures is in the form of tiny buttresses or bridges of woven bone attached to trabeculae of lamellar bone or as struts of purely woven bone in the marrow (Figure 10.6).

Whilst looking at the architecture of the bone the cellular composition of the marrow should also be scrutinized for evidence of infiltration by malignant or mast cells.

Attention may then be turned to an analysis of the bone cell population. A problem which is peculiar to osteoporosis is the effect that the decrease in bone surfaces in cancellous bone and the increase in Haversian surfaces resulting from the bone loss has on the apparent population of cells (Darby, 1981). In cancellous bone, the surface available for osteoblastic activity will be reduced, a fact more easily appreciated if the number of trabeculae per unit area of section is reduced. When the Haversian canals in cortical bone enlarge in the early phase of bone loss the bone surfaces increase in area, so that the proportion of surface occupied by active osteoblasts will be reduced even if the absolute number of cells remains constant. Subjective assessment of cell populations should take this into account.

Assessment of the rate of bone resorption by, and the duration of activity of, individual osteoclasts is not possible by direct measurement and it is not known if there is a consistent change in osteoclastic activity which contributes to bone loss in age-related osteoporosis. Evidence has been presented, by different observers, in support of an increase, no change and a decrease in resorption in age-related osteoporosis.

10.2.8 AGE-RELATED AND POSTMENOPAUSAL OSTEOPOROSIS

Radiographic and histomorphometric evidence indicates that bone loss after the menopause and in the elderly begins in the spine and occurs later in the limb bones. Immediately after the menopause, bone loss occurs relatively quickly and then slows; measurements performed on bone samples indicate that as much as 20% of the existing bone may be lost between the fifth and sixth decades in females after which the bone mass decreases very little to the eighth decade. Such striking reductions in bone mass are not seen in the ageing male population in whom bone loss is usually evident from the sixth decade onwards. The average rate of bone loss is low (in females it is between 10% and 30% in 30 years), so that one would not expect bone cell populations to show, in the majority of samples, striking differences between biopsies from patients in the fifth or seventh decades. In a small proportion of biopsies from postmenopausal females there is an increase in the number of active osteoblasts and osteoclasts, suggesting an increase in remodelling activity. Since remodelling activity does not occur throughout the skeleton simultaneously, differences in cell populations between small biopsies may be the result of chance. Timing of the biopsy relative to the menopause could also be a significant factor. Kimmel *et al.* (1990) conclude that there are no special subsets of osteoporotic subjects.

Two pieces of evidence suggest that osteoblast function may be impaired in the elderly. Estimation of calcification rate by means of double labelling of bone with tetracycline has shown a decrease in rate, which indicates a reduction in the rate of matrix production as there is no evidence of failure of mineralization of the matrix (Meunier *et al.*, 1983). The analogy is the decrease in subcutaneous fibrous tissue which is seen in the elderly (Hayflick, 1976). Measurement of 'mean wall thickness', an indicator of the amount of bone formed in a previous resorption cavity suggests that there is a decrease in apposition volume after resorption in a 'remodelling unit' (Darby and Meunier, 1981). For a review of the histomorphometric assessment of trabecular bone remodelling in osteoporosis the reader is referred to Compston and Croucher (1991).

The seeming contradiction in assigning oophorectomy as an identifiable cause of osteoporosis whilst listing postmenopausal osteoporosis as a condition of uncertain aetiology is one example of the general problem of explaining the aetiology of osteoporosis. In this particular example there is on one hand a patient who abruptly and at a precisely identified time loses ovarian hormones which can be replaced therapeutically immediately and who is also probably physically active and consumes a normal diet and on the other hand a patient who has lost oestrogen secretion for an uncertain period of time and who may also be progressively less active and taking a diet with low calcium content and whose kidneys are less effective at calcium conservation. Hormone replacement therapy may not then be as effective for the treatment of the older patient as it is for the younger.

Among the elderly population there is a small proportion who appear to have sustained a very severe loss of bone. Whether all these individuals have a common cause for this is not known. Suggested possible causes include a diminution of osteoblastic activity which is genetically determined, an excessive response by the parathyroids to a fall in plasma calcium or an increased end-organ sensitivity to parathormone. Another possible explanation is that these individuals have a low bone mass in early adult life and need only lose bone at the average rate to become severely osteoporotic. The concept of 'peak bone mass', the bone mass developed in early adult life, is discussed by Burckhardt and Michel (1989).

10.2.9 OTHER TYPES OF OSTEOPOROSIS

(a) Idiopathic juvenile osteoporosis

Idiopathic juvenile osteoporosis is a rare, self-limiting, condition occurring around the time of puberty (Smith, 1980). Vertebral involvement may lead to structural collapse. In the limbs bone loss is usually most obvious in the metaphyseal zone and may be complicated by fracture. Histological studies of affected bone are few; both increased osteoclastic activity and decreased bone formation are recorded and the aetiology and pathogenesis of the condition is unknown. The clinical differential diagnosis is mild osteogenesis imperfecta and a bone biopsy will assist only if the osteocyte population is found to be increased or there is an abnormality of the cement (reversal) line pattern which resembles that seen in Paget's disease (section 10.5.4), features of some types of osteogenesis imperfecta.

(b) Osteoporosis in young adults

Ostoporosis in young adults occurs as an idiopathic event and as a consequence of identifiable disorders (Bordier *et al.*, 1973). Osteogenesis imperfecta is one of them and may be recognized in a bone biopsy by the features described above. Hypopituitarism, hypogonadism in the male, hyperthyroidism and hypercorticosteroidism have to be excluded by the clinician by physical examination and biochemistry; histology is not helpful.

(c) Pregnancy-related osteoporosis

Pregnancy-related osteoporosis is a rare condition (Smith *et al.*, 1985) which is manifest in the last months of pregnancy or shortly after delivery, usually by evidence of vertebral collapse although localized osteoporosis in limb bones also occurs. The cause is unknown; it is possible that all cases do not have the same aetiology. The few bone biopsy studies available are non-contributory apart from confirming reduced bone mass in some of the biopsies. Bone cell populations have been in the normal range. This may be because the biopsies were obtained at different phases of the natural history and with a minimum delay of weeks after the onset of symptoms. Restoration of bone at the end of the process is partial and collapsed vertebrae remain deformed. There is no association with a particular pregnancy and patients have had subsequent uncomplicated pregnancies.

(d) Pituitary dysfunction and osteoporosis

Hypopituitarism in children is a cause of retarded skeletal development with late fusion of growth plates and inadequate bone mass, the latter predisposing to fracture in adult life. Acromegaly, the result of continued growth hormone activity after skeletal maturity, leads to the production of a skeleton of larger volume than normal without a corresponding increase in bone mass. Trabecular bone mass may therefore appear reduced in a histological section. However, the total mass of bone in the skeleton is not reduced and this is not, by definition, osteoporosis and is not included in Table 10.1.

(e) Skeletal changes in thyrotoxicosis

The activity of bone cells is stimulated by thyroid hormone and in thyrotoxic patients both osteoblast and osteoclast populations are increased. Biochemical evidence of increased bone cell activity is also present. Overall the mass of bone is reduced and, if treatment is delayed, the patient may become severely porotic. Histomorphometric studies have confirmed the increase in active cell populations on the bone surfaces (Mosekilde and Melsen, 1978). A described feature is the random distribution of resorption within the cortical bone.

(f)　Hypercorticoidism and osteoporosis

Corticosteroid administration and excess secretion inhibit bone matrix and cartilage growth plate formation (Sissons and Hadfield, 1955). Calcium absorption from the gut is also depressed. Increased parathormone and vitamin D metabolite levels in plasma are also reported in 'Cushingoid' patients (Hahn *et al.*, 1974) with evidence of increased osteoclastic activity in bone biopsies. These changes may be a response to changes in plasma calcium, whereas the decreased chondroblastic and osteoblastic activity are thought to be direct effects of the steroids. The severity of bone loss or of growth retardation which occurs in patients treated with corticosteroids is related more closely to the duration of treatment than to the dose level (Hahn *et al.*, 1974). Bone biopsies from patients with symptomatic osteoporosis after years of treatment with steroids may not show any significant difference in cell populations, possibly because a steady state has been reached.

(g)　Vitamin C deficiency

Vitamin C is required for hydroxylation of proline without which osteoid (and other collagens) cannot be produced. In young children with scurvy, deficient bone formation is usually most obvious in the limb bone metaphyses and there may be splaying of the growth plates due to mechanical failure of bone. Severe vitamin C deficiency sufficient to cause skeletal abnormalities is commonly part of the consequences of malnutrition and protein deficiency probably contributes to the inadequate bone formation. The haemorrhagic features of scurvy are usually also evident in the presence of bone disease and biopsy of bone is not required to establish the diagnosis.

(h)　Immobilization

Immobilization is a primary cause of bone loss and the converse has also been demonstrated by comparison of bone mass in men taking regular exercise with those who did not (Nilsson and Westlin, 1971). Rubin and Lanyon (1987) also discuss the relationship between mechanical stress and bone mass. Many studies of people acutely immobilized because of paralysis following spinal cord injuries attest the fact that bone is lost after such injuries and at a rate sufficient to cause increases in urinary output of calcium and hydroxyproline and hypercalcaemia. One study records a loss of 33% of bone mass over a period of 25 weeks (Minaire *et al.*, 1974). By analogy, a reasonable speculation would be that any disease which led the patient to rest, be it in bed or not, might cause bone loss. Radiographic examination of astronauts has demonstrated significant bone loss as a consequence of weightlessness (Tilton *et al.*, 1980). Limbs which are immobilized following fracture (Nilsson, 1966) or because of a painful disease of bone or joint (Ng *et al.*, 1984) also become demonstrably osteoporotic. In those cases where the primary disease has an inflammatory component (e.g. rheumatoid arthritis), the change in blood supply to the bone may promote bone resorption. Radiographic examination of parts of the skeleton which have lost bone during a temporary period of immobility indicates that the density of the bone is not always restored to normal afterwards. It appears that the skeleton can stabilize at a new, lower, level of bone mass at any age. That there is a relationship between physical activity and change in bone mass can be clearly seen in the situations cited above; they reflect striking differences operating continuously during the period of observation. The more difficult situation to analyse is the changes in loading applied to the skeleton by the majority of people over the course of their lifetimes. There has been much speculation as to the link between load and bone modelling; the most frequently expressed theory is that piezo-electric charges are produced on bone surfaces as the result of applied forces deforming crystalline structures within the bone tissue and that the polarity of the charge will dictate whether formation or resorption of bone occurs (Bassett and Becker, 1962). Studies of the effects of induced electromagnetic fields on bone formation have not produced clear cut results (Lavine and Grodzinsky, 1987).

(i) Skeletal changes in liver disease

Abnormality of liver function, when it has any effect on the skeleton, is usually associated with osteomalacia because of failure of hydroxylation of vitamin D. In a small series of bone biopsies of patients with biliary cirrhosis examined by the author the only abnormality found was osteoporosis, the explanation for which is not clear.

(j) Malignant cell infiltration

Infiltration of the bone marrow by malignant cells commonly, but not invariably, induces uncompensated osteoclastic resorption of bone. The resulting osteoporosis may be local or general depending on the extent of skeletal involvement. Myelomatosis occasionally produces radiographic changes which are indistinguishable from those of age-related osteoporosis. There is more than one possible reason for increased bone resorption adjacent to malignant cell infiltrates. The mechanisms which have been suggested will not be discussed here; they have no bearing on recognition of the situation in a bone sample. Bone resorption may be at a very high rate and cause clinically significant hypercalcaemia, especially in the patient with widespread disease.

(k) Systemic mastocytosis and heparin administration

Osteoporosis occurs in some patients with systemic mastocytosis (Fallon *et al.*, 1981) and after long-term heparin administration (Jaffe and Willis, 1965). It is thought that osteoporosis occurring in patients with chronic renal failure being treated by haemodialysis is due to heparin but this is not proven. Localized increase in mast cells occurs in the marrow in proximity to areas of osteoclastic activity in a variety of bone diseases, postmenopausal osteoporosis, osteitis fibrosa of renal disease and Paget's disease of bone included. Open thin-walled vascular channels increase in number adjacent to foci of resorption and mast cells are found close to these vessels. The significance of the mast cell and heparin in the process of bone resorption is difficult to understand in the face of the evidence.

(l) Osteoporosis and inherited diseases

Abnormalities of skeletal development resulting from chromosomal and genetic defects are discussed in Chapter 5. Osteoporosis occurring in other metabolic bone disease is described in later sections. Localized osteoporosis during immobility and associated with acute inflammatory conditions of joints is discussed above.

(m) Transitory osteoporosis

Transitory osteoporosis is a disorder of unknown aetiology which affects the juxta-articular regions usually of the large limb joints of elderly people. The patient complains of local pain but does not have any demonstrable intra-articular disease. With conservative treatment the symptoms resolve in a few weeks.

(n) Sudek's atrophy

Sudek's atrophy affects the distal parts of the limbs, usually after trauma. The part is swollen and painful and there is rapid loss of bone. Disturbance of vasomotor activity is the postulated cause. Histological sections of affected bone show irregular thinning of trabeculae and a marked increase in number of both osteoclasts and osteoblasts sometimes associated with a minimal fibrous replacement of the marrow (Figure 10.7). The appearances bear a resemblance to those seen in hyperparathyroid bone disease but lack the irregularity in cement line pattern observed in that condition.

10.3   RICKETS AND OSTEOMALACIA

10.3.1   INTRODUCTION

Rickets and osteomalacia are both consequences of failure of physiological mineralization of skeletal matrix, the former term being used when the condition occurs while the growth plates are still active and the latter when adults are affected. This, in histological terms, defines the condition as that in which skeletal matrix (cartilage or bone) which should mineralize fails to do so. To avoid undue repetition 'osteomalacia' will be used in this chapter to include both conditions unless particular circumstances dictate otherwise.

The term 'rickets' was used to describe malnourished children in whom growth was stunted and who had deformities of spine and ribs and bowed limb bones in the first half of the 17th century. It was derived from the Greek 'rachitis' (literally inflammation of the spine) before either the pathology or the pathogenesis of the condition could have been known. Osteomalacia, derived from Greek words meaning soft bones, was described in the 19th century when microscopic information was available. For 300 years after rickets was recognized the disease was thought to occur only as the result of malnutrition or, after the discovery of vitamin D, as a result of vitamin D deficiency.

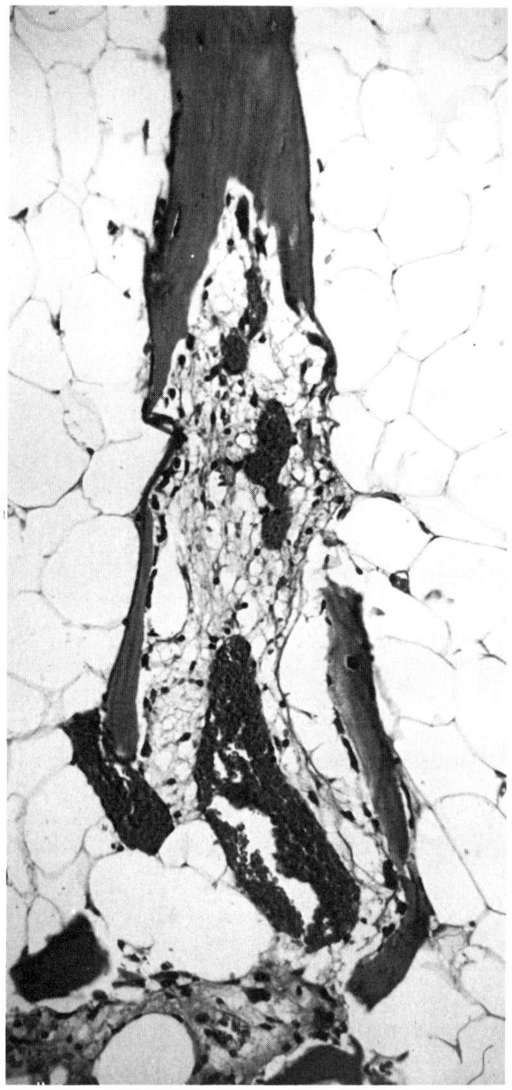

Figure 10.7 Acute osteoporosis. Decalcified, paraffin embedded section.

10.3.2   CAUSES OF OSTEOMALACIA

During the second half of the 20th century metabolic abnormalities, other than vitamin D deficiency, which cause mineralization failure in the skeleton have been described (Frame and Parfitt, 1978), and are included in Table 10.3. Some of the conditions listed are very rare and vitamin D deficiency is still the single most common cause, worldwide.

Table 10.3 Causes of rickets and osteomalacia

Vitamin D deficiency
  Dietary deficiency
  Inadequate skin synthesis

Malabsorption
  Gluten-sensitive enteropathy
  Gastrectomy and small intestine resection

Disturbance of di-hydroxylation of vitamin D_3
  Failure of 1-hydroxylation in kidney
    Chronic renal failure
    Inherited enzyme defect (vitamin D-dependent rickets)
    Parathyroid hormone deficiency
    Tumour-related rickets and osteomalacia (?)
  Failure of 25-hydroxylation in liver
    Prematurity
    Neonatal hepatitis
    Chronic hepatitis and cirrhosis

Excessive inactivation of vitamin D metabolites
  Anticonvulsant drugs, especially barbiturates
  Renal tubular defects
  Familial hypophosphataemia (vitamin D resistant rickets)
  Adult onset hypophosphataemic osteomalacia
  Fanconi syndrome (multiple renal tubular defects)
    Cystinosis
    Oculocerebrorenal syndrome
    Wilson's disease
    Galactosaemia
    Cadmium poisoning
    Multiple myeloma
  Renal tubular acidosis
    Inherited proximal or distal defect
    Ureterocolic anastomosis

Phosphate deficiency
  Antacids, especially aluminium

In-situ inhibition of mineralization
  Diphosphonates
  Sodium fluoride
  Aluminium

Miscellaneous
  Hypophosphatasia
  Fibrogenesis imperfecta ossium
  Axial osteomalacia

10.3.3 CLINICAL PRESENTATION

Regardless of the primary cause the affected child will grow more slowly and show degrees of deformation of spine, ribs and limb bones which are related to the time over which the abnormality has operated. Affected adults are more likely to be deformed if the disease began in childhood but all are susceptible to pathological fracture regardless of age of onset. Muscle weakness is a feature of osteomalacia due to abnormality of vitamin D and calcium metabolism but is not seen when hypophosphataemia is the primary abnormality.

10.3.4 BIOCHEMISTRY

As discussed in detail elsewhere (Chapter 18) the process of mineralization of bone and growth cartilage matrix is not fully understood. The conditions which lead to an osteomalacic skeleton embrace changes in the composition of extracellular fluid and the effects of localized abnormalities on the mineralization process at the tissue and cellular levels. The wide variety of combinations of biochemical abnormalities which have been recorded in patients with osteomalacia present problems of interpretation for most histopathologists and collaboration with clinical colleagues in resolving the cause in any particular case is mandatory. Unwarranted importance is attached, by some clinicians, to an elevated plasma alkaline phosphatase level as an indicator of osteomalacia in older adults in the absence of any other biochemical abnormalities related to bone disease.

10.3.5 RADIOLOGY

The epiphyses of rachitic children are increased in both length and width and the metaphyseal bone is deformed to a saucer

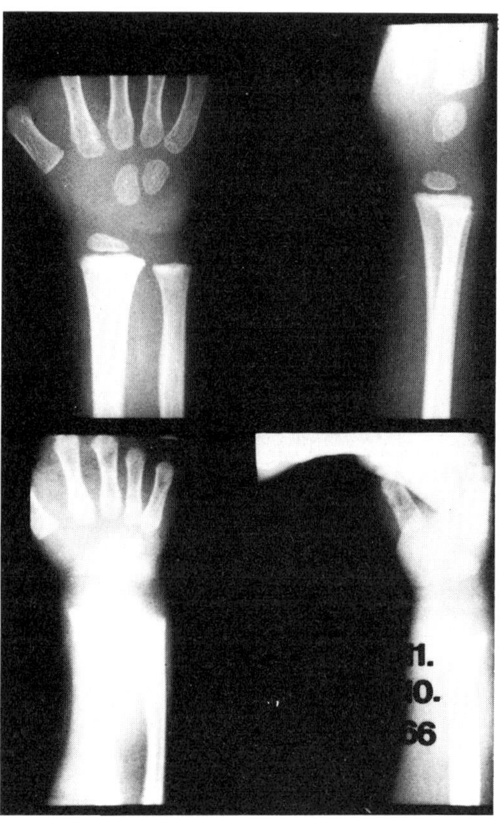

Figure 10.8 Radiographs of normal and rachitic wrists. The rachitic physis is wider and deeper than normal.

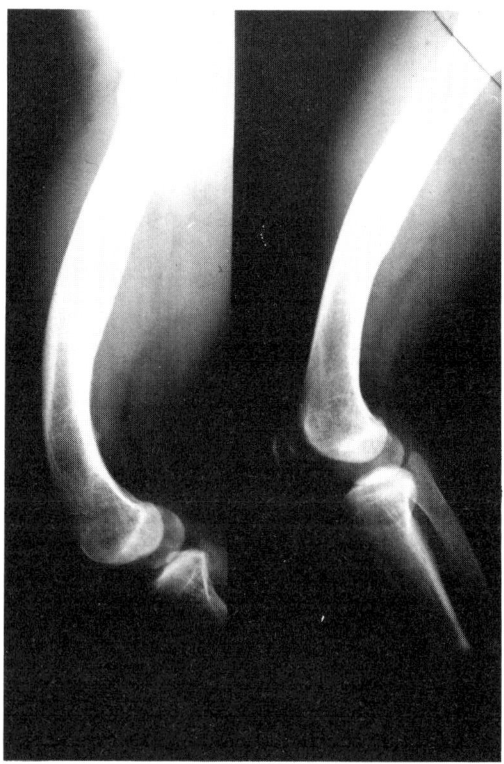

Figure 10.9 Rickets. Radiographs showing bowing of femur in X-linked hypophosphataemic rickets.

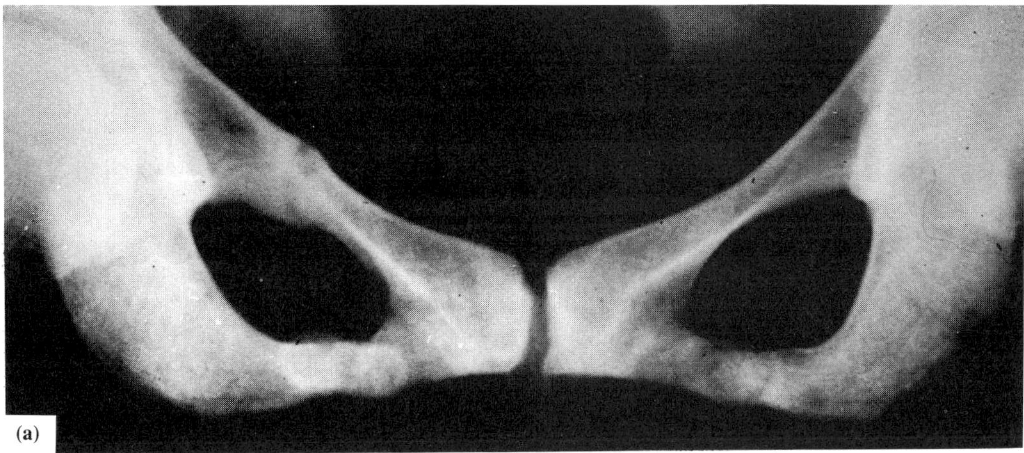

Figure 10.10 Osteomalacia. Looser's zones. (a) Radiograph of pelvis.

shape (Figure 10.8). Wrists, knees, ankles and ribs show the changes most clearly. Bowing deformities of long bones occur, usually most marked in proximity to the metaphyseal–diaphyseal junction (Figure 10.9). Spinal deformities may also be evident. In the long bones there is loss of the normal sharp definition between cortex and medulla. If osteomalacia begins in adult life loss of corticomedullary definition is the commonest feature and the bones may also be more radiolucent. Incomplete fractures, involving the cortex on one side of the bone, appear as transverse linear lucencies – 'Looser's zones' (Figure 10.10). They are found most often on the axillary border of the scapula, in the pubic rami, in the ribs and in the lower limb long bones usually adjacent to metaphyses, but no appendicular bone is exempt. Complete fractures may also be found in pelvis and ribs. Both complete and incomplete fractures may be multiple. Radionuclide scanning (McFarlane *et al.*, 1977) will identify both types of lesion (Figure 10.11). Deformity occurs without fracture, especially of the pelvis, and causes protrusio acetabuli or a more serious medial collapse of the ilia producing the 'tri-radiate' pelvis. Collapse of vertebral body end plates, together with an appearance described as 'fish vertebrae', is another feature.

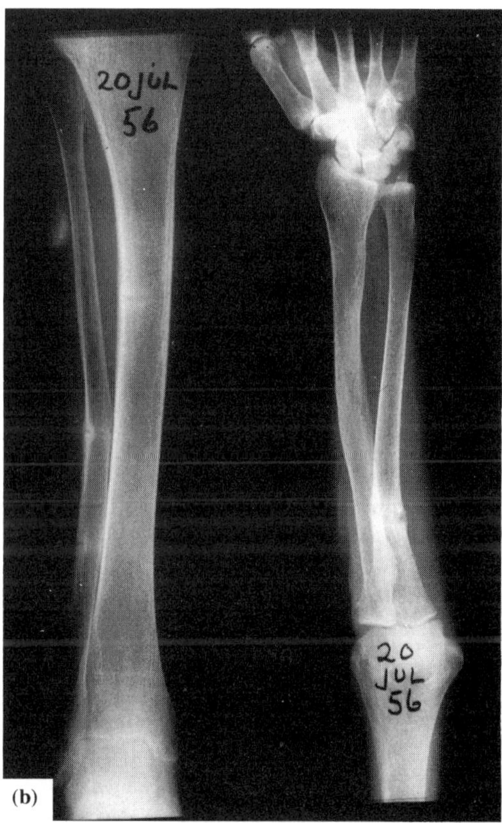

Figure 10.10 Osteomalacia. Looser's zones. (b) One Looser's zone in the ulna and two in the fibula.

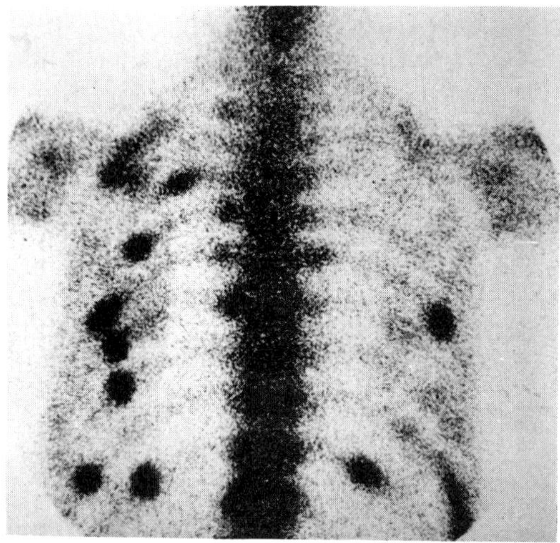

Figure 10.11 Osteomalacia. Multiple rib fractures identified by isotope scan.

When osteomalacia is a continuation from rickets the residual deformities of childhood are added to the above changes. Hyperparathyroidism secondary to the osteomalacia will introduce further radiographic changes as described in sections 10.4.7 and 10.4.11.

10.3.6 HISTOLOGY

With rare exceptions, osteomalacia is a truly generalized disease and a bone biopsy from any site may be used for diagnostic purposes. Histological examination of bone samples from a case of suspected osteomalacia requires the preparation of sections in which the calcified matrix can be reliably stained and differentiated from unmineralized osteoid. It may also be advantageous to examine sections prepared from decalcified bone and such sections should be made if the size of the bone sample permits. Electron microscopy is not required for diagnosis. A systematic examination of the bone tissue and marrow should be undertaken as outlined in the section on osteoporosis; evidence of primary diseases, for example, cystinosis and myeloma, may be found in the marrow.

What has to be demonstrated to establish a diagnosis of osteomalacia is that osteoid is not being mineralized and is accumulating on the bone surfaces in layers of excessive thickness (Figure 10.12). Osteoid of excessive thickness may cover only part or the whole of the bone surfaces. When only part of the bone surface is covered by excess osteoid other surfaces may bear osteoid of normal thickness. Measurement of the thickness of every osteoid seam is mandatory. When all bone surfaces are covered by excessively thick osteoid there may be zones of unmineralized matrix around some of the osteocytes (Figure 10.13). This appearance, the cause of which is uncertain, is not, in the author's experience, peculiar to any particular type of osteomalacia. The matrix produced is predominantly of lamellar type. Woven osteoid will be formed as a response to fracture and may also be found when osteomalacia is complicated by hyperparathyroidism. An abnormal matrix which is poorly birefringent is formed in the condition 'fibrogenesis imperfecta ossium', the early stages of which produce an histological appearance which resembles other types of osteomalacia and will only be distinguishable if the section is examined in polarized light. In those forms of osteomalacia which result from conditions leading to a fall in plasma ionized calcium or to a stimulation of parathormone secretion for some other reason there may be histological evidence of hyperparathyroidism (secondary hyperparathyroidism) and such evidence must be sought as it gives a guide as to primary cause. The method used by the author to assess osteoid thickness (counting lamellae in polarized light) usually reveals a larger number of lamellae (11 or more) in osteomalacia and secondary hyperparathyroidism due to vitamin D deficiency than in cases where the primary cause is renal failure (no more than 10). Those forms of osteomalacia which result from hypophosphataemia alone or from a local inhibition of mineralization are not complicated by hyperparathyroidism unless there is another cause; for example in the case of aluminium intoxication in a patient with chronic renal failure.

In uncomplicated osteomalacia, the osteoblast population will be found reduced relative to the extent of the osteoid surface and, in some specimens, there will be no osteoblasts. This feature is in itself a strong indication that

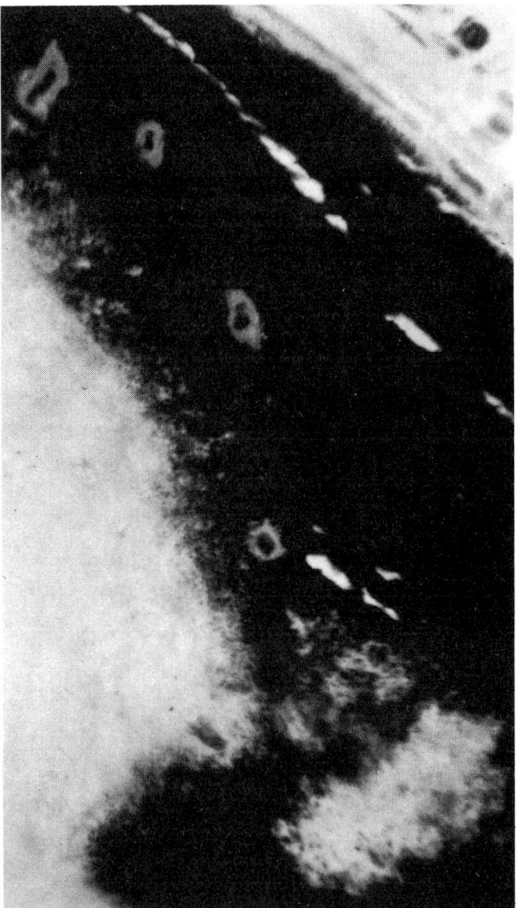

Figure 10.13 Osteomalacia. Unmineralized periosteocytic zones. Undecalcified section, von Kossa stain.

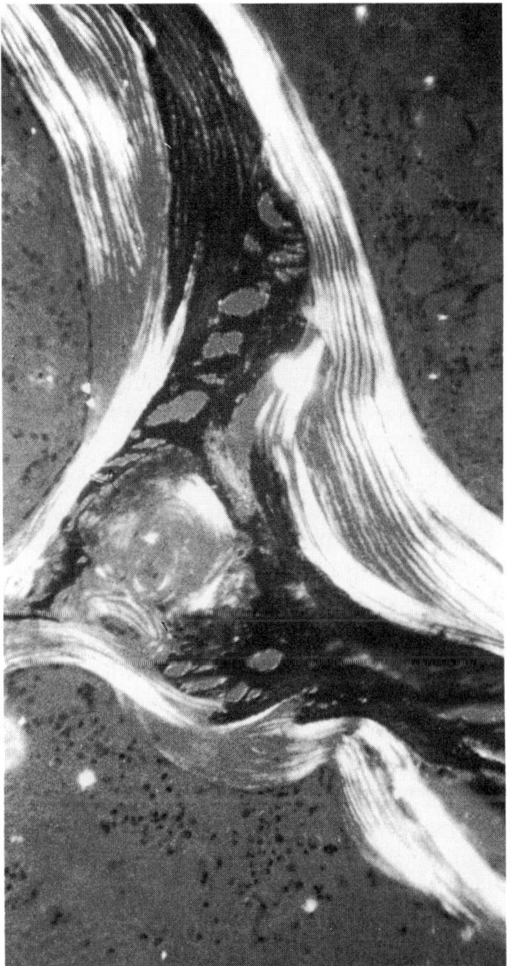

Figure 10.12 Osteomalacia. Osteoid covers all bone surfaces and some consists of five or more birefringent lamellae. Undecalcified section, von Kossa stain. Polarized light.

the osteoid is not being mineralized in the proper time sequence of bone formation. There is a close correlation between the proportion of osteoid which is undergoing mineralization as identified by the calcification front and the osteoblast count (Woods, 1976). The number of osteoclasts will also be reduced and if the entire surface of the bone is covered by osteoid there will be no osteoclasts.

When osteomalacia is complicated by hyperparathyroidism osteoblasts will be present, sometimes covering the majority of the osteoid. Osteoclasts will also be active and characteristically located on surfaces of mineralized matrix which are buried under osteoid, giving rise to the appearance described as 'dissecting' or 'tunnelling' resorption (Figure 10.14).

Osteomalacic bone may have a total matrix area (or volume) which is less than, equal to or greater than normal. In the first two of these cases the mass of true bone will be, of necessity, less than normal, and it has been suggested that this state should be described as 'osteomalacia with osteoporosis'. The reduction of true bone mass will predispose the bone to fracture. In severe osteomalacia the true bone will be in the form of islands in a sea of osteoid and this also has an adverse effect on mechanical stability (Figure 10.15).

Reference is made above to the possibility

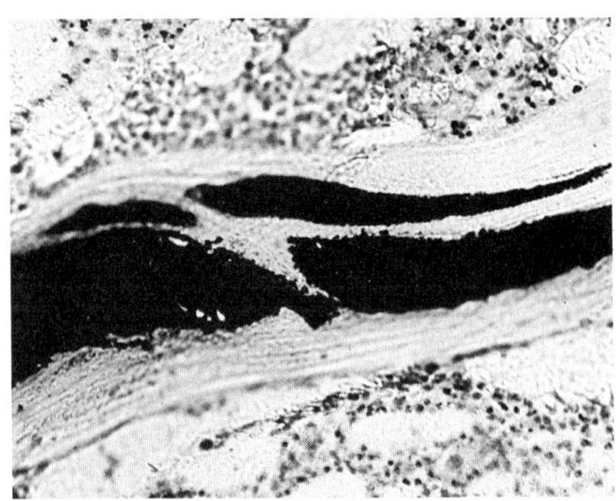

Figure 10.15 Osteomalacia. Severe form of the disease with mineralized tissue reduced to disconnected fragments within the osteoid. Undecalcified section, von Kossa stain.

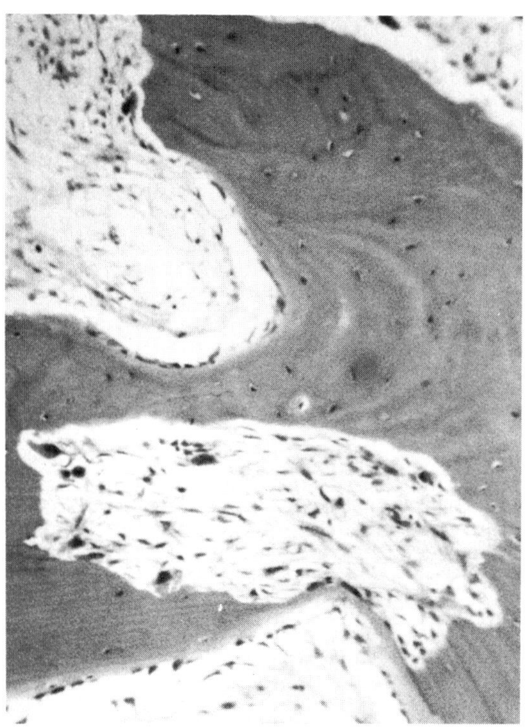

Figure 10.14 Osteomalacia with secondary hyperparathyroidism. Dissecting (tunnelling) resorption. Decalcified, paraffin embedded section.

that the total matrix mass may be greater than normal. In some cases of osteomalacia radiographs may show areas of increased density, the zone adjacent to the end plates of vertebral bodies being one such. This does not invariably mean that the mass of mineralized bone is increased; osteoid is radiopaque relative to marrow tissue.

The commonest appearance in an histological section of osteomalacic bone is of a sandwich with a centre of mineralized tissue and osteoid on the outside. Sometimes the sandwich is a 'multi-decker' with two or more strips of bone separated by osteoid (Figure 10.16). This variant of the histological appearance may be found in patients with vitamin D deficiency due to malabsorption who temporarily experience exposure to long hours of sunlight or those in chronic renal failure who are given 1_α-(OH)D$_3$. From this one may speculate that the multi-layer sandwiches are the result of partial or temporary correction of the primary cause of the disease.

When vitamin D deficiency is effectively treated the plasma alkaline phosphatase rises during the second week of treatment. Bone biopsy at that time will show large osteoblasts on the surface of the osteoid (Figure

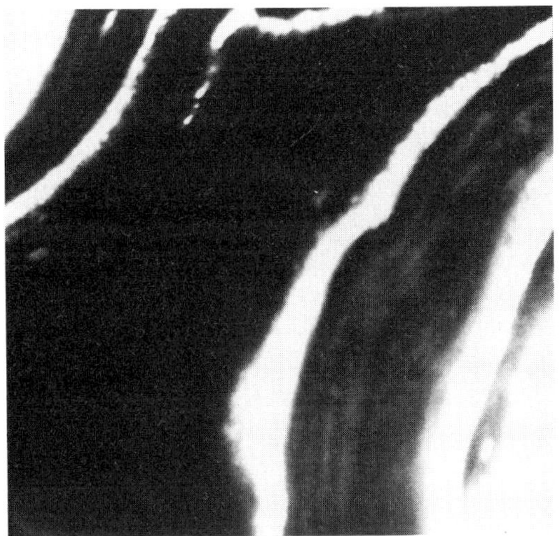

Figure 10.16 Osteomalacia. The 'multi-decker' sandwich appearance. Undecalcified section, von Kossa stain.

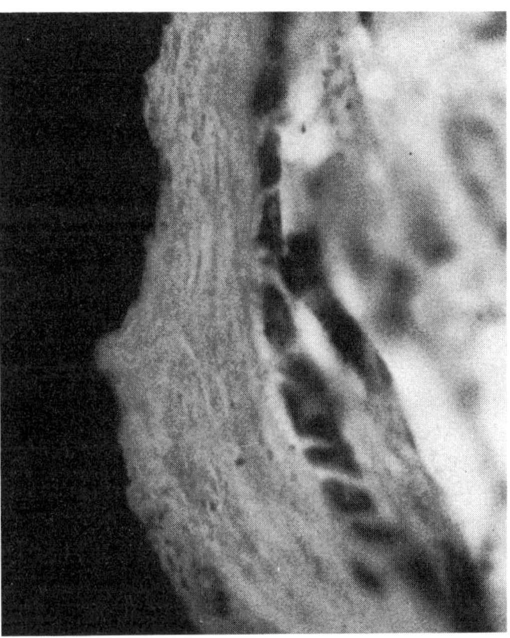

Figure 10.17 Osteomalacia. Active osteoblasts on an osteoid surface. Vitamin D deficiency osteomalacia 14 days after starting treatment. Undecalcified section, von Kossa stain.

10.17) and a thin layer of mineralized tissue may be seen, occasionally, lying immediately beneath the cells. There may also be osteoclasts lying against what appears to be an osteoid surface. Whether, with better resolution than is possible with the light microscope, one would see mineral in the matrix next to the osteoclast has not been tested. Observations on the effect of vitamin D therapy and the phenomenon of the multi-sandwich suggest a mode of healing of osteomalacia due to vitamin D deficiency. The hypothesis is that the osteoid formed during the time of deficiency is removed in sequences of surface mineralization and resorption; normal bone formation resumes on the mineralized cores of bone when they are exposed. The alternative suggestion that the excess osteoid is mineralized from the deep surface outwards would lead one to expect a striking increase in radiographic density of bone, and the physis in children, after treatment, but these are not recognized signs of healing.

Looser's zones are the result of unhealed incomplete fractures. The radiolucent area contains fibrous, cartilaginous and osseous matrix in various combinations but without evidence of mineralization. Complete fractures are followed by the usual sequence of changes to the time when mineralization would normally occur. Mineralization of a small proportion of both bone and cartilage callus occurs. The size of the callus bridge may be excessive.

10.3.7 RENAL DISEASE AND METABOLIC BONE DISEASE

(a) Glomerular disease and renal failure

Chronic glomerular disease with cortical destruction and comprehensive renal failure is associated with variable combinations of derangement of calcium and phosphate metabolism together with failure of hydroxylation of vitamin D and stimulation of parathormone secretion. Renal tubular acidosis also ensues. Abnormality of other endocrine functions, for example, gonadal steroids, calcitonin and thyroxine, may also contribute to the skeletal changes. Radiographic and histological examination of the skeleton of patients with chronic renal failure before haemodialysis treatment is started shows some to be apparently normal and the others to be osteoporotic or osteomalacic with or without hyperparathyroid changes. Some descriptions of the skeletal abnormalities in chronic renal failure group all of them together as 'renal osteodystrophy'. This is not acceptable as a term for histological reports because it gives no indication to the clinician as to what supplementary treatment could be added to correct specific abnormalities nor does it give room for a change of diagnosis if the histological appearances change, as commonly happens in both untreated and treated chronic renal failure. Haemodialysis alone does not restore bone remodelling to normal and the skeletal complications of chronic renal failure are a significant cause of morbidity among patients maintained on haemodialysis. Supplementary treatments can also influence the state of the skeleton. Administration of 1_α-(OH) cholecalciferol will correct the mineralization defect whereas aluminium hydroxide given to lower plasma phosphate level may make osteomalacia worse. Parathyroidectomy is required to control hyperparathyroid bone disease. Haemodialysis may make bone disease worse if heparin is a cause of osteoporosis and if aluminium is accumulated in the body from dialysis fluid. The histological appearances in a bone biopsy from a patient with chronic renal failure on maintenance haemodialysis are dependent on many variables that the histologist will either not be aware of or will not fully understand the significance of. In many instances the clinician will not be able to provide a certain answer as to why the bone appears as it does.

(b) Disorders of tubule function

Abnormalities of renal tubule function without comprehensive renal failure affect vitamin D hydroxylation, plasma phosphate conservation and acid–base balance. Vitamin D-dependent rickets is a rare inherited disorder in which the skeletal changes of rickets and osteomalacia occur without evidence of vitamin D deficiency. In most cases the cause is a failure of 1_α-hydroxylation in the kidney (Fraser *et al.*, 1973); other cases are ascribed to decreased tissue sensitivity to normal plasma levels of 1,25-dihydroxy vitamin D_3 ($1,25(OH)_2D_3$) (Brooks *et al.*, 1978). The histological appearances are those of osteomalacia sometimes with superadded hyperparathyroid bone disease. Large doses of vitamin D or of $1,25(OH)_2D_3$ are curative. Vitamin D-resistant rickets is an X-linked inherited disorder which results in excess loss of phosphate in the urine and a low plasma phosphate (Glorieux *et al.*, 1980). Rickets occurs in some of the patients and they present all the radiographic and histological changes of severe rickets but without changes of hyperparathyroidism. Administration of phosphate alone does not correct the skeletal abnormalities but in combination with $1,25(OH)_2D_3$ is reported to be effective treatment. There are also forms of hypophosphataemic osteomalacia resulting from tubular dysfunction which are manifest after skeletal maturity, some of them apparently inherited as an autosomal recessive characteristic and others associated with the presence of a tumour. Tumour-related hypophosphataemic osteomalacia has been described as a consequence of a variety of lesions including benign skeletal and soft tissue tumours (Evans and Azzopardi, 1972), meningioma and prostatic carcinoma (Lyles *et al.*, 1980). The link between the primary lesion and the renal defect has not been established but is thought to be due to a failure of 1_α-hydroxylation. Removal of the lesion corrects the tubule malfunction. Osteomalacia has been described in some patients with hypoparathyroidism (Drezner *et al.*, 1977) as a condition in which the plasma calcium level is below normal and the conversion of 25-hydroxy D to 1,25-dihydroxy D is impaired (Lund *et al.*, 1980). Failure to conserve phosphate is part of the multiple tubular deficiencies of Fanconi's syndrome, which has several causes (Table 10.3) the most common of which is cystinosis. Acidosis may also result from the tubular defects. The situation may be further complicated by progressive destruction of the kidney due to cystine deposition and comprehensive renal failure.

10.3.8   METABOLIC ACIDOSIS

Acidosis occurs as the result of inherited renal tubular defects or after ureterocolic anastomosis. Osteomalacia associated with acidosis has been ascribed to a direct effect on bone mineral, an increased response to parathormone by bone and hypophosphataemia because of a change in renal handling of phosphate also induced by parathormone. The histological changes are those of uncomplicated osteomalacia and these changes can be eliminated by correction of the acidosis with bicarbonate. Vitamin D is commonly given in addition.

10.3.9   DIPHOSPHONATES

Diphosphonates are compounds in which the oxygen of the phosphate radical is replaced by carbon. They are absorbed when ingested and are incorporated into bone mineral. The first compound produced for therapeutic use, ethane 1-hydroxy-1, 1-diphosphonate, when administered in effective dosage for the treatment of Paget's disease, interferes with mineralization. Within the course of a few weeks the bone surfaces are covered by a thick layer of osteoid; at the same time the intense cellular activity characteristic of Paget's disease is totally suppressed (Figure 10.18). Plasma phosphorus levels are elevated while the drug is being taken. The other biochemical changes reflect the reduced bone cell activity. Subsequently developed compounds do not appear to have the same effect on mineralization.

10.3.10   FLUORIDE

Fluoride is ingested in large quantities as a consequence of industrial pollution (aluminium smelting), naturally occurring high water concentrations and the treatment of osteoporosis. The quantities added to drinking water and to toothpaste to protect teeth against caries do not present a risk of excessive intake. After long exposure to a high dosage of fluoride, structural changes occur in the skeleton as the result of new bone formation under the periosteum and in ligamentous insertions into bone. Active remodelling is seen in both cortex and medulla. Haversian canals are enlarged and apposition occurs with widening of bone trabeculae. Some of the new bone is of immature type. Mineralization is impaired and osteoid accumulates over much of the bone in abnormally thick layers. Zones of unmineralized matrix around osteocytes have also been described. Fluoride treatment of osteoporosis was supplemented with vitamin D and calcium to prevent the mineralization failure although there is no evidence that fluoride adversely affects the metabolism of either of these substances.

10.3.11   ALUMINIUM

Ingested aluminium salts inhibit absorption of phosphate and may reduce the level of plasma phosphate sufficiently to inhibit bone mineralization. Aluminium hydroxide is an antacid and if taken in large quantities

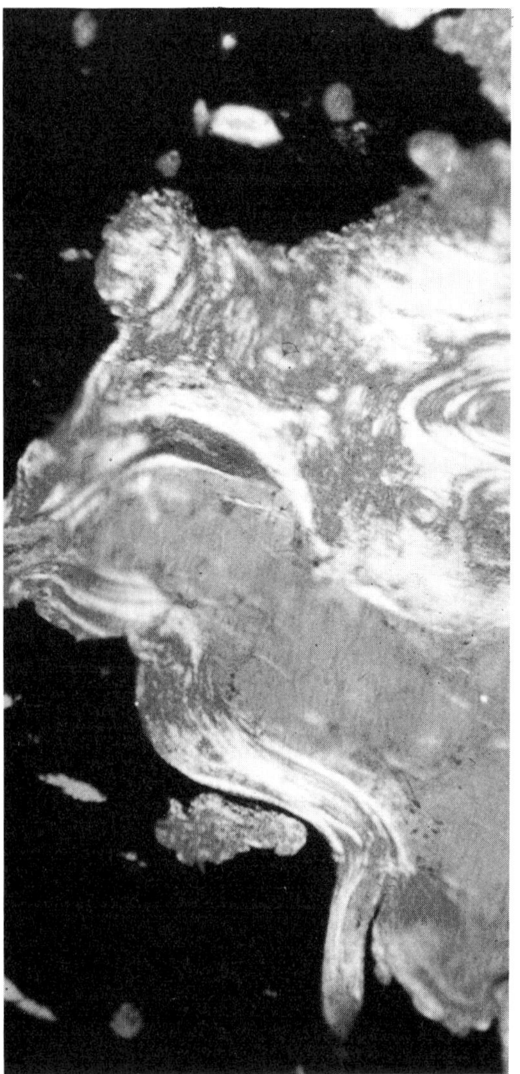

Figure 10.18 Mineralization failure induced by diphosphonate treatment of Paget's disease. Undecalcified section, von Kossa stain. Polarized light.

can cause hypophosphataemia, hypercalcaemia, muscle weakness and osteomalacia. Aluminium hydroxide has been given to patients with chronic renal failure maintained on haemodialysis in order to reduce the level of plasma phosphate. A small proportion of ingested aluminium is absorbed. During the process of purification of drinking water aluminium sulphate is added to the water to precipitate particulate matter. If dialysis solution contains aluminium some will pass into the patient's blood and from there to the extracellular fluid to be incorporated into sites of bone mineralization. The presence of aluminium inhibits the mineralization process. Undecalcified sections of bone embedded in plastic and stained for aluminium will show the distribution of the incorporated metal (Figure 10.19). In a large number of bone biopsies from patients on maintenance haemodialysis examined by the author the aluminium has been seen in cement lines, at the interface between bone and osteoid and, sometimes, in mineralized matrix. The osteoid covering a line of aluminium incorporation is not always of abnormal thickness and not every osteoid layer which is abnormally thick has aluminium in the underlying bone surface. These observations indicate that the presence of local aluminium may inhibit mineralization only in the immediate vicinity and that the florid histological osteomalacia is the consequence of lowered plasma phosphate. Local inhibition of mineralization occurs when other 'foreign' substances which are permanently incorporated into mineralizing matrix are administered; tetracyclines are a case in point.

10.3.12 HYPOPHOSPHATASIA

Hypophosphatasia is a rare familial disease inherited as a recessive characteristic and expressed by a failure of skeletal mineralization together with a low plasma alkaline phosphatase and the excretion of phosphoethanolamine in the urine. Pyrophosphate, which inhibits mineralization, has been found to be increased in the plasma. Whether all cells in the tissues and particularly the osteoblasts have a reduced alkaline phosphatase activity and to what degree is not known. Nor is the reason for the excretion of phosphoethanolamine. The

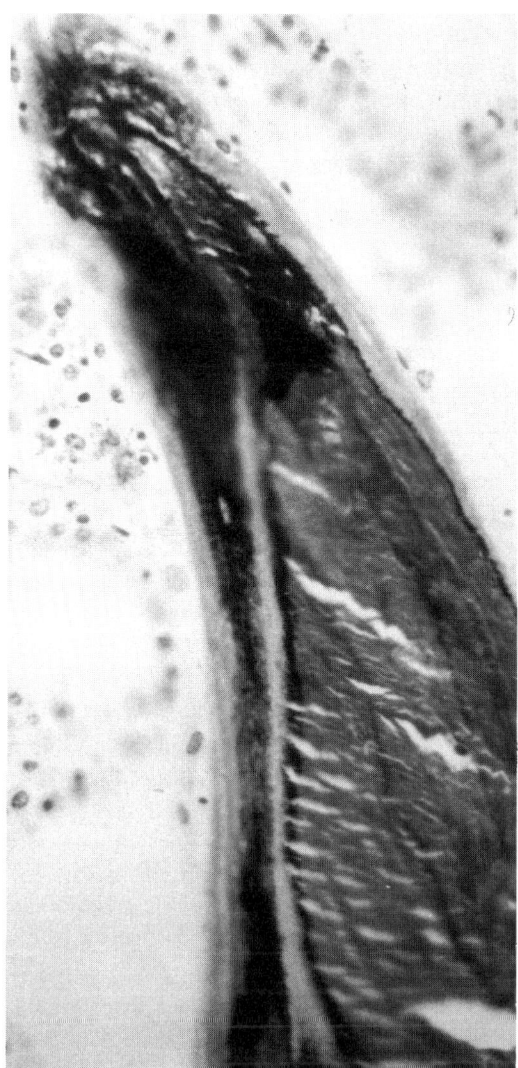

Figure 10.19 Aluminium deposition demonstrated by solochrome stain. Chronic renal failure treated by haemodialysis. Undecalcified, plastic-embedded section.

abnormality may be first manifest at any age from birth to adult life (Beighton, 1978), early expression being associated with the most severe skeletal problems. Failure of mineralization of both growth cartilage and bone matrix produces the skeletal deformities of rickets and osteomalacia plus virtual absence of ossification of the skull in an affected neonate and poor development with premature loss of deciduous and permanent teeth in any patient in childhood. Radiographic changes are similar to those seen in rickets but often very much more severe and there may also be ragged areas of lucency in the metaphyses of long bones (Figure 10.20). Those patients who present with disease after the neonatal period may have temporary remissions for reasons unknown. During remissions the mineralization process will be normal, the alkaline phosphatase level in the plasma may rise but phosphoethanolamine excretion will persist. Histological appearances in bone sections may vary with timing and site of sampling. For example, unequivocal evidence of osteomalacia may be found in an area of radiographic lucency of the metaphysis whilst the adjacent growth plate appears to be adequately mineralized. The primary disorder cannot be corrected.

Fibrogenesis imperfecta ossium is described in section 10.6.

10.3.13   AXIAL OSTEOMALACIA

Axial osteomalacia (or familial axial osteomalacia) is a rare condition of unknown aetiology which affects children and adults of either sex. Patients complain of pain in the spine, ribs or pelvis and radiographs show sclerosis of bone and coarse irregularity of trabeculae in these areas. Levels of plasma calcium, phosphorus, alkaline phosphatase and vitamin D metabolites are normal. Iliac bone biopsies show accumulation of osteoid and delayed mineralization (Whyte *et al.*, 1981). The osteoid is of lamellar type, which distinguishes the disorder from fibrogenesis imperfecta ossium and from fluorosis. Whyte *et al.* (1981) report an affected mother and son but the majority of recorded cases appear to be sporadic. The natural history of the disease and the effects of any form of treatment are not known.

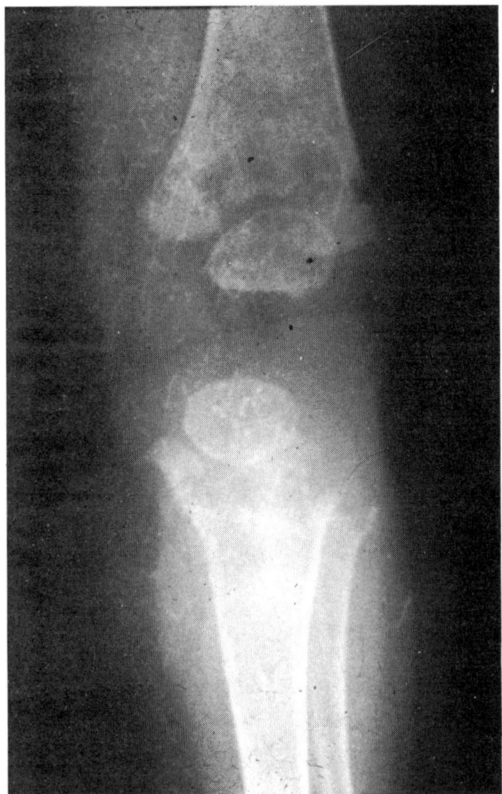

Figure 10.20 Hypophosphatasia. Radiograph of knee joint. Note, in addition to saucer-shaped deformity of physis, the translucent areas extending through the metaphyses.

10.4 HYPERPARATHYROID BONE DISEASE

10.4.1 INTRODUCTION

Parathormone overproduction may occur as the result of idiopathic cellular proliferation of one, or rarely more, parathyroid glands or in response to a metabolic change which results in a persistent lowering of the level of ionized calcium in the plasma. These situations are described as primary and secondary (and sometimes tertiary) hyperparathyroidism respectively.

10.4.2 PRIMARY HYPERPARATHYROIDISM

The usual cause is a solitary adenoma; multiple adenomata and hyperplasia of all glands are uncommon and carcinoma is rare. A parathyroid adenoma may be part of a multiple endocrine neoplasia syndrome. Females are more often affected than males and the peak incidence is in middle adult life, but the disease can occur at any age.

10.4.3 BIOCHEMISTRY

The principal biochemical consequence is an elevated plasma calcium. Hypophosphataemia may also be found whilst the plasma alkaline phosphatase and the urinary hydroxyproline levels will be raised only if the skeleton is affected, which it is in a minority of patients (Byers and Smith, 1971).

10.4.4 CLINICAL PRESENTATION

Most patients present because of problems caused by the elevated plasma calcium and many are now discovered to have hyperparathyroidism as a result of biochemical screening. Those patients presenting because of skeletal abnormalities do so because of pain or pathological fracture.

10.4.5 HISTOLOGY

The skeletal changes produced by increased parathormone secretion are generalized but not uniform and, especially in elderly females, random sampling may show areas of bone which do not have all the histological features necessary to make an unequivocal diagnosis. Subperiosteal bone resorption tends to be more marked in some bones than others, a situation best appreciated in radiographic studies of the skeleton and described below. In some patients areas of the medulla are cleared of bone and occupied by giant-cell rich tissue which, because there is usually abundant haemosiderin pigment also present, is described as the 'brown tumour' of hyperparathyroidism. The primary effect of hyperparathyroidism on bone is an increase in osteoclastic activity and bone resorption. Bone formation also increases as does the number of osteoblasts (Mosekilde and Melsen, 1978). This increase in cellular activity is accompanied by the appearance of fibrous tissue separating the active bone cells from the adjacent marrow (Figure 10.21), usually as a thin layer and not replacing large areas of marrow as occurs in Paget's disease. The increased turnover of bone is reflected in the disorganization of the cement line pattern, which is usually easily recognized but rarely is so marked as to be confused with the 'mosaic' appearance of Paget's disease. In male patients and females under the age of 40 years, the increased cellular activity does not produce a significant generalized change in skeletal mass provided that the patient remains constitutionally well and ambulant. Apart from areas occupied by 'brown tumour' deviations from normal both higher and lower may be found in a small proportion of biopsies. Middle-aged and elderly females may have a significantly lower bone mass than is normal for their age (Coupron *et al.*, 1976). In some biopsies there will be trabeculae of immature bone between the lamellar struts and in those cases the mature bone area will usually be less than normal.

An increased population of active osteoblasts results in an increase in the proportion of bone surfaces covered by prominent osteoid seams which are within the normal range of thickness (Figure 10.22). By some histomorphometric criteria this state might be categorized as osteomalacic but primary hyperparathyroidism does not *per se* cause mineralization failure. An abnormally high proportion of osteoid which is the result of an increase in osteoblastic activity should be termed 'hyperosteoidosis'. If the osteoid is abnormally thick (i.e. if there are both hyperparathyroid changes and true osteomalacia) then one has to consider the possibilities that

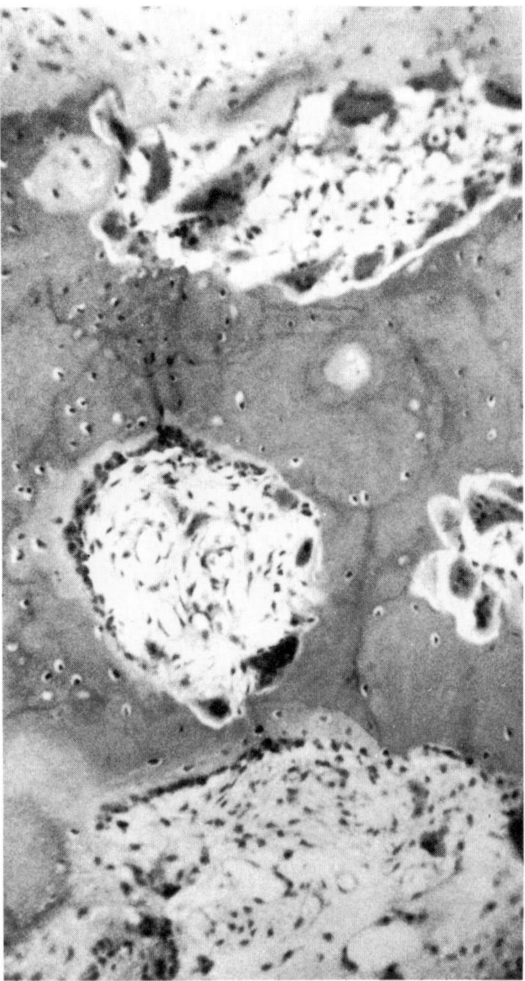

Figure 10.21 Hyperparathyroid bone disease. Increased numbers of both osteoblasts and osteoclasts affecting cortical bone including subperiosteal zone (top). Decalcified, paraffin-embedded section.

the hyperparathyroidism is secondary to the cause of the osteomalacia, or that there is a cause for the osteomalacia (e.g. dietary) which may or may not be connected with the parathyroid disorder.

The 'brown tumour' is composed of a mass of mononuclear spindle and ovoid cells among which is scattered a variable, sometimes large, number of multinucleated cells

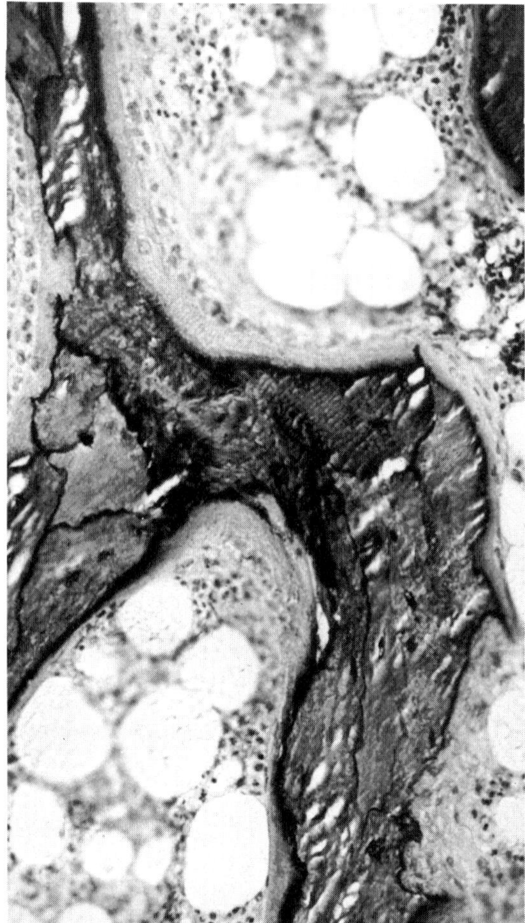

Figure 10.22 Hyperparathyroid bone disease. Increased numbers of osteoblasts with increase in the proportion of bone covered by osteoid which is of normal thickness. Undecalcified, plastic-embedded section. Toluidine blue.

which closely resemble osteoclasts. Characteristically there is also haemosiderin pigment in sufficient amount to give the tissue a macroscopical brown colour (Figure 10.23). The pigment is both intra- and extracellular. At the periphery of the lesion there will often be scattered trabeculae of woven bone. The lesion resembles, in histological appearance, and may be confused with giant cell tumour or reparative giant-cell granuloma. The cor-

rect diagnosis can be established if the margin of the lesion and enclosing bone are available for histological examination or by the abnormal biochemistry associated with the 'brown tumour'. Other evidence which should make one suspect that an osteoclast-rich lesion is hyperparathyroid related includes location in diaphysis, jaw or skull, multiple lesions, the characteristic radiographic changes in the hands and the patient being over 60 years old and female.

Removal of abnormal parathyroid tissue is very quickly followed by a reversion of bone cell activity to a normal level. The disordered

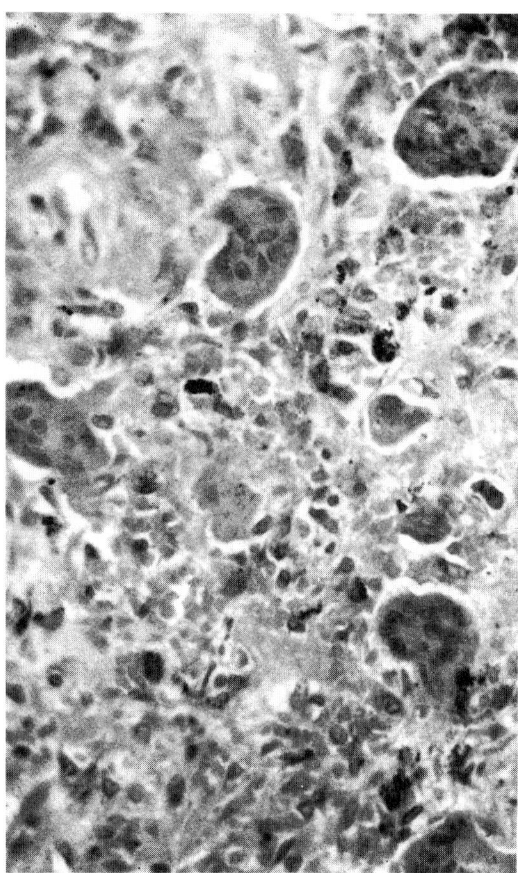

Figure 10.23 Hyperparathyroid bone disease. 'Brown tumour'. Decalcified, paraffin-embedded section.

arrangement of cement lines and structural alterations in the bone persist for months or several years after treatment (Collins, 1966).

10.4.6 RADIOLOGY

The radiographic changes associated with hyperparathyroidism are related to the focal concentration of areas of resorption and the generalized disturbance of bone remodelling. Intramedullary areas of osteolysis produce 'cystic' lesions which may be in any part of any bone and are the 'brown tumours' described above (Figure 10.24). Subperiosteal bone resorption may also be detected in any tubular bone but is usually looked for in the metacarpals and phalanges (Figure 10.25). Diaphyseal subperiosteal erosions occur most frequently on the radial side of the bone. Erosion in the terminal phalanx may lead to complete loss of the distal end (the clinical appearance resembles clubbing). Erosion of the lamina dura around the roots of teeth may be valuable evidence in the investigation of a focal lesion in the jaw, provided that the patient is not edentulous. The generalized changes may be subtle and consist of a loss of the normally sharp definition between the cortex and medulla of tubular bones and a hazy texture in cancellous bones such as vertebral bodies.

10.4.7 SECONDARY HYPERPARATHYROIDISM

The major causes of reactive parathyroid hyperplasia are chronic renal failure and vitamin D deficiency due to malabsorption.

10.4.8 BIOCHEMISTRY

The biochemical abnormalities will include raised levels of plasma calcium, alkaline phosphatase and parathormone together with any other abnormalities associated with the primary disorder.

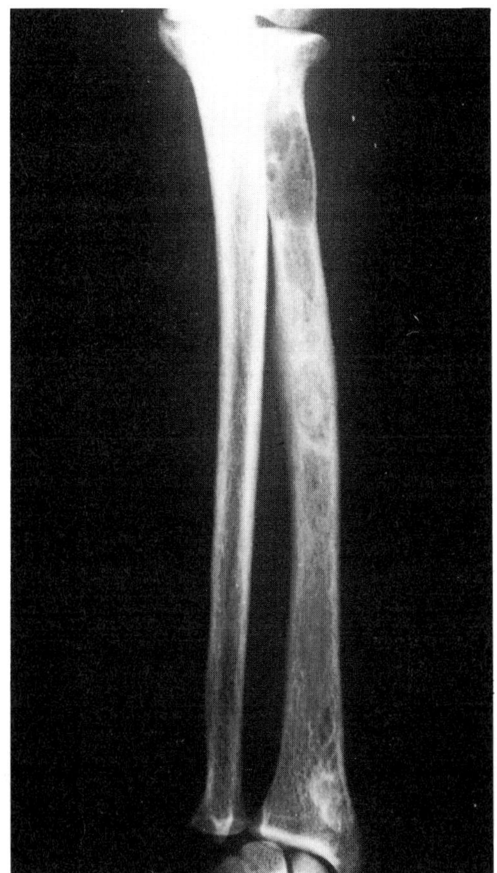

Figure 10.24 Hyperparathyroid bone disease. Radiograph of forearm. Osteolytic foci in radius.

10.4.9 HISTOLOGY

In all cases of vitamin D deficiency the histological appearances will be a combination of osteomalacia and the increased bone cell activity of hyperparathyroidism, the latter commonly modified by the osteoclastic activity being directed along the centres of bone trabeculae, an appearance described as 'tunnelling' or 'dissecting' resorption (Figure 10.14). A possible cause of confusion is the increase in osteoblastic and osteoclastic activity which occurs shortly after vitamin D deficiency is corrected and enquiry should always be made regarding this possibility

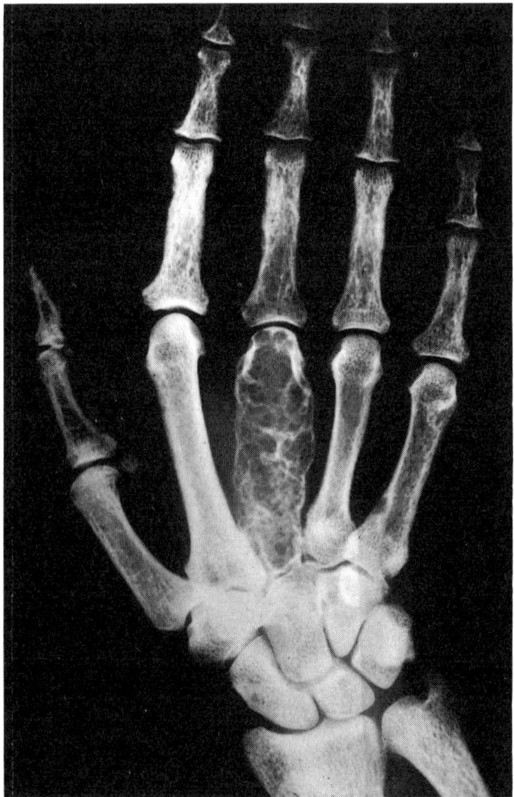

Figure 10.25 Hyperparathyroid bone disease. Radiograph of hand. Periosteal resorption of diaphyses of phalanges and metacarpals and 'brown tumour' in third metacarpal.

before reporting a bone biopsy as showing 'osteomalacia with secondary hyperparathyroidism'.

The untreated patient with secondary hyperparathyroidism associated with chronic renal failure will have the combined features of osteomalacia and hyperparathyroidism with 'dissecting' resorption as described above. This appearance is the only one to which the term 'renal osteodystrophy' should be attached. It is now common for patients with renal osteodystrophy to be given 1α(OH) D_3 and this may remove the osteomalacic component from the histological appearances. Because evidence of present

or previous 'dissecting' resorption will usually be found, a diagnosis of 'secondary hyperparathyroidism' may still be possible.

The degree of distortion of the cement line pattern is usually greater in secondary than in primary hyperparathyroidism but rarely to the extent of a true 'mosaic'.

Osteosclerosis occurs commonly in renal osteodystrophy (Ellis and Peart, 1973) but is not a feature of dietary vitamin D-deficiency-related secondary hyperparathyroidism. The reason for this difference is not certain but may be related to the higher levels of circulating parathormone found in patients with osteosclerosis (Teitelbaum *et al.*, 1980).

10.4.10 RADIOLOGY

The abnormalities seen will be essentially the same as those described for primary hyperparathyroidism. In secondary hyperparathyroidism another area which seems particularly liable to excessive erosion is the outer ends of the clavicles. There is also a greater incidence in the appearance of areas of bone sclerosis and these are usually best seen in lateral radiographs of the spine where sclerotic vertebral body end-plates contrast with porotic central areas of bone and lucent intervertebral discs to produce a pattern described as 'rugger jersey' spine (Figure 10.26).

10.4.11 TERTIARY HYPERPARATHYROIDISM

This is a clinical term applied when reactive hyperparathyroidism persists after the primary cause has been corrected. A common example is the patient with chronic renal failure who has been maintained on haemodialysis for several months or more and then has a successful renal transplant before hyperplastic parathyroid glands have been completely removed. There are no radiographic or histological features peculiar to the condition.

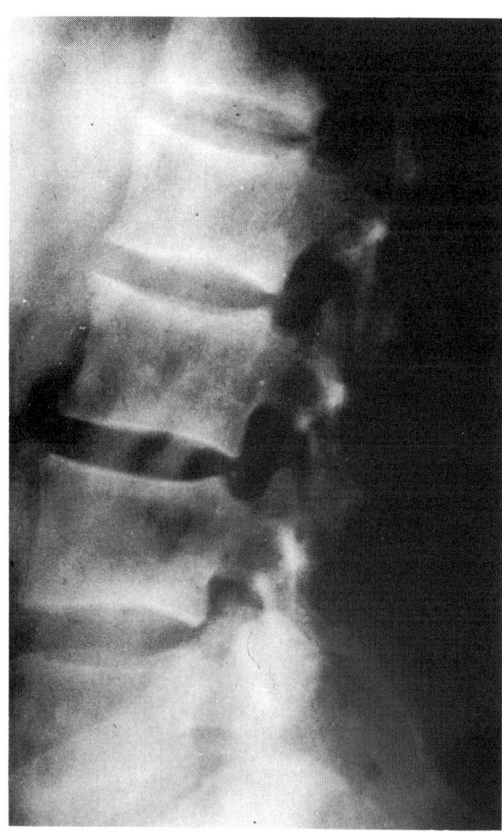

Figure 10.26 Hyperparathyroid bone disease. Lateral radiograph of lumbar spine showing 'rugger jersey' appearance.

10.5 PAGET'S DISEASE

10.5.1 INTRODUCTION

Osteitis deformans was the name given by Paget in the late 1870s to a disease of the skeleton which occurred in middle-aged and elderly people and resulted in enlargement of the skull, curvature of the spine and bowing of the legs. The name was coined in the belief that the changes in the bone were an inflammatory reaction. Now the condition is commonly called Paget's disease of bone and the abbreviated form, Paget's disease, will be used here.

This is not a generalized affection of the skeleton and the biochemical abnormalities which occur are the result of the disordered and excessive osteoclastic and osteoblastic activity which characterize the disease rather than the cause. The aetiology of the disease is unknown although there are suggestions as to possible causes, some of which will be discussed later.

10.5.2 INCIDENCE

Paget's disease occurs relatively commonly in some countries and extremely rarely in others (Rosenbaum and Hanson, 1969). Two explanations, not necessarily antagonistic, have been offered for this finding. Populations most at risk are those of Anglo-Saxon descent and a genetic factor may predispose to the disease (McKusick, 1972). However, there are differences in the incidence of disease in different countries with the same races of people (Detheridge *et al.*, 1982) and even in different areas of one country, and environmental factors, as yet unidentified, may also be important. Radiological surveys have disclosed a higher incidence in the north-west than in other areas of England and a lower incidence in British immigrants to Australia than occurs in England but being more common than in the indigenous people. Estimates of incidence of disease are difficult to make in Paget's disease because only a small proportion of those affected (less than 10%) present with symptoms. Post-mortem studies and radiographic surveys (Barker *et al.*, 1977) indicate that, where the disease is prevalent, it is present in more than 5% of people over 50 years of age and that more men than women are affected. Although it is a disorder affecting predominantly the over 40 age group young adults occasionally present with the disease. True Paget's disease has not been found in children.

10.5.3 DISTRIBUTION OF LESIONS

Every bone has at some time been observed as affected by Paget's disease. Those most frequently involved are the skull, vertebrae, ilium, ribs, femora and tibiae (Jaffe, 1977). At time of presentation there may be one bone only affected or several. Only one side of the pelvis or one limb may be affected. Within any one bone there may be partial or complete involvement.

10.5.4 SYMPTOMS AND SIGNS

Pain is a common cause of presentation. In some patients, especially those with disease in the pelvis or proximal femur, there will be osteoarthritic changes in the adjacent joint (Altman, 1980) and that may be the source of the pain. It is postulated that pain may be the result of microfractures in the abnormal bone or, alternatively, arise from periosteum covering areas of active bone deposition. Malignant change may be signalled by the onset, or increased intensity, of pain.

Pathological fracture occurs in an estimated 8% of patients with Paget's disease. As is characteristic of pathological fractures, the break in a long bone is usually transverse (Figure 10.27). The bone may break close to the advancing edge of an active lesion where the resorptive phase of the disease is dominant or through an area in which the bone is significantly more dense than normal. In the latter case two factors may contribute to mechanical failure, the disorganized arrangement of the trabeculae and the loss of continuity of the collagenous framework within the bone tissue, both of which impair the distribution of loads applied to the bone. Fractures heal at a normal rate but there is a significant incidence of non-union (Barry, 1980). There is a potential problem of hypercalcaemia attendant on the immobilization of someone with extensive active disease. The occurrence of a pathological fracture should alert the clinician to the possibility of malig-

nant change in the Pagetic bone. Partial fractures involving one side of the cortex also occur.

Deformity is a striking feature in some cases, with bowing of long bones, kyphosis and enlargement, with sclerosis, of the skull vault and facial bones (Figure 10.28) and may be the major complaint. The enlarged vault may appear to spread over the ears and back of neck like a 'tam-o-shanter'.

Neurological problems (Feldman *et al.*, 1979) particularly deafness can be the cause of considerable disability. Enlargement of bone around foramina may lead to nerve compression and together with vertebral collapse can cause paraplegia. Deformity of the

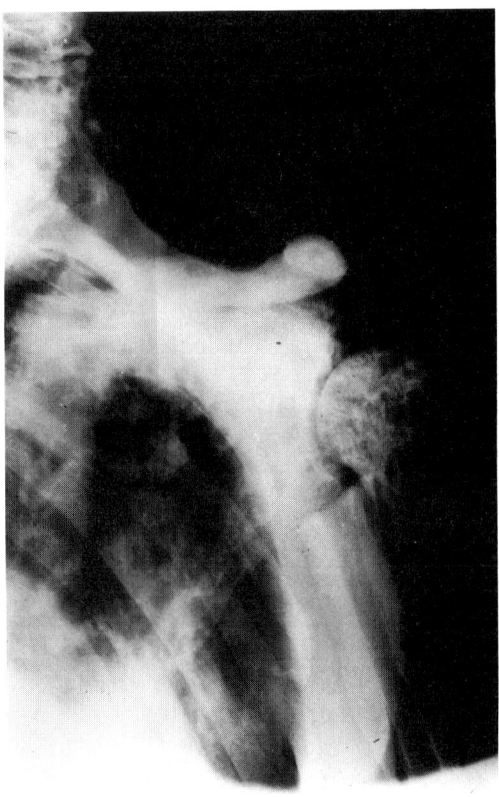

Figure 10.27 Paget's disease. Radiograph of affected proximal humerus with pathological fracture.

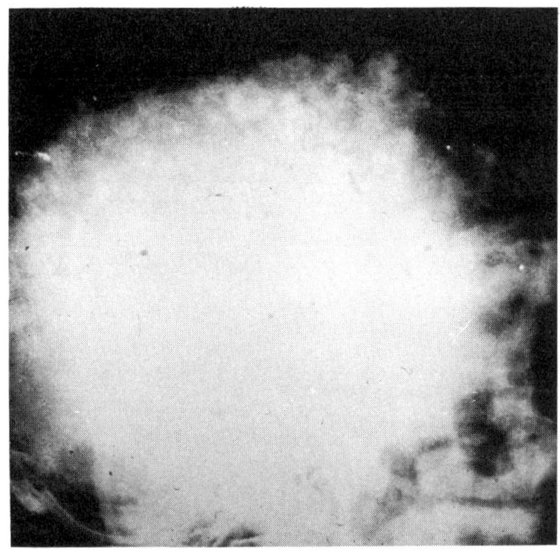

Figure 10.28 Paget's disease. Radiograph of extensively affected calvarium and facial bones.

skull may, in addition to cranial nerve palsies, produce basilar invagination.

Heart failure is said to result from the greatly increased blood flow through Pagetic bone. There is no evidence that there are arteriovenous shunts in abnormal bone and cardiac failure is common in the elderly making the relationship between bone disease and heart failure unclear.

Sarcoma develops in less than 1% of patients with Paget's disease and may present because of pain, swelling, pathological fracture or a combination of these. At time of presentation pulmonary and systemic metastases may be detected. Detailed description of sarcoma in Pagetic bone is given in Chapter 13.

In addition to the physical signs which can be anticipated from the presenting symptoms, it is usual to find that the skin over subcutaneous bones in which there is active disease is warm.

10.5.5 BIOCHEMISTRY

When Paget's disease is active the plasma alkaline phosphatase is elevated, usually to

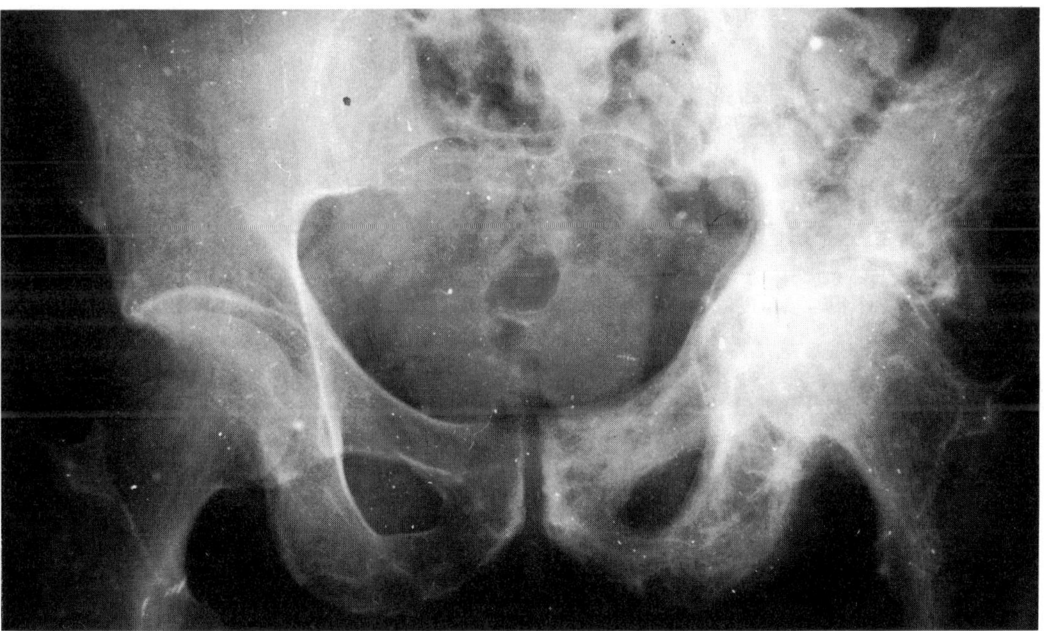

Figure 10.29 Paget's disease. Radiograph of pelvis with unilateral involvement. Note the irregular texture and widening of the pubic rami (right in figure) and reduced size of the obdurator foramen.

several times the normal level, and both plasma and urinary hydroxyproline are also raised (Woodhouse, 1972). Plasma acid phosphatase is not commonly significantly higher than normal and plasma calcium and phosphorus levels are normal in the ambulant patient. Immobilization of the patient may lead to clinically significant hypercalcaemia. Hyperuricaemia, with clinical gout occurs in a significant number of patients (Altman, 1980).

10.5.6   RADIOLOGY

The characteristic appearance of Pagetic bone is the irregular increase in overall size of the affected bone (Figures 10.29 and 10.30). Other features include the porosis at the advancing edge of a lesion and the mixed sclerotic and porotic appearance in areas of established disease (Milgram, 1977). The porosis of the early phase of a lesion in a long bone may be so marked as to simulate the changes associated with an expansile tumour. A characteristic appearance of the advancing edge of a lesion is a flame-shaped area of porosis. In the skull a large area of porosis may persist in the vault (osteoporosis circumscripta cranii) (Figure 10.31). The benign 'giant cell tumour-like' lesion described below will appear as a well-defined osteolytic lesion possibly producing an expansile mass covered by bone. Sarcomatous lesions are usually predominantly osteolytic with irregular medullary and cortical destruction and extension into the soft tissues (Figure 10.32). Multifocal sarcoma is sometimes evident at time of presentation with malignant change, not always with radiographically demonstrable pulmonary lesions.

10.5.7   GROSS AND MICROSCOPIC PATHOLOGY

An affected bone is irregularly increased in diameter or thickness and has a rough, pitted external surface. Long bones may be bowed and the skull vault flattened. The cortex is irregularly thickened and shows areas of

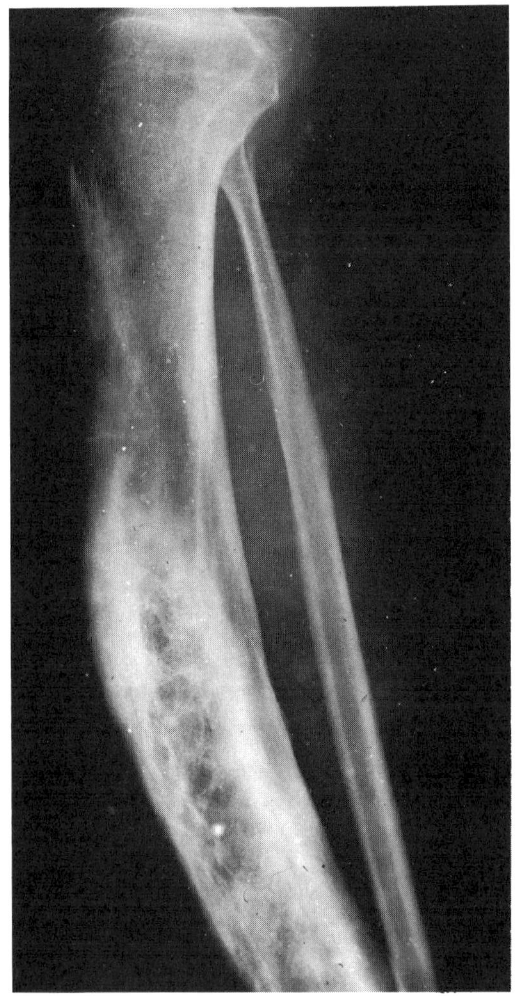

Figure 10.30 Paget's disease. Radiograph of tibia showing areas of sclerosis and lysis in the diaphysis, widening of the bone and bowing.

increased vascularity (Figure 10.33). Cancellous bone is made up of trabeculae of markedly differing diameters in disarray, an abnormality which is most easily recognized in the femoral neck (Figure 10.34). The sequence of changes which occur in Paget's disease can be summarized as excessive osteoclastic resorption followed by bone formation occurring over an unpredictable period of time. Microscopic examination may consequently show

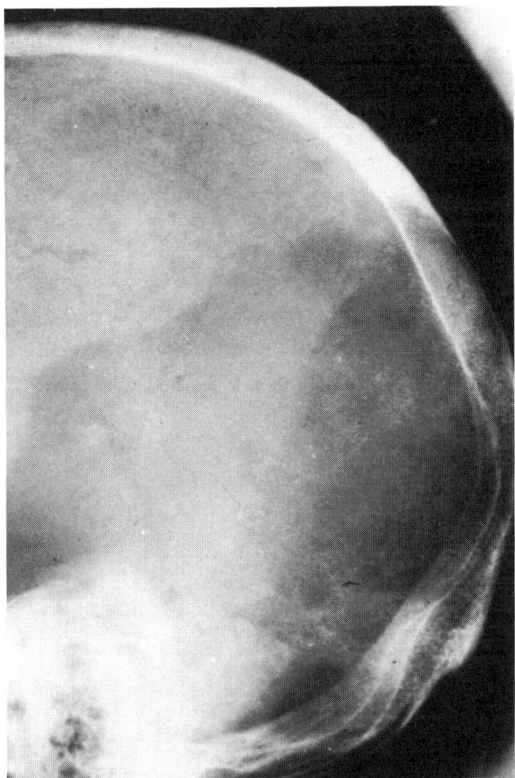

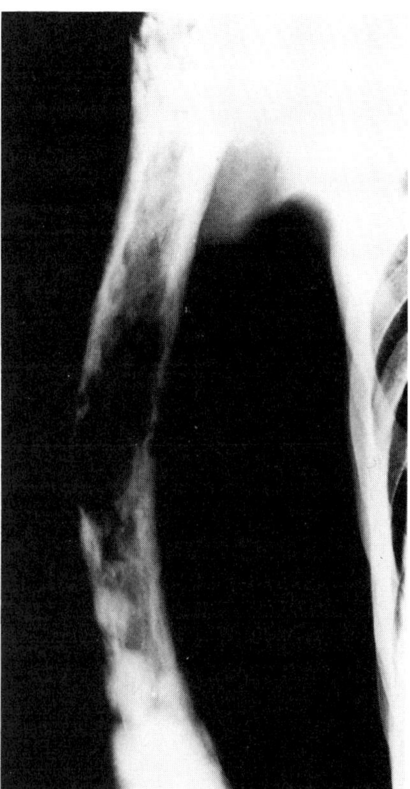

Figure 10.31 Paget's disease. Radiograph of skull. Osteoporosis circumscripta cranii (occipital area).

Figure 10.32 Paget's disease. Radiograph of humerus. The area of lucency in the mid-diaphysis and the rounded opacities in the lower half indicate the extent of sarcoma complicating Paget's disease.

one of a variety of possible combinations of populations of osteoblasts and osteoclasts, a wide range of bone mass and of the amount of osteoid and the possible presence of woven bone which may occasionally be the predominant type of bone (Figure 10.35). For diagnostic purposes histomorphometry is not required and sections of decalcified bone are adequate. Electron microscopic examination is not essential but will be discussed later in the context of aetiology.

Histological examination of bone in which the disease is active will usually show a great variation in the dimensions of Haversian canals, poor definition of the transition between cortex and medulla and great variation in both shape and width of trabeculae. Some of the wider trabeculae may include

small vascularized spaces resembling Haversian canals. Subperiosteal new bone formation will be occurring. The cement (reversal) lines will be abnormally disposed in both cortex and medulla, separating the lamellar bone into small fragments. This abnormal internal structure is described as 'mosaic' and is characteristic, if not absolutely specific, of Paget's disease (Figure 10.36). When examined in polarized light the orientation of the collagen matrix in each fragment will be seen to be different from that in adjacent fragments. There will be an increased number of osteoclasts in Howship's lacunae with the intervening bone surfaces covered by osteoblasts (Figure 10.37). Many of the osteoclasts will have numerous nuclei (50 or more). If an (optional) undecalcified section is examined osteoid will be found to be increased in total area (or volume) compared with normal. With rare exceptions the osteoid is not excessive in thickness. In the exceptional circumstance when the author has found small areas of osteoid which are abnormally thick there has not been any biochemical evidence to suggest that the patient might have osteomalacia, a subsequent biopsy has not shown the abnormality and it is assumed that this is a localized and probably temporary aberration of the mineralization process. When there is a high level of cellular activity, normal marrow will be completely displaced by fibrous tissue in which there are numerous distended thin-walled vascular channels. Trabeculae of woven bone may be found either isolated in the fibrous tissue or attached to lamellar bone, sometimes there is more woven than lamellar bone.

The evolution of the disease process is believed, because of the radiographic appearance of porosity in small lesions, to begin with a phase of pure osteoclastic resorption (Collins, 1966) but, even at an interface between abnormal and normal

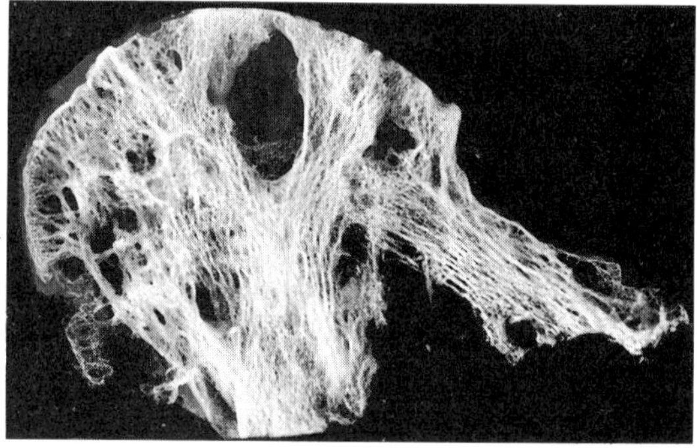

Figure 10.34 Paget's disease. Specimen radiograph of resected Pagetic femoral head.

bone, some osteoblasts will always be found.

A rare variation of the cellular processes leads to the formation of a circumscribed and sometimes expansile lesion composed of a large number of osteoclasts amongst which are dispersed fibroblastic and histiocyte-like mononuclear cells, the whole appearance resembling that of a giant cell tumour. These lesions are benign, as careful examination of the cellular morphology and the absence of infiltration will show. If the cellular activity ceases in Pagetic bone, the marrow reverts to fatty and haematopoietic tissue. The irregularity of size and shape of cortex and medulla persists as does the 'mosaic' structure.

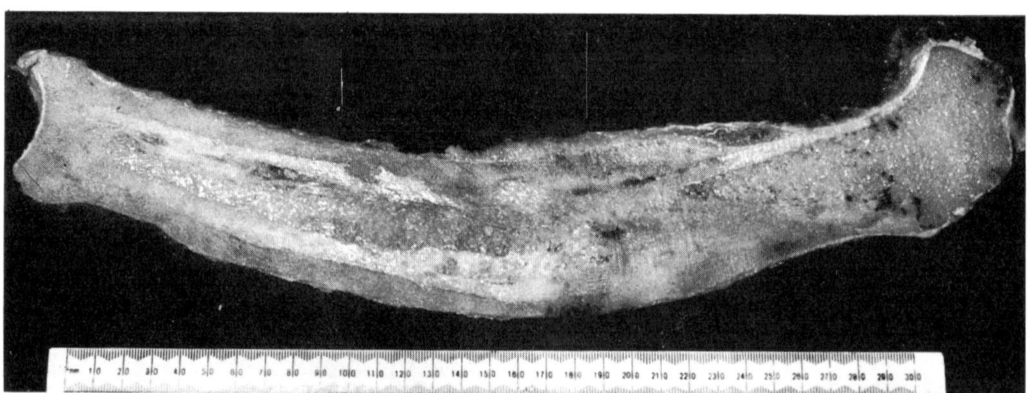

Figure 10.33 Paget's disease. Bisected tibia. Note irregular thickening of cortices in lower half and mass of bone occupying marrow in upper half. The latter is entirely benign, reactive bone.

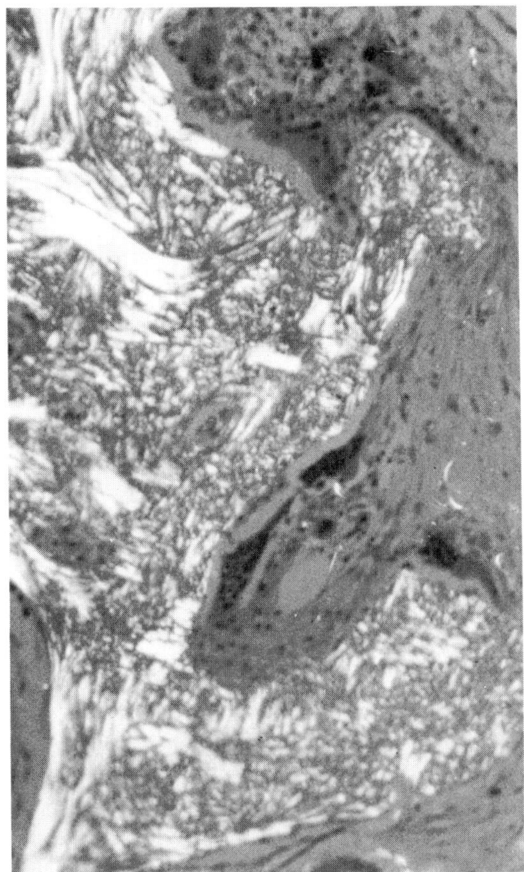

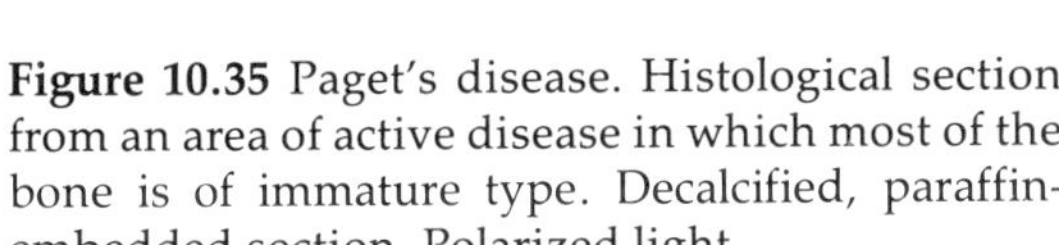

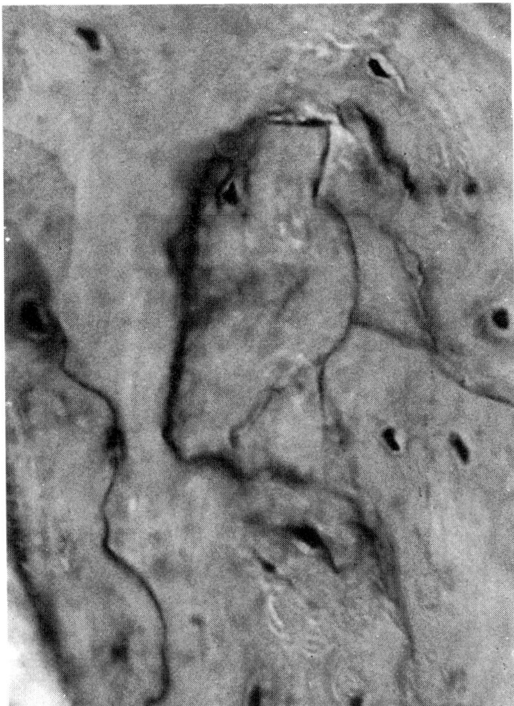

Figure 10.36 Paget's disease. Irregular cement lines producing a mosaic appearance. Decalcified, paraffin-embedded section.

Figure 10.35 Paget's disease. Histological section from an area of active disease in which most of the bone is of immature type. Decalcified, paraffin-embedded section. Polarized light.

10.5.8   ELECTRON MICROSCOPY

Electron microscopic studies of the bone cells in Pagetic bone have shown intra-nuclear and, less commonly, intracytoplasmic inclusions composed of randomly arranged microcylinders producing an appearance unlike any known cell organelle (Harvey *et al.*, 1982). Similar structures have been described in the multinucleate cells of a giant cell tumour which was not part of the Pagetic process, but otherwise appear to be a feature peculiar to Paget's disease. The nature of the inclusions has been the cause of much speculation, focused on the possibility that they are derived from a virus, and that Paget's disease is a 'slow virus' disease. This would be the environmental factor which could explain the geographical distribution of the disease in genetically susceptible people. The first suggestion, that the virus was the measles virus, has not been confirmed nor the alternative postulate of a respiratory syncytial virus. The evidence for a viral aetiology and other possible causes of Paget's disease is discussed by Singer and Mills (1983). More recent work suggests that a paramyxovirus, canine distemper virus, is the candidate virus (see Chapter 7) (Cartwright *et al.*, 1993).

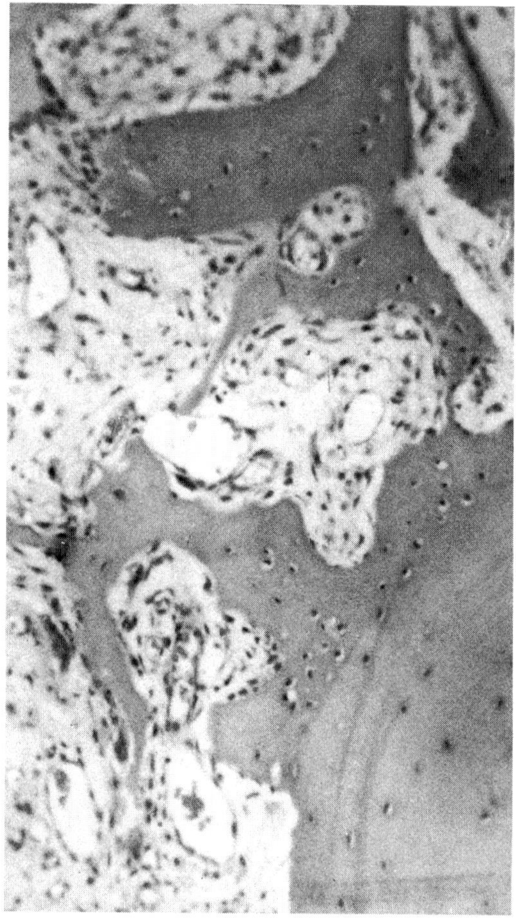

Figure 10.37 Paget's disease. Increased numbers of osteoblasts and osteoclasts, total replacement of normal marrow by fibrous tissue in which there are dilated, thin-walled, vascular channels. Decalcified, paraffin-embedded section.

10.5.9 DIFFERENTIAL DIAGNOSIS

Before considering those diseases which may have features in common with Paget's disease, it should be remembered that, where a disease is common it may coexist with some other condition, including those mentioned below. Metastatic carcinoma, especially of prostatic origin, and fibrogenesis imperfecta ossium produce changes in the radiographic appearances of bone which resemble those of Paget's disease except that neither cause irregular widening of bone and the presence of this feature will resolve the radiological differential diagnosis.

An elevated plasma alkaline phosphatase in a middle-aged or elderly patient may lead a clinician to suppose that the patient is osteomalacic. The rare finding of delayed mineralization in Paget's disease is described above and does not have the degree of osteoid accumulation usually seen in osteomalacia.

Increased osteoblastic and osteoclastic activity, with resultant changes in the histological appearances which may be confused with Paget's disease, occurs in a variety of bone disorders. The effect of excessive parathyroid hormone secretion is described in section 10.4, suffice to say here that, in hyperparathyroidism, the degree of fibrosis of the marrow and of abnormality of cement line arrangement are both less severe than in Paget's disease and that the biochemical abnormalities are different.

Lesions of fibrous dysplasia when presenting in adult life can closely mimic Pagetic bone including the presence of irregular blocks of lamellar bone in which cement lines produce a mosaic appearance. This problem can be a most difficult one when Paget's disease presents in a young adult. Only if the biochemical changes of active Paget's disease are present can this differential diagnosis be resolved as both conditions can be monostotic and confined to the diaphysis.

Non-specific reactions in bone such as may occur in the juxta-articular zone when the articular cartilage has been eroded or in the periphery of erosive tumours can also be confused, histologically, with Paget's disease. Radiographic and, less frequently required, biochemical information will clarify the situation.

10.5.10 LEONTIASIS OSSEA

Virchow thought that hyperostoses of cranio-facial bones were the analogue in the skeleton of leontiasis in the soft tissues, the latter being a particular manifestation of elephantiasis of connective tissue which, in turn, he considered to be a basic pathological process in subcutaneous tissue responsible for a number of clinical conditions. On this basis he introduced the term leontiasis ossea (Virchow, 1869). Knaggs (1924) wrote comprehensively on the subject, recording cases from several centres. He commented that the label was only descriptive and no longer diagnostic. It was dropped from Index Medicus in 1984, and reference is to hyperostosis frontalis interna, a not very satisfactory substitute, where is to be found a mixed bag.

The known diseases that form external hyperostoses, to coin a phrase, are Paget's disease of bone (Byers and Jones, 1969), renal disease (Dantas *et al.*, 1991), yaws (Botreau-Roussel, 1925), and fibrous dysplasia (many references). In addition there have been several historic cases of unknown aetiopathogenesis which are well documented in Knaggs (1924). It is to be noted that fibrous dysplasia usually affects only one side of the face and that in as far as leontiasis ossea has had any descriptive function it has been for symmetrical affections.

Thus, there is no single entity to describe. The pathological processes of the known disease entities sometimes cause enlargement of the maxilla in particular, and sometimes it is the only bone affected in a case. The result can vary from a thickened ridge of bone arising on either side of the nose and bridging it, or separate maxillary swellings with the nose between. Of passing interest is a case of cherubism reported by Khalifa and Ibrahim (1988) in which the maxilla was affected, giving rise to the bridging deformity. Many of the yaws-associated cases have the separate maxillary prominences, which gave rise to a description of the horned men of Africa (Lamprey, 1887; Byers and Jones, 1969). The fact that East Africa is the only region of the worldwide distribution of yaws in which these bony enlargements are found raises doubts about the role of yaws in their aetiology. The involvement of the skull and other facial bones in cases of both recognized disease processes and of unknown pathogenesis can result in grotesque deformities (Byers and Jones, 1969; Knaggs, 1924). Rarely, the mandible is involved; Knaggs (1924) illustrates cases where this has been the case.

The diagnosis in a case of hyperostosis of craniofacial bones is established by the usual forms of patient investigation, which may include histological study of tissue samples, which must be judged by the established criteria for the disease processes under consideration.

10.5.11 HYPEROSTOSIS FRONTALIS INTERNA

As the name of the condition indicates this is a thickening of the frontal bone confined to the inner table. The term has been applied, incorrectly, when there is a general thickening of skull and facial bones (leontiasis ossea and heritable cranial dysplasias).

Hyperostosis frontalis interna is part of the Morgani–Stewart–Morel syndrome, the other features of which are virulism, obesity and neuropsychiatric symptoms; a disorder presenting almost exclusively in older women. The full clinical syndrome is uncommon but hyperostosis frontalis interna is not rare if looked for at autopsy and may be found in men also. The cause is unknown but hyperprolactinaemia has been frequently demonstrated in affected patients and hyperostosis frontalis interna may occur as part of acromegaly in both males and females (Fulton *et al.*, 1990).

When an affected frontal bone is sawed in

the horizontal plane the thickening of the inner table is seen to be irregular, the endocranial surface being bosselated. The bone is of mature type and there are no distinctive histological features by which the condition can be identified.

Imaging techniques (Jacobson and Haverling, 1988) show that the bone deposition may begin in early adult life and that the rate of deposition slows with advancing years.

10.6 FIBROGENESIS IMPERFECTA OSSIUM

10.6.1   INTRODUCTION

Fibrogenesis imperfecta ossium (FIO) is a very rare disorder (Swan *et al.*, 1976). Of the few cases reported in the literature most of the patients have been more than 50 years old. Males and females appear to be equally susceptible. The cause of the condition is unknown. There is a general involvement of the skeleton but the degree of abnormality varies even within the same bone.

The skeletal abnormality is the result of the irregular replacement of normal bone collagen matrix by a matrix which is both non-birefringent and incompletely mineralized. In consequence the bone fractures more easily.

10.6.2   CLINICAL PRESENTATION

Patients present with bone pain or because of fracture and may become totally immobile because of the extreme fragility of their bones.

10.6.3   RADIOLOGY

The characteristic feature is the coarse appearance of trabecular bone, usually with reduced bone mass (Figure 10.38). There is no widening of bones and that distinguishes the radiographic appearances from those of Paget's disease. Collapsed vertebral bodies and fractures of ribs and long bones are invariably seen at some time in the evolution of the disease.

10.6.4   BIOCHEMISTRY

An unexpected finding is the presence of an abnormal globulin such as is found in patients with myeloma and since that observation was made all patients tested have shown that abnormality. The cells producing the globulin have not been identified; plasma cells are not conspicuous in the bone marrow. There are no other consistent biochemical abnormalities.

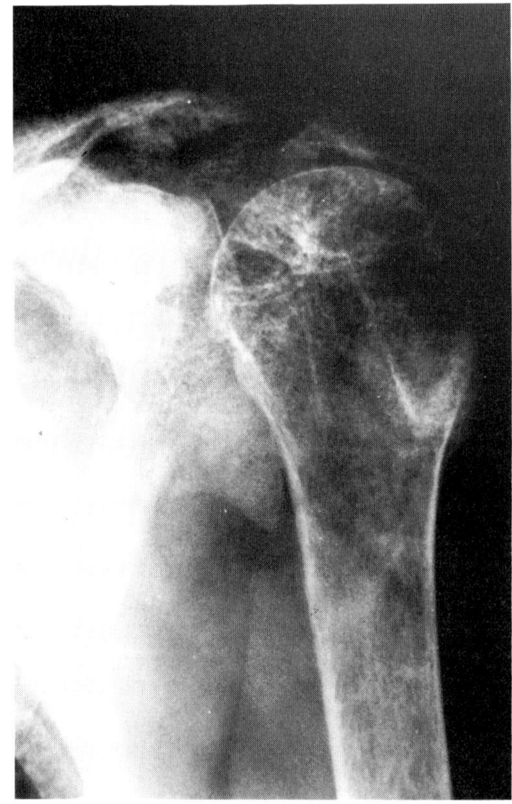

Figure 10.38 Fibrogenesis imperfecta ossium. Radiograph of shoulder. The bones are irregular in texture and the humeral cortices are thin. There is no increase in the overall diameter of the humerus. Note the avulsion of the acromion.

10.6.5 HISTOLOGY

The condition can be positively identified by the presence of thick layers of non-birefringent matrix on the surface of trabeculae or Haversian canals (Figure 10.39). This type of matrix may be on the whole or only part of the bone surfaces, presumably reflecting the duration of the disease. In addition there may be a marked variation in the thickness of trabeculae. The numbers of both osteoblasts and osteoclasts may be normal or slightly increased: the increase is not so great as in hyperparathyroidism or Paget's disease. If undecalcified sections are examined the relative volume of unmineralized matrix and the proportion of bone surface covered by it are both greater than normal, an appearance which mimics osteomalacia. The mineralization process will also be abnormal in that the non-birefringent matrix will have areas of spotty calcification within it (Figure 10.40). Electron microscopy also shows the abnormal pattern of mineralization associated with the abnormal fibrillary matrix. Ossification may occur in periosteal fibrous insertions.

10.6.6 DIFFERENTIAL DIAGNOSIS

The possibility of confusion with osteomalacia is mentioned above and is most likely to arise in the early phase of the disease before the overall structure of the bone has become disorganized.

The combination of abnormal and irregularly mineralized bone matrix together with exosteophytes at ligamentous insertions might be misinterpreted as the result of excessive fluoride ingestion.

Examination of the section in polarized light will reveal the true nature of the condition; the osteoid in osteomalacia will have a lamellar structure and in fluorosis a woven arrangement.

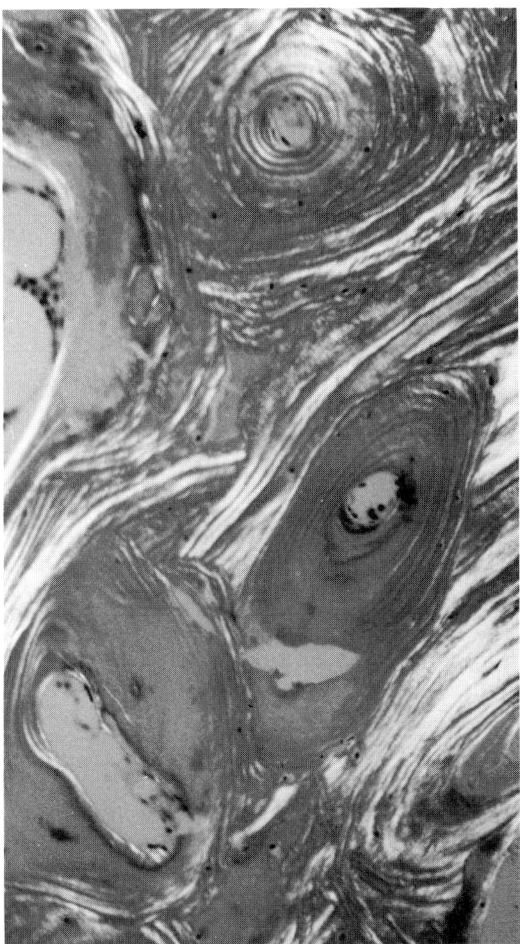

Figure 10.39 Fibrogenesis imperfecta ossium. Histological section viewed in polarized light. Some of the bone is of lamellar type and there are areas of non-birefringent matrix. Decalcified, paraffin-embedded section. Polarized light.

10.7 APPLICATION OF TECHNIQUES TO THE STUDY OF METABOLIC BONE DISEASE

Osteoporosis, Paget's disease, hyperparathyroid bone disease and fibrogenesis imperfecta ossium can all be diagnosed using decalcified sections stained with haematoxylin and eosin (H & E). Infiltrations of the marrow are most easily identified in H & E stained decalcified sections. Decalcified sec-

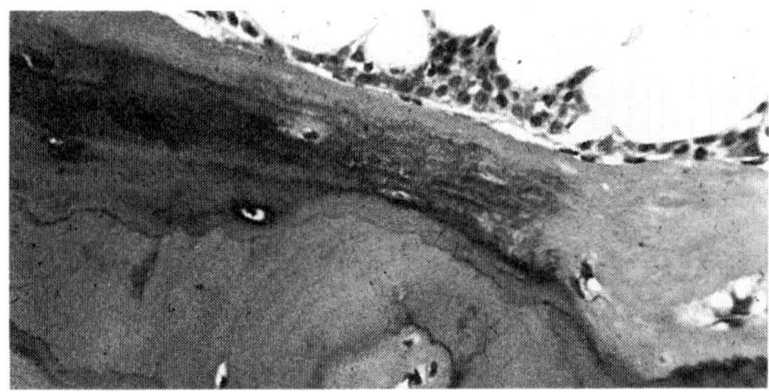

Figure 10.40 Fibrogenesis imperfecta ossium. In the upper part of the matrix there is a band of granular basophilic staining corresponding with an area of incomplete calcification in non-birefringent tissue. Decalcified, paraffin-embedded section.

tions give more reliable results with immunocytochemical methods because the schedules used for soft tissue sections can be followed without modification.

Undecalcified sections are required for quantitation of osteoid, for assessment of calcification front and for aluminium detection using the solochrome stain.

Identification of bone cells and cement lines is not affected by the method of tissue processing nor by most staining methods except for the von Kossa technique which masks both cement lines and the birefringence of mineralized collagen.

10.8 HISTOMORPHOMETRY

10.8.1 INTRODUCTION

The interest in bone and its diseases escalated after the Second World War providing an impetus for the quantitation of the skeleton, particularly with respect to osteoporosis (Rodahl *et al.*, 1960). The concept of bone turnover had been enunciated by Hunter in 1837, and the role of osteoblasts was established between 1845 and 1867 by Goodsir, Koelliker, Virchow and Gegenbauer and of osteoclasts by Koelliker in 1873 (Sissons, 1960). It was recognized that an imbalance in

the activity of those cells altered skeletal mass, and brought about its decline with age. The discovery and clinical application of X-rays revealed the changes in the skeleton with age, but there were limitations to determination of bone density by X-ray imaging (Lachmann, 1955; Barnett and Nordin, 1960). However, microradiographs (undecalcified sections radiographed with soft X-rays on fine grain film (Engstrom, 1951) could be quantitated for their mineral content (Engstrom and Amprino, 1950), for some of the same features as histological sections (Jowsey *et al.*, 1965), and autoradiographed for radioisotopes (Leblond *et al.*, 1950). Moreover, the incorporation and turnover of radioisotopes in the skeleton offered an indirect quantitative assessment of the skeleton (Bauer and Ray, 1958), which was actively developed and pursued during the 1950s and 1960s in parallel with direct methods. Volumetric measurements, weighing and ashing of whole, or parts of, bones were employed (Arnold, 1960, 1973). However, there were limitations to these, and the use of histological sections was more practicable. Technical progress depended on developing methods for preparing undecalcified sections (Arnold, 1951), needed to avoid shrinkage artefact and enable recognition of osteoid, and on a simple means of quantitation, point and line sampling (Chalkley, 1943; Chalkley *et al.*, 1949; Hennig, 1958; Weibel, 1963; Merz, 1968).

The quantitative analysis of histological sections of bone has become part of the routine examination of biopsies from patients with known or suspected metabolic bone disease. Most analyses provide information about the situation at the point in time of the biopsy, 'static' data, and are of most value when performed on sequential biopsies or on large populations. Other analyses will provide, either directly or indirectly, evidence of previous cell (usually the osteoblast) activity, 'dynamic' data. During the 1960s and 1970s several methods of

Table 10.4 Abbreviated symbols of terms used in bone histomorphometry

A	apposition(al)	Cp	cytoplasm(ic)	Ex	external		
G	grow(th)(ing)	Lc	lacuna(r)	N	number (profiles/structures)		
On	osteon(al)	Sa	sample	Vd	void		
Ab	absolute	Cr	cortex	F	formation		
H	Haversian	Le	length	Nc	nucle(us)(ar)		
Ot	osteocyt(e)(ic)	Se	section	Vk	Volkmann's		
Ac	activation	Cy	cycle	Fa	fatty		
Hm	haemopoietic	Li	lining	Nd	node		
P	period	Sg	sigma	Vt	vertical		
Aj	adjusted	D	dimension(al)	Fb	fibro(sis)(us)		
Hp	hypertrophic	Lm	lamellar	n	number sampling units		
Pf	profile	Sm	seam	W	wall		
Al	aluminum	De	depth	Fe	iron		
Ht	height	Ln	line	O	osteoid		
Pl	plate	Sn	spongiosa	Wi	width (2D)		
Ar	area (2D)	Dg	degenerat(ive)(ion)	Fr	front		
Hz	horizontal	Lo	longitudinal	Ob	osteoblast(ic)		
Pm	perimeter (2D)	Sp	separation	Wo	woven		
a	activ(e)(ity)	Dm	diameter	f	frequency		
h	hit	1	lag	Oc	osteoclast		
Po	por(e)(ous)(osity)	St	structur(e)(al)	Z	zone		
B	bone	Dn	density				
I	interface (3D)	M	mineral(iz)(ing)(ation)				
Ps	periost(eal)(eum)	s	single				
BMU	basic multicellular unit	Do	domain				
Ia	intra	Ma	marrow				
Pt	point	T	tissue				
Bd	boundary (2D)	Dp	diaphys(is)(eal)				
Ic	intercept	Md	mineralized				
Q	quiescent	Tb	trabecula(r)				
C	core	Dt	delta				
Il	initial	Me	medullary				
R	rate	Th	thickness				
Ca	canalicul(a)(r)	d	double				
In	internal	M l	modelling				
Rd	radi(al)(us)	Tm	termin(al)(us)				
Cd	corrected	E	ero(ded)(sion)				
Ir	inter	Mo	mononucle(ar)(ated)				
Rf	referen(t)(ce)	Tr	transitional				
Ce	cell	Ec	endocortical				
Is	instantaneous	Mp	metaphys(is)(eal)				
Rm	remodelling	Tt	total				
Cg	cartilage	En	envelope				
It	interstitial	Mu	multinucle(ar)(ated)				
Rs	resorption	t	time				
Cm	cement	Ep	epiphysis				
I	intersection	Mx	matrix				
Re	reversal	U	unit				
Cn	cancellous	Es	endost(eal)(eum)				
L	label(led)	m	maturation				
S	surface (3D)	V	volume (3D)				

Table 10.5 Primary measurements in bone histomorphometry

	Measurement	Abbreviation	
Type	name	3D	2D
Area	Bone volume	B.V	B.Ar
	Osteoid volume	O.V	O.Ar
	Mineralized volume	Md.V	Md.Ar
	Void volume	Vd.V	Vd.Ar
	Marrow volume	Ma.V	Ma.Ar
	Fibrosis volume	Fb.V	Fb.Ar
	Canal volume	Ca.V	Ca.Ar
	Cell volume	Ce.V	Ce.Ar
	Cytoplasmic volume	Cy.V	Cy.Ar
	Nuclear volume	Nc.V	Nc.Ar
Length	Bone interface	BI	B.Bd
	Bone surface	BS	B.Pm
	Osteoid surface	OS	O.Pm
	Eroded surface	ES	E.Pm
	Quiescent surface	QS	Q.Pm
	Mineralized surface	Md.S	Md.Pm
	Osteoblast surface	Ob.S	Ob.Pm
	Single-labelled surface	sL.S	sL.Pm
	Double-labelled surface	dL.S	dL.Pm
	Osteoclast surface	Oc.S	Oc.Pm
	Reversal surface	Rv.S	Rv.Pm
Distance	Cortical thickness	Ct.Th	Ct.Wi
	Wall thickness	W.Th	W.Wi
	Mineralized thickness	Md.Th	Md.Wi
	Osteoid thickness	O.Th	O.Wi
	Label thickness	L.Th	L.Wi
	Trabecular thickness	Tb.Th	Tb.Wi
	Trabecular diameter	Tb.Dm	–
	Canal radius	Ca.Rd	–
	Cell height	Ce.Ht	–
	Nuclear height	Nc.Ht	–
Number	Osteoblast number	–	N.Ob
	Osteoclast number	–	N.Oc
	Osteocyte number	–	N.Ot
	Nuclear number	–	N.Nc
	Canal number	–	N.Ca
	Seam number	–	N.Sm
	Erosion number	–	N.E
	Profile number	–	N.Pf
	Node number	–	N.Nd
	Terminus number	–	N.Tm

analysis were proposed and, more confusingly, different ways of expressing the results were adopted. Because no consensus was reached as to which methods of analysis and mathematical manipulation of results should be generally applied there is now a large body of literature much of which is intelligible only to those who are conversant with the methods of the authors. The American Society of Bone and Mineral Research undertook to establish a unified system of terminology through the agency of an international committee of experts who consulted widely as part of their deliberations. Their recommendations have been widely published (Parfitt *et al.*, 1987; Parfitt, 1988) and are a source of valuable information and of a wide range of references to the literature. A nomenclature was agreed for the terms used in histomorphometry, with abbreviations and symbols (Table 10.4) and a list of the primary measurements (Table 10.5) and the derived indices (Table 10.6).

Histomorphometry is time consuming especially if it is undertaken with graticules inserted into a routine microscope and manual counting. Semi- and fully automated systems are available to speed the process but are expensive and bulky. In this generally confusing and highly unsatisfactory situation the only course is to look critically at all the options and adopt those which are appropriate to one's needs and

suggestions about this are made at the end of this section. What follows is a brief outline of the principles and the results of analyses of normal bone. Original papers relating to the principles, rationale and results of morphometry are contained in the published proceedings of three bone histomorphometry workshops (Jaworski, 1976; Meunier, 1976; Jee and Parfitt, 1980). A review of methods and results is presented by Revell (1986) and an analysis of the function of osteoblasts and derived cells in 'optimal' and 'non-optimal' conditions, based mainly on histomorphometric analyses, given by Parfitt (1990).

10.8.2 BONE BIOPSY

Most histomorphometry is concerned with remodelling bone and it is usual to focus analysis on cancellous tissue. For practical reasons of accessibility and patient safety the ilium has become the preferred site of biopsy in patients with generalized bone disease. Comparative studies indicate that the results

Table 10.6 Derived indices in bone histomorphometry

Indices	Name	Abbreviation	Formula
Structural	Trabecular number	Tb.N	(BV/TV)/Tb.Th
	Trabecular separation	Tb.Sp	(1/Tb.N)-Tb.Th
Kinetic	Mineralizing surface	MS	(dLSLS/2)/BS
	Mineral apposition rate	MAR	Ir.L.Th/Ir.L.t
	Adjusted apposition rate	Aj.AR	MAR*(MS/OS)
	Osteoid apposition rate	OAR	same
	Mineral formation rate	MFR	MAR*(MS/BS)
	Bone formation rate	BFR	same
	Bone resorption rate	BRs.R	
	Mineralization lag time	Mlt	O.Th/Aj.AR
	Osteoid maturation time	Omt	O.Th/MAR
	Formation period	FP	W.Th/Aj.AR
	Resorption period	Rs.P	FP*(Oc.S/OS)
	Reversal period	Rv.P	FP*(ES-Oc.S)/OS
	Remodelling period	Rm.P	FP/(ES+OS9/OS
	BMU lifespan (sigma)	Sg	
	Quiescent period	QP	FP*(qS/OS)
	Total period	Tt.P	FP*(BS/OS)
	Activation frequency	Ac.f	(1/Tt.P)

obtained from iliac bone, rib, vertebral body and proximal tibial metaphysis are very similar. It is usual for biopsies to be obtained with a trephine through a small skin incision and using local anaesthesia. Some operators take a core of bone through the ilium 2 cm below the crest and 2 cm behind the anterior superior spine whereas others prefer to go into the bone vertically from the iliac crest 3 cm from the anterior spine. Whichever route is selected should be used consistently because differences in values have been obtained from different sites in the same ilium. A core 1 cm long and 5 mm diameter is required to provide sections large enough for adequate analysis.

10.8.3 SECTION PREPARATION

Various methods of preparing and staining histological sections are described in Chapter 21 and at this point the application of some of those methods for histomorphometric purposes must be considered. Most histomorphometric analyses are expressed as ratios of lengths, areas or volumes. At different stages in the processing of the tissue from the unfixed state to the stained and mounted section there are occasions when the volume or area of the specimen are changed. Decalcified tissue is susceptible to shrinkage during dehydration and all types of embedded section may be compressed by microtomy or distorted whilst being flattened on the slide. It is therefore important that only one method of section preparation be used (especially if sequential examinations are made) and that some means of assessment of artefactual distortion be devised. This author is not aware of any article in which the effect of tissue distortion on the accuracy of analyses is discussed whereas there is a surfeit of information on other sources of error. The only practicable method known to this author is to prepare a contact radiograph of the fixed tissue block and, in the case of a cylindrical biopsy,

measure the long axes of the radiograph and of the stained, mounted, section. The method is relatively crude but it enables the rejection of sections which are outside the usual range of distortion. Internal disruption of the tissue with separation of osteoblasts and osteoclasts from bone surfaces occurs almost only with paraffin-embedded sections and was relieved by the introduction of plastic embedding.

Decalcified sections are satisfactory for the analysis of quantity of total matrix, widths of trabeculae, diameters of Haversian canals, cell populations, 'mean wall thickness' and degrees of marrow fibrosis. The Tripp and McKay technique (section 21.4.3) is satisfactory for the assessment of surface osteoid.

Undecalcified sections are mandatory for precise visualization and the accurate measurement of osteoid and rates of bone apposition using *in vivo* tetracycline labels. Plastic embedding materials are best for this purpose; sections prepared from blocks embedded in a nitrocellulose/paraffin sequence are suitable only for identification of osteoid and measurement of ranges of its thickness.

Haematoxylin and eosin-stained sections are adequate for measurements of total trabecular matrix and for the identification of osteocytes, osteoblasts and multinucleate osteoclasts. The von Kossa technique is best for the discrimination between osteoid and mineralized bone and can be used with any of several counterstains of which toluidine blue is the most popular for general purposes. Trichrome stains are used as alternatives to the von Kossa technique and Goldner's recipe is said to give the best approximation to the results obtained with silver nitrate. Solochrome cyanin and cobalt nitrate staining methods were used for detection of the 'calcification front'. The former does not discriminate osteoid from calcified bone as reliably as the von Kossa technique and the latter relies on the same principle as silver nitrate, which demonstrates 'calcification front' as effectively as either. The proponents of tetracycline labelling claim it to be superior to any *in vitro* method for the detection of bone mineralization. Mononuclear osteoclasts and osteoblasts can be directly identified by their staining with acid and alkaline phosphatase respectively although most histologists would make the distinction on the basis of the nature of the adjacent matrix, a cell in contact with osteoid being designated as osteoblastic.

10.8.4 MEASUREMENT; EQUIPMENT AND TECHNIQUES FOR MANUAL METHODS

The ability to quantify any feature in an histological section is dependent upon the observer being able to see the object. Provided that the magnification of the eyepiece is in the range 8× to 20× the critical factor for the discrimination of objects in a microscope image is the resolving power of the objective lens which is a function of the numerical aperture (resolution = wavelength of light × 0.6/numerical aperture). The magnification number inscribed on the barrel of the objective only loosely approximates to the resolving power and the calculated total magnification of the microscope image gives no information about what can be seen in the section. This is not very important when quantifying bone mass or counting cells, any 20× or 40× objective will clearly reveal all that is necessary. The purpose in making the above comments is to alert the reader to the fact that some osteoid seams are so thin as to be detectable only with the electron microscope and the use of different light microscope objectives will produce significant differences in the measured area of osteoid. Although published results may include a statement of the total magnification it is rare to be told what the limit of resolution of the osteoid was. To obviate this problem some observers have chosen to ignore all seams which are less than 1 µm thick.

Reproducibility of results requires that a minimum number of the particular feature be counted. What that number is can be calculated provided that the frequency of the feature in the specimen is known. As this can be ascertained only by a preliminary analysis of several specimens it is just as easy to construct a graph of the relationship between the average number of the feature per microscopic field and the number of fields examined and to determine the number of fields to be examined from that part of the graph where the plot becomes horizontal.

The microscope should have polarization attachments, an alternative source of UV light (epi-illumination for choice) and, ideally, a centrable rotating mechanical stage. Graticules should be mounted in Kellner eyepieces, not laid on the field stop of a standard eyepiece.

Point counting involves the use of an eyepiece graticule upon which a number of dots or small crosses (usually 25) are marked within a defined area. The image of the graticule is superimposed on the image of the section and the number of dots overlying the feature of interest is compared with the total number of dots. This gives an area as a proportion of the total area. If the size of the defined area of the graticule is calibrated using a stage micrometer the area can be expressed in absolute terms. This method is used for determining areas of osteoid and mineralized matrix either as a relationship to each other or to the area of section scrutinized.

Linear intercept counting makes use of a graticule on which are inscribed parallel equidistant lines (usually 10). Where any line crosses a bone surface the type of cell on the surface is recorded and the type of surface (i.e. osteoid, mineralized and 'inactive' or mineralized and part of a resorption surface). Graticules are available which combine points and parallel lines, one in common use is that developed by Schenk *et al.* (1969).

Measurements of widths of trabeculae and

of osteoid seams, the spacing of double tetra-cycline labels and the distance between the surface of a trabecula and the cement line nearest to it ('mean wall thickness') are made with an eyepiece micrometer which is calibrated from a stage micrometer.

The shape and orientation of trabeculae and the thickness and distribution of osteoid on the bone surfaces, as seen in histological sections, are random. Particularly with regard to the osteoid, which is normally less than 5% of the total matrix, the relatively large variation in apparent thickness which is possible depending on whether a seam is cut through the diameter or a chord can cause errors of interpretation with some methods of measurement. For this reason the author prefers to determine whether osteoid seams are normal by the appearance in polarized light. In polarized light a section stained by the von Kossa technique with any simple counterstain will show the lamellar structure of mature osteoid ranging from a single band of birefringence to a multilayered seam composed of alternating bright and dark bands. The number of bright bands in each seam is counted. Five or more bright bands in any seam indicates mineralization failure and this is independent of total amount of osteoid however that is calculated (Woods *et al.*, 1967).

Examining osteoid seams in this way will, incidentally, show how the apparent thickness of an osteoid seam can vary at different points along a bone surface whilst still consisting of a fixed number of lamellae. If the 'true' thickness of an individual birefringent lamella or of an osteoid seam is required the thinnest lamella or seam can be taken as being that which has been cut through a diametric line. This technique is not applicable to trichrome or solochrome cyanin-stained sections because the birefringence of calcified matrix is not quenched by these methods. Artefactual variations in the distance between double tetracycline labels and the measurement of mean wall thickness also occur because of the unsymmetrical shape of trabeculae. A mathematical correction to take this into account was suggested by Frost (cited in Meunier, 1976).

What is directly measured is numbers, lengths or areas either absolute or proportionate. The preference of the author is to express them in that form but many investigators manipulate the primary data so that, for example, lengths become surface areas and areas become volumes.

10.8.5   NORMAL VALUES

The values quoted below are intended as a guide only and unless otherwise indicated are those used by the author. Measurements of osteoid were made with an objective discriminating 0.5 µm. From the comments previously made it is evident that the only normal values of real use to the reader will be those obtained by local investigation.

Trabecular bone area (as a percentage of section area).

Age (years)	Males	Females
18–40	18–25	18–25
41–50	16–22	16–22
51–60	16–22	15–22
61–70	12–22	11–20
71–80	12–21	11–17

Osteoid area (as a percentage of the combined areas of bone and osteoid).

Maximum 5% in all age groups. A zero score has no diagnostic significance and is not unusual in subjects over 60 years of age.

Osteoid surface (as a percentage of length).

Maximum 20% in all age groups. Zero scores occur (see Osteoid area above)

Osteoblast population (the proportion of length of osteoid surface covered by columnar or cuboidal osteoblasts).

Maximum 25% in all age groups. When the osteoid is not more than one lamella thick 'active' osteoblasts may not be present.

Osteoid thickness (by counting birefringent lamellae).

Maximum four lamellae. Most osteoid is one lamella thick and multiple lamellae are indicators of apposition activity.

Resorption surface (the proportion of length of bone surface formed by the base of a Howship's lacuna).

Maximum 4% in all age groups. Surfaces distinguished as 'active' if an osteoclast is present at the intercept.

Osteoclast population (the number of cells identified whilst analysing 400 intercepts using any 40× objective).

Maximum two at all ages. Examination of the cortical bone will often show a greater osteoclast population relative to bone surface than is present in the cancellous bone.

Calcification front (the interface between bone and multilamellated osteoid which has a granular appearance when stained by the von Kossa technique).

Between 50 and 75% of surface length of multilamellate osteoid. This approximates to the extent of cover of the osteoid by 'active' osteoblasts. Information relating to calcification detected by tetracycline label is available in Revell (1986).

Rate of apposition

This is calculated by measuring the distance between markers provided by tetracycline administered at known intervals. Duration and timing of the labels and the correction factor required to convert the actual measurement into the 'true' measurement are given by Revell (1986). The rate is variously reported as between 0.65 and 0.7 µm/day which approximates the width of a birefringent osteoid lamella when measured through a diameter.

Mean wall thickness (the mean of distances between cement lines and adjacent bone surfaces).

Coupron *et al.* (1980) give the distances as 50.2 ± 8.71 µm for adult males and 59 ± 9.1 µm for adult females. Method of tissue processing, section thickness and staining can make significant differences to the measurements.

Osteocyte density (the number of osteocyte lacunae per unit area of bone).

Quoted by Parfitt (1990) as $940/mm^2$ for cortical bone and $1870/mm^2$ for cancellous bone but best determined by the observer counting lacunae in the small squares of a squared graticule using a fixed magnification.

The above are the basic measurements which are made on bone sections. They will appear in the literature under other terms (there are at least six terms applied to trabecular bone volume calculations) but the raw data are all that is required. Although it is theoretically possible to construct an equation which describes a cement line it is not a practicable undertaking and subjective assessment is required to distinguish normal from abnormal.

In some pathological states fibrous tissue is laid down adjacent to active bone cells and may occupy the whole marrow space. There is some correlation between the amount and distribution of the fibrous tissue and the primary abnormality and some means of describing and quantifying this feature may be useful. For example a +, ++, +++ system could indicate fibrous tissue in resorption cavities only, fibrous tissue on both apposition and resorption surfaces and fibrous tissue extending completely across marrow spaces respectively. Hyperparathyroid bone disease will usually merit a ++ score and active Paget's disease will be rated +++. Numerical quantification is not required.

10.8.6 APPLICATIONS

An histological diagnosis requires no more than the measurement of trabecular bone quantity and a technique which will detect excessive thickness of osteoid. Manual methods will be satisfactory for both purposes. Histomorphometry alone will not distinguish hyperparathyroidism from Paget's disease. Investigation of the effects of treatment may necessitate counting cell populations, measuring apposition and resorption surfaces, extent and rate of mineralization in addition to the basic measurements indicated above. Whether investment in a semi- or fully automated counting system is justifiable will depend on the number of specimens that is anticipated. A student of the dynamics of bone modelling and remodelling will use all the methods of analysis mentioned above and others as quoted in Parfitt (1990). Computer assistance will be required.

REFERENCES

Altman, R.D. (1980) Musculoskeletal manifestations of Paget's disease of bone. *Arthritis Rheum.*, **23**, 1121–7.

Arnold, J.S. (1951) A method for embedding undecalcified bone for histologic sectioning and its application to radioautography. *Science*, **114**, 178–80.

Arnold, J.S. (1960) Quantitation of bone as an organ and tissue in osteoporosis. *Clin. Orthop.*, **17**, 167–75.

Arnold, J.S. (1973) Some early volumetric quantification of human trabecular and cortical bone recalled. In *Proceedings of the First Workshop on Bone Histomorphometry* (ed. Z.F.G. Jaworski). University of Ottawa Press, Ottawa, pp. 94–6.

Barker, D.J.P., Clough, P.W.L., Guyer, P.B. *et al.* (1977) Paget's disease of bone in 14 British towns. *Br. Med. J.*, **1**, 1181–3.

Barnett, E. and Nordin, B.E.C. (1960) The radiological diagnosis of osteoporosis. A new approach. *Clin. Radiol.*, **11**, 166–74.

Barry, H.C. (1980) Orthopedic aspects of Paget's disease of bone. *Arthritis Rheum.*, **23**, 1128–30.

Bassett, C.A.L. and Becker, R.O. (1962) Generation of electrical potentials in bone in response to mechanical stress. *Science*, **137**, 1063–4.

Bauer, G.C.H. and Ray, R.D. (1958) Kinetics of strontium metabolism in man. *J. Bone Joint Surg.*, **40A**, 171–86.

Beighton, P. (1978) Inherited disorders of the skeleton. *Genetics in Medicine and Surgery Series.* Churchill Livingstone. Edinburgh.

Bordier, P.H.J., Miravet, L. and Hioco, D. (1973) Young adult osteoporosis. *Clin. Endocrinol. Metab.*, **2**, 272–92.

Botreau-Roussel. (1925) *Osteites Pianique Goundou.* Masson and Cie, Paris.

Brooks, M.H., Bell, N.H., Love, L. *et al.* (1978) Vitamin D-dependent rickets type II. Resistance of target organs to 1,25 di-hydroxy vitamin D. *N. Engl. J. Med.*, **298**, 996–9.

Burckhardt, P. and Michel, C. (1989) The peak bone mass concept. *Clin. Rheumatol.*, **8 Suppl. 2**, 16–21.

Byers, P.D. and Jones, A.N. (1969) Leontiasis ossea. *Br. J. Surg.*, **56**, 262–7.

Byers, P.D. and Smith, R. (1971) Quantitative histology of bone in hyperparathyroidism. Its relation to clinical features, X-ray and biochemistry. *Q. J. Med.*, **40**, 471–86.

Cartwright, E.J., Gordon, M.T., Freemont, A.J. *et al.* (1993) Paramyxovirus and Paget's disease. *J. Med. Virol.*, **40**, 133–41.

Chalkley, H.W. (1943) Method for the quantitative morphologic analysis of tissue. *J. Natl. Cancer Inst.*, **4**, 47–53.

Chalkley, H.W., Cornfield, J. and Park, H. (1949) A method for estimating surface to volume ratios. *Science*, **110**, 295–7.

Collins, D.H. (1966) *Pathology of Bone.* Butterworths, London.

Compston, J.E. and Croucher, P.I. (1991) Histomorphometric analysis of trabecular bone remodelling in osteoporosis. *Bone Miner.*, **14**, 91–102.

Coupron, P., Meunier, P.J., Bressot, C. *et al.* (1976) Amount of bone in iliac crest biopsy. Significance of the trabecular bone volume. Its values in normal and pathological conditions. In 2nd International Workshop, *Bone Histomorphometry* (ed. P.J. Meunier) Armour Montagu, Paris.

Coupron, P., Lepire, P., Arlot, M. *et al.* (1980) Mechanisms underlying the reduction in age of the mean wall thickness of trabecular bone basic structure unit (BSU) of human iliac bone. In *Bone Histomorphometry,* 3rd international workshop (eds W.S.S. Jee and A.M. Parfitt). *Metab. Bone Dis. Relat. Res.*, **2**, (suppl).

Dantas, M., Costa, R.S., Jorgetti, V. *et al.* (1991) Facial leontiasis ossea: a rare presentation of hyperparathyroidism secondary to renal insufficiency. *Nephron*, **58**, 475–8.

Darby, A.J. (1981) Bone formation and resorption in post-menopausal osteoporosis (letter). *Lancet*, **ii**, 536.

Darby, A.J. and Meunier, P.J. (1981) Mean wall thickness and formation periods of trabecular bone packets in idiopathic osteoporosis. *Calcif. Tissue Int.*, **33**, 199–204.

Detheridge, F.M., Guyer, P.B. and Baker, D.J.P. (1982) European distribution of Paget's disease of bone. *Br. Med. J.*, **285**, 1005–8.

Drezner, M.K., Neelon, F.A., Jowsey, J. *et al.* (1977) Hypoparathyroidism: a possible cause of osteomalacia. *J. Clin. Endocrinol. Metab.*, **45**, 114–22.

Ellis, H.A. and Peart, K.M. (1973) Azotaemic renal osteodystrophy: a quantitative study on iliac bone. *J. Clin. Pathol.*, **26**, 83–101.

Engstrom, A. and Wegstedt, L. (1951) Equipment for microradiography with soft Roentger rays. *Acta Radiol.*, **35**, 345–5.

Engstrom, A. and Amprino, R. (1950) X-ray diffraction and X-ray absorption studies of immobilised bones. *Experientia*, **6**, 267–9.

Evans, D.J. and Azzopardi, J.G. (1972) Distinctive tumours of bone and soft tissue causing acquired vitamin D-resistant rickets. *Lancet*, **i**, 353–4.

Fallon, M.D., Whyte, M.P. and Teitelbaum, S.L. (1981) Systemic mastocytosis associated with generalised osteopaenia: histopathological characterisation of the skeletal lesion using undecalcified bone from two patients. *Hum. Pathol.*, **12**, 813–20.

Feldman, R.G., Culebras, A. and Schmideck, H.H. (1979) Paget's disease and the nervous system. *J. Am. Geriatr. Soc.*, **27**, 1–8.

Frame, B. and Parfitt, A.M. (1978) Osteomalacia: current concepts. *Ann. Intern. Med.*, **89**, 966–82.

Fraser, D., Koch, S.W., Kind, H.P. *et al.*, (1973) Pathogenesis of hereditary vitamin D-dependent rickets. An inborn error of vitamin D metabolism involving defective conversion of 25-hydroxy vitamin D to 1,25-dihydroxy vitamin D. *N. Engl. J. Med.*, **289**, 817–24.

Fulton, J.D., Shand, J., Ritchie, D. *et al.* (1990) Hyperostosis frontalis interna, acromegaly and hyperprolactinaemia. *Postgrad. Med. J.*, **66**, 16–9.

Genant, H.K., Block, J.E., Steiger, P. *et al.* (1989) Appropriate use of bone densitometry. *Radiology*, **170**, 817–22.

Glorieux, F.H., Marie, P.J., Pettifor, J.M. *et al.* (1980) Bone response to phosphate salts, ergocalciferol and calcitrol in hypophosphataemic vitamin D-resistant rickets. *N. Engl. J. Med.*, **303**, 1023–31.

Hahn, T.J., Boisseau, V.C. and Avioli, L.V. (1974) Effect of chronic corticosteroid administration on diaphyseal and metaphyseal bone mass. *J. Clin. Endocrinol. Metab.*, **39**, 274–82.

Harvey, L., Gray, T., Beneton, M.N.C. *et al.* (1982) Ultrastructural features of the osteoclasts from Paget's disease of bone in relation to a viral aetiology. *J. Clin. Pathol.*, **35**, 771–9.

Hayflick, L. (1976) The cell biology of human aging. *N. Engl. J. Med.*, **295**, 1302–8.

Hennig, A. (1958) A critical survey of volume and surface measurement in microscopy. *Zeiss Werkzeitschr.*, **30**, 78–87.

Jacobson, H. and Haverling, M. (1988) Hyperostosis cranii. Radiology and scintigraphy compared. *Acta Radiol.*, **29**, 223–6.

Jaffe, H.L. (1977) The classic Paget's disease of bone. *Clin. Orthop.*, **127**, 4–23.

Jaffe, M.D. and Willis, P.W. (1965) Multiple fractures associated with long-term sodium heparin therapy. *J. Am. Med. Assoc.*, **193**, 152–4.

Jaworsky, Z.F.G. (ed.) (1976) First workshop on bone histomorphometry. University of Ottawa Press, Ottawa.

Jee, W.S.S. and Parfitt, A.M. (eds) (1980) *Bone Histomorphometry*. 3rd international workshop. *Metab. Bone Dis. Relat. Res.*, **2, (suppl)**.

Jowsey, J., Kelly, P.J., Riggs, B.L. *et al.* (1965) Quantitative microradiographic studies of normal and osteoporotic bone. *J. Bone Joint Surg.*, **47A**, 785–806.

Khalifa, M.C. and Ibrahim, R.A. (1988) Cherubism. *J. Laryngol. Otol.*, **102**, 568–70.

Kimmel, D.B., Recker, R.R., Gallagher, J.J. *et al.* (1990) A comparison of iliac bone histomorphometry in post menopausal osteoporotic and normal subjects. *Bone Miner.*, **11**, 217–35.

Knaggs, R.L. (1924) Leontiasis ossea. *Br. J. Surg.*, **11**, 347.

Lachmann, E. (1955) Osteoporosis: potentialities and limitations of its radiological diagnosis. *Am. J. Roentgenol*, **74**, 712–5.

Lamprey, J.J. (1887) Horned men of Africa. *Br. Med. J.*, **2**, 1273.

Lavine, L.S and Grodzinsky, A.J. (1987) Electrical stimulation of repair of bone. *J. Bone Joint Surg.*, **69**, 626–30.

Leblond, C.P., Wilkinson, G.W., Belanger, L.F. *et al.* (1950) Radio-autographic visualization of bone formation in the rat. *Am. J. Anat.*, **86**, 289–341.

Lund, Bj., Sorenson, O.H., Lund, B. *et al.* (1980) Vitamin D metabolism in hypoparathyroidism. *J. Clin. Endocrinol. Metab.*, **51**, 606–10.

Lyles, K.W., Berry, W.R., Haussler, M. *et al.* (1980) Hypophosphataemic osteomalacia: association with prostatic carcinoma. *Ann. Intern. Med.*, **93**, 275–8.

McFarlane, J.D., Lutkin, J.E. and Burwood, M.A. (1977) The demonstration by scintography of fractures in osteomalacia. *Br. J. Radiol.*, **50**, 369–71.

McKusick, V.A. (1972) *Heritable Disorders of Connective Tissue*. C.V. Mosby, St Louis.

Merz, W.A. (1968) Streckenmessung an gerichteten strukturen im mikroskop und ihre anwendung zur bestimmung von oberflachenvolumen-relationen im knockengewebe. *Mikroskopie*, **22**, 132.

Meunier, P.J. (ed.) (1976) *Bone histomorphometry*. 2nd international workshop. Armour Montagu, Paris.

Meunier, P.J., Briancon, D., Sellami, S. *et al.* (1983) Dynamic bone histomorphometry in primary osteoporosis. In *Osteoporosis. A Multidisciplinary Problem* (eds A. St J. Dixon, R.G.G. Russell and T.C.B. Stamp), International congress and symposium series **No.55**, 67–73.

Milgram, J.W. (1977) Radiological and pathological assessment of the activity of Paget's disease of bone. *Clin. Orthop.*, **127**, 43–54.

Minaire, P., Meunier, P.J., Edouard, C. *et al.* (1974) Quantitative histological data on disuse osteoporosis. *Calcif. Tissue Res.*, **17**, 57–73.

Mosekilde, L. and Melsen, F. (1978) A tetracycline based histomorphometric evaluation of bone resorption and bone turnover in hyperthyroidism and hyperparathyroidism. *Acta Med. Scand.*, **204**, 97–102.

Ng, K.C., Revell, P.A., Beer, M. *et al.* (1984) The incidence of metabolic bone disease, rheumatoid arthritis and osteoarthritis. *Ann. Rheum. Dis.*, **43**, 370–7.

Nilsson, B.E. (1966) Post-traumatic osteopaenia. A quantitative study of the bone mineral mass in the femur following fracture of the tibia in man using americum-241 as a photon source. *Acta Orthop. Scand.*, **37 (91)**, 1–55.

Nilsson, B.E. and Westlin, N.E. (1971) Bone density in athletes. *Clin. Orthop.*, **77**, 179–82.

Parfitt, A.M. (1988) Bone histomorphometry; proposed system for standardisation of nomenclature, symbols and units. *Calcif. Tissue Int.*, **42**, 284–6.

Parfitt, A.M. (1990) Bone forming cells in clinical conditions. In *Bone* (vol. 1) (ed. B.K. Hall), Telford Press. Caldwell, NJ, pp. 351–429.

Parfitt, A.M., Drezner, M.K., Glorieux, F.H. *et al.* (1987) Bone histomorphometry: standardisation of nomenclature, symbols, and units. Report of the ASBMR histomorphometry nomenclature committee. *J. Bone Miner. Res.*, **2**, 595–610.

Revell, P.A. (1986) *Pathology of Bone*. Springer-Verlag, Berlin.

Rodahl, K., Nicholson, J.T. and Brown, E.M. (1960) *Bone as a Tissue*. McGraw-Hill, New York.

Rosenbaum, H.D. and Hanson, D.J. (1969) Geographic variation in the prevelance of Paget's disease of bone. *Radiology*, **92**, 959–63.

Rubin, C.T. and Lanyon, L.E. (1987) Osteoregulatory nature of mechanical stimuli. Function as a determinant of adaptive remodelling in bone. *J. Orthop. Res.*, **5**, 300–10.

Schenk, R.K., Mertz, W.A. and Muller, J. (1969) A quantitative histological study on bone resorption in human cancellous bone. *Acta Anat.*, **74**, 44–53.

Singer, F.R. and Mills, B.G. (1983) Evidence for a viral etiology of Paget's disease of bone. *Clin. Orthop.*, **178**, 245–51.

Sissons, H.A. (1955) The structural pathology of osteoporosis. *Proc. R. Soc. Med.*, **48**, 566–78.

Sissons, H.A. (1960) Osteoporosis of Cushing's syndrome, In *Bone as a Tissue* (eds K. Rodahl, J.T. Nicholson and E.M. Brown), McGraw-Hill, New York, pp. 3–17.

Sissons, H.A, and Hadfield, G.J. (1955) The influence of cortisone on the structure and growth of bone. *J. Anat.*, **89**, 69–79.

Smith, R. (1980) Idiopathic osteoporosis in the young. *J. Bone Joint Surg.*, **62B**, 417–27.

Smith, R., Winearls, C, G., Stevenson, J.C. *et al.* (1985) Osteoporosis of pregnancy. *Lancet*, **i**, 1178–80.

Swan, C.H.J, Shah, K., Brewer, D.B. *et al.* (1976) Fibrogenesis imperfecta ossium. *Q.J. Med.*, **45**, 233–53.

Teitelbaum, S.L., Bergfeld, M.A., Freitag, *et al.* (1980) Do parathyroid hormone and 1,25-dihydroxy vitamin D modulate bone formation in uraemia? *J. Clin. Endocrinol. Metab.*, **51**, 247–51.

Tilton, F.E., Degioanni, T.T.C. and Schneider, V.S. (1980) Long-term follow-up of Skylab bone demineralisation. *Aviat. Space Environ. Med.*, **51**, 1209–13.

Virchow, R. (1869) *Pathologie des Tumeurs. Traduit par Paul Arossohn*. Germer Baillière, Paris, Vol 2, pp. 20–4.

Weibel, E.R. (1963) Principles and methods for the morphometric study of the lung and other organs. *Lab. Invest.*, **12**, 131–42.

Whyte, M.P., Fallon, M.D., Murphy, W.A. *et al.* (1981) Axial osteomalacia. Clinical, laboratory and genetic investigation of affected mother and son. *Am. J. Med.*, **71**, 1041–9.

Woodhouse, N.J.Y. (1972) Paget's disease of bone. *Clin. Endocrinol. Metab.*, **1**, 125–41.

Woods, C.G., Morgan, D.B., Paterson, C.R. *et al.* (1967) Measurement of osteoid in bone biopsy. *J. Pathol. Bacteriol.*, **95**, 441–7.

Woods, C.G. (1976) Why count osteoblasts? In *Bone Histomorphometry*, 2nd International Workshop (ed. P.J. Meunier), Armour Montagu, Paris.

PART THREE

Neoplasia

INTRODUCTION 11

Jonathan R. Salisbury and Paul D. Byers

Cancer is concerned with the control of cell proliferation. An abundance of readily accessible information can be found in Alberts *et al.* (1989) and Watson *et al.* (1988) from which the following has been prepared. The approximately 10^{13} cells that form a human body are differentiated into many types, some of which never divide at all, but others must divide at appropriate rates to replace the billions of cells that die each day, and do so for a lifetime. Elaborate control systems, exercised by social control genes, promote and restrain growth. A single cell which no longer responds to these controls forms a localized neoplastic growth. If the controls that keep the cells *in situ* are also overcome, entry of cells into the circulation and colonization of a distant site is possible. The acquisition of these new behavioural patterns is by alterations in DNA which comes about through the action of environmental carcinogens, or viral infection, or defects in its replication, repair and recombination. More than one mutation must occur before transformation to a malignant cell takes place in a normal individual. The number of mutations is estimated to be from 2 to 7. For these to accumulate takes time, so that most cancers increase in incidence with age. The normal cellular genes that can be altered so as to cause cancer are called proto-oncogenes, and in their altered state are known as oncogenes.

The knowledge that underlies those brief statements has accumulated at an increasing rate over many years. Studies in epidemiol-ogy and the many disciplines involved in molecular biology have been the major sources and human and animal populations, primary cells and cell lines, viruses and the replicating and controlling constituents of cells the subject matter.

Experimental chemical carcinogenesis has demonstrated that a carcinogenic agent (a mutagen) initiates an alteration that does not produce cell proliferation until a second agent has been applied. The second agent is not a mutagen, but promotes the expression of the genetic mutation that has been initi-ated by the mutagen. Thus it requires an initiator and a promoter to establish growth, which may cease if the promoter is with-drawn. But if, among the proliferating cells there is one which undergoes a further spon-taneous mutation uncontrolled growth ensues. The viruses that are known to be tumourigenic belong to two groups: those with a DNA genetic structure and the retro-viruses containing RNA. The oncogenes of the former are virus-coded and take part in the replication of the virus. The retrovirus oncogenes are transduced cellular genes, a chance event, and are not necessary for repli-cation of the virus.

With respect to viruses, cells are either permissive, allowing the virus to enter and multiply and kill the cell by lysis, or they are non-permissive in that the virus can enter but not mutiply lytically. In a small propor-tion of non-permissive cells the chromosome of DNA viruses is incorporated into the cell's genome where it is replicated, or it forms a circular molecule that replicates without killing the cell. This sometimes transforms the cell.

RNA virus infection in a permissive cell often leads to release of progeny by budding at the cell surface and to a genetic change in the cell. The latter comes about through the insertion of a gene, picked up by the virus from a previous host cell, into the genome of the current host (Figure 11.1). The transduced gene undergoes mutation in the process, and if it was a social proto-oncogene it now acts as an oncogene and transforms the cell.

Physico/chemical mutagenic agents and viruses are recognized as acting in closely similar ways to induce cancers in that they modify individual genes to produce their effect. The study of tumour viruses has been more effective in elucidating the proto-oncogenes so far discovered which exceed 60. The methods used detect dominant mutations but there are grounds for believing that recessive mutations also occur so that a more elaborate social control gene system may yet be uncovered.

The functions of proto-oncogenes is to code for components of the normal system of social control genes, viz.:

- Growth factors
- Growth factor receptors
- Intracellular regulatory proteins for cell adhesion
- Proteins that relay signals for cell division to the nucleus

The conversion of these to oncogenes means that they function abnormally, leading to uncontrolled growth. Some of the pathways whereby this takes place are shown in Figure 11.2.

The natural events leading to cancer are more complex than are observed in many experimental systems, and they in turn are much more so than has been conveyed here. Much research uses immortal cell lines which are abnormal and are readily transformed by

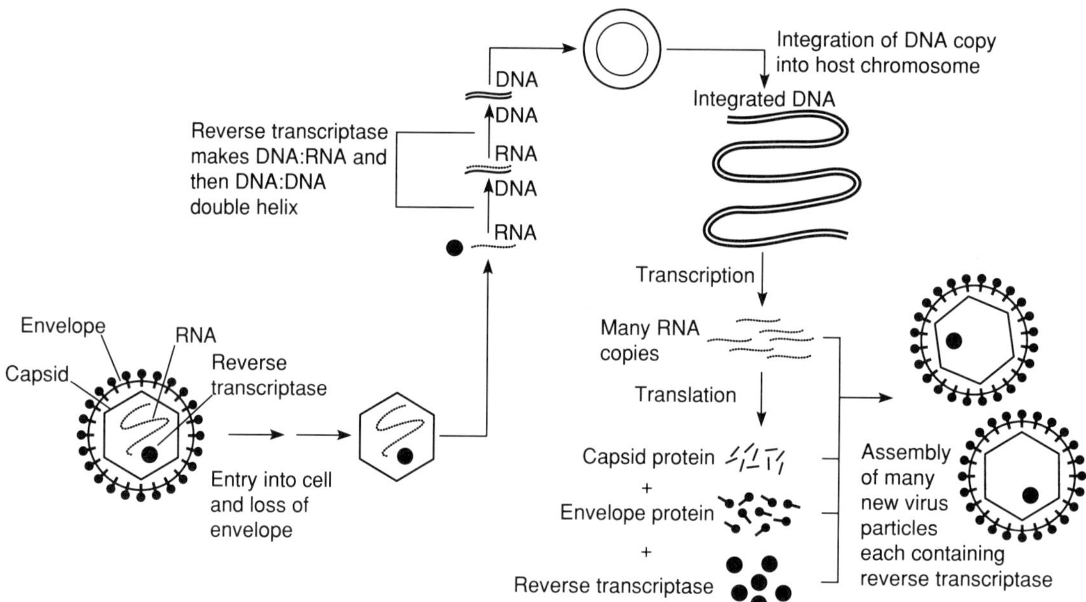

Figure 11.1 The life cycle of a retrovirus. (Reproduced from Alberts *et al.* (1989) with permission.)

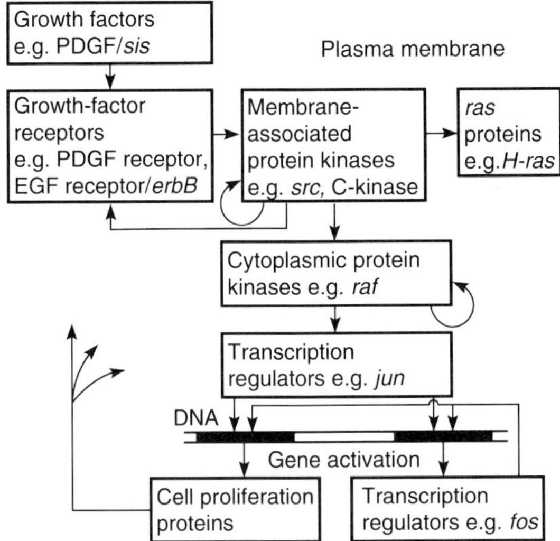

Figure 11.2 A tentative outline of the relationships of the major classes of proto-oncogenes in the intracellular control network through which external signals stimulate cell proliferation. (Reproduced from Alberts *et al.* (1989), with permission.)

a single event. But in nature a succession of events is required, and the complexity provides a fail-safe system. This appears to be enhanced by tumour suppressor genes which act to suppress excessive cell proliferation.

It appears that cancer cells not only override the regulatory system for growth and place, but are also able to affect other regulatory systems such as those of bone cell function and calcium homoeostasis (Mundy, 1990, 1991a, b), giving rise to paraneoplastic syndromes of hypercalcaemia, hypocalcaemia, hypophosphataemia and osteomalacia. Most of the observations concerning these are made in metastatic carcinoma. But cases discussed by Mirra (1989) as toxic osteoblastoma might well qualify. The effect of the cancer cells is mediated by factors produced by the cancer cells, or by normal host cells in response to the presence of the cancer cells; some act locally and some are systemic, affecting, for example, renal handling of cal-

cium. It seems a reasonable proposition that not only metastatic cancers but also primary neoplasia in bone, benign or malignant, disturb the local regulatory systems, since it is self-evident that local bone and marrow cells are affected by their presence.

For the histopathologist the local effects are an important source of information about a tumour. In most diagnostic work they are most readily perceived through the agency of radiographs and other imaging techniques. To overlook this information is to put at peril correct diagnosis and the interests of the patient. The classic example is to diagnose fibrous dysplasia in a biopsy of parosteal osteosarcoma: the tissue often supports that histological interpretation, but it is not sustainable for a lesion on the bone surface; the fact of that location is immediately discernible from the radiograph.

Bone tumours can have several effects on the host bone:

- Activate intraosseous bone cells: osteoblasts, osteoclasts
- Stimulate the periosteal bone cells
- Invade marrow

Which effect is dominant is a reflection of the character of the tumour. The resulting pattern in radiographs contributes to identification. Additionally the tumour tissue itself may have properties which can be detected radiographically: bone formation; calcification, adding to the characterization.

It is apparent that what makes a tumour (or any other bone lesion) visible in a radiograph is a change in bone density. An appreciable alteration, at least 15%, must occur to be detectable in a film. If a process is invasive but does not lead to any bone cell activity, then it will not be visible. Neoplasia in bone is primarily destructive, but tumours can permeate marrow with little disturbance of bone cells, e.g. some cartilage tumours, malignant round cell tumours, leukaemias and lymphomas, some metastatic carcinomas. In consequence it may be some time before a telltale difference in density, which may be an increase and/or decrease appears. Thus an expanding tumour induces osteoclasts to clear the way, so to speak. There may be more or less substantial osteoblastic activity accompanying this. The net effect is to produce radiographic appearances which allow assessment of the behaviour and character of the tumour. Taken in conjunction with clinical information it is possible to class a neoplasm according to one of the following categories:

- Stable
- Growing non-invasive
- Slowly destructive + or − invasion
- Rapidly destructive and invasive

A number of tumour and tumour-like lesions are clinically silent, and are only discovered incidentally or following pathological fracture. When symptoms are present these are one or more of: (a) pain; (b) swelling or (c) loss of function. The symptoms will sooner or later lead to X-ray. A pathological fracture does so promptly. But persistent pain, particularly near a joint, can for long be attributed to a common disorder such as strain, arthritis, frozen shoulder. Time may pass before an X-ray is taken, and even then a low level of textural alteration of the bone may be difficult to recognize.

Other things being equal it is also possible roughly to categorize tumours according to the treatment that is appropriate:

- None
- Limited surgery
- Radical surgery and/or adjuvant therapy

These can be seen to correspond with the behavioural categories outlined above. The correlation of the qualities of the tumour, the extent of tissue involvement at the site of origin, extensions and metastases, are used to establish the 'stage' of a tumour, which can be used as a guide to treatment. Staging is discussed in Chapter 12.

Each bone tumour has its characteristic relationship with the host bone, and this, within the limits already discussed, is seen in the radiographs. The skeletal distribution is also known, and sites can be graded as common, uncommon, rare, never affected. Because many of these observations are not specific to any one entity, frequently it is not possible to do more than list the possible causes of the radiographic findings. Experience and judgement are of great importance here, allowing some to proceed further in identification. But it seems undesirable to force a choice which is beyond the capacity of the available expertise, or which the evidence will not support, and which may in any case be unnecessary for the required decisions.

The recognition of a malignant bone tumour, or the inclusion of that category as a possibility in the initial consideration of a case, is generally not difficult. This should of course always include the possibility of metastatic carcinoma. Depending on the location of the lesion, i.e. the position in the skeleton (long bone, flat bones, vertebrae, hands and feet); the localization in a tubular bone (epiphysis, metaphysis, diaphysis); the age of the patient; radiological features (amount of periosteal reaction); the content of the lesion (uniform, loculated, mineralized); associated conditions (Paget's disease, previous radiation, etc.) a provisional diagnosis or a selection of possible diagnoses may be made. These can be drawn from a hierarchical list, the last term of which can be expanded from the classification of bone tumours:

- Malignant tumour, unspecified
- Metastatic carcinoma, unspecified or known
- Primary malignant bone tumour, unspecified
- Specific primary sarcoma of bone

To proceed to the definitive diagnosis from any list of possibilities is a matter of identification of specific criteria. These are not always necessarily histological. Thus to exclude the possibility of brown tumour of hyperparathyroidism in reaching a diagnosis of giant cell tumour it is necessary to remember that hyperparathyroidism is a biochemical diagnosis. It may be that the possibility of that condition is so improbable that appropriate tests are unnecessary, but this must be a deliberate decision and not an oversight.

Malignant neoplasms that diffusely involve the bone with irregular destruction and some periosteal reaction must be distinguished from osteomyelitis, lymphomas and leukaemias, and metastatic carcinomas. Obviously the age of the patient, the history, symptoms, physical findings, and laboratory results will help to order the possibilities. The importance of taking tissue at the time of biopsy for bacteriological examination must be stressed.

REFERENCES

Alberts, B., Bray, D., Lewis, J. *et al.* (1989) *Molecular Biology of the Cell*, 2nd edn. Garland Publishing, New York.

Mirra, J.M. (1989) *Bone Tumors: Clinical, Radiologic and Pathologic Correlations*. Lea and Febiger, Philadelphia.

Mundy, G.R. (1990) Incidence and pathophysiology of hypercalcemia. *Calcif. Tissue Int.*, **46**, suppl., S3–10.

Mundy, G.R. (1991a) Ectopic production of calcitropic peptides. *Endocrinol. Metab. Clin. North Am.*, **20**, 473–87.

Mundy, G.R. (1991b) Mechanisms of osteolytic bone destruction. *Bone*, **12**, Suppl. 1, 81–6.

Watson, J.D., Hopkins, N.H., Roberts, J.W. *et al.* (1988) *Molecular Biology of the Gene*, 4th edn. Benjamin/Cummings, California.

Jonathan R. Salisbury and Paul D. Byers

Several musculoskeletal tumour staging systems have been developed in America from the 1960s, addressing the problem of uniform reporting of the results of treatment, mainly of sarcomas, in the furtherance of therapeutic advance. In 1980 Enneking *et al.* published a system developed since 1967 in association with the Musculoskeletal Tumor Society. In a review in 1989 Enneking proposed modifications in the light of experience with its use and of developments in competing systems, recognizing at the same time the desirability and difficulty of achieving uniformity. The Musculoskeletal Tumor Society system appears to have been the one most widely adopted. This is concerned with malignant tumours, and is summarized here. Full details can be obtained from the references quoted above.

The three components of the system which require evaluation, and their symbols, are:

- the grade of the tumour = G
- the extent of the tissues involved, specified in relation to tissue compartments = T
- metastases; in the original system nodal and distant metastases were lumped; a modification is to record these separately: nodal = N, and distant = M

12.1 GRADE

In principle neoplasia can be graded as:

   benign
     inactive
     active
     aggressive

   malignant
     low-grade sarcoma
     high-grade sarcoma

In practice, the original staging system dealt only with low- and high-grade neoplasia. In the revision, an intermediate grade was introduced. The classification is based on clinical, macroscopic and microscopic observations.

1. The clinical observations are:
   1.1 presentation
   1.2 rate of growth
   1.3 relationship to adjacent tissues

2. The macroscopic observations, which in the case of bone are mainly radiographic, concern the relationship between neoplasia and the host bone.
   2.1 osteoblastic reaction
   2.2 osteoclastic reaction reflecting
   2.3 growth and invasion
   2.4 soft tissue reaction reflected in imaging modalities

3. Microscopically the features are:
   3.1 cell/matrix ratio
   3.2 maturity of matrix
   3.3 cytological features of malignancy
   3.4 extension of tumour
   3.5 reaction of contiguous tissues

Under clinical observations, the presentation of tumours (1.1 above) varies from incidental observation of asymptomatic lesions, to the rapidly growing painful examples with local reactions. Growth (1.2) is described in qualitative terms but without definition or demarcation criteria for the different rates. The relationship to adjacent tissues (1.3): for soft tissue tumours this refers to fixation to adjacent structures; in bone, the reference is to penetration of cortex and contiguity with soft tissue, and extension into and around joints.

Under macroscopic observations (2 above), confining discussion to bone tumours, the assessment is a judgement on the nature of the interface between neoplasm and bone. Basically this is what the method of radiological tumour grading by Lodwick (1964, 1966) depends on:

1. Geographic destruction
   (a) Sclerotic marginal zone, sharp edge, partial or non-penetration of cortex
   (b) Expansion of bone +/- sclerotic margin, partial or non-penetration of cortex
   (c) Total penetration of cortex

2. Geographic + moth-eaten and/or permeated destruction

3. Only moth-eaten and/or permeated destruction.

The third aspect of the grading (3 above) is the microscopic assessment. The traditional grading system for this is Broders' four-grade method (Broders *et al.*, 1939). In Enneking's original staging system only two grades were employed, low (Broders I and II) and high (Broders III and IV). In the revision this was expanded to include an intermediate grade (spanning grades II and III). The histological grading of bone tumours is considered under individual entities. The use of four grades has been discussed by Unni and Dahlin (1984); a three-grade method, for soft tissues, has been described by Enzinger *et al.* (1969). The assessment of the margin of the neoplasm is concerned with tumour invasion and the risk of incomplete local excision, and has a bearing on the next category.

Table 12.1 Compartments to be considered in the staging of a tumour

Compartments	*Non-compartmental*
Intraosseous	
Intra-articular	
Superficial to deep fascia	
(skin and subcutaneous tissue)	
Parosseous	
Intrafascial	
Ray of hand or foot	Mid and hindfoot, midhand
Posterior calf	Popliteal space
Anterolateral leg	
Anterior thigh	Groin
Posterior thigh	Interpelvic
Buttocks	
Volar forearm	Antecubital fossa
Dorsal forearm	
Anterior arm	Periclavicular
Posterior arm	Axilla
Periscapular	Paraspinal
	Head and neck

12.1.1   SITE

This category of information is location with reference to compartments. The compartments are considered to be as shown in Table 12.1

Necessarily there are conventions about some of the limits to these spaces, as in the skin and subcutaneous tissue where a margin greater than 5 cm constitutes a compartment boundary. Nevertheless, anatomical detail makes possible the definitions of margins in the surgical removal of tumours as shown in Table 12.2.

12.2   METASTASES

The final category in staging is the presence of metastases. There is now a subdivision into regional (nodal, N) and distant (M).

In summary, these three categories of information are:

G1 Low grade malignant
G2 Moderate grade malignant
G3 High grade malignant

T1 Intracompartmental
T2 Extracompartmental

N0 No node metastases
N1 Node metastases

M0 No distant metastases
M1 Distant metastases

The stages derived from these are:

Stage I
A G1 T1 N0 M0
B G1 T2 N0 M0

Stage II
A G2 T1 N0 M0
B G2 T2 N0 M0

Stage III
A G3 T1 N0 M0
B G3 T2 N0 M0

Stage IV
A G1–3 T1–2 N1 M0
B G1–3 T1–2 N0–1 M1

The application of these principles to individual cases is necessarily a question of experience. It is not possible to avoid the conclusion that such experience can only be gained, and its benefits and standards advanced, through concentrating it at specialist centres.

REFERENCES

Broders, A.C., Hargrave, R. and Myerding, H.W. (1939) Pathologic features of soft tissue fibrosarcoma. *Surg. Gynecol. Obstet.*, **69**, 267–80.

Enneking, W.F. (1986) A system of staging musculoskeletal neoplasms. *Clin. Orthop.*, **204**, 9–24.

Enneking, W.F. (1989) Musculoskeletal tumor staging. *Cancer Treat. Res.*, **44**, 39–49.

Enneking, W.F., Spanier, S.S. and Goodman, M.A. (1980) A system for the surgical staging of musculoskeletal sarcoma. *Clin. Orthop.*, **153**, 106–20.

Enzinger, F.M., Lattes, R. and Tartoni, H. (1969) *Histologic Typing of Soft Tissue Tumors*. World

Table 12.2 Definitions of margins in the surgical removal of tumours

Class of margin	Plane of dissection	Tissue of margin
Intracapsular	Within lesion	Tumour
Marginal	Within reactive zone	Reactive tissue ±extension of tumour
Wide	Intracompartmental normal tissue	Normal tissue ±skin lesions
Radical	Extracompartmental normal tissue	Normal tissue

Health Organization, Geneva.

Lodwick, G.S. (1964) Reactive response to local injury in bone. *Radiol. Clin. North Am.*, **2**, 209–19.

Lodwick, G.S. (1966) Solitary malignant tumours of bone. The application of predictor variables and diagnosis. *Semin. Roentgenol.*, **1**, 293–313.

Unni, K.K. and Dahlin, D.C. (1984) Grading of bone tumors. *Semin. Diagn. Pathol.*, **1**, 165–72.

OSTEOBLASTIC AND CARTILAGINOUS NEOPLASMS 13

Jonathan R. Salisbury and Paul D. Byers

13.1 OSTEOBLASTIC NEOPLASMS

There are many non-neoplastic osteoblastic lesions which produce tumours, i.e. swellings, of bone and in soft tissues which must be included in the consideration of osteoblastic neoplasia since their morbid anatomy and bone-forming potential can lead to difficulties in diagnosis. A primary classification of the lesions to be considered is shown in Table 13.1 (the categories of myositis ossificans, osteoid osteoma, and osteosarcoma are expanded in the sections devoted to their discussion).

13.2 REACTIVE LESIONS

The reactive lesions are discussed in some detail in Chapters 6 and 20. The lesions under consideration have been classified as shown in Table 13.2.

Age, sex and skeletal distribution are not features that figure in the matter of patho-

Table 13.1 Primary classification of osteoblastic neoplasms

	Bone		Soft
	In	*On*	*In*
I Reactive			
Callus	+	+	+
Myositis ossificans			
II Hamartoma/dysplasia			
Osteoma	+		
Enostosis	+		
Fibrous dysplasia	+		
Osteofibrous dysplasia	+		
Ossifying fibroma	+		
III Neoplasia			
Osteoid osteoma	+		
Osteoid osteoma of unusual size	+		
Multicentric osteoid osteoma	+		
Benign osteoblastoma	+		
Aggressive osteoblastoma	+		
Osteosarcoma			
Intraosseous	+		
Juxtacortical		+	
Soft tissue			+

Table 13.2 Reactive lesions

| | Bone | | Soft |
	In	*On*	*In*
Callus	+	+	+
Post-traumatic myositis ossificans			
Single major blow		+	
Multiple minor blows		+	
Avulsion injury		+	
Post-traumatic ossification of ligaments and tendons			+
Ossification after			
Bone/joint prosthetic replacement		+	+
Burns		+	
Tetanus		+	
In neurological conditions		+	
In arthropathies		+	
Pseudomalignant osseous tumour of soft tissues			+

logical diagnosis since none are exempt from trauma. The clinical detail which is important is the history. Knowledge that trauma occurred provides corroboration, not proof, that suspect tissue is reactive. Other things being equal, the absence of such a history weakens the reactive hypothesis. But reactive changes sometimes occur without apparent provocation, e.g. periostitis, pseudomalignant osseous tumour of soft tissue. Observation of the patient over time (weeks) may be required.

In summary the basis of callus is granulation tissue in which bone and cartilage differentiate. The former is generated by membrane formation, and as the trabeculae develop the osteoblasts form a single layer over the surfaces ('mantling'). The cartilage is formed in nodules and undergoes ossification. Mitoses may be present, but the cytology is benign. It is, however, an invasive tissue and will incorporate muscle fibres.

Myositis ossificans is similar regardless of cause. The underlying tissue is fibrovascular, with a range of differentiation from mainly cellular to collagenized. The bony component is trabecular; it is generated at the periphery by membrane formation and later apposition, and is remodelled throughout. Those forms attached to bone tend to mature at the base, whereas those in soft tissue are enclosed by more mature peripheral bone. In the latter there is often central highly cellular, mitotically active spindle cell tissue.

13.3   HAMARTOMA/DYSPLASIA

13.3.1   OSTEOMA

This is a smooth firm rounded swelling arising from the surface of the bones formed in membrane, nearly always the skull and nasal sinuses, composed of dense lamellar bone without much osteonal organization. Mirra (1989) illustrates spongy osteoma, a lesion of the same sites composed of cancellous rather than compact bone. Multiple osteomas occur in Gardner's syndrome (Gardner and Richards, 1953), some of which may be on long bones.

13.3.2   ENOSTOSIS

A bone island is an acquired focus of dense bone in cancellous tissue, ranging in size to a few centimetres, which is found incidentally in the bones of adults and only rarely in children. It is lamellar in structure, with an osteonal organization. One explanation is that it results from a local remodelling error.

13.3.3 FIBROUS DYSPLASIA AND OSSIFYING FIBROMA

Fibrous dysplasia is regarded as a developmental disorder, implying that it starts in childhood. In most cases a single bone is affected (monostotic). But in some there is multiple bone involvement (polyostotic); girls are more commonly affected than boys; in some there is an associated hormonal disturbance with precocious sexual development (Albright *et al.*, 1937). Historically, the polyostotic form had been confused with neurofibromatosis and with hyperparathyroidism. Lichtenstein and Jaffe (1942) established criteria for fibrous dysplasia.

(a) Clinical features

The age range is decades 1–8; 50% occur in decades 1–2. The lesion is slightly more common in females.

(i) *Skeletal distribution*

Mirra (1989) gives the percentages of 344 cases as follows:

- Jaws   11
- Skull   6
- Other flat bones
     ribs   10
     girdles
          pelvic: ilium, pubis, sacrum   3
- Spine
- Long tubular   70
     femur, tibia   55
     humerus, radius, ulna, fibula   15
- Hands and feet   3

(ii) *Radiology*

The radiology is that of a benign lesion: well demarcated, but with a limited peripheral osteoblastic reaction, and no periosteal reaction. The bone formed in the lesion mineralizes and when sufficiently dense this casts a shadow in the film. Because of the fine trabecular pattern it projects as a ground glass quality. This is relative, but at its best is characteristic to the point of being diagnostic. But even in the absence of certainty on this point, the conclusion of benign osteoblastic lesion is sufficient to give a context for the histology.

(b) Pathology

(i) *Morbid anatomy*

These lesions are nearly always solitary, arising during the growth of the skeleton. It is thought that many resolve in time. However, some are found in adults and evidence in a portion of these cases indicates that they developed in adulthood. It is not clear what the significance of that observation is. Multiple lesions also occur; Mirra (1989) states the incidence of these cases, determined radiologically, is 1/20 of the monostotic cases.

The majority of the lesions are small, metaphyseal and symptomless; they come to notice incidentally, possibly as the result of pathological fracture (Figure 13.1). Larger lesions may give rise to swelling or deformity and associated disability.

(ii) *Histopathology*

There is a benign fibrous stroma whose cells have a stellate quality (Figure 13.2). The amount of collagen is not great, but can be variable within moderate limits. Increases in it are associated with decreases in cellularity. This pattern of behaviour is seen in older lesions as they mature. There is no distinctive pattern of organization of the fibrocellular tissue; if anything it might be qualified as whorled.

The bone is formed by differentiation of stromal cells to osteoblasts who then form bone in membrane. Individual trabeculae are

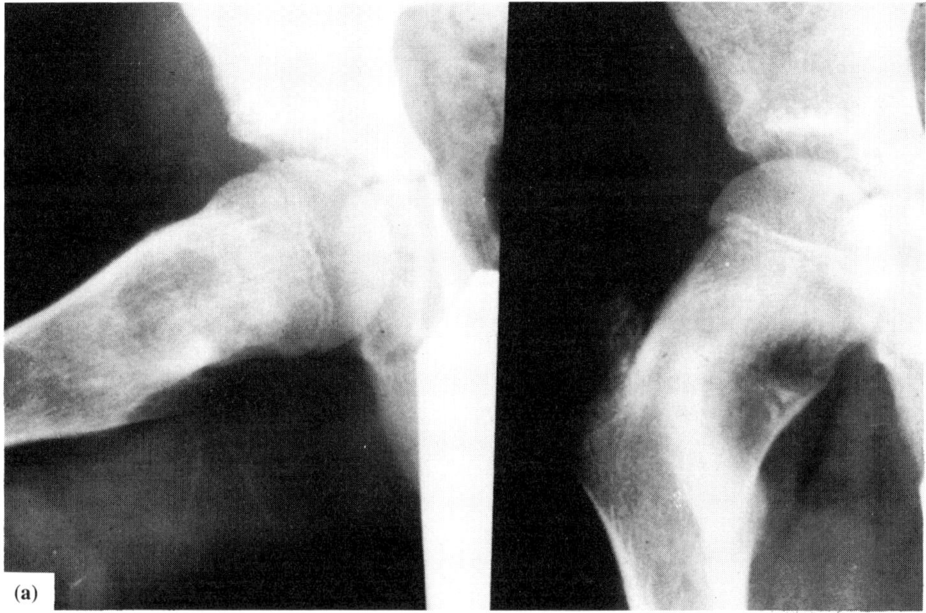

Figure 13.1 (a) Male, 9 years. Fibrous dysplasia of femoral neck with stress fracture. The limits of the lesion are not easily defined. In the lateral film (left) the clear cut edge of the lesion runs beneath the upper cortex; it can be followed inferiorly to the lower endocortex; superiorly the edge is obscured by an increase of bone density in part the result of fracture callus. There are lucent areas and zones of 'ground glass' texture. In the AP view (right) the lesion appears as a lucent area, the site of stress fracture, and a bounding dense zone. There is no periosteal reaction. The femoral neck is expanded.

short, curved and at one or both ends tend to join with contiguous trabeculae to form a distinctive network, characteristic and specific when combined with the apppropriate morbid anatomy.

In most lesions the bone cells most readily recognized are the osteocytes. The osteoblasts are not ordinarily very prominent at the surfaces of the trabeculae. However, in some lesions they 'mantle' the trabeculae. Such lesions have been distinguished with the title ossifying fibroma. They occur mainly in the skull, principally the occiput, and the jaws. Recently lesions with this feature, but which have arisen in the cortex (and may later expand into the medullary cavity) and have a more rectilinear pattern of orientation of the trabeculae, have been designated osteofibrous dys-

plasia (Campanacci, 1976). To what extent one is dealing with distinct entities remains controversial. Osteoclasts are not usually numerous. Occasional osteoclasts may be scattered here and there; in active lesions small numbers aggregate around trabeculae which are undergoing resorption. Older lesions undergo a more formal remodelling of their trabeculae as evidenced by the surface activity, and reversal lines.

Occasional associated features are (a) cartilage; (b) cysts; (c) foam cells.

The cartilaginous component generally consists of a few lobules constituting a small portion of the lesion. However, in an occasional case this element may predominate, to the point where the diagnosis of cartilage tumour seems appropriate, leading away from

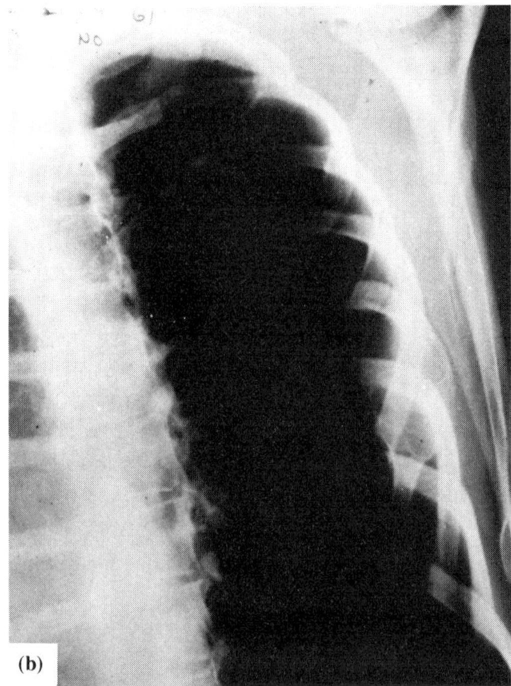

Figure 13.1 (b) Female, 28 years. Fibrous dysplasia found on mass chest radiograph. Egg-shaped lesion of the 6th rib. Well demarcated, smooth expansion, no periosteal reaction or endocortical erosion; ground glass texture from lesional bone formation.

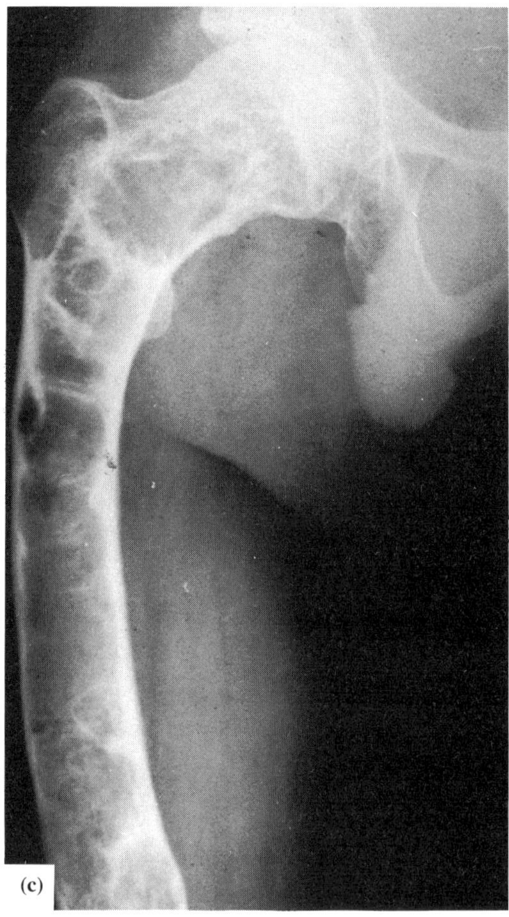

Figure 13.1 (c) Young adult male. Extensive (polyostotic) fibrous dysplasia affecting most of the femur. The bone, which is expanded with a thinned cortex, has adopted a 'shepherd's crook' deformity. Most of the lesion has a ground glass texture.

the recognition of the fibro-osseous tissue as having the features of fibrous dysplasia.

Microcysts, which are not uncommon, sometimes appear to be associated with resorption of bone. But much larger cysts can occur, which are unilocular, smooth surfaced and usually filled with clear fluid. The results of biopsy can be confused if there are several large cysts in the tissue at the site of biopsy.

Foam cells sometimes occur in substantial collections.

The prime histological feature in the diagnosis is the osseous trabeculae, both the pattern of the developed structures and their membranous formation. If they are not present in the sections recourse to the radiographs may show the ground glass appear-ance they give to the tissue.

Differentiation from ossifying fibroma is a matter of conviction, and of a decision as to how many osteoblasts make a mantle. Benign fibro-osseous lesion of bone serves both equally well. If the tissue sample is largely cystic, or mainly composed of cartilage there may be difficulty over the possibility of aneurysmal bone cyst or cartilage tumour. A thorough sampling of the specimen and close

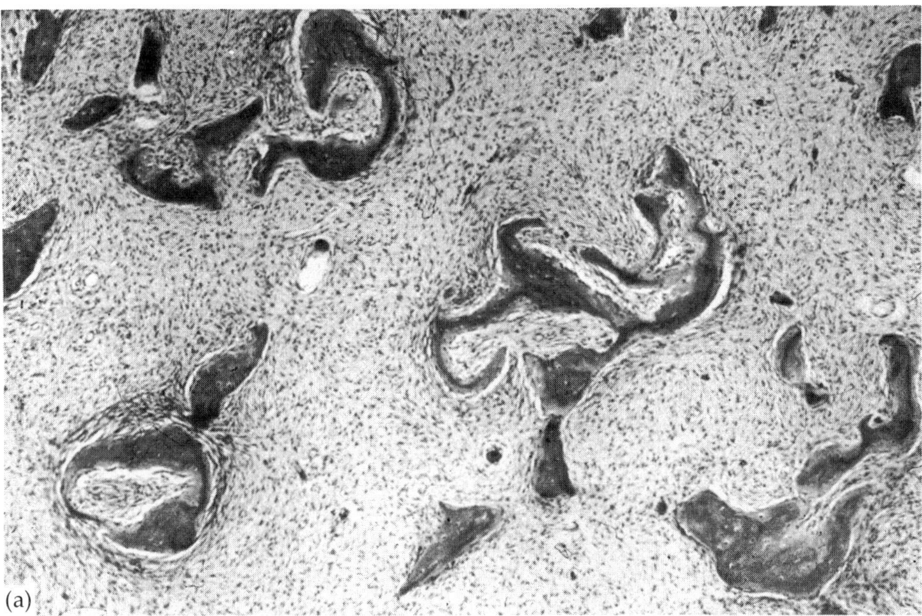

Figure 13.2 Fibrous dysplasia. (a) The typical curvilinear pattern of membrane bone formation in a pattern-free stroma of stellate and spindle cells.

consideration of the radiographs may resolve the question.

13.3.4 OSTEOFIBROUS DYSPLASIA

This is the name given by Campanacci (1976) to an intracortical lesion of the tibia and/or fibula of children under the age of ten in which the histological structure is similar to fibrous dysplasia, but in which there is prominent osteoblastic rimming of the trabecula. Campanacci and Laus (1981) have reported 40 cases and Nakashima *et al.* (1983) 12 cases. Mirra (1989) records having seen three cases and that in two of these and in two of Campanacci's cases epithelial nests, as in adamantinoma, have been found.

13.3.5 FIBROUS DYSPLASIA AND ADAMANTINOMA

There are lesions, mainly in the tibia, which resemble fibrous dysplasia, but which also contain an epithelial component as in adamantinoma. These were originally reported as a

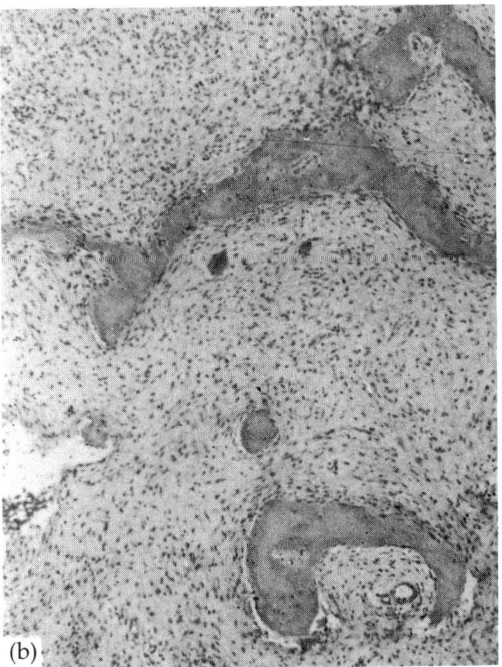

Figure 13.2 Fibrous dysplasia. (b) A variation of the pattern.

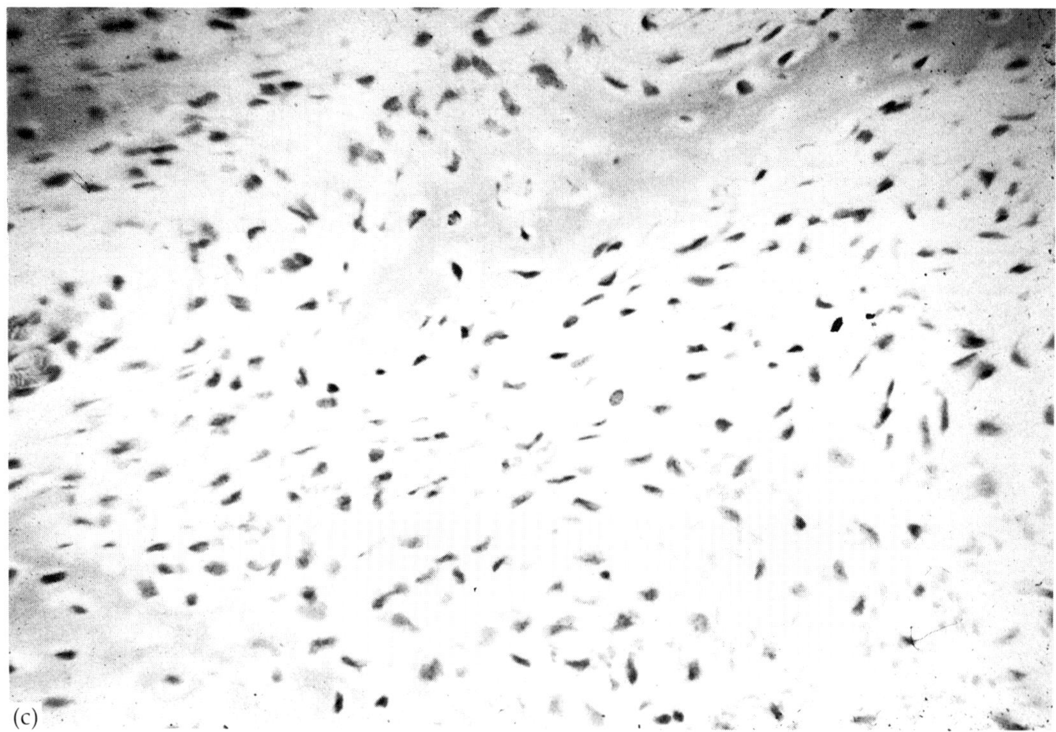

Figure 13.2 Fibrous dysplasia. (c) Early stage of bone formation. The bone increases by differentiation of osteoblasts adjacent to the bone which then enclose themselves in osteoid, becoming osteocytes in the process.

as a mixed lesion (Cohen *et al.*, 1962). Dahlin is quoted by Mirra (1989) as having concluded that the tissue of these cases does not represent classical fibrous dysplasia. Thus they are adamantinomas masquerading as fibrous dysplasia (Mirra, 1989). Personal experience leads to the conclusion that the masquerade is likely to be successful until the epithelial component is found. Thus, it is important thoroughly to study fibrodysplastic tissue from sites where adamantinoma is found, i.e. the major long bones, particularly the tibia and fibula, for an epithelial component.

'Ossifying fibroma' is a term that has been put to a number of uses, so that its use is liable to engender confusion, which is compounded by similarity to 'osteogenic fibroma'. The latter was applied to benign osteoblastoma but has now fallen out of use. In British pathology ossifying fibroma has come to be a term applied to lesions, mostly of the jaw and skull, which differ histologically from fibrous dysplasia in one respect, mantling of trabeculae by osteoblasts. The significance of this is arguable, and is argued. In 1983 Sissons *et al.* used the term for a lesion seen in two children, composed of spindle cell tissue containing rounded acellular, calcified bodies rather like those in meningioma or cementoma.

Malignant transformation in fibrous dysplasia is a recognized event (Taconis, 1988). The development of neoplasia alters the radiographic pattern of the lesion, with enlargement and loss of definition at the boundary. Pathological fracture may bring the lesion to notice; there may be soft tissue swelling. Histologically the transformed tissue is cellular, with cytological anaplasia and mitoses. The cells may form bone, osteosarcoma, or not, the lesion then being a spindle cell or fibrosarcoma.

13.4 NEOPLASIA

The initial descriptions of osteoid osteoma and benign osteoblastoma were in the 1930s by Jaffe and Jaffe and Mayer. The basic concept of two kinds of benign osteoblastic lesion, namely: a small painful lesion giving rise to abundant reactive bone, and a growing painless lesion with little reaction and with a predilection for vertebrae has been affirmed by experience. But in the course of this there has come to light a number of variants. These are osteoid osteoma of unusual size (sometimes called giant osteoid osteoma), multicentric osteoid osteoma and aggressive osteoblastoma. Most authorities tend to regard these as unrelated groups, but there is a point of view championed by Schajowicz (1981) that they are related entities.

13.4.1 OSTEOID OSTEOMA AND VARIANTS

The variants under consideration are multifocal and giant osteoid osteoma.

(a) Clinical features

The age range is from 3–80 years; most cases occur in the first three decades, the peak is in the second decade. There is a slight male preponderance.

(i) Skeletal distribution

Mirra (1989) gives the percentage, of 635 cases as:

- Jaws   <1
- Skull   <1
- Other flat bones
      Ribs   <1

      Girdles
          Shoulder: clavicle, scapula   1+
          Pelvic: ilium, pubis, sacrum   2
- Spine   6
      cervical 1, thoracic 1, lumbar 4
- Long tubular   71
      femur 34+, tibia 23, humerus 6   63+
      fibula, radius, ulna   7+
- Hands and feet   20+
      short tubular   11
          metacarpals 4, metatarsals 3,
          phalanges 4
      cuboidal   9+
          carpals <1, tarsals 9

In long bones the location is most frequently metaphyseal. In the femur, the proximal metaphysis, particularly the neck, is a common site. In the vertebral column it is more usual for the neural arch to be affected.

Apart from rare exceptions, this is a painful lesion, relieved by aspirin, but often for brief periods only. It heals spontaneously, but few patients can put up with the pain for the years this requires (Byers, 1968). It has been demonstrated that cutting the nerve supply to the bone relieves the pain (Mayer, 1958). Lesions in the spine can be a cause of scoliosis (Ransford *et al.*, 1984).

There are two variations on the classical theme in the form of multifocal and giant lesions. A few cases of the former have been described in which there have been adjacent foci in the same bone or foci in adjacent bones of osteoblastic tissue each of which has had the features of osteoid osteoma (Odell *et al.*, 1976). Giant osteoid osteoma is a rarely observed lesion which has the features of osteoid osteoma but is much larger in size (Dahlin and Johnson, 1954). On occasion such a lesion has first been observed when of small size, and has been diagnosed as osteoid osteoma. It is the presence of abundant reactive bone which establishes the diagnosis radiologically, distinguishing it from benign osteoblastoma. The histology of these is of the osteoid osteoma/benign osteo-

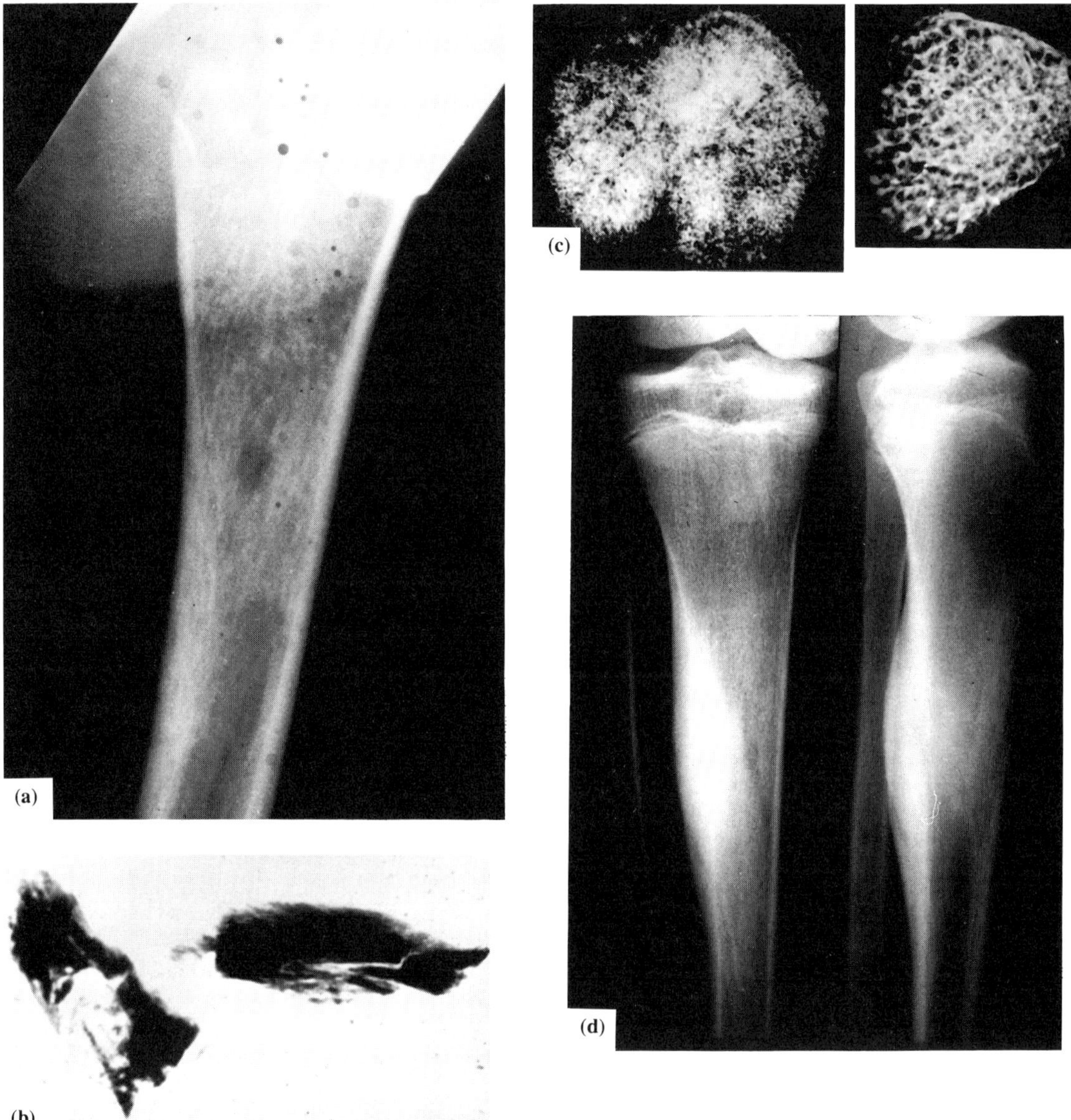

Figure 13.3 Osteoid osteoma. (a) Lesion on endocortical bone of proximal femoral metaphysis. Surrounding reactive bone is mainly cancellous, partly periosteal. (b) Fine detail radiograph of cortical fragments, one containing the non-mineralized lesion. (c) Fine detail radiograph of a heavily mineralized lesion showing the fine trabecular pattern (at the margins) compared with mixed cancellous and reactive bone. (d) Osteoid osteoma near periosteal surface giving rise to abundant periosteal reaction.

blastoma type and not that of aggressive osteoblastoma (see below).

Treatment is surgical removal of the lesion. Successful removal gives immediate relief. If removal is incomplete pain recurs shortly, and necessitates further surgery. There appear not to be sequelae if the lesion is not treated, and the pain ceases after a protracted period. A secondary scoliosis in spinal cases disappears following prompt removal.

(b)   Pathology

(i)   *Morbid anatomy* (Figure 13.3)

The lack of growth which characterizes osteoid osteoma and its potential to resolve contradicts the notion that it is a neoplasm. The size is in the range of a few mm to 2 cm, although most ascribe 1 or 1.5 cm as the maximum. The location within the bone may be cancellous or cortical; in the latter situation it may be centred anywhere from the endosteal to the periosteal surfaces. It generally provokes a substantial osteoblastic reaction, least when the location is medullary, but of increasing intensity as the position approaches the periosteal surface. At its maximum the periosteal reaction is a substantial, smooth, dense, swelling which may obscure the lesion. However, an exception to this is lesions on the neck of the talus. The lesion is osteolytic, well demarcated, and often with a radio-opaque centre where the density of the mineral can become sufficient to cast a detectible shadow. The fine detail radiograph of the tissue reveals a uniform trabecular pattern which contrasts in its delicacy with that of fracture callus (the latter, nevertheless, presenting a pattern of regularly disposed, uniform trabeculae in comparison with cancellous bone architecture). The surgeon may have to remove numerous bone chips in getting to the lesion, which creates a problem of identification in the laboratory. To avoid having to process all this material it can be spread out on radiolucent material,

radiographed, and left undisturbed until the film can be viewed. Then those fragments whose architecture is most similar to the pattern of osteoid osteoma can be processed.

(ii)   *Histopathology*

Histologically, the lesion is composed of vascular fibrous tissue containing a network of trabeculae of woven structure (Figure 13.4). Apart from varying surface coverage by osteoid, these are mineralized, but because of their delicacy the mineral density is often insufficient to show on clinical films. The central mineralization that may be evident results from aggregation of trabeculae to form a solid central mass. Osteoblasts and osteoclasts are abundant on the bone surfaces in much of the tissue and the bone is actively remodelled, although some deny this because cement lines are hard to visualize. At the extreme periphery of the lesion an insubstantial band of its fibrous tissue is free of the trabeculae, or else they are tenuous, providing a separation from the surrounding bone, but merging into the fibrous tissue of the marrow. Diligent search of sections stained for axons reveals nerves and individual axons in the fibrous tissue of marrow, zonal fibrous tissue and the fibrous tissue of the lesion itself in a proportion of cases (Byers, 1968; Schulman and Dorfman, 1970). Variation within this basic histological pattern can result from the number and activity of the bone cells. Occasional mitoses attest the production of cells; remodelling has already been referred to. The surrounding bone is subject to active turnover and shows a degree of mosaic pattern, and active surfaces.

The problem of identifying the lesion from among numerous bone fragments is discussed above. The diagnosis is established by demonstrating benign osteoblastic tissue, patterned as described above, from a small, stationary lesion in bone. The diagnosis is reinforced if there is a characteristic pattern of pain.

The radiographic appearance of the lesion

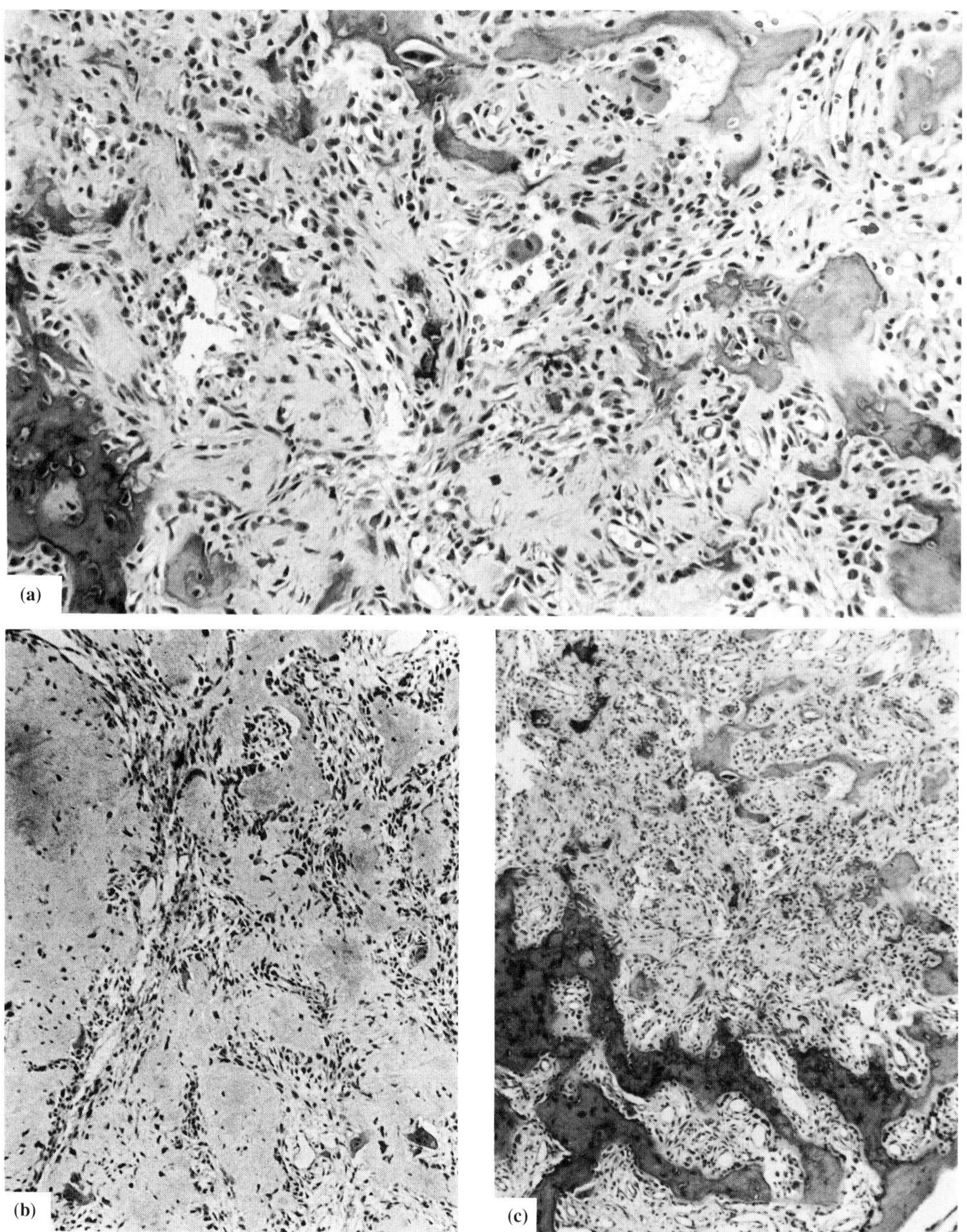

Figure 13.4 Benign osteoblastic tissue. (a, b) Fields of fine trabeculae, some mantled by normal osteoblasts, with intervening loose, sparsely cellular, fibrovascular tissue, which includes some osteoclasts. This tissue is characteristic of osteoid osteoma and benign osteoblastoma. (c) Tissue at the periphery of a lesion showing the progression to coarse trabeculae and sheets of osteoid/bone often seen in osteoid osteoma. Some tenuous shreds of perilesional fibrous tissue remain on the surface.

precludes a diagnosis of other osteoblastic lesions, but may be indistinguishable from bone abscess.

13.4.2 BENIGN OSTEOBLASTOMA

(a) Clinical features

The age range is from a few years to the seventh decade. There is a male preponderance of about 3:1.

(i) *Skeletal distribution*

Mirra (1989) gives percentage distribution of 135 cases as:

- Jaws   5.2
- Skull/nose   4.4
- Other flat bones

Ribs	4.4
Girdles	16.2
Shoulder: scapula	0.7
Pelvic: ilium 4.4, pubis 4.4,	
sacrum 6.7	15.5

- Spine   27.5

  Cervical 10.4, thoracic 10.4, lumbar 6.7
- Long tubular   30.4

Femur 10.4, tibia 9.6,	
humerus 5.2	25.2
Fibula, radius, ulna	5.2

- Hands and feet   10.4

  Short tubular 4.4

  Carpals 1.5, tarsals 4.4

Within a bone, the location is medullary, cortical, or occasionally periosteal. In long bones the location is nearly always metaphyseal.

The lesion does not produce the intense pain of osteoid osteoma. In some cases, as in the spine, the pain derives from pressure on adjacent tissues.

Curettage is the usual treatment. In inaccessible sites, such as the spinal column, radiotherapy may be employed.

Removal is curative. However, if it is incomplete ensuing recurrences can be troublesome. The question of progression to malignancy takes one into an area of controversy where there are several extant hypotheses. A discussion of this follows in section 13.1.3.

(ii) *Radiology*

The tumours are osteolytic, with well-defined margins (Figure 13.5). By definition they are in the order of 2 cm in size or larger, but even though they are growing lesions they seldom exceed 5 cm. They are often eccentrically located and expand the bone, with limited amounts of periosteal reaction. More central lesions do not cause substantial reactive bone. Mineralization is not a prominent feature.

(b) Pathology

(i) *Histopathology*

A fibrovascular stroma containing osteoid and bone trabeculae of woven structure with active, benign osteoblasts and osteoclasts at the surfaces, which field for field is similar to osteoid osteoma (Figure 13.4). Sheets of osteoid and bone are seldom present in benign osteoblastoma, which may be responsible for a sense of greater cellularity. But, in addition there can be fields free of trabeculae which also accentuate cellularity.

The diagnosis turns on the demonstration of benign osteoblastic tissue from a lesion larger than 2 cm clearly demarcated from the surrounding bone.

The differential diagnosis depends on both the radiographic and histological features. The tissue must be distinguished from that of other osteoblastic lesions. Confusion with sclerotic osteosarcoma may arise because the cells in it are neither numerous nor obviously anaplastic; but its matrix is very compact, without intertrabecular fibrovascular tissue. Confusion with giant cell tumour arises when osteoblastoma

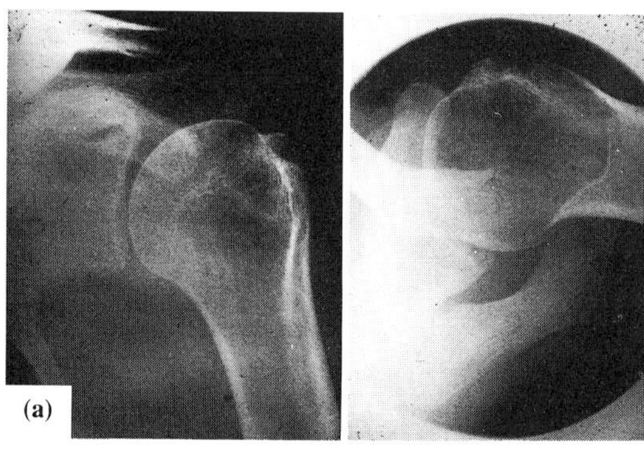

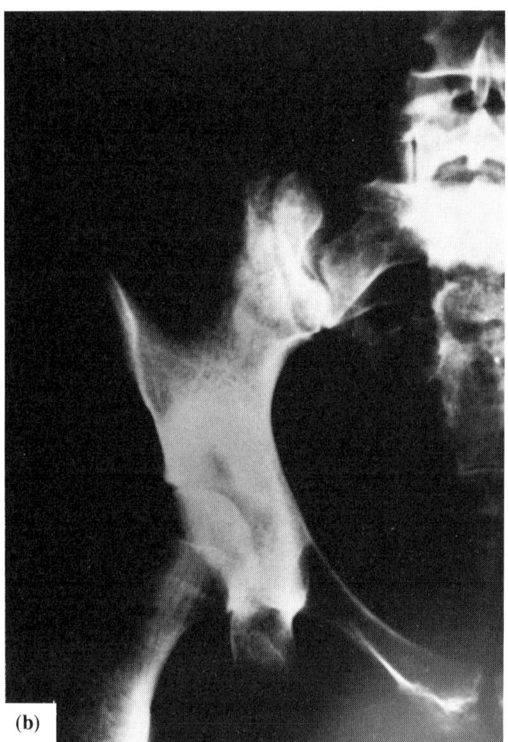

Figure 13.5 Benign osteoblastoma. (a) A well-demarcated, global, osteolytic lesion of the humeral head and metaphysis: the appearance is not specifically that of benign osteoblastoma. (b) A similar lesion in the roof of the acetabulum. Both lesions responded to curettage without recurrence. Histological features as in Figure 13.4 a,b,c.

contains a lot of osteoclasts, or a giant cell tumour has (reactive) bone formation. However, osteoblastoma is not centred on an epiphysis, which does not help with the rare vertebral giant cell tumour. Aneurysmal bone cyst of the spine is radiologically similar, but the tissues differ, unless the osteoblastoma has been subjected to aneurysmal bone cyst change; in that situation only the finding of intact osteoblastoma tissue can help. The more aggressive osteoblastomas discussed below must be suspected when any out-of-the-ordinary feature is observed by imaging or histology.

13.4.3 AGGRESSIVE OSTEOBLASTOMA (FIGURES 13.6 AND 13.7)

In 1976 Schajowicz and Lemos described eight cases, which they called malignant osteoblastoma, that had a tendency to recur rather than to metastasize, and an histology that was closer to benign osteoblastoma than to osteosarcoma. Dorfman (1973) and colleagues (Dorfman and Schiller, 1980; Dorfman and Weiss, 1984) described cases of similar behaviour but with some difference in histological detail under the name of aggressive osteoblastoma. McLeod *et al.* (1976) had recognized an osteoblastic osteosarcoma, which, in Dahlin's (1978) opinion, was the same as the entity described by the other two groups. However, Dorfman and Weiss (1984) extended their concept and proposed this group of osteoblastic lesions, intermediate between osteoblastoma and osteosarcoma, formed four distinct categories:

1. Low-grade osteoblastoma-like osteosarcomas
2. Pseudomalignant osteoblastoma
3. Malignant transformation of benign osteoblastoma
4. True aggressive osteoblastoma (malignant osteoblastoma)

Mirra (1989) advocates the subdivision of the last category into:

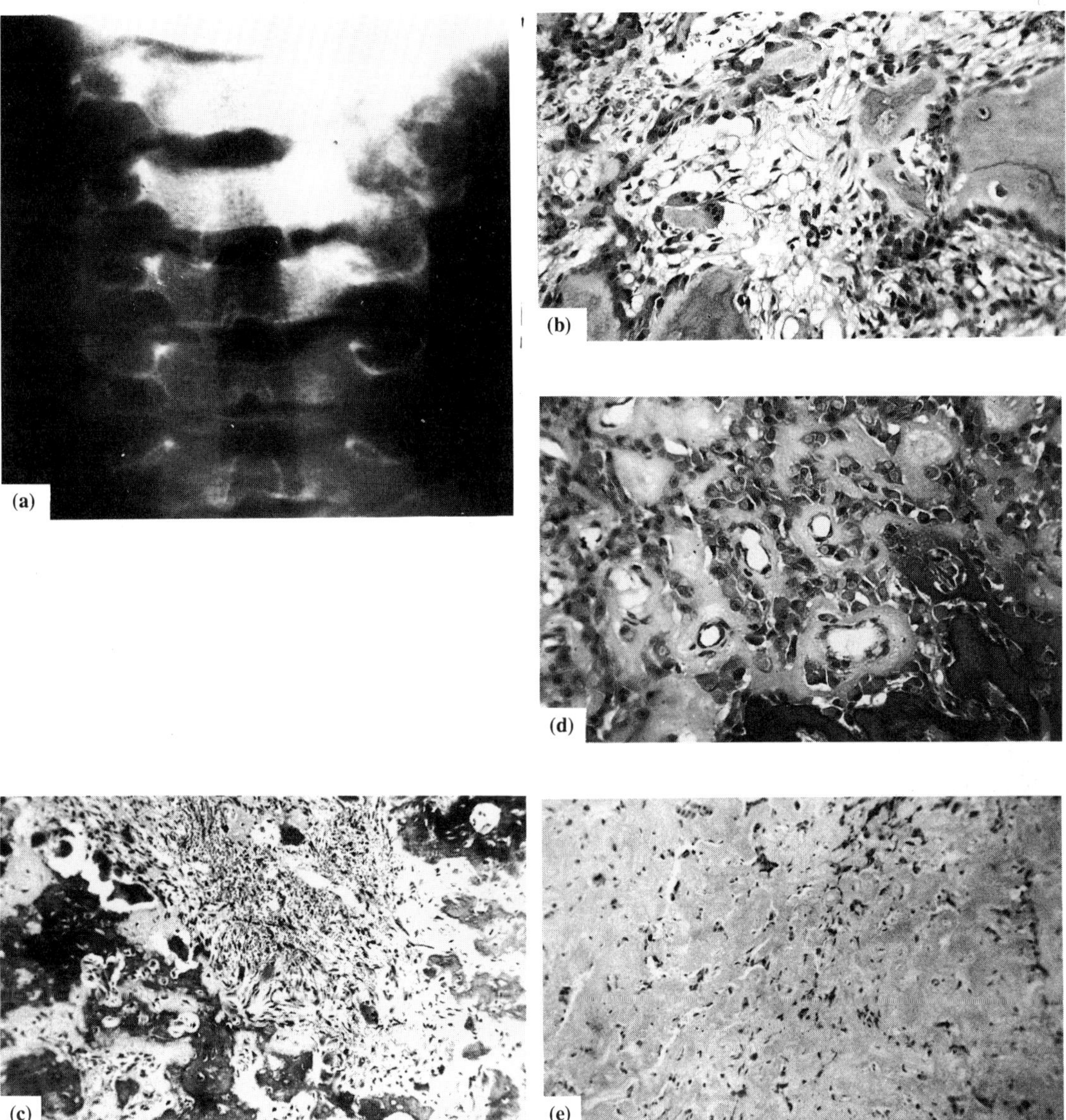

Figure 13.6 Aggressive osteoblastoma (a) Male 7 years. Stiff neck. A large round lesion arising from the transverse process of C3. Its limit is marked in part by a shell of bone. The cloudy mineralization is osteoblastic. The demarcation, diffuse bone formation (as opposed to graded development), the site point to osteoblastoma rather than osteosarcoma. The size raises the possibility of aggressive osteoblastoma. (b) Benign osteoblastic tissue. (c) A mixed field of very cellular tissue, without significant anaplasia, surrounded by sheet osteoid with trabecular mineralization. (d) A close trabecular pattern with room only for plump osteoblasts. (e) A trabecular tissue from which nearly all cells are excluded. The variegated tissue, and local recurrence after the first resection, support the diagnosis of aggressive osteoblastoma. The child remained well following a second removal.

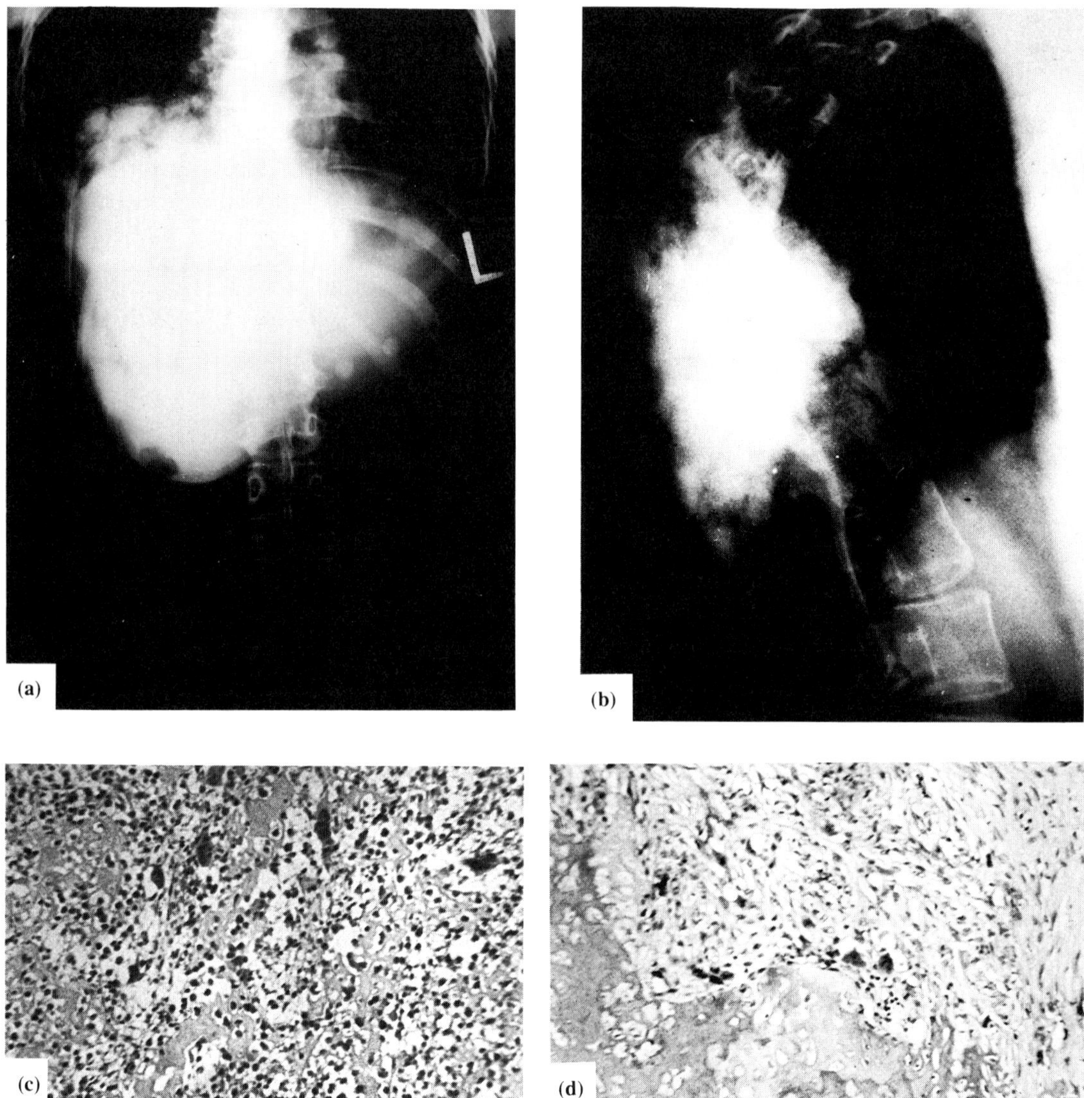

Figure 13.7 Aggressive osteoblastoma. Female aged 25 years at onset of illness; (a,b) radiograph 8 years later after four attempts at excision. Large osteoblastic mass attached to lower thoracic vertebrae. Patient died two years later with massive involvement of diaphragm. No metastases. (c) One of several patterns of osteoblastic tissue; abundantly cellular, but no significant anaplasia. (d) A field of benign fibrovascular tissue encroaching on sheet osteoid/bone.

1. True aggressive osteoblastoma, including toxic osteoblastoma
2. *In situ* osteosarcoma

The basis for these categories are summarized below.

(a)   Low-grade osteoblastoma-like osteosarcoma

This was described by Dahlin and colleagues and was reviewed by them in 1985 (Bertoni *et al.*, 1985). In some osteosarcomas there is abundant bone formation. The effect of this is to reduce greatly the space available to cells, and those that remain lose their malignant characteristics and appear benign. Jaffe (1958) commented on this 'normalizing' influence. Seen early, while still within the medulla and without periosteal reaction, they invite consideration as osteoblastoma (although the fluffy margin is a counterindication). If that diagnosis is made then later events will raise the possibilities of malignant osteoblastoma or transformation of osteoblastoma. There are histological features that lead to the diagnosis of osteosarcoma: invasiveness of the tumour; solid bone and osteoid with no intertrabecular fibrovascular tissue; no osteoblastic rimming; the presence of cartilage is indicative of osteosarcoma; cell clusters will show anaplasia.

(b)   Pseudomalignant osteoblastoma

Mirra *et al.* (1976) reported a case of osteoblastoma in which there were numerous cells with multiple, large bizarre nuclei and osteoblasts with similar nuclear features indicative of anaplasia. However, radiologically the lesion was small and well demarcated, and histologically no mitotic activity was found. Mirra (1989) has since seen a second case and believes two cases referred to by Dahlin are similar. Since similar pseudomalignant change is described in other neoplasias he presents this as a diagnostic category.

(c)   Malignant transformation of benign osteoblastoma

Mirra (1989) suggests that the foregoing categories account for instances of this kind, but acknowledges that the possibility of such an occurrence cannot be excluded.

(d)   True aggressive osteoblastoma according to Dorfman and Weiss (1984)

Observations have been made on 15 cases (no details given of the basis of selection). The radiographic appearance was presumably the usual features of conventional osteoblastoma. Histological features were as follows:

- Wider and more irregular trabeculae; cement lines not usually present
- Non-trabecular osteoid in seven cases
- Lace-like osteoid in four cases
- Osteoclastic foci prominent in nine, less so in six cases
- Epithelioid osteoblasts were the most prominent feature (twice the size of normal osteoblasts; rounded; large vesicular nuclei; abundant cytoplasm; scattered or in sheets)
- Stroma of well-differentiated fibroblasts
- Low mitotic activity, no abnormal forms
- Seven lesions recurred within two years of therapy, but no metastases

(e)   Malignant osteoblastoma according to Schajowicz and Lemos (1976) and Schajowicz (1981)

There were the usual features of conventional osteoblastoma: blue spiculated bone; immature, small trabeculae staining dark blue in H & E sections; similar to bone in osteosarcoma. Mitoses were more numerous than in osteoblastoma, including atypical forms. There were local recurrences if not completely removed.

No metastases were found.

(f)   Toxic osteoblastoma

Mirra *et al.* (1976) encountered an osteoblastoma causing such severe constitutional symptoms (fever, clubbing of the fingers, anaemia, hypergammaglobulinaemia, cachexia, grave morbidity) that the affected leg was amputated. The patient immediately recovered. The lesion had given rise to abundant reactive bone and was surrounded by large numbers of plasma cells and lymphocytes. But the histology of the lesion was similar to benign osteoblastoma. It is proposed that an inappropriate immune response was responsible for the systemic reaction. Dorfman and Schiller (1980) described a similar case.

(g)　*In situ* osteosarcoma

This is Mirra's (1989) concept of aggressive osteoblastoma, of malignant osteoblastoma, and of osteoblastoma-like osteosarcoma. He cites lipoma-like liposarcoma as an example: an inexorably recurring lesion if not completely removed, which will only metastasize if there is transformation to a high grade. For him aggressive osteoblastoma is an equivalent lesion. He acknowledges the difficulties that surround the subject, and that they will be resolved only by continued study of cases and discussion. The foregoing discussion concerns a small proportion of osteoblastomas, lesions bordering on malignancy, culled over time from the larger group because of behaviour, or some inconsistency with the recognized pattern of osteoblastoma, or both. The panoply of pattern of most neoplasms is difficult to convey in words or to depict in pictures. The selection of each, words and pictures, will be biased by beliefs, with the result that it can be difficult to know if the things are the same and only the beliefs differ or if more than one thing is under discussion. Personal experience has been of a group of osteoblastic lesions in the middle ground between benign and malignant, recognizable by combining careful radiographic and histological scrutiny in the light of clinical data. This experience is summarized here (Figures 13.6 and 13.7).

(h)　Clinical features

(i)　*Skeletal distribution*

The axial skeleton and the major long bones are all affected. Lesions are mainly centred on the medulla.

Where possible the lesion should be removed surgically. Otherwise radiotherapy is used.

For surgically amenable cases the prognosis is good. Otherwise there is a protracted course of partially successful treatments with death resulting from local complications.

(i)　Pathology

(i)　*Morbid anatomy*

Two tissue patterns are manifest, one sclerotic and poorly cellular and the other cellular with a variable but limited amount of bone. This results in two radiological patterns: a round, dense demarcated lesion with a lucent line separating it from the bone; and one with irregular bone formation, also demarcated. In both instances there is little osteoblastic reaction, and no cortical invasion. The latter lesion may extend well beyond the anatomical limits of the host bone, but remains within the periosteum. Growth is slow.

(ii)　*Histopathology*

The first type is a very poorly cellular neoplasm, with growth occurring at the periphery by membrane formation in the thin layer of cellular tissue by which it is enclosed and separated from the bone. The pattern of the tissue that results is very distinctive with its radially oriented trabeculae. Already poorly cellular at the periphery, there is a progressive diminution in their number towards the centre and a proportionate increase in the bone volume, accounting for the radiological appearance. In the other pattern of development the picture is more variable. The tissue is cellular with bone-free zones and others in which bone formation is variable to the point of producing small foci similar to those of the first type. These form the evidence that they are related. Lesions of this more cellular type can grow to a large size, and may be difficult to remove when they occur in a vertebra. As they grow larger the tissue becomes more variable as the result of tissue remodelling in which foci of old tissue are replaced by new, giving rise to a somewhat lobulated appearance. The remodelling is effected at least in part by osteoclasts which are common throughout.

Despite some variation in cytology, which can extend to pleomorphism, hyperchromatism and occasional mitoses, the tissue pattern is not that of osteosarcoma. However, it does in part resemble benign osteoblastoma.

In a typical case the age, site and morbid anatomy will positively support the histological recognition of non-malignant osteoblastic tissue. The distinctive zoning features of the tissue are also diagnostic.

The differentiation from benign osteoblastoma and osteosarcoma can often be established histologically. However, when this is not apparent the clinical and radiological findings give guidance.

13.4.4 OSTEOSARCOMA

Osteosarcoma is a malignant neoplasm whose cells have the capacity to form osteoid and bone. In a given case the recognition of malignancy is based on the morbid anatomy, as demonstrated by radiograph, and the pattern and cytology of the tissue. The bone-forming potential is also a morbid anatomical and histological decision. Given that there is radiographically detectible mineral, the pattern of its disposition will often indicate that it is bone rather than cartilage, as discussed in Chapter 4. The histological recognition and assessment of bone has been

Table 13.3 Osteosarcoma and its variants

Osteosarcoma	Malignant grade		
	High	*Medium*	*Low*
Intraosseus (in bone)			
Primary			
1 Unqualified	+		
2 Osteoblastic	+		
3 Chondroblastic	++		
4 Fibroblastic	+		
5 Fibrohistiocytic (MFH)	+		
6 Telangiectatic	+		
7 Osteoclast rich	+		
8 Small cell	+		
9 Epithelioid	+		
10 Intracortical	+		
11 Central		+	
Secondary			
Paget's	++		
Irradiation	+		
Multicentric			
Synchronous		+	
Metachronous		+	
Jaw		+	
Juxtacortical			
Parosteal			+
Periosteal		+	
Soft tissue (in soft)		+	
Variants unusual but may be 1–6 as for intraosseous			

discussed in Chapter 2.

A number of categories of osteosarcoma have been established on the basis of features in one or more of the morbid anatomy, the histological structure or the grade of malignancy (Unni and Dahlin, 1989). As indicated in Table 13.3 most of the variants are high grade with a poor prognosis. The few lower-grade types are important to recognize on the grounds of their differing treatment and outcome.

Anatomically the principal division is intraosseous and juxtacortical, i.e. in and on bone. Soft tissue osteosarcoma is a third anatomical division.

Subclassification within these is by tissue structure. In the period just prior to the advent of chemotherapy it was the fashion to play down the subdivisions of intraosseous osteosarcoma since there was little or no difference in prognosis to be detected by the treatments then available. But the need for assessment of the immediate and long-term response to chemotherapeutic treatment brought attention to the subcategories and the problem of the criteria to be used in their recognition. The definition of osteosarcoma remained unaltered, namely: a sarcoma whose cells had the potential to make osteoid. But the development of fine-needle aspiration biopsy posed a problem in the recognition of this potential, which ordinarily depended on the association of osteoid/bone and malignant cells in a pattern persuasive of the former having been formed by the latter. The solution was the application of the histochemical reaction for alkaline phosphatase to tissue films on glass slides prepared at the time of biopsy. A positive reaction is indicative of osteoblasts, the assessment of malignancy being by the usual criteria.

Variability of tissue pattern is a feature of osteosarcoma. This may be limited to the degree of bony differentiation and development or it may involve the presence of a number of connective tissue elements: cartilage, fibrous/spindle cell tissue, vascular spaces, osteoclasts. Moreover, the degree to which the cells are developed or differentiated can also vary. These variations can combine to produce many patterns, and since there is now potential advantage in recognizing variants their number has been slowly growing.

It must be recognized, however, that not all neoplasms are going to be differentiated and that some neoplasms in bone may not be classifiable histologically, even to the point where primary or secondary must be decided on clinical grounds (Figure 13.8).

The advantage concerns differences in behaviour of some variants, which influences the choice of the slowly extending treatments that are available, and the prognosis.

However it must be realized that not all of these variants behave differently from what can be called unqualified, or perhaps, primary high grade osteosarcoma; that the significance of the pattern is not known, and that the usefulness of annotating them lies in the realm of diagnosis in pointing to potential pitfalls.

The term unqualified in Table 13.3 implies that there are osteosarcomas which do not manifest features requiring the use of a qualifying term. Consideration of such cases is a useful start for discussing osteosarcoma. The variants, whose hallmarks will be mentioned at appropriate points, have been listed in Table 13.3.

(a)   Osteoblastic sarcomas; in bone; unqualified osteosarcoma

(i)   *Clinical features*

The age range is 2–50 years with the peak in the 2nd and 3rd decades.

Skeletal distribution The percentage distribution of all high-grade osteosarcomas from the Latin American Registry of Bone Pathology (Schajowicz, 1981) is as follows:

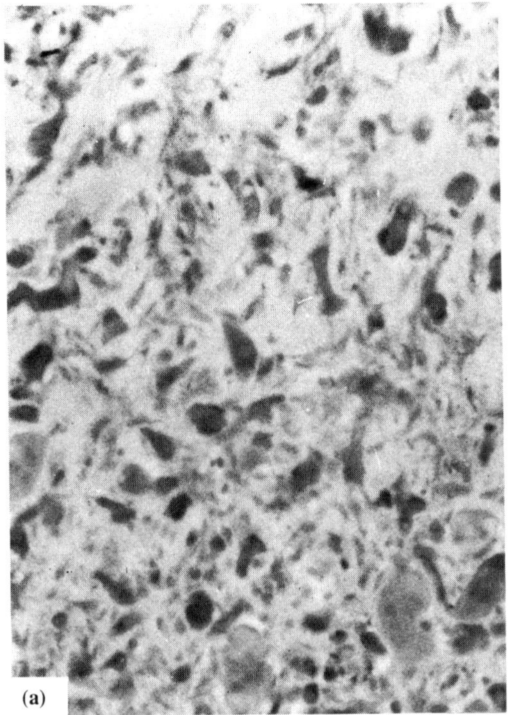 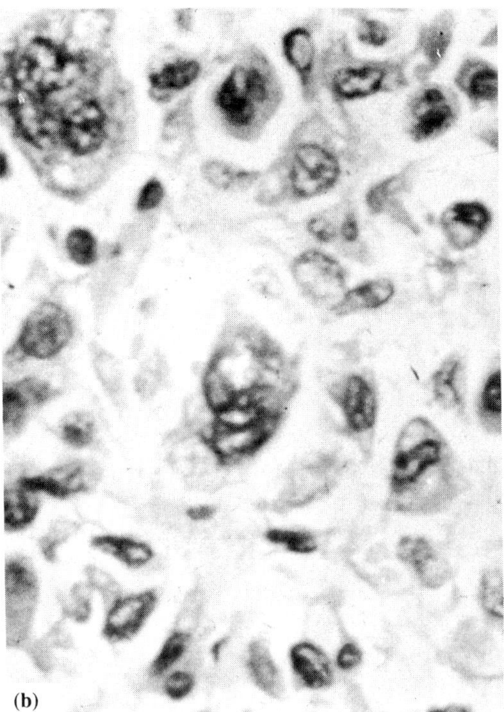

(a) (b)

Figure 13.8 (a,b) Malignant tumour. Biopsies of tumours in bone sometimes present undifferentiated tissue in a variety of patterns, such as the illustrations. There are no objective criteria in the tissue here to go beyond malignant tumour unspecified. Clinical and radiographic information, and special procedures may help to move the diagnosis along the scale of metastatic, primary, or specific malignancy.

- Jaws   3
- Skull   2
- Other flat bones
  - Ribs
  - Girdles   5
    - Shoulder: clavicle, scapula   1.5
    - Pelvic: ilium, pubis, sacrum   3.5
- Spine   1
  - Cervical, thoracic, lumbar (sacral)
- Long tubular   85
- Hands and feet   1.5

Details of the lesions found in the long tubular bones are shown in Table 13.4.

References to osteosarcomas at uncommon sites are given by: craniofacial osteosarcoma, Lee *et al.* (1988); vertebral osteosarcoma, Tigani *et al.* (1988), Miller *et al.* (1992); hand, Carroll (1957); toe phalanx, Mirra *et al.* (1988).

Clinical presentation is with pain of varying severity, accompanied by local swelling and heat.

(ii) Pathology

Morbid anatomy (Figure 13.9) About two-thirds of tumours in long bones are metaphyseal, usually eccentric. In its earliest stages, the tumour is cellular with little differentiation, a condition which persists at the periphery, whereas, with time and enlargement, bone production increases towards the centre at the expense of the cells. The tumour is invasive, but sooner or later

Table 13.4 Skeletal distribution of unqualified osteosarcoma in long tubular bones

	Metaphyseal		*Diaphyseal*	*Totals*
	Proximal	*Distal*		
Humerus	47	2	3	52
Femur	30	192	25	247
Tibia	102	15	6	123
Radius	1	8	9	18
Ulna	1			1
Fibula	17			17
Totals	397		61	458 (knee=294)

leads to bone resorption. Thus, in the beginning and at the margins tissue of little differentiation is invading the marrow, provoking minimal or no resorption: the lack of differentiation means little or no bone formation and hence none or insufficient contrast material (calcium) to be visible on radiograph. However, towards the centre there is increasing density as the amount of bone builds up. The physis resists penetration by the tumour, so that epiphyseal involvement is late. But penetration of the cortex along vascular routes, with or without the aid of resorption, brings tumour to the outside. A periosteal response, which may be lamellar, spicular or nondescript occurs early; rarely, it may be the first radiographic sign that a lesion is present. This response is accentuated as the tumour accumulates externally, but becomes confined to the angle between the swelling and the cortex (Codman's triangle).

Histopathology In keeping with the graded density there is a wide range of osteoid and bone formation (Figures 13.10 and 13.11). Peripherally there are purely cellular expanses of tumour. These give way centripetally to increasing amounts of bone, at first in the form of delicate trabeculae, then progressively broader trabeculae which eventually form sheets of bone with diminishing cell spaces. The cellular component is in inverse proportion to the bone. As the cells diminish in number so does their anaplastic features, to the point where they appear normal. Jaffe

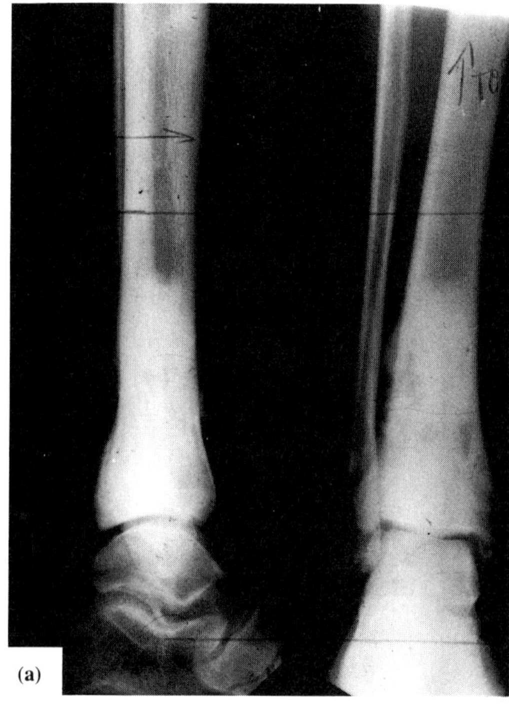

Figure 13.9 Osteosarcoma. (a) Clinical radiograph of 14-year-old male. Osteoblastic tissue involves the lower third of the tibia, obliterating landmarks. The lateral cortex has been penetrated: the limits of the soft tissue swelling are marked by Codman triangles.

(1958) referred to this as 'normalization', and is followed in this by Mirra (1989).

Immunohistochemistry has not been performed to any extent in osteosarcomas; some results have been published by Hasegawa *et al.* (1991).

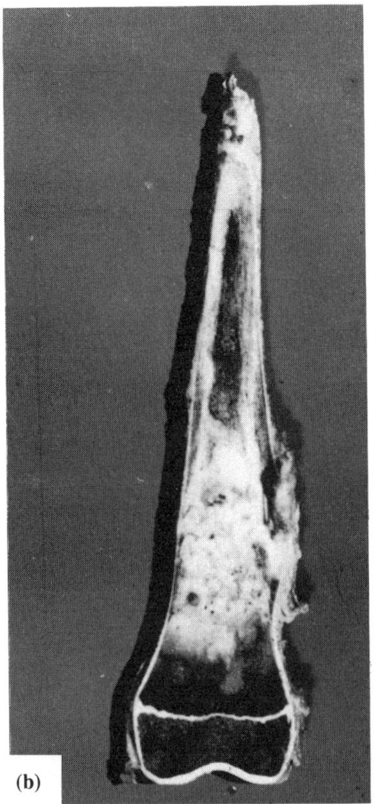

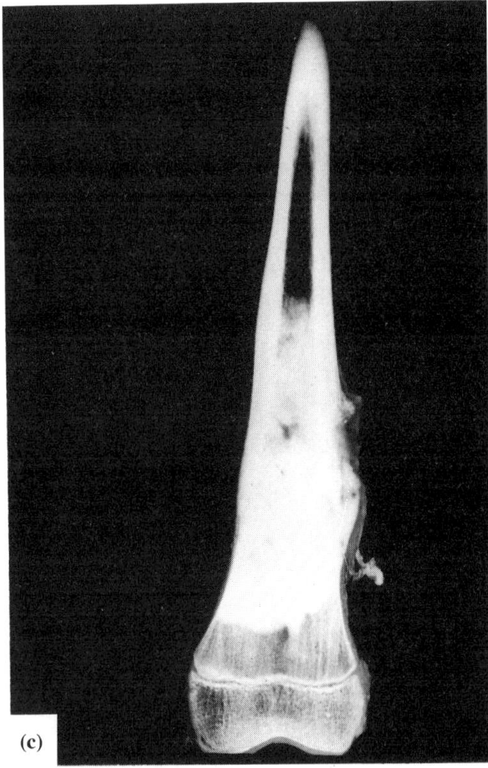

Figure 13.9 Osteosarcoma. (b, c) Cut surface and slab radiograph of distal femur occupied by osteosarcoma. There are signs in each that tissue extends in both directions beyond the main mass of the tumour. Histological sections show cellular tissue extending through marrow down to the physis.

(b) Variants of intraosseous osteosarcoma

The features which lead to the use of qualifying terms concern cell differentiation and the quality and quantity of the matrix component.

The lesion described above is clearly osteoblastic, but it is one in which there is a substantial cellular component. There are osteosarcomas where the matrix predominates leading to the ready use of the description 'sclerotic'. For many this is the meaning of osteoblastic osteosarcoma, and the level of sclerosis at which it is used is subjective (Bertoni *et al.*, 1985). An alternative use of the term is as a way of emphasizing that the lesion does not have a component of one of the other variants. Those are principally fibroblastic and chondroblastic, and are used to indicate that the tumour is composed of striking amounts of those tissues. There are no absolute values for 'striking amount', but at least a dominant amount of the tissue must be of the category. Given that the diagnosis is being made on a biopsy, sampling may determine the histological decision. Some degree of corroboration can be looked for in the radiographs. Since fibrous tissue does not mineralize, and cartilage does so in recognizable patterns, these variants will have radiolucent regions proportional to the volume of these tissues. Radiologically

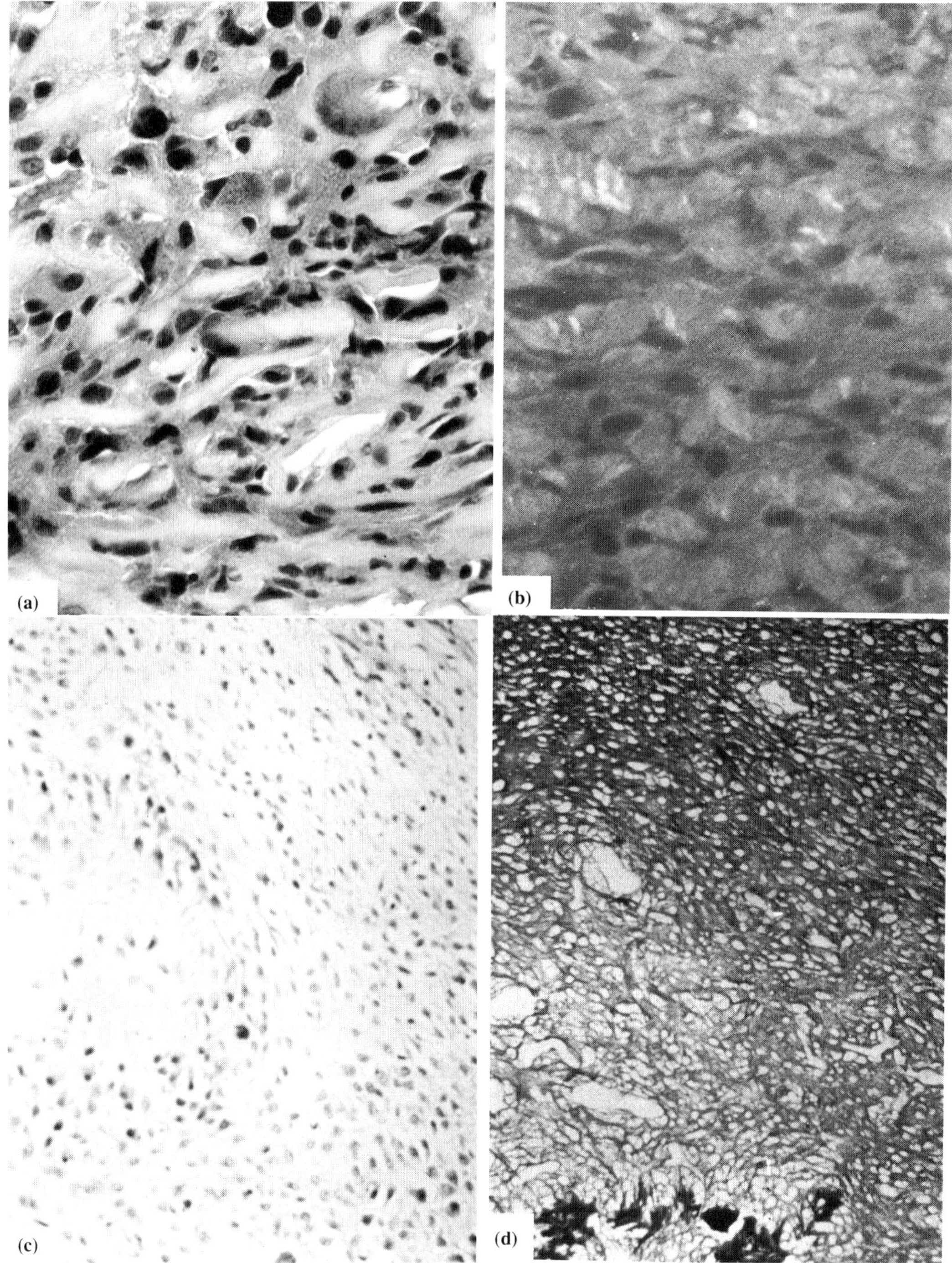

Figure 13.10 Minimal bone formation in osteosarcoma. Sites of suspect osteoid formation in H&E stains (a, c) are readily studied in polarized light (b), which will reveal collagen aggregation in a woven pattern if it is osteoid. Collagen or reticulin (d) stains will identify the collagen but not the woven pattern.

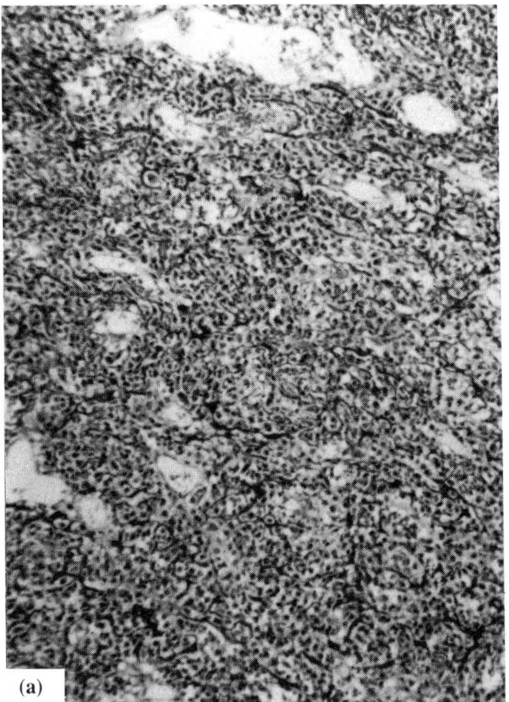 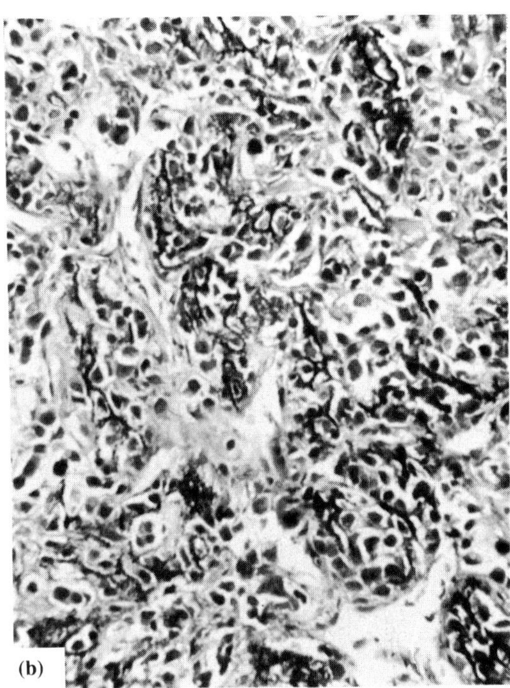

Figure 13.11 Osteosarcoma. Patterns of bone formation. (a) Very cellular tissue, with rounded cells; the threads of bone are dark due to the mineral, creating a pattern suggestive of chondroblastoma. (b) Focal 'chicken wire' ossification enhances that suggestion; but note the anaplasia.

there is no way to distinguish these from one another, nor from volumes of undifferentiated osteoblastic tissue. The diagnosis requires evidence that the tumour has osteoblastic potential and that more than half the tissue is fibroblastic or chondroblastic. Given a biopsy sample and a radiograph it is clear that some assumptions must be made to arrive at a definitive diagnosis that goes beyond primary malignant bone tumour unspecified.

The fibroblastic component is spindle celled, cellular and usually with limited collagen matrix. Sometimes there is an admixture of other mononuclear cells in addition to the spindle cells resulting in an appearance similar to malignant fibrous histiocytoma (Ballance *et al.*, 1988). The chondroblastic element is relatively more variable in its degree of differentiation ranging from a hyaline matrix with round chondroblasts, with features of malignancy, to a mucinous matrix with stellate cells. Total loss of differentiation, with round, oval or spindle cells, pleomorphism and mitotic activity renders impossible the recognition of these features. And if this also affects the osteoblastic component then the only diagnosis possible is primary malignant bone tumour unspecified. But it is necessary again to emphasize that the histological diagnosis of osteosarcoma depends on the persuasive demonstration of bone matrix formed by malignant cells or of connective tissue cells positive for alkaline phosphatase. But there can be combinations of radiographic appearances and non-osteoblastic malignant tissue which

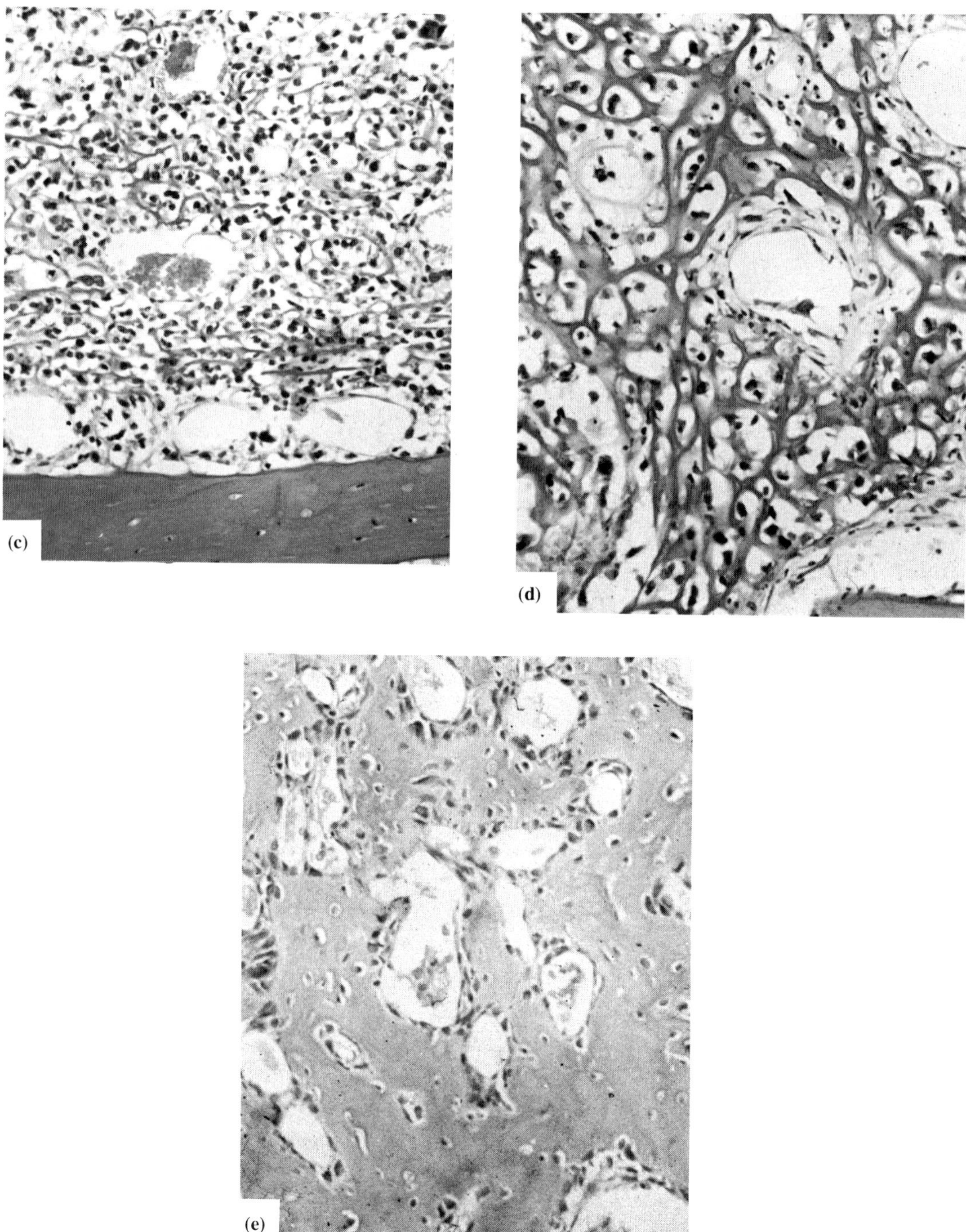

Figure 13.11 Osteosarcoma. Patterns of bone formation. (c, d) Lacework of osteoid; the cellularity reduces as the osteoid increases, but anaplasia is still evident. (e) Massive bone formation, with normalization of cells; the tissue resembles that the other osteoblastic tumours can produce.

will lead to a diagnosis of an osteosarcoma variant.

Some of the variants of osteosarcoma have attracted such interest that data relating to them individually have been assembled.

(i)   Telangiectatic variant (Matsuno *et al.*, 1976; Kyriakos and Hardy, 1991)

Age: decades 1 to 3
Site: long tubular bones are the most usual sites.
Clinical: pain and rapidly progessing swelling.
Morbid anatomy: permeative destruction of bone, involving cortex and medulla, extension to soft tissue early and extensive, little or no reactive bone or tumour bone formation (Figure 13.12).
Histopathology: this tissue is dominated by large thin-walled vascular spaces, greater in volume than can be accounted for by vascular congestion. Although the distribution of the vessels can vary, well over half the tissue volume is occupied by them. At the extreme it can be very difficult to identify the osteoblastic component, and the diagnosis may appear to rest in the category of vascular neoplasia, with aneurysmal bone cyst (ABC) a prime candidate. Thus the diagnosis could rest on a judgement of this possibility.
Diagnosis: as in all osteosarcoma the diagnosis turns on demonstrating tumour bone and/or malignant osteoblasts (alkaline phosphatase).
Differential diagnosis: vascular neoplasia, and possibly ABC. An extensive permeative pattern of destruction is not a feature of ABC, nor cells with a malignant cytology. In the poorly cellular tissue it may be difficult to establish the nature of the cells.
Treatment: responds to chemotherapy.
Prognosis: an aggressive lethal variant that is apparently controlled by chemotherapy.

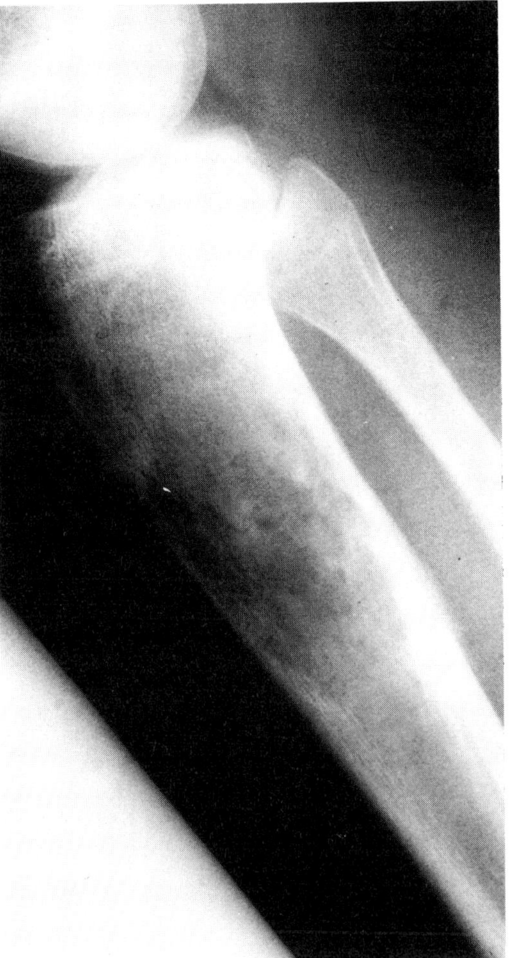

Figure 13.12 Radiograph of telangiectatic osteosarcoma.

(ii)   Giant cell rich variant (Sanerkin, 1989)

Age: decades 1 to 3.
Site: femoral and tibial diaphyses are usual.
Clinical: slowly developing pain and swelling; pathological fracture is frequent.
Morbid anatomy: metaphyseal location, global destruction, expansion with cortical thinning, little or no periosteal reaction. Looks more like giant cell tumour (GCT) or aneurysmal bone cyst (ABC).

Histopathology: these are cellular tumours in which osteoclasts are prominent, and bone formation not always strikingly apparent. A strong resemblance to GCT exists, because of the numerous osteoclasts, and the problem is to avoid this diagnosis. This is perhaps most easily done by careful search for tumour bone.

Diagnosis: the usual criteria.

Differential diagnosis: the problem is to avoid diagnosing ABC and GCT. Age may help, the finding of malignant cells forming bone – a task of some difficulty.

Treatment: as for conventional disease.

Prognosis: poor.

(iii)   Central low-grade osteosarcoma (Kurt *et al.*, 1990)

Age: decades 1 to 5, with peak in 2–4.

Site: long bones of lower limb.

Clinical: chronic low level pain.

Morbid anatomy: metaphyseal or diaphyseal. Global destruction, well demarcated. Expansion, thinning of cortex, or periosteal apposition. Tumour mineralization not obvious.

Histopathology: the cellular component is fibrocellular with cytological evidence of malignancy. Within this are coarse trabeculae of immature bone with a disposition reminiscent of fibrous dysplasia.

Diagnosis: cytological malignancy and tumour bone formation = malignant osteoblastic lesion = OS.

Differential diagnosis: the problem is to avoid fibrous dysplasia.

Treatment: surgical ablation.

Prognosis: good, if adequately treated at first attempt.

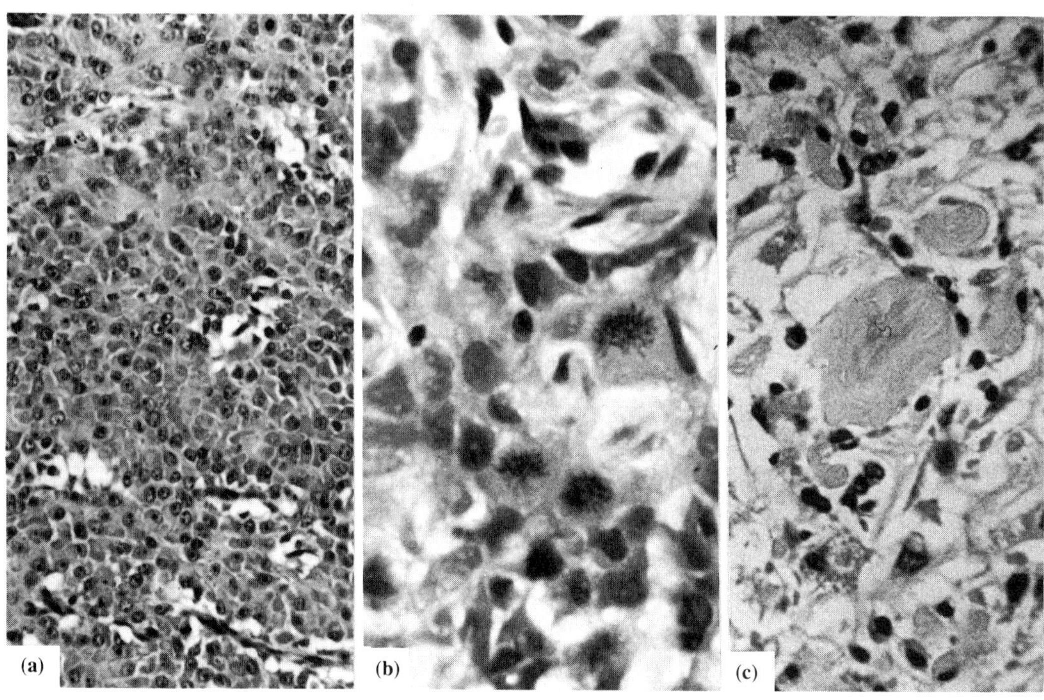

Figure 13.13 Epithelioid osteosarcoma. (a) A field composed mainly of large cells with abundant opaque cytoplasm. (b) In other areas a mixture of epitheliod and spindle cells was present. (c) Other areas provided the evidence of bone formation essential to the diagnosis.

(iv) Intracortical osteosarcoma (Lopez-Barea
   et al., 1991; Mirra *et al.*, 1991; Kyriakos
   et al., 1992)

Age: decades 1 to 4.
Site: diaphyseal cortex of tibia or femur
(Kyriakos *et al.*, 1992).
Clinical: the rarest form of osteosarcoma
(OS). Pain and swelling.
Radiographic appearance: early: small
intracortical osteolytic focus with some
reactive bone; a non-specific pattern, often
of benign appearance. Late: extension to
medulla (? and soft tissue) and appearances
of OS.
Histopathology: all reported lesions have
been of sclerotic type, with one exception
(Kyriakos *et al.*, 1992) which was a small cell
variant.
Diagnosis: the diagnosis is determined by
site and histology.
Differential diagnosis: the residual cells of
a sclerotic osteosarcoma can appear normal
and this might deflect the diagnosis
towards osteoblastoma (q.v.).
Treatment: as for conventional OS.
Prognosis: as for conventional OS.

(v) Small cell osteosarcoma (Ayala *et al.*,
   1989; Kyriakos *et al.*, 1992)

This variant affects the same age group and
occurs in the same sites as conventional
osteosarcoma, and has the same prognosis. It
is distinctive because of the small uniform
cells which suggest Ewing's sarcoma, lymphoma or chondroblastoma. The last is
accentuated by the pattern of bone formation, matrix always being present in these
tumours, and by the occasional presence of
cartilage.

(vi) Epithelioid osteosarcoma (Yoshida *et al.*,
   1989) (Figure 13.13)

Another group distinctive by reason of its
structure but equally malignant as the others.
Cells with a distinctly epithelial cast are
gathered in compact groups and sheets
within which delicate trabeculae of osteoid
are formed. This may form only part of the
structure of a lesion.

(vii) Osteosarcoma in Paget's disease (Price
   and Goldie, 1969) (Figure 13.14)

Age: decades 5 to 8.
Site: in order of frequency: pelvis, femur,
skull, tibia.
Clinical: pain and swelling.
Morbid anatomy: global destructive lesion
with irregular, wide transition. A small
proportion have OS patterns of mineral
deposition.
Histopathology: primary sarcomas of bone
in this condition are often poorly differentiated and the evidence for a diagnosis of
OS may be wanting, or else there may be
fibroblastic or chondroid features.
Diagnosis: evidence of Paget's disease of
bone (this may be radiological), and of primary
malignant connective tissue neoplasia, with or
without evidence of differentiation.
Differential diagnosis: little difficulty.
Prognosis: whatever the character of the
tumour the prognosis is bad.

(viii) Post-irradiation sarcoma (Weatherby *et al.*,
   1981; Huvos, 1986)

Age: decades 5 to 8.
Site: of previous irradiation.
Clinical: pain and swelling at site of previous
irradiation. Criteria for the diagnosis were
postulated by Cahan *et al.* (1948):

   site was originally normal or had a benign
   lesion.

   radiation was sufficient: >60 Gy.

   latent period 5–30 years.

   histological proof of tumour.

Morbid anatomy: destructive lesion with
wide transition zone.

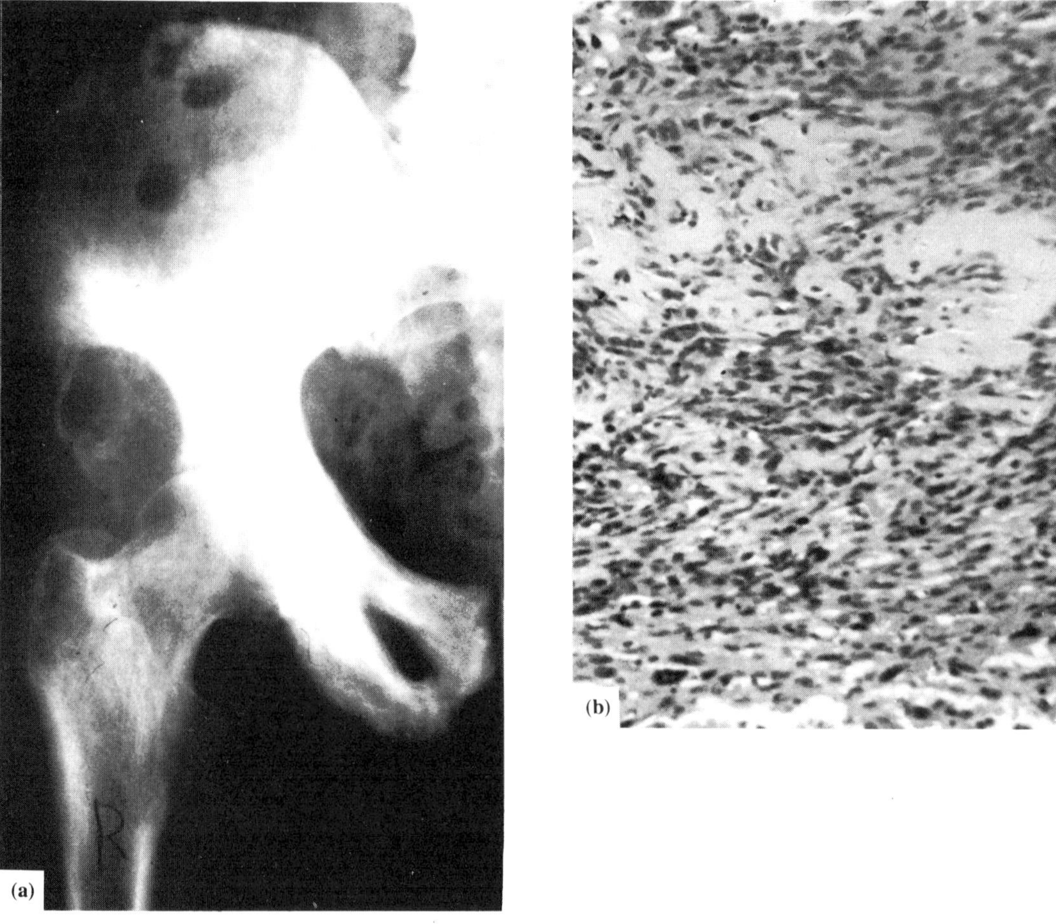

Figure 13.14 Paget's sarcoma. (a) Paget's disease of pelvis and right femur. A mass of tumour tissue, bulging externally from the ilium, has cloudy mineralization. (b) The neoplasm was composed of pleomorphic spindle cell tissue which produced small foci of osteoid/bone.

Histopathology: the resulting neoplasms are a variety of primary malignant connective tissue tumours, only a small proportion of which are an osteosarcoma. However, it has long been usage to refer to them as osteosarcoma.
Diagnosis: discussed above.
Differential diagnosis: beyond recognizing malignancy there is no problem.
Prognosis: poor.

(ix)   Multicentric osteosarcoma (Mahoney *et al.*, 1979)

Age: decades 1 to 4.
Site: disseminated distribution, usually long bones and axial skeleton.
Clinical: pain and/or swelling. There are two categories of case: synchronous – those in which multiple lesions are present when the patient is first seen (which increases the likeli-

hood of separate origins); metachronous – lesions appear at intervals over months or years. In both instances the patient must be free of pulmonary metastases.

Morbid anatomy: generally sclerotic lesions. Cortical erosion and soft tissue swelling occur.

Histopathology: more matrix than cells.

Diagnosis: the problem which must be confronted in these cases is whether the multiple lesions are metastases. The longer the patient remains free of pulmonary lesions the greater the probability of true multicentricity.

Differential diagnosis: metastatic carcinoma, particularly from renal carcinoma with osteogenic differentiation (Macke *et al.*, 1985) or osteosarcoma, taking account of the possibility of skip metastases (Enneking and Kagan, 1975).

Treatment: excision and chemotherapy.

Prognosis: better than conventional disease and for metachronous type.

(x) Osteosarcoma in jaw (Kragh et al., 1958; Dahlin and Unni, 1988; Lee et al., 1988)

Age: decades 2 to 6.

Site: mandible more than maxilla.

Clinical: slowly growing swelling.

Morbid anatomy: little bone destruction, sclerotic swelling.

Histopathology: much bone, few cells, chondroid tissue, which may predominate.

Diagnosis: recognition of osteoblastic lesion with the clinical and radiological features of the condition. The malignant potential of the osteoid forming cells might not be obvious.

Differential diagnosis: if there is abundant cartilage then confusion with chondrosarcoma is possible, and the diagnosis would depend on identifying and classifying as malignant, rather than reactive, an osteoblastic component.

Treatment: excision.

Prognosis: good if the removal is complete.

(c) Osteosarcoma on bone: Juxtacortical, or surface osteosarcoma (Schajowicz *et al.*, 1988; Raymond, 1991)

These lesions are classified as: parosteal, periosteal or high-grade surface osteosarcoma.

'Juxtacortical' can be used as a generic term to imply proximity to the cortex, the relationship with the periosteum remaining undefined. Used in this way the term can qualify any lesion in this location. The forms of osteosarcoma found there will be discussed here. This discussion must be in the context both of osteosarcoma and of reactive lesions on bone (section 13.2). In the first case it is necessary to establish the categories of lesion, and in the second to establish the features which distinguish between neoplastic and reactive.

The categories are:

1. A low-grade osteoblastic neoplasm, with a tendency to recur as a progressively more aggressive lesion that will ultimately metastasize, nearly always located on the metaphysis. These constitute about 5% of malignant neoplasms of bone (Mirra, 1989).

2. A higher-grade neoplasm, primarily arising on the diaphysis, predominantly cartilaginous but with some bone formation variously interpreted as neoplastic or reactive, leading to categorization as chondrosarcoma or osteosarcoma (with appropriate qualification to specify the location 'on bone'). These form a much smaller percentage than category 1.

3. Osteoblastic neoplasms which conform closely with the histological structure of conventional osteocarcoma, and behave similarly. These are least common of all.

(i) Distinguishing neoplastic from reactive

This problem only exists in the case of category 1. In summary it may not be possible to decide histologically, and this must be done on the basis of behaviour: reactive lesions consolidate or regress; neoplastic are progressive.

Category 1. Juxtacortical or parosteal osteosarcoma (Figure 13.15) Age: nearly all are over the age of 20 years.

Site: mainly long tubular bones distribution as shown in Table 13.5.

Clinical: protracted natural history, as long as 10 years. Few symptoms – mild pain. Swelling may be palpable.

Morbid anatomy: the lesion is closely applied to the outer surface of the cortex. In its early stages it is a sessile swelling with a smooth contour. It is fairly dense in its radio-opacity, with some falling off towards the periphery. If there is a cartilaginous component (see below) there will be radiolucent foci. Growth gives rise to a more or less lobulated contour, and the lateral expansion overgrows the periosteum which appears as a radiolucent line between the lateral lobules and the bone. Growth accentuates the contrast in density between the superficial and deeper parts. Histopathology: growth of the lesion takes place at its periphery where there is a band of fibrocellular tissue which forms woven bone as an extension of that already present. The cellular band, which is narrow and lies beneath encapsulating fibrous tissue, does not have features of malignant tissue. The bone architecture is trabecular, with an orientation roughly perpendicular to the surface. The fibrocellular tissue continues into the marrow spaces. The proportion of bone to marrow space is variable, but in the outer regions is 50:50, but tending to favour bone. Progressively, in the direction of the base, the bone is remodelled, producing ever more substantial trabeculae, and reduction in the marrow space. At the junction with the cortex of the host bone the bone component will be approaching 100%. In structure and cytological detail the lesion is a fibro-osseous condition, without overt features of malignancy, and in many fields bears a close resemblance to fibrous dysplasia.

In some lesions there is a chondroid component in the form of lobules of cartilage. These are located at or near the surface, and are benign in character.

Diagnosis: Given the morbid anatomy the lesion cannot be an intraosseous condition such as fibrous dysplasia. The only possibilities are parosteal osteosarcoma or a reactive lesion. The latter can be eliminated on the grounds of cause and course: a significant cause is required; under treatment the lesion will resolve in time either by maturation or regression if it is reactive.

Differential diagnosis: reactive lesion on the benign side and periosteal sarcoma on the malignant side. The latter is discussed

Table 13.5 Distribution of parosteal osteosarcoma

| | Metaphysis | | Diaphysis |
	Proximal	Distal	
Femur	5	1	3
Tibia	4	7	
Humerus	2		7
Fibula	7	7	
Radius			
Ulna			
Metatarsal			6
Ilium		7	

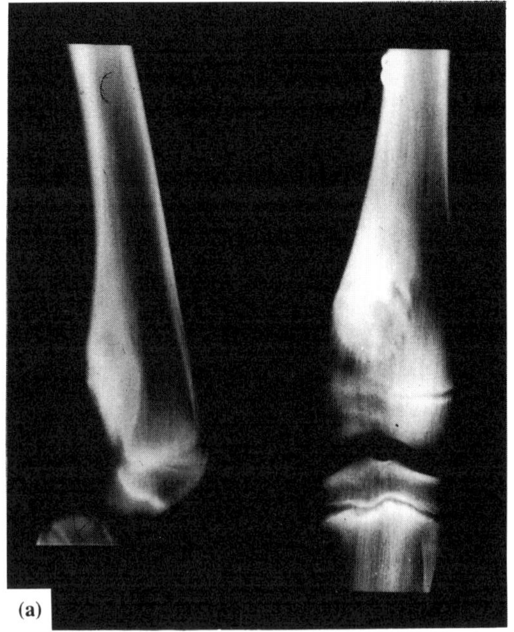

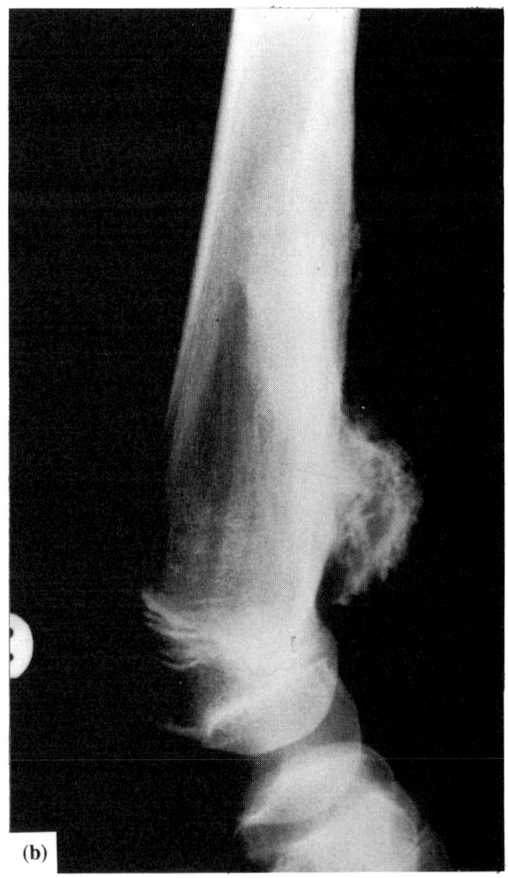

Figure 13.15 Parosteal osteosarcoma. (a) Male aged 14 years. Osteoblastic mass on the posteromedial aspect of the distal femoral metaphysis. Without reference to the radiograph a diagnosis of fibrous dysplasia was made on a biopsy. (b) Male aged 16 years. Mass arising from posterior aspect of distal femoral metaphysis. There is also a wisp of periosteal reaction higher up. The excised lesion had the histological appearance of reactive tissue.

below under periosteal sarcoma.

Treatment: local resection.

Prognosis: good, if surgery is adequate. There is a risk of recurrence, and with it of progression towards a more malignant state, eventuating in a sarcoma (spindle cell or osteoblastic), and metastasis.

Category 2: Periosteal osteosarcoma (Figure 13.16) Age: decades 2 and 3.

Site: most usual in long bones of lower limb.

Clinical: pain and swelling.

Morbid anatomy: a diametaphyseal lesion resting on outer surface of cortex. Peripherally the lesion is predominantly radiolucent, with either of both spicular mineral or spotty calcification. Deeper, the spicular (bony) component becomes more pronounced, but irregularly distributed. In more advanced lesions the cortex may be breached and the medulla invaded.

Histopathology: there is a large cartilage component, responsible for the lucency and the spotty calcification. The spicular element is due to woven bone formation.

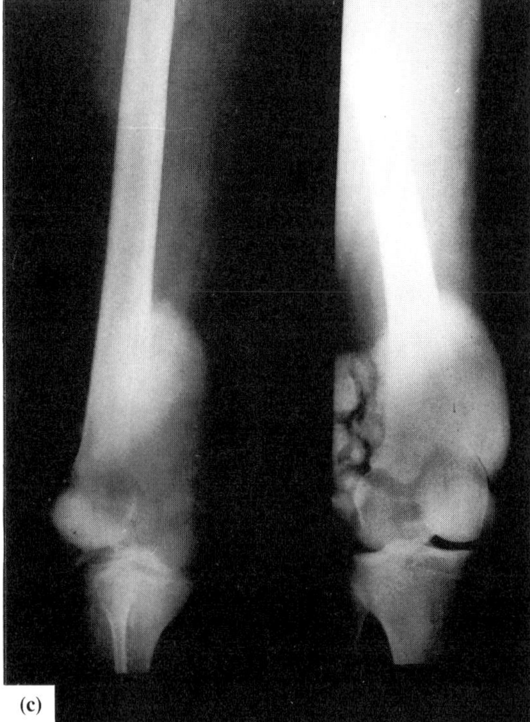

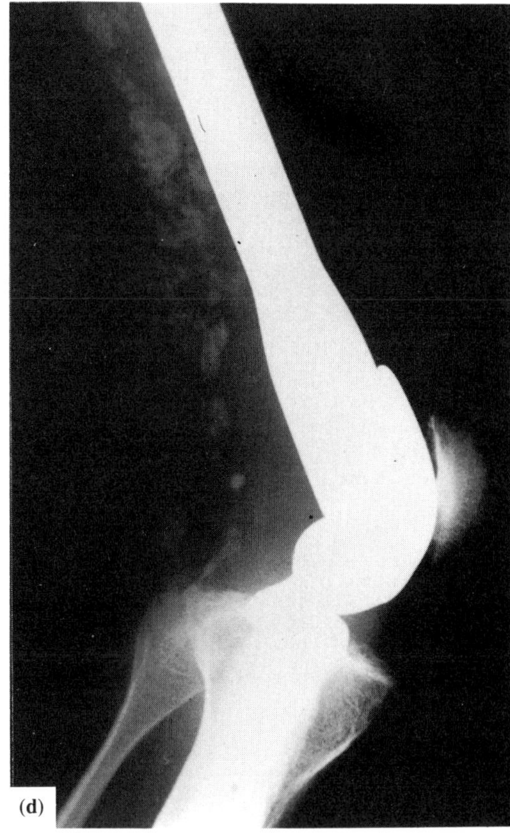

Figure 13.15 Parosteal osteosarcoma. (c) Several years later the lesion had recurred massively. (d) Prosthetic replacement was followed after two years by the appearance of bone nodules in soft tissue. Several of these were removed. Ten years on the patient is a university graduate, with some stable ossified soft tissue lesions.

Owing to the mingling of the osseous and cartilaginous tissues it is not always clear whether the bone is resulting from ossification of the cartilage or membrane formation by osteoblasts. In the latter case differentiation between reactive and neoplastic cells must be made. It is the presence of neoplastic osteoblasts which establishes the diagnosis. The cytology of the tissue shows the features of malignancy. These are not necessarily blatant, but in the classical case there is no difficulty in ascertaining that both chondroid and osteoblastic elements are suspect.

It is necessary to emphasize the range of variation within both this category and parosteal OS. The former can be so extensively cartilaginous that chondrosarcoma is being considered, but the proportions of bone and carilage can alter to the point where it becomes arguable that the lesion is a *parosteal* osteosarcoma. There is a concomitant shift in the cytological features, causing more or less difficulty in the adjudication of malignancy.

Diagnosis: when the classical features are present both anatomically and histologically there is no difficulty in reaching a diagnosis,

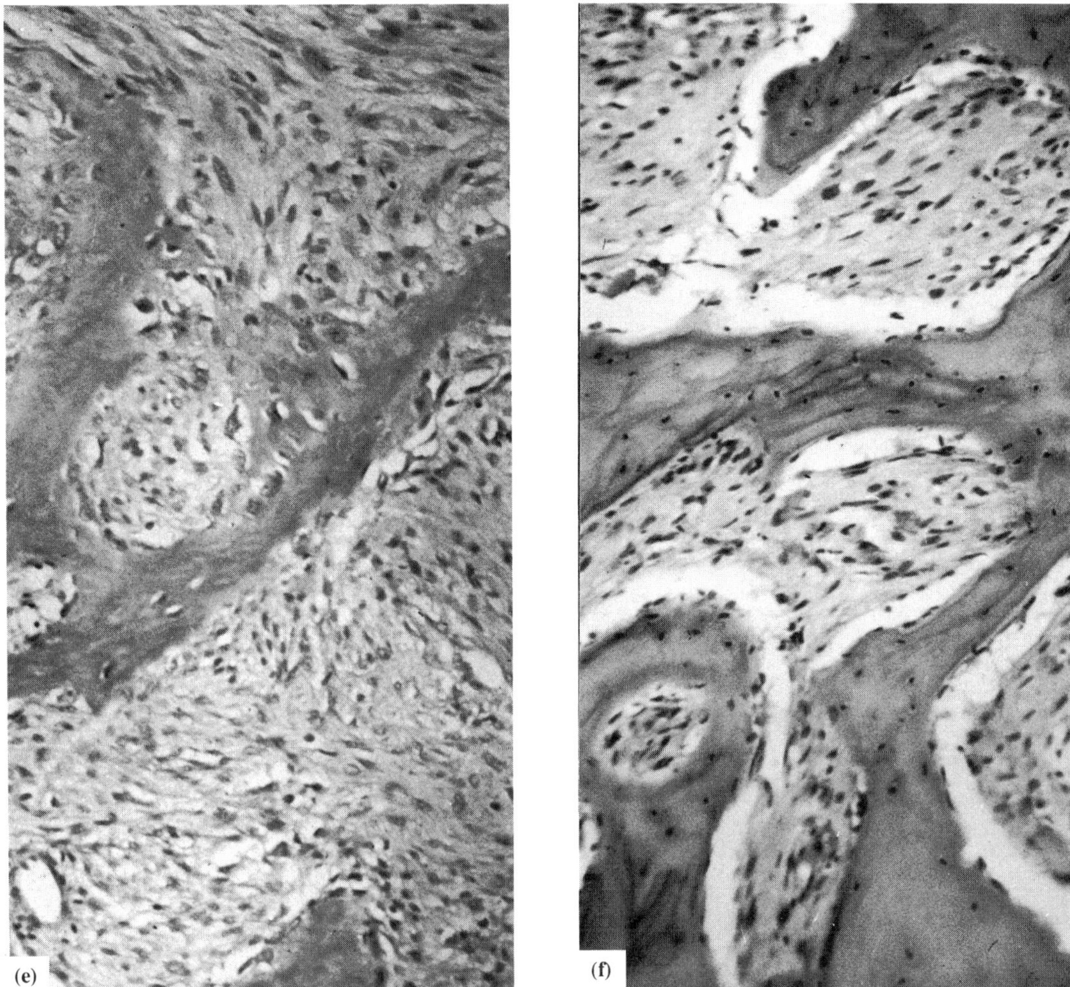

Figure 13.15 Parosteal osteosarcoma. (e) Histology of the tumour near its surface shows spindle celled tissue with developing woven bone trabeculae, a pattern reminiscent of fibrous dysplasia. (f) A deeper section with more mature, less cellular, fibrous tissue in which bone trabeculae are well developed and show evidence of past remodelling.

particularly if the specimen is large. Differential diagnosis: as discussed. Treatment: surgical. Prognosis: fair.

Category 3. High grade surface osteosarcoma (Wold *et al.*, 1984) These are rare tumours, only nine cases were reported from the Mayo Clinic (Wold *et al.*, 1984). By definition they are, *ab initio*, highly malignant osteoblastic lesions on the bone surface. There must not have been a preceding lesion (a parosteal osteosarcoma which has become high grade), and there must be no question of intraosseous origin. The last point may be hard to decide if there is appreciable tumour both inside and on the surface. In addition to the above requirements, the histology must be of a high-grade neoplasm with osteoblastic potential.

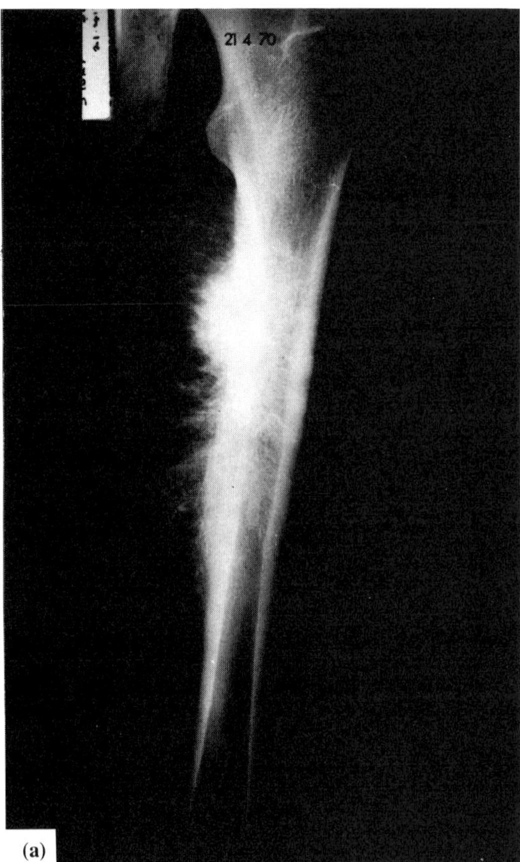

(a)

Figure 13.16 Periosteal osteosarcoma. Male 33 years. Discomfort and mass in thigh. (a) A lesion arising from the medial aspect of the diaphysis. The length of the vertical spiculation indicates the size of the soft tissue component. The spicules are periosteal reactive bone incorporated into the tumour, which is composed principally of cartilage. There is a distinct osteoblastic element responsible for the low rounded densities.

Treatment: as for high grade osteosarcoma. Prognosis: seven of the cases reported by Wold *et al.* (1984) died within two years.

(d)   Soft tissue osteosarcoma

These are uncommon tumours. For example, between 1950 and 1987 there were 26 cases seen at the M.D. Anderson Cancer Centre in Houston (Bane *et al.*, 1990). The common sites were: thigh, 11; upper extremity, 3; retroperitoneum, 3.

There was a wide range of tissue patterns: osteoblastic, chondroblastic, fibroblastic, MFH, giant celled, telangiectatic, small cell. These occurred in various combinations, but a malignant bone-forming component was always present.

Seven patients were living free of disease at 30 to 122 months, and two with disease at 28 and 54 months; 16 had died of disease at 2 to 54 months; there was one unrelated death. The main prognostic factor was tumour 5 cm or more in size.

REFERENCES

Albright, F., Butler, A.M., Hampton, A.O. *et al.* (1937) Syndrome characterised by osteitis fibrosa disseminata, area of pigmentation and endocrine dysfunction, with precocious puberty in females. *N. Engl. J. Med.*, **216**, 727.

Ayala, A.G., Ro, J.Y., Raymond, A.K. *et al.* (1989) Small cell osteosarcoma. A clinico-pathological study of 27 cases. *Cancer*, **64**, 2162–73.

Ballance, W.A., Mendelsohn, G., Carter, J.R. *et al.* (1988) Osteogenic sarcoma: malignant fibrous histiocytoma sub-type. *Cancer*, **62**, 763–71.

Bane, B.L., Evans, H.L., Ro, J.Y. *et al.* (1990) Extraskeletal osteosarcoma. *Cancer*, **65**, 2762–70.

Bertoni, P., Unni, K., McLeod, R. *et al.* (1985) Osteosarcoma resembling osteoblastoma. *Cancer*, **55**, 416–26.

Byers, P.D. (1968) Solitary benign osteoblastic lesions of bone. Osteid osteoma and benign osteoblastoma. *Cancer*, **22**, 43–57.

Cahan, W.G., Woodward, H.Q., Higinbotham, N.L. *et al.* (1948) Sarcoma arising in irradiated bone. Report of 11 cases. *Cancer*, **1**, 2–39.

Campanacci, M. (1976) Osteofibrous dysplasia of long bones. A new clinical entity. *Ital. J. Orthop. Traumatol.*, 2, 221–37.

Campanacci, M. and Laus, M. (1981) Osteofibrous dysplasia of tibia and fibula. *J. Bone Joint Surg.*, **63A**, 367–75.

Carroll, R.E. (1957) Osteogenic sarcoma in the hand. *J. Bone Joint Surg.*, **39A**, 325–31.

Cohen, D.M., Dahlin, D.C and Pugh, D.C (1962) Fibrous dysplasia associated with adamantinoma of long bones. *Cancer*, **15**, 515–21.

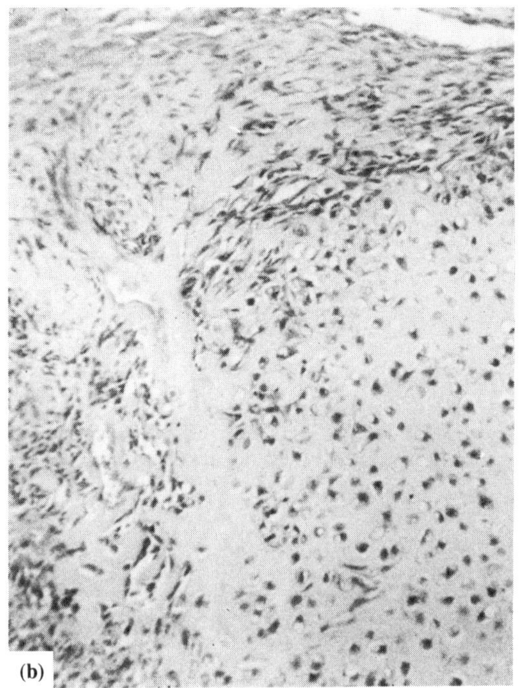 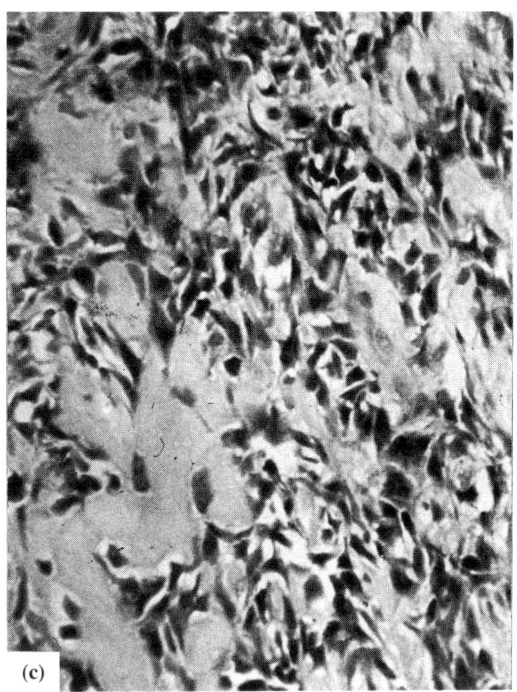

Figure 13.16 Periosteal osteosarcoma. Male 33 years. Discomfort and mass in thigh. (b) Low power view near the surface showing the field to be divided between malignant cartilage and neoplastic bone. (c) High power view of the malignant bone forming tissue.

Dahlin, D.C. (1978) *Bone Tumors*, 3rd edn, Charles C. Thomas, Springfield, IL.

Dahlin, D.C. and Johnson, E.W. (1954) Giant osteoid osteoma. *J. Bone Joint Surg.*, **36A**, 559–72.

Dahlin, D.C. and Unni, K.K. (1988) *Bone Tumors*. 4th edn. Charles C Thomas, Springfield, IL.

Dorfman, H.D. (1973) Malignant transformation of benign bone lesions. *Proceedings Seventh National Cancer Conference.* pp. 901–13.

Dorfman, H.D. and Schiller, A. (1980) Aggressive osteoblastoma, ilium, with secondary aneurysmal bone cyst. *N. Engl. J. Med.*, **303**, 866–73.

Dorfman, H.D. and Weiss, S. (1984) Borderline osteoblastic tumours: problems in the differential diagnosis of aggressive osteoblastoma and low grade osteosarcoma. *Semin. Diagn. Pathol.*, **1**, 215.

Enneking, W.F. and Kagan, A. (1975) 'Skip' metastases in osteosarcoma. *Cancer*, **36**, 2192–205.

Fairbank, H. and Baker S.L. (1948) Hyperplastic callus formation with or without evidence of a fracture in osteogenesis imperfecta. *Br. J. Surg.*, **36**, 1–16.

Gardner, E. and Richards, R. (1953) Multiple cutaneous and subcutaneous lesions occuring simultaneously with hereditary polyposis and osteomatosis. *Am. J. Hum. Genet.*, **5**, 139–17.

Hasegawa, T., Hirose, T., Kudo, E. *et al.*, (1991) Immunophenotypic heterogeneity in osteosarcoma. *Hum. Pathol.*, **22**, 583–90.

Huvos, A. (1986) Osteogenic sarcoma of bones and soft tissues in older persons. A clinicopathologic analysis of 117 patients older than 60 years of age. *Cancer*, **57**, 1442–9.

Jaffe, H.L. (1958) *Tumors and Tumorous Conditions of Bones and Joints*. Lea and Febiger, Philadelphia.

Klenerman, L. and Townsend, A. (1967) Osteosarcoma occurring in osteogenesis imperfecta. A report of two cases. *J. Bone Joint Surg.*, **49B**, 314–23.

Kragh, L.V., Dahlin, D.C. and Erich, J.B. (1958) Osteogenic sarcoma of the jaws and facial bones. *Am. J. Surg.*, **96**, 496–505.

Kurt, A.M., Unni, K.K., McLeod, R.A. *et al.* (1990) Low grade intraosseous osteosarcoma. *Cancer,* **65**, 1418–28.

Kyriakos, M. and Hardy, D. (1991) Malignant transformation of aneurysmal bone cyst, with an analysis of the literature. *Cancer,* **68**, 1770–80.

Kyriakos, M., Gilula, L.A., Becich, M.J. *et al.* (1992) Intracortical small cell osteosarcoma. *Clin. Orthop.,* **279**, 269–80.

Lee, Y.Y., Van Tassel, P., Hauert, C. *et al.* (1988) Craniofacial osteosarcoma: plain film, CT, and MR findings in 46 cases. *Am. J. Roentgenol.,* **150**, 397–402.

Lichtenstein, L. and Jaffe, H.L. (1942) Fibrous dysplasia of bone. *Arch. Pathol. Lab. Med.,* **33**, 777.

Lopez-Barea, F., Rodriguez-Peralto, J.L., Gonzalez-Lopez, J. *et al.* (1991) Intracortical osteosarcoma: a case report. *Clin. Orthop.,* **268**, 218–22.

Macke, R.A., Hussain, M.R., Imray, T.J. *et al.* (1985) Osteogenic and sarcomatoid differentiation of a renal cell carcinoma. *Cancer.* **56**, 2452–7.

Mahoney, J.P., Spanier, S.S. and Morris, J.L. (1979) Multifocal osteosarcoma. A case report and review of the literature. *Cancer,* **44**, 1897–1907.

Matsuno, T., Unni, K.K., McLeod, R. *et al.* (1976) Telangiectatic osteosarcoma. *Cancer,* **38**, 2538–47.

Mauer, L. (1958) Osteoid osteoma of the 12th rib: resection under local anaesthesia. A case report. *Milit. Med.,* **122**, 194.

McLeod, R.A., Dahlin, D.C. and Beabout, J.W. (1976) The spectrum of osteoblastoma. *Am. J. Roentgenol.,* **126**, 321–35.

Miller, T.T., Adelwahab, I.F., Hermann, G. *et al.* (1992) Case report 735. Vertebral osteosarcoma. *Skeletal Radiol.,* **21**, 277–9.

Mirra, J.M. (1989) *Bone Tumors: Clinical, Radiologic and Pathologic Correlations.* Lea and Febiger, Philadelphia.

Mirra, J.M., Kendrick, R.A. and Kendrick, R.E. (1976) Pseudomalignant osteoblastoma versus arrested osteosarcoma. A case report. *Cancer,* **37**, 2005–14.

Mirra, J.M., Kameda, N., Eckardt, J. *et al.* (1988) Osteosarcoma of toe phalanx: first reported case. *Am. J. Surg. Pathol.,* **12**, 300–7.

Mirra, J.M., Dodd, L., Johnson, W. *et al.* (1991) Case report 700. Primary intracortical osteosarcoma of femur, sclerosing variant, grade 1 to 2 anaplasia. *Skeletal Radiol.,* **20**, 613–16.

Nakashima, Y., Yamamuro, T., Fujiwara, Y. *et al.* (1983) Osteofibrous dysplasia (ossifying fibroma of long bones). A study of 12 cases. *Cancer,* **52**, 909–14.

O'dell, C.W., Resnick, D. and Niwayama, G. (1976) Osteoid osteoma arising in adjacent bones. *J. Can. Assoc. Radiol.,* **27**, 298–300.

Price, C.H.G. and Goldie, W. (1969) Paget's sarcoma of bone. A study of 80 cases. *J. Bone Joint Surg.,* **51B**, 205–24.

Ransford, A.O., Pozo, J.L. and Hutton, P.A.N. *et al.* (1984) The behaviour pattern of the scoliosis associated with osteoid osteoma or osteoblastoma of the spine. *J. Bone Joint Surg.,* **66B**, 16–20.

Raymond, A.K. (1991) Surface osteosarcoma. *Clin. Orthop.,* **270**, 140–8.

Sanerkin, N.G. (1980) Definitions of osteosarcoma, chondrosarcoma and fibrosarcoma of bone. *Cancer,* **46**, 178–85.

Schajowicz, F. (1981) *Tumors and Tumorlike Lesions of Bone and Joints.* Springer, New York.

Schajowicz, F. and Lemos, C. (1976) Malignant osteoblastoma. *J. Bone Joint Surg.,* **58B**, 202–11.

Schajowicz, F., McGuire, M.H., Santini Araujo, E. *et al.* (1988) Osteosarcoma arising on the surface of long bones. *J. Bone Joint Surg.,* **70A**, 555–64.

Schulman, L. and Dorfman, H.D. (1970) Nerve fibres in osteoid osteoma. *J. Bone Joint Surg.,* **52A**, 1351–6.

Sissons, H.A., Kancherla, P. and Wallace, B. (1983) Ossifying fibroma of bone. Report of two cases. *Bull. Hosp. Joint Dis. Orthop. Inst.,* **43**, 1–14.

Taconis, W.K. (1988) Osteosarcoma in fibrous dysplasia. *Skeletal Radiol.,* **17**, 163–70.

Tigani, D., Pignatti, G., Picci, P. *et al.* (1988) Vertebral osteosarcoma. *Ital. J. Orthop. Traumatol.,* **14**, 5–13.

Unni, K.K. and Dahlin, D.C. (1989) Osteosarcoma: pathology and classification. *Semin. Roentgenol.,* **24**, 143–52.Benjamin/Cummings, California.

Weatherby, R.P., Dahlin, D.C. and Irins, J.C. (1981) Postradiation sarcome of bone. Review of 78 Mayo Clinic cases. *Mayo. Clin. Proc.,* **56**, 294–306.

Wold, L.E., Unni, K.K., Beabout, J.W. and Pritchard, D.J. (1984) High grade surface osteosarcoma. *Am. J. Surg. Pathol.,* **8**, 181–6.

Yoshida, H., Yumoto, T., Adachi, H. *et al.* (1989) Osteosarcoma with prominent epithelioid features. *Acta Pathol. Jpn.,* **39**, 439–45.

13.5 CARTILAGE TUMOURS

This section discusses cartilage tumours classified as shown in Table 13.6.

13.6 INTRAOSSEOUS CARTILAGE NEOPLASIA

Multiple cartilage tumours are much less common than solitary lesions. Multiplicity and size apart, however, the morbid anatomy and the histological features are much the same. For descriptive purposes discussion will be concerned with solitary lesions, and where necessary multiple lesions will be specifically referred to.

Cartilage tumours are the most common primary neoplasm in bone. The great majority, benign or malignant, have the architecture and structure of hyaline cartilage. Most intraosseous chondrosarcomas present in adults, and are low-grade, well-differentiated lesions that cause death by slow inexorable growth. The assessment of growth is very important in their diagnosis. But with higher grade malignancy the hyaline pattern becomes less apparent. In addition, the uncommon mesenchymal and clear cell chondrosarcomas are less recognizably cartilaginous on ordinary grounds, but their morbid anatomy and/or histology are reasonably distinctive. The pathologist's most frequent problems therefore are concerned with the ordinary intraosseous cartilage tumours – chondroma and chondrosarcoma. The main difficulty is in distinguishing between benign and low-grade cartilage neoplasia.

Any bone that is formed in cartilage can be affected by intraosseous benign or malignant cartilage neoplasms. The skeletal distribution of these lesions as recorded by Mirra (1989), from a large literature survey of benign and malignant cartilage tumours, is in close accord with Dahlin and Unni (1988) (Table 13.7).

However, Mirra's (1989) personal experience leads him to conclude that the order of sites according to the frequency with which they are affected by endochondroma is:

- Common sites
  Femoral diaphyses and metadiaphyses (about 40% of cases)
  Humerus
  Tibia
  Short tubular bones of hand and foot (< 15%)
- Less common sites
  Ribs
  Radius
  Fibula
  Ulna
  Pelvis (about 3% of cases)

He explains these differences from the more conventional figures by predicting that more enchondromas will be discovered by radionuclide scanning, and that enchondromas of long and flat bones over the age of 40 years with increased cellularity and double-nucleated chondrocytes are being overdiagnosed as low-grade chondrosarcomas because these criteria are regarded as sufficient in themselves. The similarity of the cases culled from the literature and the Mayo Clinic cases leads to reservations about this thesis; admittedly, the predicted scanning effect will not have had time to influence the Mayo figures, but it is improbable that they will have been biased by overdiagnosis. Nevertheless, it must be recognized that there is bias, sometimes difficult to identify and often difficult to assess, in the incidence data from any source. But, taking all that into account, the basic principle, on which all authorities are agreed, that chondrosarcoma is rare in the hands and feet, is not disturbed.

The WHO definition of these two classes of neoplasm (Schajowicz *et al.*, 1972) is as follows:

Chondroma: a benign tumour characterized by the formation of mature cartilage but lacking the histological characteristics of

Table 13.6 Classification of cartilage tumours

In bone: intraosseous
Benign
  Chondroma
    Solitary
    Multiple (calcifying chondroma, Schajowicz)
Malignant
  Chondrosarcoma
    Primary of hyaline cartilage
    Secondary of hyaline cartilage
    Dedifferentiated primary or secondary
    Mesenchymal
    Clear cell

On bone: juxtacortical
Benign
  Osteochondroma
    Solitary
    Multiple
  Juxtacortical (periosteal) chondroma
Malignant
  Chondrosarcoma
    Primary periosteal
    Secondary to osteochondroma
(see also parosteal and periosteal osteosarcoma)

In soft: extraskeletal
Benign
  Chondroma
Malignant
  Chondrosarcoma
    Myxoid
    Mesenchymal

In joint (and tendon sheath)
Benign (metaplasia)
  Synovial (osteo)chondromatosis
Malignant
  Secondary to synovial chondromatosis

chondrosarcoma (high cellularity, pleomorphism and presence of large cells with double nuclei or mitosis).

Chondrosarcoma: a malignant tumour characterized by the formation of cartilage, but not of bone, by the tumour cells. It is distinguished from chondroma by the presence of more cellular and pleomorphic tumour tissue, and by appreciable numbers of plump cells with large or double nuclei.

Mitotic cells are infrequent.

Inadvertently these definitions raise the expectation that the diagnosis of chondrosarcoma is made by histological criteria alone. However, the features which must be brought into the assessment are age, site, clinical history and radiographic findings (size and signs of growth). The histological criteria are judged in the light of these factors.

Table 13.7 Skeletal distribution of lesions in cartilage

Site	Dahlin (nos) Chondroma	Sarcoma	Mirra (%) Chondroma	Sarcoma
Jaws		+		1
Skull		+		2
Other flat bones	10	38	11	42
Girdles	5		6	31
Shoulder	7		2	(8)
Pelvic		24	4	(23)
Spine	+	3	+	2
Long tubular	18	51	23	49
Femur, tibia, humerus	15	49	19	46
Fibula, radius, ulna			5	3
Hands and feet	70	6	66	4
Short tubular	70	5		
Cuboidal	+	1	1	1

+ = recorded but <1%

13.6.1 BENIGN CARTILAGE TUMOURS

(a) Enchondroma

(i) Clinical features

The majority are solitary, a few are multiple, and of these a small proportion are unilateral. This last group was described by Ollier (1900) as dyschondroplasia, and is widely referred to eponymously, although there seems not to be any significant difference between uni- and bilateral disease. Rarely, multiple enchondromas are associated with soft tissue haemangiomas, a combination named after Maffucci, who described the syndrome in 1881.

The multiple lesions arise as the result of dysplasia in the physis: a portion fails to mineralize, and persists as a column or nodule of cartilage in marrow, sometimes in cortex or periosteum (Milgram, 1983). The mechanism of separation from the physis is not known; 'pinching off' is suggested (Mirra, 1989).

Possibly all chondromas are formed in this way. If this were the only source of cartilage tissue in the marrow space all chondrosarco-mas could be seen as secondary to them. But there are inducible cells in the marrow that form the cartilage of callus. Potentially these too could be an origin of chondrosarcoma.

Enchondromas are found over a wide age range, the first to seventh decade, with a peak around the fourth. Thus, in contrast to many bone tumours, they are predominant in adults.

Most cases are found incidental to other investigations. A few undergo pathological fracture with acute onset of pain; these are most often in fingers. A small number have symptoms of stress fracture (pain on exercise, relieved by rest). In yet a smaller number, pain is spontaneous; some have another local condition to account for it; in very few it seems to be generated within the lesion. As one descends through this catalogue of presentations there is increasing concern over the possibility of chondrosarcoma.

The prognosis is good in solitary lesions.

(ii) Pathology

Morbid anatomy These tumours are located within the marrow cavity (a location usually referred to as central) in the metaphysis or at one end of the diaphysis. But they occupy much of the cavity of small bones such as phalanges (Figure 13.17). They are well demarcated lesions, without signs of erosion, with limited marginal or periosteal reaction. Most are quiescent at presentation. They may grow and expand the bone, although the periosteal apposition often fails to keep up with the resorption, leading to a breach of the cortex. This is especially true of lesions in small bones such as those of hands and feet, where small tumours are relatively large compared to the size of the bones. An important feature is that the endosteal surface is smooth, without signs of scalloping. The largest benign tumours are found in patients with multiple lesions, giving rise to gross deformity, mainly of the limbs.

In the absence of mineral deposition there is not a great deal that is specific about the radiological appearance, and a variety of diagnoses can be entertained. Characteristic calcification of the matrix can occur which then allows a confident statement about diagnosis.

Table 13.8 presents a widely accepted descriptive terminology of the patterns of mineral deposition in a variety of tissues.

In well differentiated, benign or low-grade tumours the mineral deposits are distinct, often dense. A common description is popcorn-like. In higher grade tumours the mineral, if present, is less well delineated and less dense; descriptive terms such as hazy, cloudy, windblown are used.

Histopathology (Figures 13.17–13.22) All the material from a biopsy or curettage should be processed, including bone fragments from the periphery.

The tissue of these tumours is hyaline cartilage, which presents no difficulty in recognition, present in the form of nodules. They vary in size, scattered or clustered. However, since some both mineralize and ossify the picture may appear confused at first glance, but, given that clinical and radiological information is available, further examination leaves little alternative to cartilage tumour. The possibility of mistaking fracture callus exists, but ancillary information should secure the right interpretation.

The relationship of the cartilage nodules to the surrounding tissue must be assessed for its behaviour, since benign and grade 1 sarcomas can be cytologically indistinguishable. In non-growing tumours many nodules of cartilage will be invested with a layer of lamellar bone, appearing as an integral part of the nodule (Figure 13.21). These are the circles observed in radiographs. Cartilage abutting on trabeculae

Table 13.8 Patterns of mineral deposition in bone and cartilage

	Bone			
	Reactive	*Dysplasia*	*Neoplasia*	*Cartilage*
Flecks/spots				+
Rings				+
Floccules	+			+
Ground Glass	+	+		
Lumpy			+	
Cloudy			+	
Solid			+	
Netted			+	

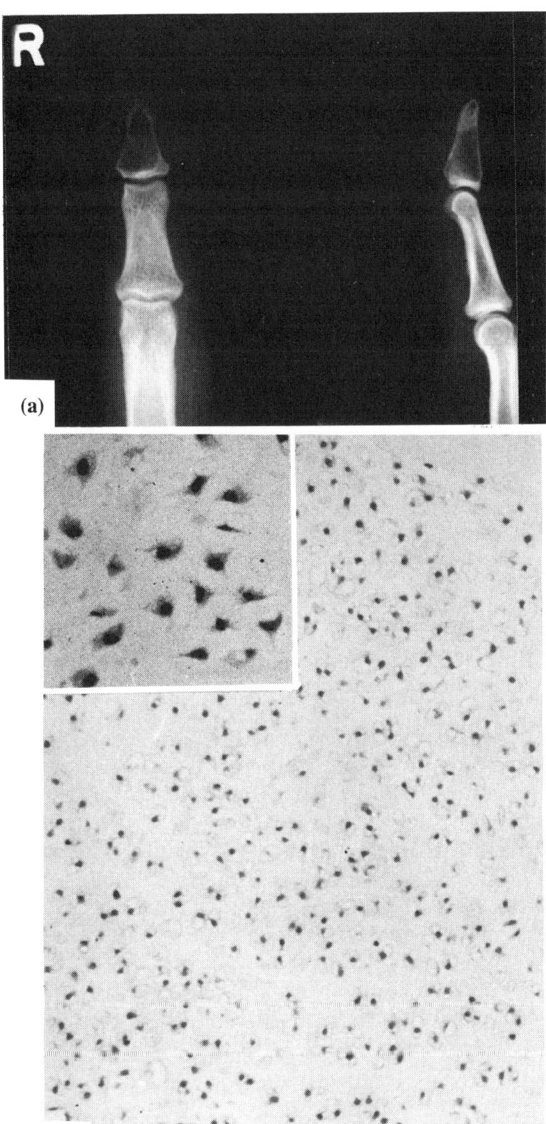

Figure 13.17 Female, adult. The commonest form of enchondroma, sudden pain in finger. (a) The osteolytic lesion in the terminal phalanx has caused slight expansion of the bone, with uniform thinning of the cortex. There is fine, irregular stippling of the contents, indicative of cartilage. One cortex has an infarction. (b) Histological sections of curetted fragments of hyaline cartilage showed moderately cellular tissue, well-defined nuclei verging on plump and with occasional binucleate cells. The matrix is well formed, and the tissue is orderly.

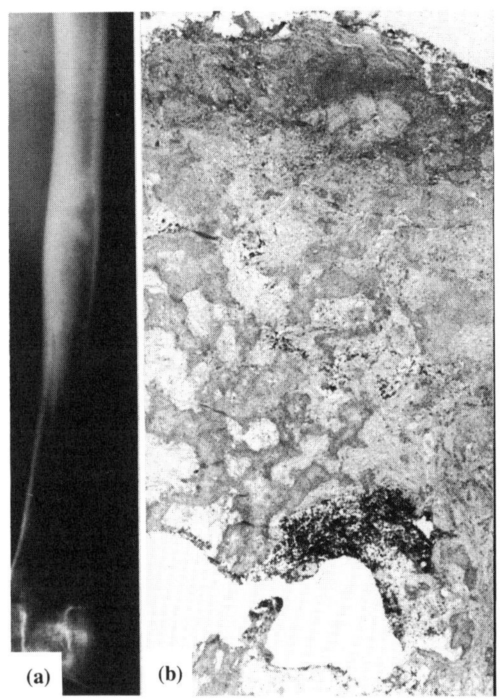

Figure 13.18 Female aged 49 years. A lesion comparable in some respects to Figure 13.3. (a) There is an expanding lesion, focally calcified in the pattern of cartilage tissue, in the mid-shaft of femur. The expansion is uniform without endosteal erosion (scalloping). The fact that growth of a cartilaginous tumour had occurred in the long bone of an adult warranted biopsy (curettage). (b) This revealed totally necrotic, extensively calcified and ossified tissue. Radiograph courtesy of Mr I.B.M. Stephen.

with a resorption surface is indicative of growth. The presence of 'naked' nodules between trabeculae is indicative of permeation of tumour (Figures 13.20b and 13.22e). Reactive bone trabeculae (woven bone) are also suggestive. Clusters of tumour nodules separated by fibrous bands are growing and compressing the marrow stroma (Barnes and Catto, 1966). Such growth indicators call for careful judgement.

Cellularity is variable from sparse to abundant, even within one lesion. There

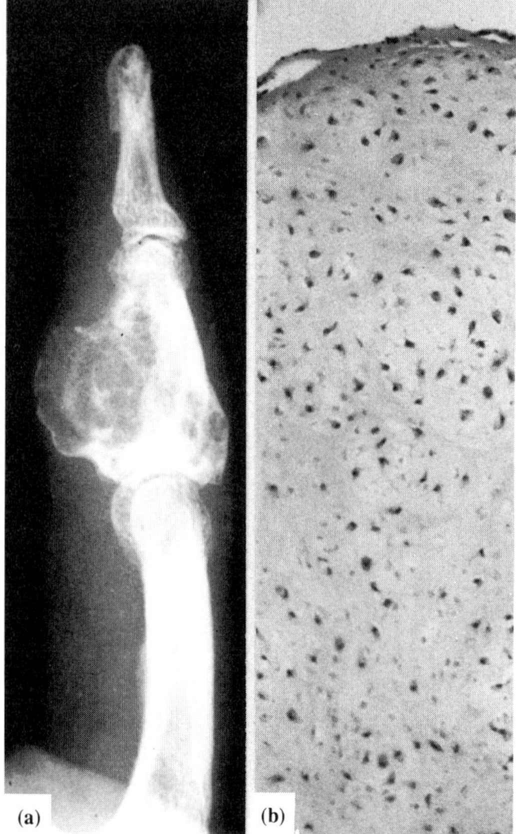

Figure 13.19 Female aged 53 years. Enlarging phalangeal enchondroma. Complaint: swelling of finger, sometimes painful. (a) The neoplasm is recognized as cartilaginous from the stippled mineral deposition. The phalanx is expanded on the palmar and dorsal apects, with a uniformly thin cortex, which may be fractured at several points. There is no soft tissue swelling. (b) Histologically the tissue is benign: in keeping with finger lesions it is cellular, with clustering, but free of features of anaplasia; binucleate cells are present. Mineralization and ossification are present. Consideration must be given to chondrosarcoma, but there is nothing to support that diagnosis. Radiograph courtesy of Mr D.J. Klugman.

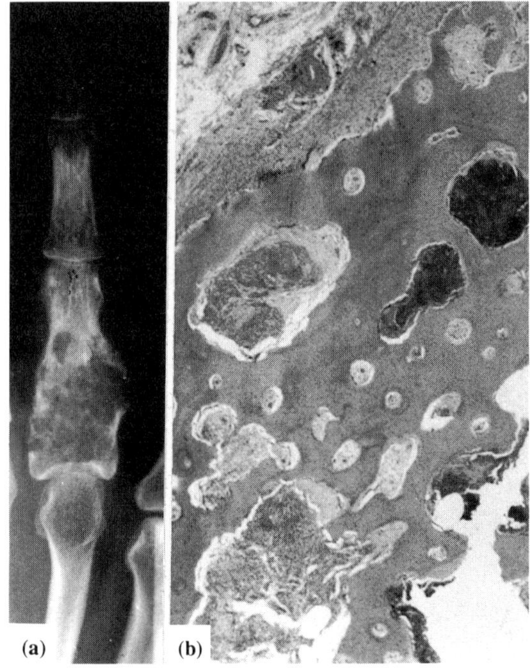

Figure 13.20 Male aged 59 years. Phalangeal chondrosarcoma. Moderately painful enlarging lesion of finger. (a) The initial radiograph shows an expanding lesion occupying the proximal half of the marrow of a proximal phalanx. The cortex is irregularly eroded, and breached near the base and in the middle of one margin, bulging the periosteum. Curettage was carried out, producing fragments of cartilage and of bone. All the tissue was processed. There were no cytological features demanding a diagnosis of chondrosarcoma after making allowance for the site. (b) The significance of the invasion of the cortex in one of the bony fragments was not recognized. Not only are several osteonal canals filled by tumour, but there is active resorption of the bone surfaces, indicating growth.

are no features of anaplasia. Occasional doubly nucleated cells are not unusual. Multiple lesions and those of the extremities tend to be more cellular, and this must

be discounted. It is also necessary to recognize that 'plump' cells do not include swollen, vacuolated degenerate cells. Some cells of this kind bear a distinct resemblance to physaliphorous cells. These are all relative criteria, which place a burden on anyone, but especially those seeing few cases, and reinforces the necessity to have all the

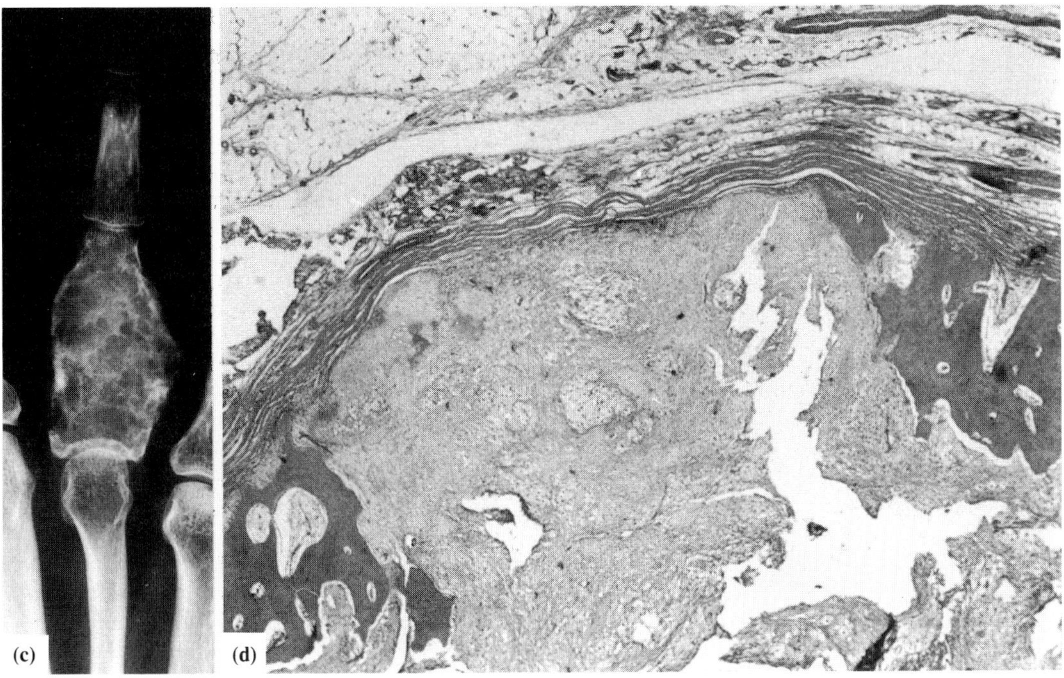

Figure 13.20 Male aged 59 years. Phalangeal chondrosarcoma. Moderately painful enlarging lesion of finger. (c) No further treatment was undertaken until there was a recurrence. (d) The tumour now fills the entire marrow cavity, and there are breaches of the cortex. One of these is shown in the photomicrograph, demonstrating the active erosion of bone induced by the tumour, and the invasion of the cortex. Radiographs courtesy of Mr H.D. Smith.

information available, and to review it in consultation. One of the strengths of a Bone Tumour Panel is that diagnoses are reached in the presence of all parties, a practice that can be emulated by any.

Criteria whereby benign and low-grade malignant cartilage tumours can be distinguished are discussed below.

Diagnosis depends on an acceptable radiograph of a small lesion (for a major long bone 5 cm is a helpful, but not absolute, demarcation) in an acceptable site in a patient of an acceptable age; confirmation that the lesion is composed of hyaline cartilage free of cytological features of malignancy.

The differential diagnosis is low-grade chondrosarcoma: other things being equal, the decision can turn on the interpretation of radiographs.

13.6.2 INTRAOSSEOUS CHONDROSARCOMA

The classification of these lesions is shown in Table 13.6.

Intraosseous (or medullary) chondrosarcomas of hyaline cartilage are mainly of low grade, but, by conventional criteria, grade 2, or rarely grade 3 tumours occur. These central tumours sometimes undergo 'dedifferentiation', producing more malignant tissue of another type. Clear cell and myxoid chondrosarcomas begin as high-grade tumours.

Some hyaline chondrosarcomas are regarded as primary, that is there is no antecedent enchondroma, and the others as secondary, arising in a benign cartilage tumour at the site. The classical secondary is in multiple enchondromatosis. But there are also cases of solitary enchondroma which

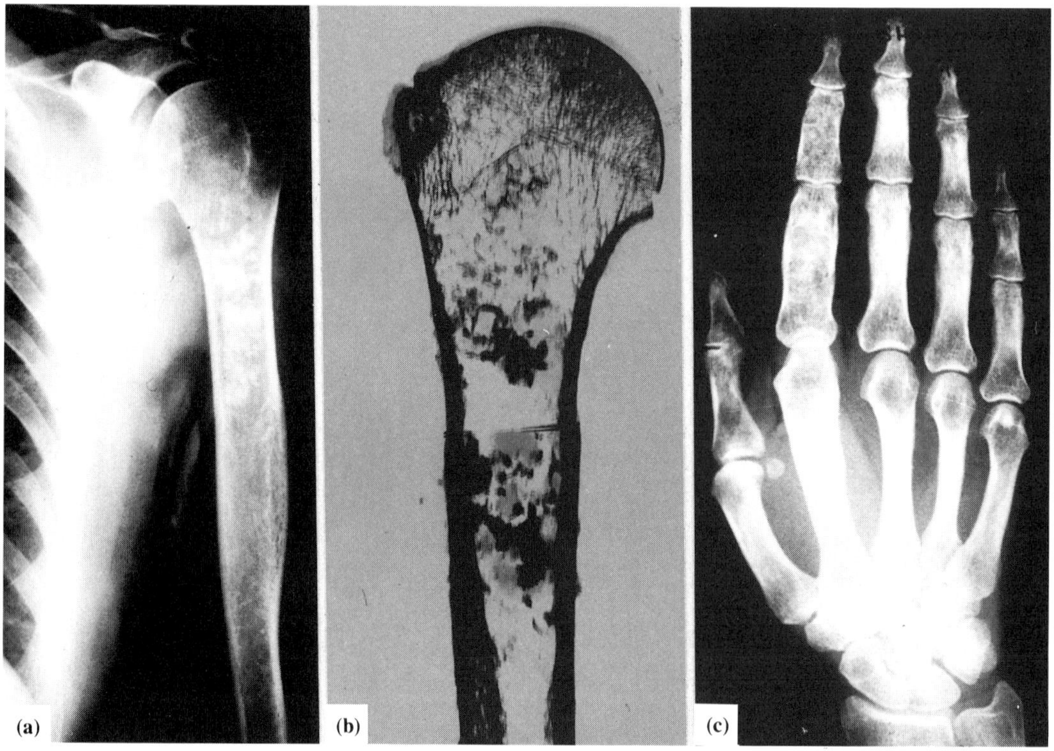

Figure 13.21 Female aged 57 years. Benign enchondromata in Ollier's disease. Pain in 'shoulder'. (a) Radiograph of the humerus shows scattered dense calcified foci in the upper third (the descriptive term 'popcorn' is apposite). There is no significant radiolucency. The shape of the humerus is normal and the endosteal surface is unaltered. The diagnosis of Ollier's disease, and the absence of anything else to account for the pain led to a clinical decision to do prosthetic replacement. (b) Fine detail radiograph of a slab (reversed) confirms the normal cortex; endosteal irregularities are due to calcified and ossified cartilage nodules in contact with it. Small and large mineralized foci are scattered through the marrow; some in the metaphysis have a ring contour. (c) Skeletal survey had also revealed smooth expansion of the metacarpal and phalanges two and three of the index finger with many small calcific foci.

transform to chondrosarcoma. The case illustrated in Figure 13.22 might qualify. The incidence of this is uncertain: if clear cut radiographic evidence is used, it is not very prevalent; if histological evidence of benign tissue in the presence of chondrosarcoma is accepted the incidence rises (with an equal fall in the incidence of primary cases) (Mirra, 1989). Dahlin (1978), using radiographic criteria, recognized 12% secondary chondrosarcoma. Mirra (1989), advocating histological criteria, suggests an incidence of 55%. For him this means that all large enchondromas must be curetted and all the tissue examined histologically for the presence of chondrosarcoma. Given the uncertainty of the statistics, the histological difficulty, the morbidity of the procedure and the necessity for continued follow-up it seems that a justifiable option is to do only the follow-up. The choice is a matter of judgement in each case.

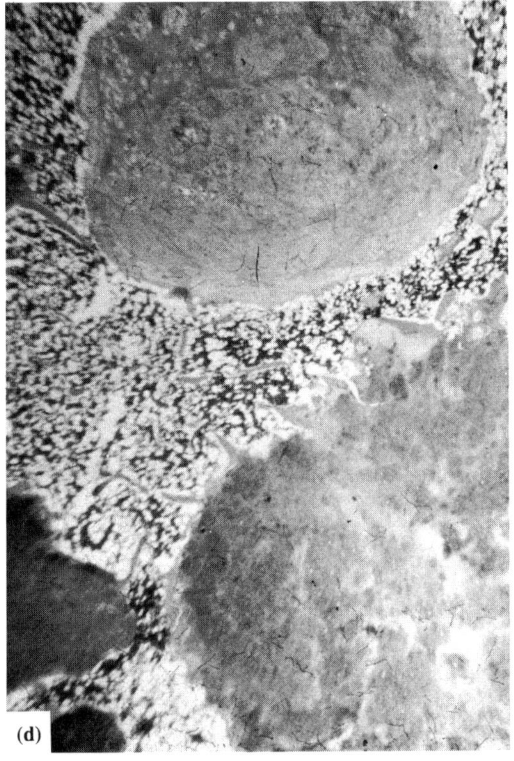

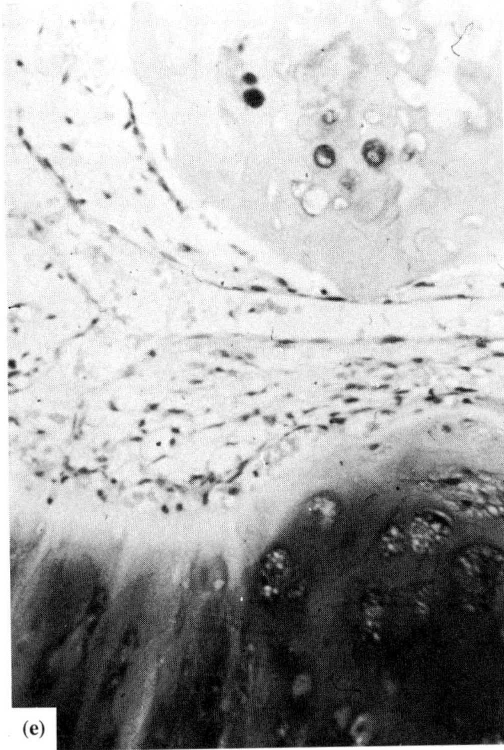

Figure 13.21 Female aged 57 years. Benign enchondromata in Ollier's disease. Pain in 'shoulder'. (d) Small and large nodules of cartilage encased by a thin sheet of bone, continuous with some trabecula, sit inertly in normal marrow. (e) Two nodules, one calcified, in close proximity but with no compression of marrow.

(a)   Hyaline intraosseous chondrosarcoma

(i)   Clinical features

The age range is the 2nd to 7th decades, most prevalent in decades five and six. It is distinctly unusual for children to have low grade cartilage tumours as do adults. Young *et al.* (1990) reported 47 cases under 17 years of age from the Mayo Clinic. Of these 47, 17 were Mayo Clinic cases and were drawn from a total 634 Clinic cases of chondrosarcoma.

Skeletal distribution The bones which are most affected, in decreasing prevalence, are: major long bones (especially the femur), the pelvis (notably the ilium) and the flat bones

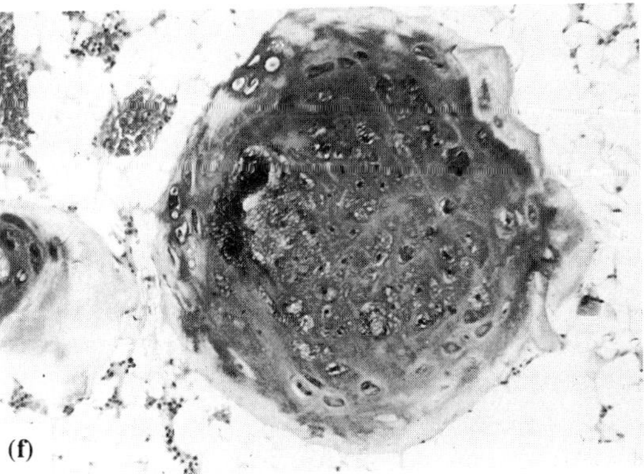

Figure 13.21 Female aged 57 years. Benign enchondromata in Ollier's disease. Pain in 'shoulder'. (f) A small nodule partly enclosed by bone, lying in normal marrow. The more central cells are well preserved, modest in number, and cytologically normal; there is one doubly nucleated cell.

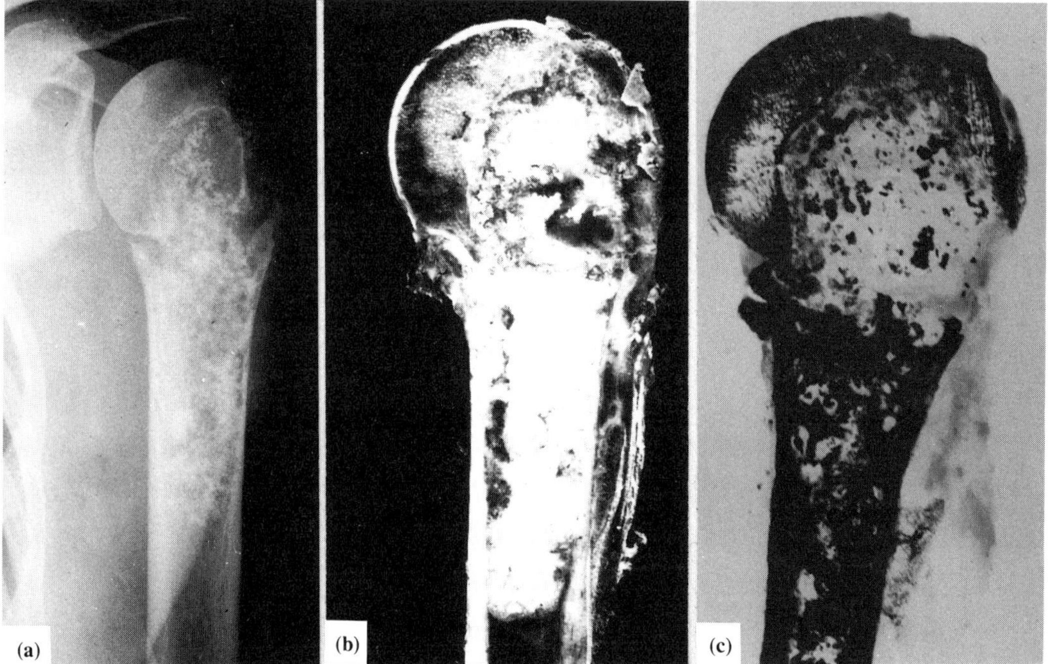

Figure 13.22. Female aged 60 years. Low-grade chondrosarcoma of humerus. Chronic pain in shoulder with acute exacerbation. (a) Clinical radiograph with densities similar to Figure 13.21a. But here there is a distinct lower edge indicating a tumour mass, endosteal erosion, a pathological fracture through the metaphysis, which terminates at a breach in the cortex on the lateral margin (not well reproduced), below which there is a thin soft tissue shadow extending down the periosteal cortical surface. (b) and (c) These features can be identified in the specimen photograph and the slab radiograph. The cortical breach was enlarged during biopsy. The marrow space is filled by solid tumour, a mixture of soft and mineralized cartilage. Although there appears to be a sclerotic upper margin in the clinical radiograph, a comparison with the specimen photograph and the slab radiograph shows that tumour has infiltrated (permeated, invaded) the marrow with a variable resorptive response.

of the trunk. Other sites are less common, and it is rare in hands and feet.

Differences of opinion over the prevalence of sarcoma secondary to solitary enchondroma have been discussed above. But all are agreed that in cases with multiple lesions (Ollier's disease and Maffuci syndrome), the risk of secondary chondrosarcoma is high. The figures quoted for Ollier's are: Mirra (1989) 43%; Schajowicz (1981) 30%; Liu *et al.* (1987) 29%. Lewis and Ketchum (1973) reported 15% of chondrosarcomas in 105 Maffuci cases. According to Mirra (1989) 5% of all chondrosarcomas are in cases with Ollier's disease.

Regardless of whether these tumours arise *de novo*, or as secondary change in a chondroma, the natural history of low-grade chondrosarcoma is persistent but slow growth over months to years. The danger to the patient comes more from the persistent growth than from metastasis (see prognosis). Untreated they grow to massive size. Inadequately treated they recur and spread, killing the patient when they reach strategic sites, such as the thoracic inlet, the spinal canal, the pelvic organs. Tumours of the flat bones are particularly difficult to deal with because they expand into soft tissue early on. In long bones they are contained for a long

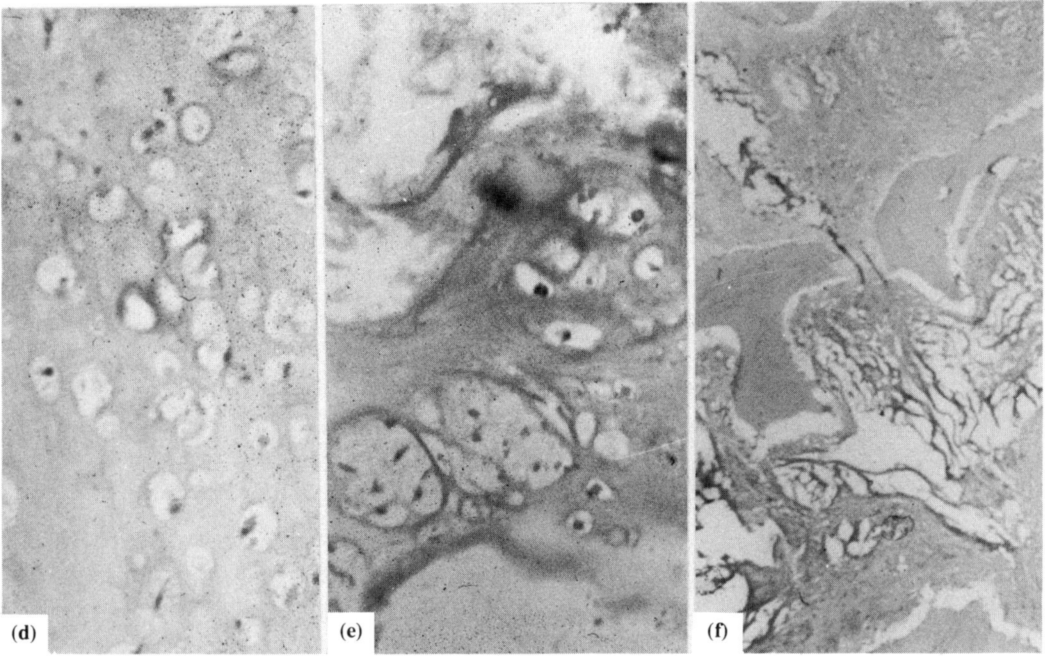

Figure 13.22. Female aged 60 years. Low-grade chondrosarcoma of humerus. Chronic pain in shoulder with acute exacerbation. (d) and (e) Viable non-mineralized tissue is not particularly cellular; many lacunae are empty, but the remaining cells have deeply stained nuclei and significant numbers are binucleate. Some cell clones are becoming degenerate. (f) Tissue from the epiphysis shows marrow invasion by cartilage of modest cellularity and poor matrix formation; there is active resorption of pre-existing trabeculae.

period during which time prosthetic replacement is very effective.

In most sites swelling is not obvious early on. Pain is the usual symptom, but may at first be attributed to another lesion, such as osteoarthritis, trauma, frozen shoulder. There is a risk that radiographs taken to investigate these diagnoses do not include the lesion, leading to a delay in recognition. In some cases there is not much change in aggressiveness over time and metastasis does not occur. In others there is a progression in malignancy with a risk of metastasis. In a few cases there is dedifferentiation of the neoplasm with growth of much more malignant tissue (see below).

The only effective treatment is extra-lesional surgical removal.

Mirra (1989) gives the following metastatic rates for grades of tumour: grade 1 <15%; grade 2 15–50%; grade 3 >50%.

The outcome is affected by conditions at the time of treatment: lesions contained within bone have a better prognosis following excision. In situations where operation is difficult recurrence rate is high, death due to local causes resulting from tumour growth, or metastasis.

Radiology (Figures 13.22–13.24) In long bones these are medullary lesions of the metaphysis or metadiaphysis, sometimes extending to the epiphysis (Figure 13.24). They are generally in excess of 5 cm in size, globally lytic lesions, patchily mineralized in a more diffuse pattern than the flecks, spots and circles of chondroma; these may be locally present if the sarcoma is secondary to solitary chondroma. Expansion of the bone is usual, but the periosteal response is less constant. The cortex may be thickened uniformly, thinned in part by erosion, or altogether reduced to a thin expanded shell. Pathological fracture in the latter instance is common. Penetration of the cortex occurs more at thinned points, but is not restricted to them. A soft tissue swelling is evident at these points. Extension of the tumour into the marrow cavity from the main mass is not

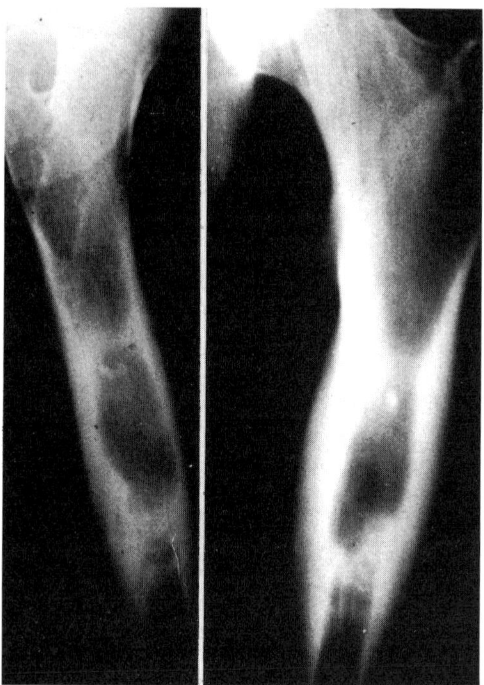

Figure 13.23. Female aged 45 years. Low-grade chondrosarcoma. A patient under observation for a slowly expanding osteolytic lesion of the femoral diaphysis for 10 years. Radiographic and histological interpretation of curettage on two occasions were interpreted as benign, the sections revealed only benign cartilage. After a further period of growth another curettage produced similar tissue but now a fragment of bone revealed invasion (permeation) by this tissue, an appearance similar to Figure 13.22 (f).

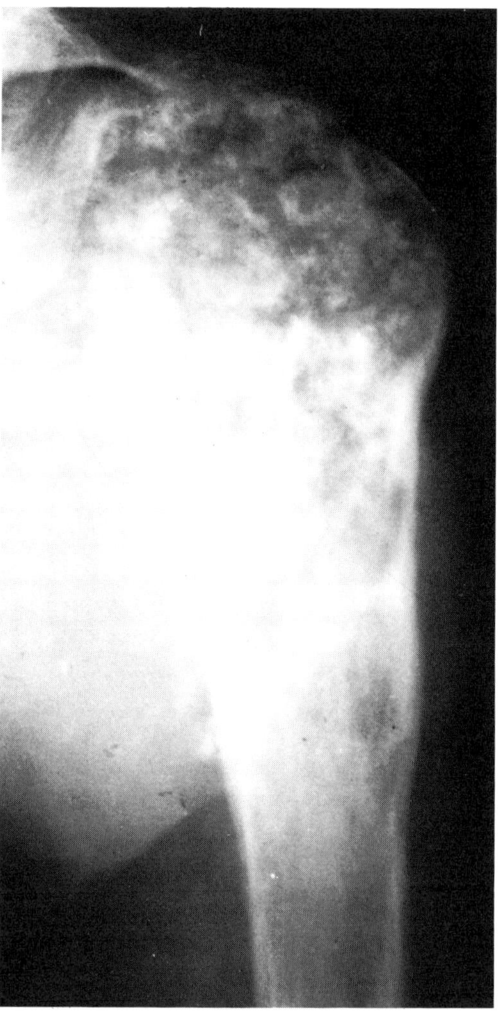

Figure 13.24. Male aged 48 years. Low-grade chondrosarcoma. Intermittent discomfort of shoulder for 'years'; gradual enlargement more recently. Diagnostic mineral pattern in tissue causing expansion of upper humerus. The cortex is irregularly eroded laterally, and is thinned to vanishing superiorly where there is the beginning of a soft tissue shadow. The endosteal irregularity extends down the shaft beyond the limits of the film indicating potential tumour extension; additional imaging would be required. Tissue from the amputation specimen had a structure similar to Figure 13.22 (d).

uncommon. This may give rise to little disturbance of the bone and not be immediately obvious; confirmation of its limits may require tomography. A further development which may occur is the formation of sequestra as the result of loss of blood supply to trabecular bone following marrow invasion by the tumour. This mechanism is the same in principle as in osteomyelitis, where the invading tissue is inflammatory.

Chondrosarcomas of flat bones have the same basic pattern, but, since the bones are small, extension to soft tissues is earlier and very large extraosseous masses can occur unnoticed, particularly from the ilium.

Sarcomas in multiple enchondromatosis give rise to an alteration of radiographic tissue pattern at the affected site (Liu *et al.*, 1987; Mirra, 1989). This precedes the onset of pain, usually by a long interval. The tumours are aggressive, particularly if they dedifferentiate.

(ii)   Pathology

Histopathology (Figures 13.22 and 13.27) These tumours are large and tend to be variable so that sampling is a consideration in the diagnosis. All curettings or biopsy fragments should be processed. Contact radiographs of slabbed intact specimens are helpful in identifying critical areas for examination: those where resorption or invasion of contiguous bone has occurred, and viable non-mineralized tissue.

If the tumour is secondary to a chondroma, benign tissue may be encountered (see above). If it is a grade 1 sarcoma the tissue may be indistinguishable from benign tumour and it will be its behaviour which is critical (Figure 13.20). This is judged from what is happening where the tumour tissue lies against host bone: resorption of the bone at the interface; permeation (infiltration, invasion) of the marrow; satellite nodules without investment by lamellar bone. Within the tumour, compression of fibrous tissue between contiguous tumour nodules is significant. These are indicative of growth, and in an adult are presumptive evidence of malignancy. With other features of the case, clinical and radiological, they can establish the diagnosis.

If the lesion is of grade 2 or 3 the histological assessment is relatively straightforward following conventional criteria for anaplasia (Figures 13.25 and 13.27).

The cytological features of cartilage tumours are listed in Table 13.9, with an indication of their relative incidence in different categories.

It must be emphasized that there are no agreed objective criteria, such as numbers per field or dimensions, by which to recognize cellularity, plumpness, numbers of binucleate cells or mitoses. Nevertheless, Mirra *et al.* (1985) in a study of 51 cases reached the following conclusions about the features of the most concentrated fields:

Table 13.9 Cytological features and relative incidence of cartilage tumours

	Hand and foot		*Axial and long bone*		
Malignancy	*Benign*	*High*	*Benign*	*Low*	*High*
Cellularity	+/+++	+++	+/++	+/++	+++
Pleomorphism	0	+++	0	+	+++
Plump cells	0/+	++	0/+	0/+	++
Large nuclei	0	++	0	0/++	++
Binucleate	0/+	++	0/+	0/++	++
Mitosis	0	+	0	0	+

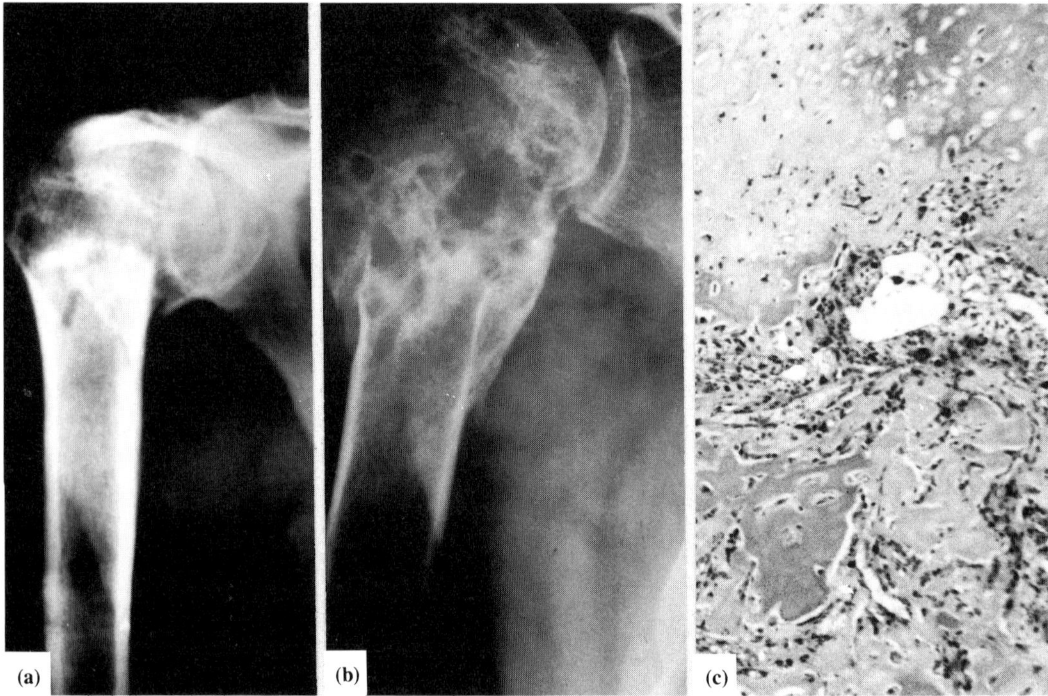

Figures 13.25 Male aged 45 years. Dedifferentiated chondrosarcoma. (a) Fractured humerus in road traffic accident. The radiolucent lesion in the metaphysis was not recognized. The detail is not sufficient for radiological diagnosis, but is consistent with the chondrosarcoma shown in (b). Two years later he had a pathological fracture. There is heavy mineralization with many ring structures. The fracture allowed the tumour to grow around the shaft, but within the periosteum, to produce an unusual expansion. In the centre of the tumour there is an irregular radiolucent zone which indicates more aggressive growth; this is present laterally as well where the mineralized tissue has been replaced, leaving irregular margins and some fluffy mineralization in the replacement tissue. These changes might be due to a local increase in grade of the tumour or to dedifferentiation. The extremely thin cortex of the distal shaft may be the effect of osteoporosis, but extension of tumour could be excluded by further imaging. (c) Biopsy of the lateral destructive focus. Chondrosarcomatous tissue at the top: moderately cellular but the nuclei are pleomorphic, hyperchromatic and often double. Below there is malignant osteoblastic tissue, highly cellular at the left margin.

Cells/0.159 mm^2 (1 high power field, $\times$ 400)

    more than 60 – 90% probability of chondrosarcoma

    more than 100 – 95% probability of chondrosarcoma

    more than 200 – 100% probability of chondrosarcoma

Doubly nucleated cells/3.1859 mm^2 (20 high power fields)

    more than 26 – 90% probability of chondrosarcoma

Mitoses/7.96 mm^2 (50 high power fields)

    two or more – malignancy

In most cases the radiographs provide sufficient evidence for the diagnosis. Histological confirmation may not be forthcoming; but since the overlap in the histology of benign and low-grade chondrosarcoma is well recognized the radiological/morbid anatomical evidence of growth of the lesion in a skeletal site other than hands and feet in an adult takes precedence and calls for a diagnosis of chondrosarcoma. In hands and feet a diagnosis of chondrosarcoma requires careful evaluation.

(b) High-grade chondrosarcoma (Figures 13.26 and 13.27)

Low-grade chondrosarcomas may progress to high-grade lesions, affecting only a portion of the tissue. But others arise as high-grade neoplasia and progress rapidly to death by metastasis. There is little about the latter group, clinically or radiologically, that is distinctive; they are destructive and invasive with no sign of calcification. They have a strong propensity to invade blood vessels, extending into major veins from where they may give rise to large emboli. Macroscopically they tend to be gelatinous rather than hyaline. Histologically they are variable in structure but unequivocally malignant. In less differentiated regions, where they are often highly pleomorphic, it is not easy to recognize their chondroid character.

The principal differential diagnosis in younger patients is osteosarcoma of the chondroblastic type. Probability greatly

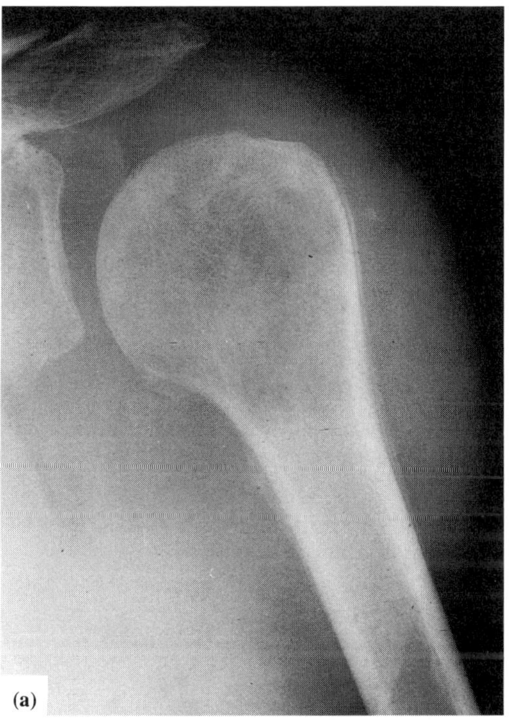

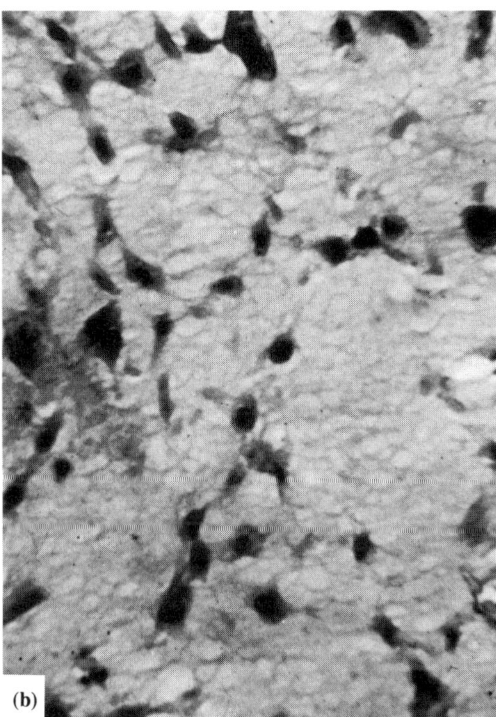

Figure 13.26 Male aged 47 years. High-grade chondrosarcoma. A short history of pain and swelling of shoulder. (a) There is a lytic lesion of the head and neck of the humerus in which there is patchy survival of cancellous bone. The endocortex is not obviously eroded. A delicate periosteal reaction is present, forming Codman triangles on the medial side of the metaphysis. But there is a much more extensive soft tissue swelling than is suggested by this, enveloping the whole of the upper end of the humerus, and causing widening of the joint space. Forequarter amputation revealed that tumour was growing in the subclavian vein. (b) The tumour was a poorly differentiated chondrosarcoma, giving rise to massive pulmonary metastasis.

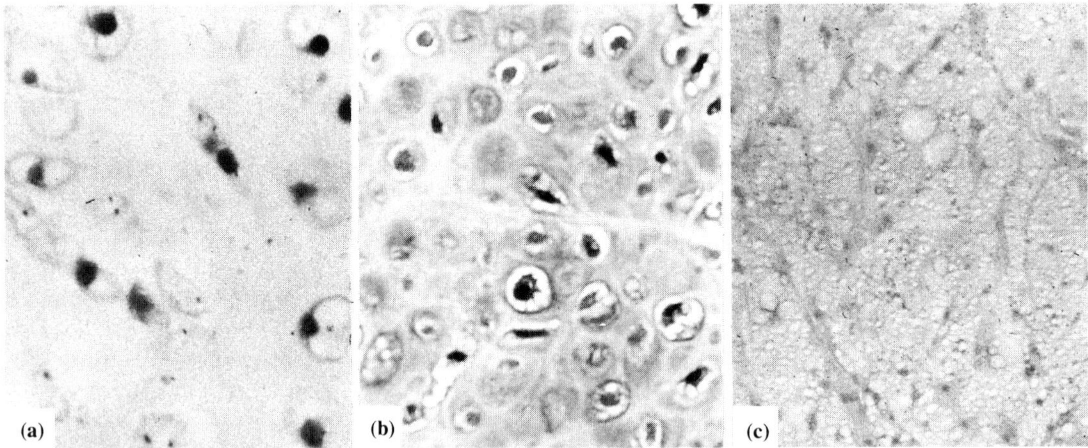

Figure 13.27 High-grade chondrosarcomas. Tissue from three tumours which gave rise to pulmonary metastases. (a) Moderately cellular with plump hyperchromatic nuclei, and scattered binucleate cells, characterless matrix. (b) A cellular hyaline matrix with many cells showing considerable pleomorphism; the larger nuclei are hyperchromatic and their cytoplasm is clear. (c) Moderate cellularity, with many spindle forms. But some cells are round and situated in lacunae. Slight hyperchromatism, and a good few binucleate cells.

favours this possibility and it should receive the most careful consideration taking all the evidence into account.

(c)   Dedifferentiated chondrosarcoma
(Figure 13.25)

(i)   Clinical features

The development of highly malignant tissue in low-grade chondrosarcoma was described by Dahlin and Beabout in 1971. Mirra (1989) has assembled data on 102 cases, including his 19 cases. In his estimate 10–20% of conventional chondrosarcomas are complicated by dedifferentiation.

The age range is 29–85 years, averaging 60 years.

Skeletal distribution These tumours occur mainly at the same sites as low-grade chondrosarcoma (see above); most occur in the pelvis (32%), femur (proximal 10%, distal 17%), proximal humerus (17%). The scapula (10%), ribs, proximal tibia, vertebrae and metacarpal follow.

Clinical presentation is with exacerbation of symptoms or, sometimes, pathological fracture.

Whatever the treatment for the more malignant component, the chondrosarcoma will require surgical removal.

The five-year survival is 10–15%.

Radiology In addition to the changes of the antecedent cartilage tumour there is lysis of bone by non-mineralized tissue with extension into soft tissue.

(ii)   Pathology

Histopathology The existing tumour is supplemented by additional, clearly demarcated neoplastic tissue. This was usually spindle celled, showing features of fibrosarcoma/fibrous histiocytoma in 60%; of osteosarcoma in 30%; of rhabdomyosarcoma in 3%; of a giant cell tumour look-alike in 2%; or undifferentiated sarcoma in 5%. Diagnosis requires the finding of high-grade malignant connective tissue in the presence of a conventional chondrosarcoma. In the case of a biopsy in which only the former appears the latter may be established from the morbid anatomy of the lesion.

There is no differential of the primary diagnosis given that the pathologist is made aware or finds out for himself, from the radiographs or the histological material, that there is a chondrosarcoma. The secondary diagnosis, of the dedifferentiated tissue, may present difficulties in classification.

(d)   Mesenchymal chondrosarcoma (Figure 13.28)

This tumour was recognized as a primary bone tumour in 1959 by Lichtenstein and Bernstein (1959). Goldman identified it as also occurring in soft tissues in 1967. Salvador *et al.* (1971), reported 30 cases from the Mayo Clinic; and in Huvos *et al.* (1983) a further 35 cases. In addition, papers based on one or a few cases are regularly published. Dahlin and Unni (1988) consider 19 cases involving bone. Published experience indicates that the incidence is roughly three times more frequent in bone. The tissue has a resemblance to that of benign chondroblastoma, and some have wondered about their relationship. However, as the result of ultrastructural studies, a similarity to fetal chondrogenic tissue has been widely supported and a connection with chondroblastoma is not favoured (Swanson *et al.*, 1990).

(i)   Clinical features

The age range is decades one to six, with more than 50% in decades two and three.

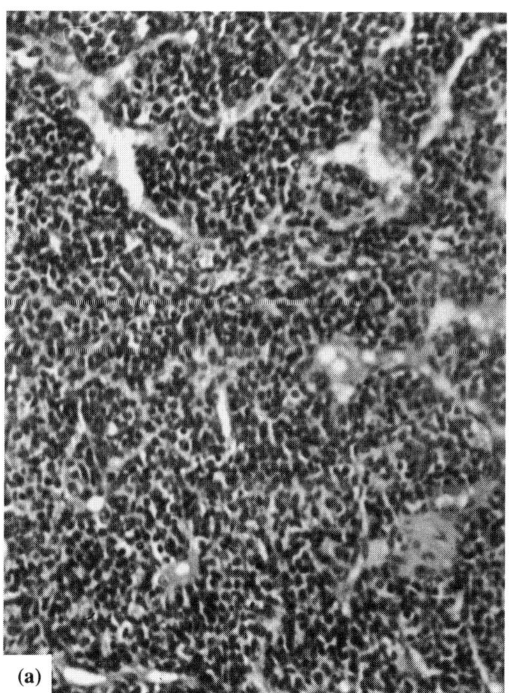
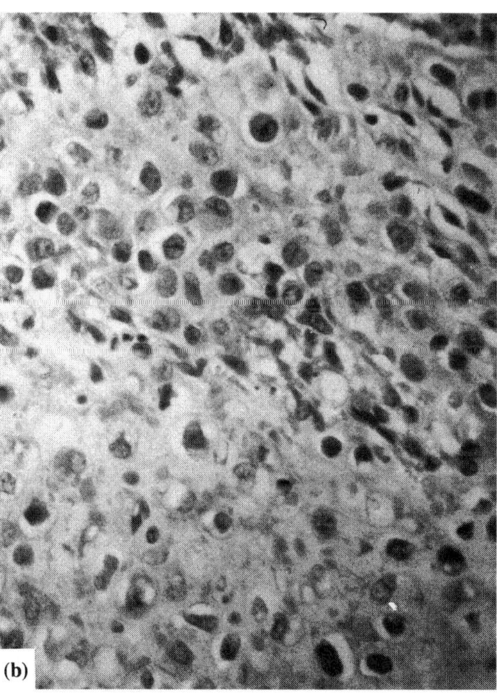

Figure 13.28 Mesenchymal chondrosarcoma. (a) Low power view showing a sheet of small round cells broken up by the vascular pattern. (b) Zone of transition between the small round cells and malignant hyaline cartilage.

Skeletal distribution The facial bones (16%), ribs (18%) and femoral diaphysis (15%) are most common: 32% are distributed through the the other flat bones, includng the skull. The remainder (18%) are in the other long and short (foot) tubular bones. In soft tissue the most common sites are in the head and neck, but the range of sites is broad.

There is no particular clinical presentation; pain and swelling are the principal complaints.

The treatment depends on site: resection/amputation is appropriate where possible; chemotherapy as adjunctive or sole treatment is used.

The prognosis is poor; the tumours metastasize early, and to somewhat unusual sites.

Radiology The lesion in bone is globally destructive, with a variable zone of transition, but without marginal reaction. About half the tumours have small, well-developed focal calcification.

(ii)   Pathology

Histopathology (Figure 13.28) The bulk of the neoplasm is formed of close packed round to oval cells, with little cytoplasm, free from pleomorphism and overt mitotic activity. Notwithstanding that the pattern of the vasculature is reminiscent of haemangiopericytoma, there is nothing specific about these stromal cells in paraffin, H & E sections, and they qualify as small round cells. The diagnostic feature is focal chondroid tissue, reasonably well differentiated, which is frequently calcified and sometimes ossified. The presence of calcified matrix should be anticipated if calcification is evident on the radiograph; since it can be widely dispersed it may require several levels and/or several blocks to locate. Cells conforming to osteoclasts may be present in proximity to the cartilage.

The diagnosis requires the demonstration

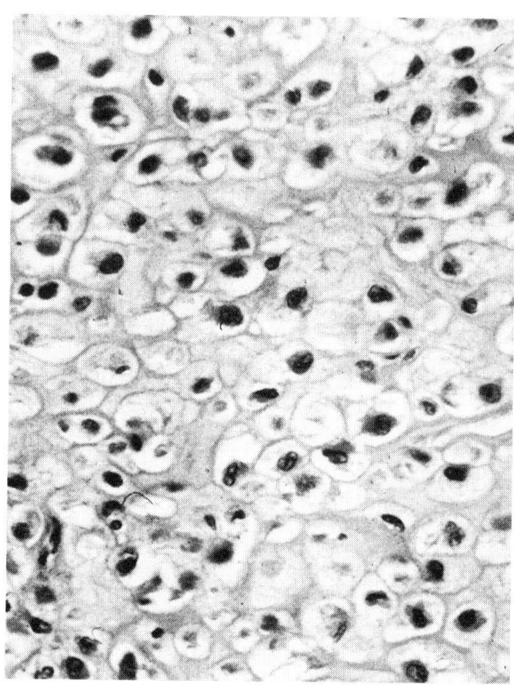

Figure 13.29 Clear cell chondrosarcoma. Very many closely packed cells, with hyperchromatic pleomorphic nuclei, some with double nuclei. The beginning of bony metaplasia is occurring at the sites where the matrix is more dense.

of chondroid tissue in an otherwise round celled neoplasm.

The cellular element carries no specific feature and might lead to consideration of round or spindle cell neoplasias (see differential diagnosis of soft tissue mesenchymal chondrosarcoma below). The morbid anatomy would be indicative of cartilage tumour if it is calcifying. Otherwise diagnosis depends on finding islands of cartilage.

(e)   Clear cell chondrosarcoma (Figure 13.29)

This was first recognized by Unni *et al.* (1976). Since then series of cases have been published (Bjornson *et al.*, 1984; Campanacci *et al.*, 1980). With his own and cases from the literature, Mirra (1989) presented details on 68 cases with a 2:1 male preponderance.

(i) Clinical features

The age range is decades two to nine, with about 45% in the third and fourth decades.

Skeletal distribution About 90% of lesions are in the major long bones, where they affect the epiphyses (proximal femur 59%; proximal humerus 17%; knee 10%). About 10% are distributed in vertebrae, ribs, pelvis and skull.

Clinical presentation is with low-grade pain over a year or more, usually referred to a joint. Pathological fracture was not uncommon.

The treatment is adequate removal by excision or amputation.

The prognosis is that most patients survive, but around 15% have recurrences or metastases leading to death.

Radiology There is a global osteolytic lesion of the epiphysis, which, in some cases, extends into the metaphysis. The bone tends to be expanded. The transition zone is nar-

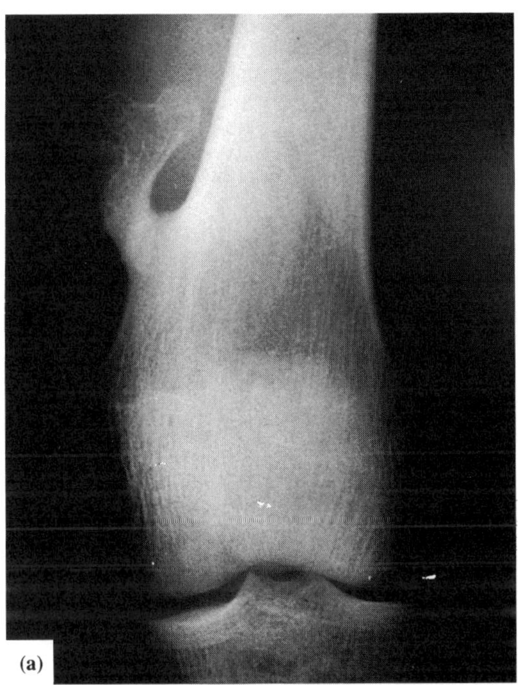

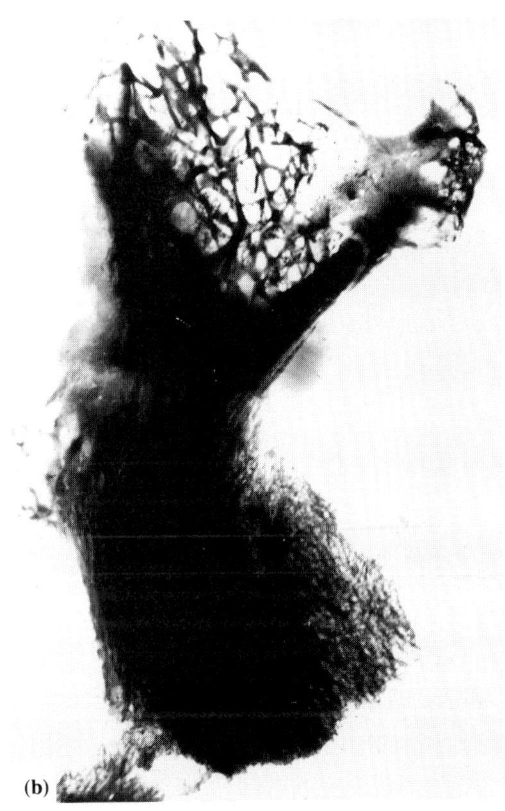

Figure 13.30 Male aged 25 years. Solitary osteochondroma, discovered following fracture of stalk. (a) Clinical radiograph: the lesion has grown out from the medial aspect of the distal femoral metaphysis, and towards the centre of the bone. There is continuity between the cortices, and between the marrow cavities. The metaphysis beyond and on the side of the lesion is abnormally wide. The cartilage cap is not demonstrated in either the clinical or fine detail radiograph. (b) The latter shows a network of indistiguishable cartilage and bony calcified structures at the top which are stages in the ossification process. Angulation at the mid-point of the stalk is the site of fracture; associated callus is present.

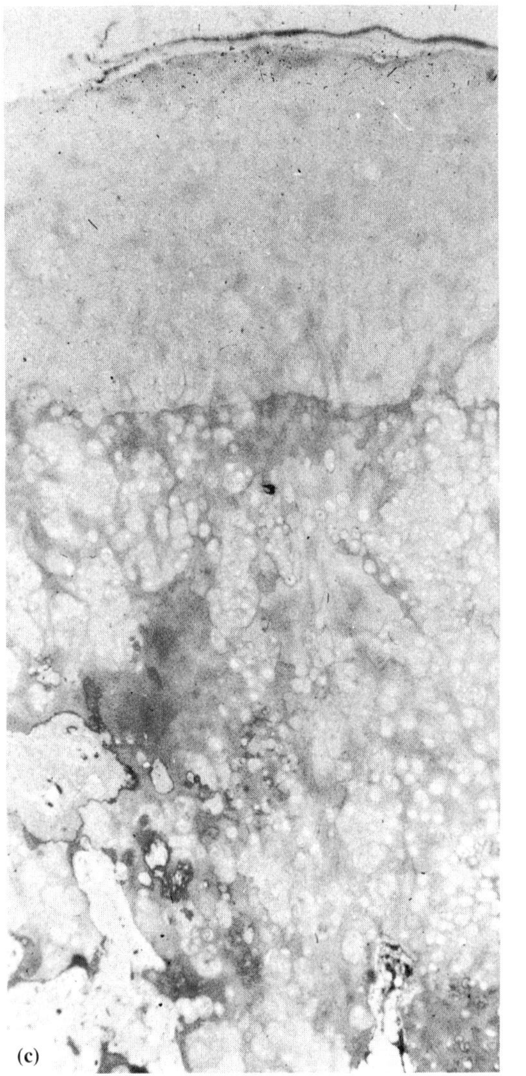

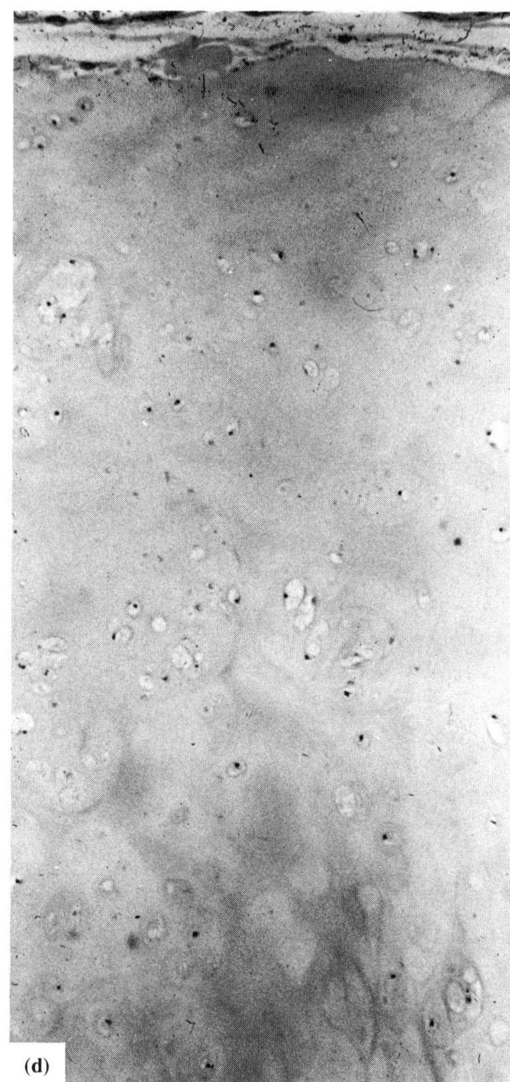

Figure 13.30 Male aged 25 years. Solitary osteochondroma, discovered following fracture of stalk. (c) The cartilage cap is not unduly thick, and rests on a wide zone of calcified, necrotic cartilage. At the bottom fingers of resorption extend into this; deposition of bone on these surfaces will follow. The completion of ossification is often irregular, leaving islands of calcified cartilage marooned in the stalk. (d) The viable surface cartilage is the tissue that must be assessed for malignant potential. The criteria are the same as for enchondroma: here the cartilage is well structured, moderately cellular, without anaplastic features, with only occasional binucleate cells.

row with a tendency to be sclerotic. Spotty calcification is evident in about half the cases. The appearance bears a close resemblance to benign chondroblastoma.

(ii)   Pathology

Histopathology (Figure 13.29) The tissue is composed of close packed clear cells, contain-

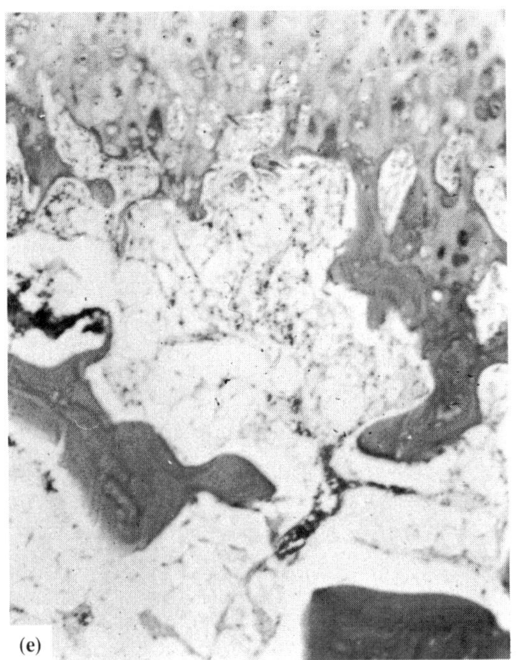

Figure 13.30 Male aged 25 years. Solitary osteochondroma, discovered following fracture of stalk. (e) The manner of ossification is epiphyseal, not physeal.

ing glycogen. In some of the tissue the cells may not be vacuolated. Cytologically there is little anaplasia, and mitoses are rare. Lobulaton is sometimes a feature. There is little intercellular chondroid matrix, but there may be osseous trabeculae of woven bone in a pattern resembling osteoblastoma, and is responsible for the mineral distribution. The cells are usually S-100 positive, and have features of cartilage cells on electron microscopy (Charpentier *et al.*, 1979).

The diagnosis requires a lesion in an adult with radiographic and histological resemblance to benign chondroblastoma which is the basis for segregating the tumour as chondroblastic. Large clear cells and osseous trabeculae are hallmarks. If this pattern is not registered the diagnosis is by exclusion of metastasis.

In the differential diagnosis chondroblas-

toma is the principal alternative. But confusion with osteoblastoma may arise if the osseous element is particularly prominent; however, it is not an epiphyseal tumour. Metastatic carcinoma can be a problem, particularly with a small biopsy.

13.7 CARTILAGE TUMOURS ON THE SURFACE OF BONES

13.7.1 OSTEOCHONDROMA AND ITS MALIGNANT TRANSFORMATION (FIGURES 13.30 AND 13.31)

This is a bony outgrowth from the metaphysis formed from a cartilage cap, which is generally accepted as being derived from the physis (Milgram, 1983). The lesion develops in childhood, grows during this period, and usually ceases to grow after puberty, or does so very slowly.

(a) Clinical features

These lesions come to attention in the first to fifth decades, but mainly in decades two, three and four.

(i) Skeletal distribution

Any non-membranous bone, but the great majority are around the knee (about 40%) and upper humerus (about 20%). Much less common are the flat bones, and vertebrae. They are rare in the hands and feet. The location within a bone is metaphyseal or diametaphyseal.

According to Mirra (1989) between 1% and 2% of individuals who have had extensive radiographic surveys show an asymptomatic osteochondroma.

In the majority of cases the lesion is solitary. But there are cases with multiple lesions (Figure 13.32), for which there is a genetic basis; the condition is known as diaphyseal aclasia. The lesions are symptomless, but can give rise to a swelling. Some are sessile and

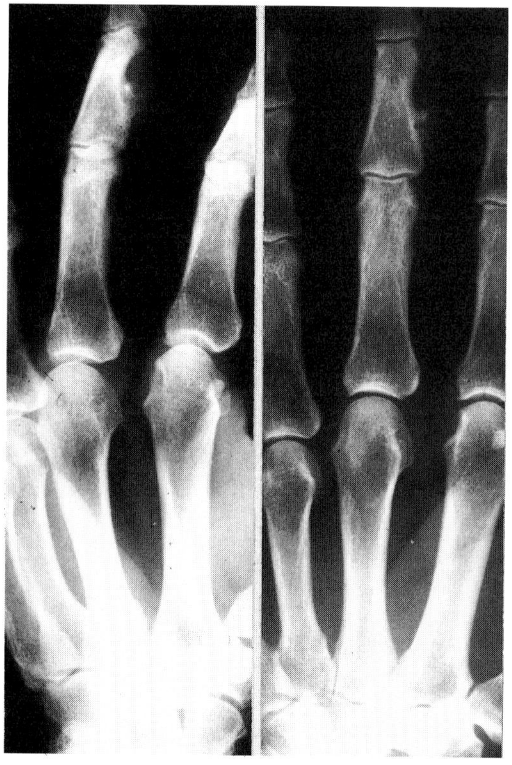

Figure 13.31 Female aged 56 years. Osteochondroma of middle phalanx of middle finger. The metaphysis is flared, and its cortex runs into the projecting lesion. Further details of the lesion are not clear, but these are sufficient for diagnosis, which was confirmed from the excised tissue. Radiograph courtesy of Mr C.E.A. Holden.

are responsible for a widening of the metaphysis (flask shaped), a feature common in patients with multiple lesions, in whom deformity can be substantial. Prominent lesions are prone to injury in some sites, particularly fracture of the stalk. Persistent growth of the lesion after puberty, or its resumption in an adult, especially where there are multiple lesions, always causes a sense of concern about malignancy (see below).

Quiescent lesions found by chance need no treatment and can be kept under surveillance. Active lesions must be removed with-

out exposing the cap and without previous biopsy.

The prognosis is good if inactive or if excision is adequate in active lesions.

(ii)   *Radiology* (Figures 13.30–13.32)

The cap grows and ossifies. The resulting bone is remodelled to produce a cortical and cancellous architecture, which are continuous with the respective elements of the bone from which the lesion arises. This feature is pathognomonic, and serves to differentiate osteochondroma from all other surface lesions. Many of the lesions have long stalks, which turn in the direction of the diaphysis as the result of the remodelling. Others are sessile, particularly those on the flat bones.

(b)   **Pathology** (Figure 13.30)

The active constituent of the lesion is the cartilage cap. Presumptively derived from the physis, it nevertheless grows and ossifies like the epiphysis (see Chapter 19). The bone is remodelled to form a cortex and medulla

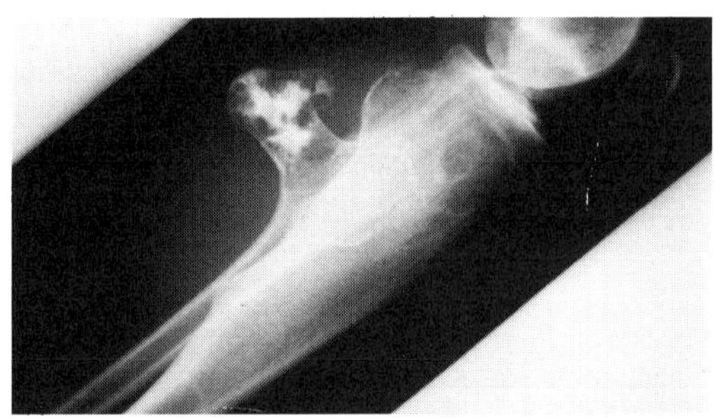

Figure 13.32 Female aged 27 years. Multiple osteochondromatosis. Lateral radiograph of the leg. A large lesion extends from the tibia and is seen in profile; the irregularity of the ossification is manifested by the focal calcification below the cap. Other lesions are seen end on, appearing as holes in the cortex where the marrow cavities are in continuity; their edge is accentuated by the cortex of the stalk. Radiograph courtesy of Mr P.W. Skinner.

each continuous with the parent structure: this is specific for the lesion. However, this may be less strikingly clear in sessile lesions, which can then be read as some other lesion on bone (parosteal osteosarcoma, myositis ossificans, avulsion injury). The quiescent lesion has a thin sparsely cellular cap, or in some cases no discernible cartilage. If growth resumes the cartilage becomes thicker, or reappears, to a thickness of 2–3 cm, and again grows and ossifies. The zones of mineralization and ossification can be very irregular, and the remodelling disorderly, leaving areas of mixed mineralized, necrotic cartilage, and bone intermingled with adipose marrow. Some benign lesions, both solitary and in osteochondromatosis, can become very large, up to 10–15 cm. The substance of these, apart from the cartilage cap, is often very dense as the result of extensive mineralization and irregular ossification of the cartilage growth. Radiographic assessment of the thickness of the cartilage cap may be difficult, but possible by CT and

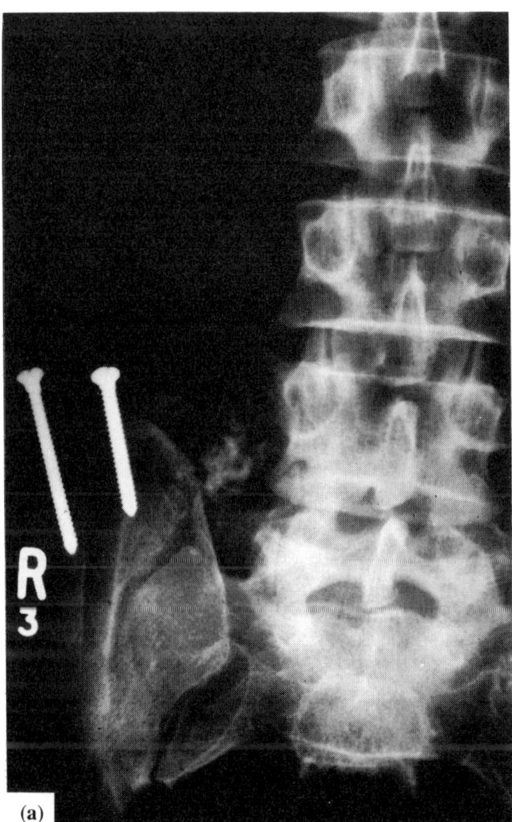
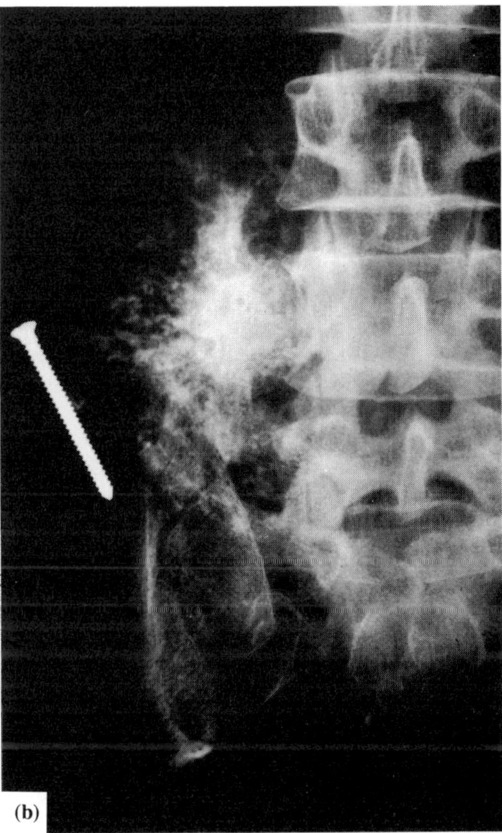

Figure 13.33 Male aged 26 years. Chondrosarcoma in multiple osteochondromatosis. (a) Radiograph of osteochondroma arising from ilium. The anatomical detail is not clear: the external focally calcified mass fixed to the ilium in a patient with osteochondromatosis is strong presumptive evidence, confirmed by other views. (b) Eight years later a very large calcified mass has developed at the site. Its surface is irregular with sinuous calcified filaments extending from it for distances of several centimetres. These are in the cartilage cap and are an indicator of its thickness, and of gross irregularity in calcification and ossification, indicative of malignancy. Radiographs courtesy of Mr T.R. Morley.

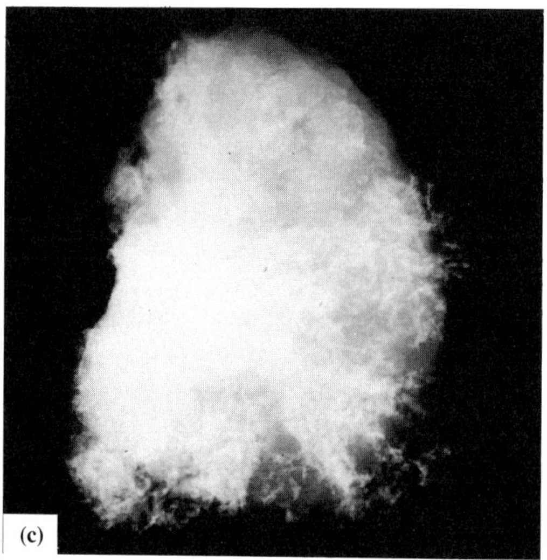

Figure 13.33 Male aged 26 years. Chondrosarcoma in multiple osteochondromatosis. (c) Slab radiograph of excised specimen showing extensive mineralization, diminishing towards the periphery, and conforming with the appearances in (b).

MRI. Norman and Sissons (1984) found the presence of flecks of mineral in the site of the cartilage cap to be indicative of malignancy (see below).

The diagnosis is established by demonstration of the morbid anatomy and a benign cartilage cap.

Alternatives to a classical osteochondroma do not exist. But this depends on demonstrating the pathognomonic morbid anatomy.

13.7.2 MALIGNANT TRANSFORMATION OF OSTEOCHONDROMA (FIGURE 13.33)

This occurs in less than 1% of solitary lesions and in the order of 10–20% of patients with multiple lesions (Jaffe, 1958). Mayo Clinic experience suggests that about 8% of chondrosarcomas arise in osteochondromas (Garrison *et al.*, 1982).

(a) Clinical features

The majority, about 85% of 168 cases (Mirra, 1989), occur between 30 and 70 years.

(i) *Skeletal distribution*

In the same report lesions were located in femoral metaphyses (27%), proximal metaphysis of tibia (8%) and humerus (9%), ilium (23%). Ribs, scapula, pubis, sacrum and vertebrate had each 4–7%. The foot, hand and clavicle were also affected.

Onset of growth in a known quiescent lesion, or swelling, and pain are the usual presentation.

Treatment is extralesional excision, which might mean amputation.

Solitary lesions undergoing transformation tend to be on long bones where they are more readily accessible and have a better prognosis. Lesions of pelvis and vertebrae are more difficult to remove and most of these patients die from the complications of local recurrence.

(ii) *Radiology*

Unless the tumour is excessively large, heavily mineralized or sessile an underlying osteochondroma may be demonstrated. Otherwise the primary lesion may be inferred on clinical grounds or from the presence in images of soft tissue overlying a mineralized mass. The important assessment is the cartilage cap, whose thickness and mineral content may be determinable by imaging.

A thickness above 3 cm is regarded as a sign of malignancy (Kenney *et al.*, 1974), although some say 2 cm is the limit (Mirra, 1989). Norman and Sissons (1984) demonstrated that the presence of mineral in a thickened cap is also an indicator of malignancy.

(b) Pathology

If there is a shift to malignant activity this takes place in the cartilage, which becomes thicker, lobulated (i.e. nodular) and assumes features of malignant cartilage. These, which are the same as for intraosseous lesions, may

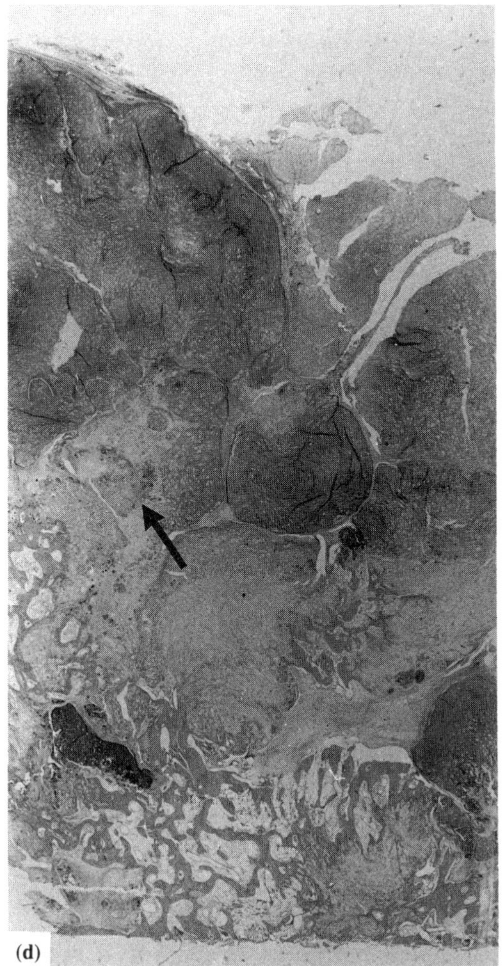

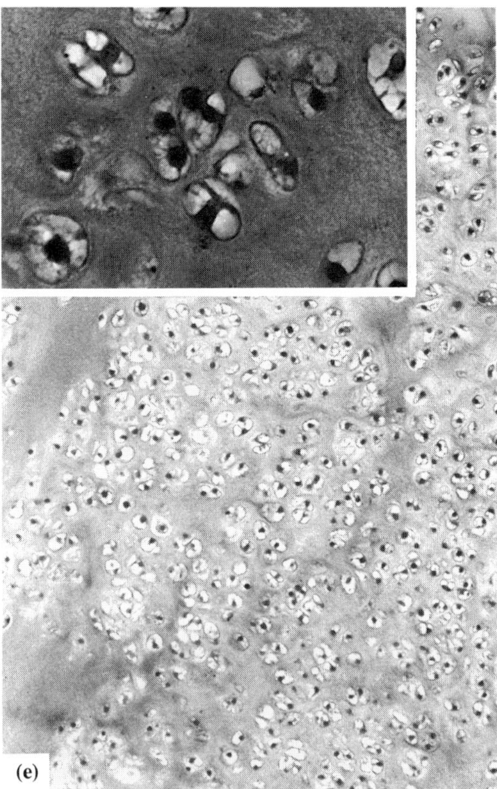

Figure 13.33 Male aged 26 years. Chondrosarcoma in multiple osteochondromatosis. (d) Low power photomicrograph of the cartilage cap. It interfaces irregularly with the bone of the stalk at the bottom; a finger of bone extends into the cartilage; beyond that there is a focus of mineralization (arrow). The cartilage is lobulated and abnormally thick; nevertheless, most of the tissue is sparsely cellular. (e) Higher magnification. Only one nodule in the several sections is very cellular with plump, well-stained nuclei and occasional binucleate cells. The thick lobulated cartilage is diagnostic of low-grade chondrosarcoma; the cellular tissue demonstrates the potential for active growth.

be more or less obvious, with proportional difficulties in reaching the diagnosis. Lobulation (formation of nodules) of the cartilage, even in the absence of other features, is a danger sign.

Given confirmation of chondrosarcoma and of an underlying osteochondroma there is no other diagnosis. If evidence of the primary lesion is wanting, an arrangement of malignant cartilage overlying mixed calcified cartilage and bone would still be circumstantial evidence for malignant change in osteochondroma. What is important for the patient is the correct assessment of malignancy.

In a few cases dedifferentiation of the chondrosarcoma has been observed (Mirra,

1989). An increase in the rate of growth of the lesion, a focus of distortion in the pattern of the lesion, and an additional soft tissue mass composed of spindle cell sarcoma were the main features.

13.7.3 PERIOSTEAL CHONDROMA (FIGURE 13.34)

These are benign cartilage tumours arising in the periosteum, which are not known to undergo malignant transformation (Lewis *et al.*, 1990).

(a) Clinical features

The age range is the second to fifth decades. Periosteal chondroma is a rare lesion, estimated by Mirra (1989) to be about 0.5% of bone tumours studied histologically.

(i) Skeletal distribution

Most occur on short and long tubular bones; the location may be metaphyseal or diaphyseal. A few occur on bones of the trunk – ribs, pelvis, vertebrae.

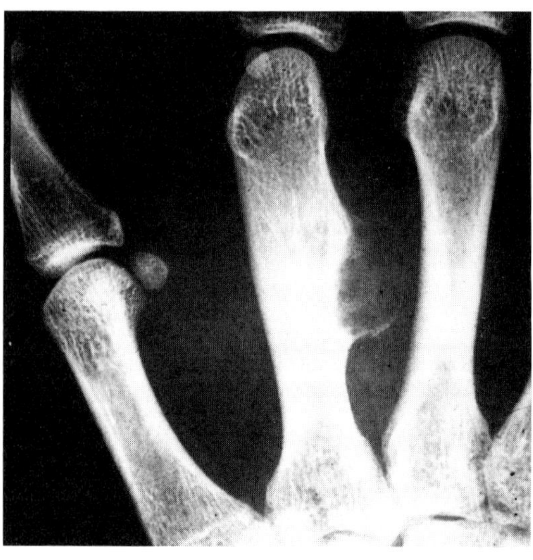

Figure 13.34 Periosteal chondroma of metacarpal. A round soft tissue nodule with spotty calcification has eroded the cortex and caused some periosteal buttressing which accentuates the depression in the cortex.

If the lesions are small and painless, as many are, they may only be detected incidentally. Swelling, often with pain, may draw attention.

Extralesional local excision is the ideal treatment.

Incomplete removal can lead to recurrence. None have been reported to become malignant.

(b) Pathology

(i) Morbid anatomy

These are radiolucent lesions, lying in a shallow depression on the surface of the bone resulting from pressure resorption. The size is in the range 1–10 cm. Spotty calcification of the tissue occurs in many, which identifies cartilage. Macroscopically the tissue is usually hyaline cartilage, sometimes with myxoid foci. There may be an osteoblastic reaction on the contiguous bone surface forming Codman triangles which accentuate the depth of the depression. Small lesions are beneath the periosteum, but this may be less apparent in larger lesions. The deep surface rests on sclerotic bone.

(ii) Histopathology

Mainly lobulated, hyaline cartilage of variable cellularity, which can be high. However, the cells are uniform, and mitoses are not seen. Doubly nucleated cells can be fairly numerous.

The morbid anatomy and the absence of cytological malignancy are diagnostic.

Of the other surface lesions only parosteal chondrosarcoma could present a problem in differential diagnosis. Factors entering into assessment are size, density of underlying bone and cytology.

13.7.4 PAROSTEAL CHONDROSARCOMA

There has been controversy and confusion over the entities parosteal chondrosarcoma and periosteal osteosarcoma. Jaffe (1958) recorded a case he considered to be a parosteal chondrosarcoma. Unni *et al.* (1976) described periosteal osteosarcoma, a lesion of bone and cartilage which they considered to be an osteosarcoma. But Schajowicz (1981) thought the latter cases were chondrosarcomas and advocated the qualification juxtacortical. He also advocated the term peripheral osteosarcoma for surface osteosarcomas of high-grade malignancy. The report by Bertoni *et al.* (1982) in which they convincingly separated seven cases of chondrosarcoma from 20 cases of periosteal osteosarcoma was convincing evidence for the entity.

Mirra (1989) describes the condition based on cases from four sources: his own (4), Jaffe (1958) (1), Bertoni *et al.* (1982) (7), Nojima *et al.* (1985) (14).

(a) Clinical features

The age range is decades two to seven; half were in decades two to four.

(i) Skeletal distribution

- Femur 54% (proximal 11%, mid 8%, distal 35%)
- Humerus 23% (proximal 19%, mid 4%)
- Tibia 4% (mid 4%)
- Pelvis 11%
- Rib 4%
- Foot 4%

Clinical presentation is with swelling, and pain in 35%.
Treatment is radical removal of the lesion.
None of 10 patients followed for 2–22 months had recurrence or metastasis.

(ii) Radiology

Round to ovoid masses, with minimal mineral deposits (punctate, granular, curvilinear), but none with a perpendicular orientation as in periosteal osteosarcoma.

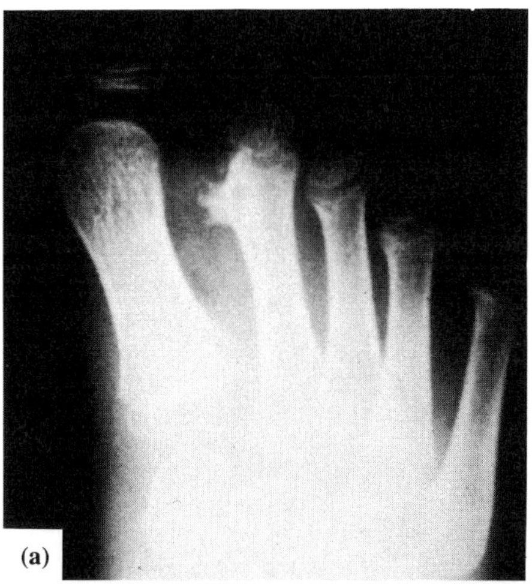

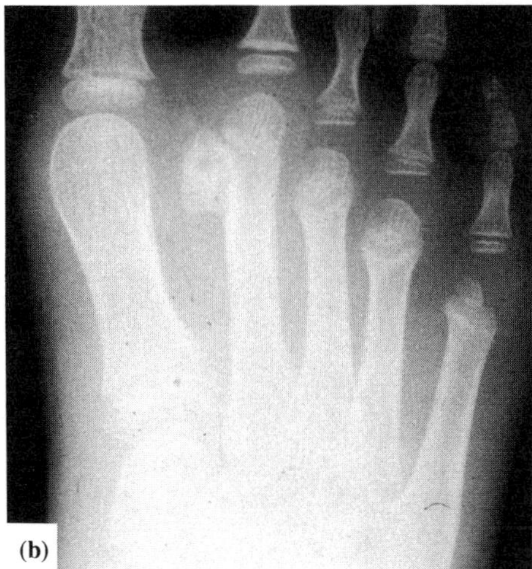

Figure 13.35 Male aged 6 years. Bizarre parosteal osteochondromatous proliferation of second right metatarsal. (a) Radiograph at presentation. Rounded radiolucent tissue, with stippling, rests on a dense, short stalk arising from the periosteum. It was confirmed that the cortex was intact on surgical removal. The lesion recurred, had a similar appearance and was again removed. (b) Radiograph at second recurrence. An ovoid calcified mass, with a satellite nodule, lies adjacent to the second metatarsal. There was no further recurrence after 15 months, follow-up. Radiographs courtesy of Mr E.M. Thomas.

The underlying bone may be eroded, and the depression accentuated by marginal reactive bone.

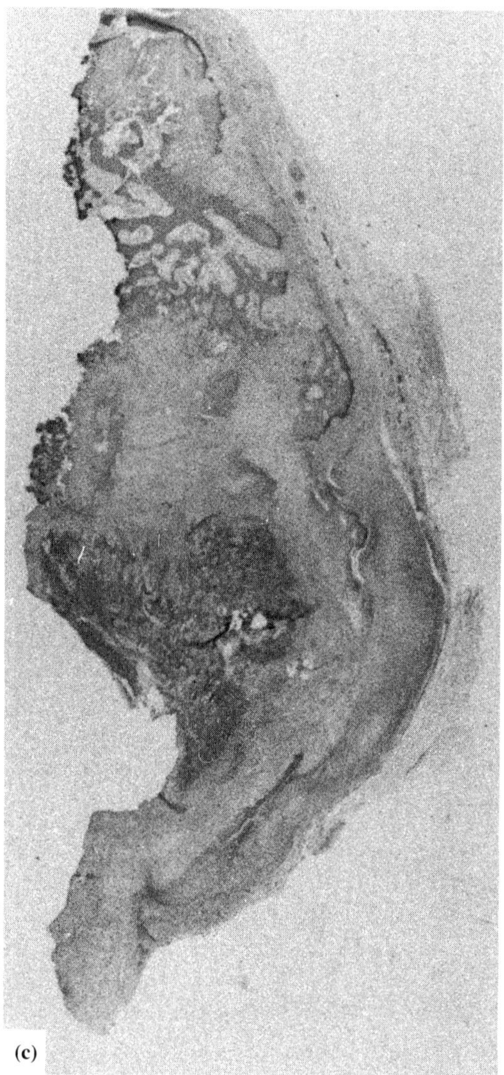

(c)

Figure 13.35 Male aged 6 years. Bizarre parosteal osteochondromatous proliferation of second right metatarsal. (c) The tissue from the three operations was similar. Panoramic view of a slice from the tissue removed at first operation. Irregular ossification in chondroid tissue with formation of nodular extensions at the surface.

(b)   Pathology

Hyaline to myxoid lobules of cartilage of malignant character, although the grade is variable.

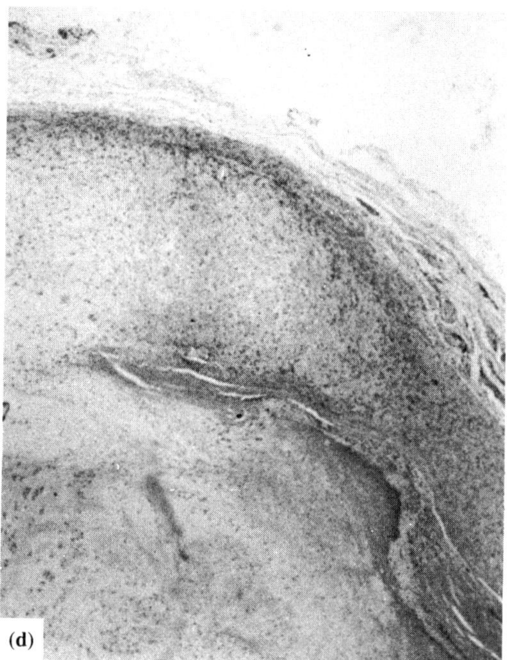

(d)

Figure 13.35 Male aged 6 years. Bizarre parosteal osteochondromatous proliferation of second right metatarsal. (d) The more superficial chondroid tissue. This is most cellular at the surface suggesting active growth at this site.

13.7.5   REACTIVE LESIONS ON THE SURFACE OF BONE AND BIZARRE PAROSTEAL OSTEOCHONDROMATOUS PROLIFERATION (FIGURE 13.35)

There are a few non-neoplastic entities that cause tumours (swellings) on the surface of bone. Heterotopic bone formation is dealt with in Chapter 6 (e.g. myositis ossificans) and periosteal reactions in Chapter 20. Stress fractures also might be considered. These are entities for which there is usually an underlying cause or associated conditions, although the pathogenesis may be far from clear. But there are other lesions where at first the reactive nature was not clear or, if it was, the provocation was not. Some such lesions, occurring in hands and feet, have been described as florid reactive periostitis

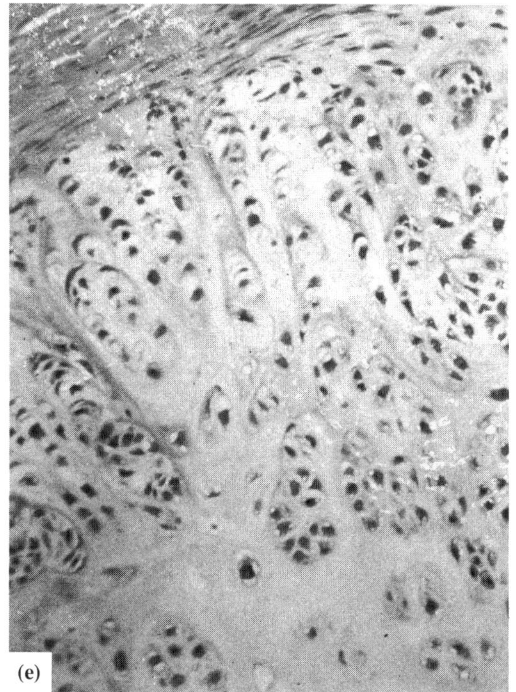

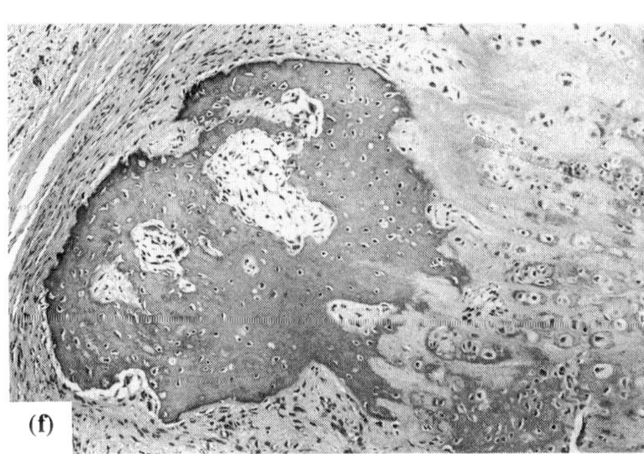

Figure 13.35 Male aged 6 years. Bizarre parosteal osteochondromatous proliferation of second right metatarsal. (e) The cellular zone of a chondroid lobule with the cells in clusters radially orientated at the surface. The nuclei are slightly pleomorphic and somewhat hyperchromatic. There are no mitoses but a few cells are binucleate. (f) The process of ossification is very irregular and difficult to explain. However, the formed bony nodule is undergoing active remodelling.

(Spujt and Dorfman, 1981), as bizarre parosteal osteochondromatous proliferation (Nora *et al.*, 1983), and as fibro-osseous pseudotumour (Dupree and Enzinger, 1986). It seems probable that these are different terms for the same thing.

(a) Clinical features

Fewer than 100 cases have been reported, mainly in the tubular bones of the hands. Swelling is usually accompanied by pain and tenderness. Rapid growth sometimes occurs. The age range of patients is the second to eighth decades.

Radiologically these are partly mineralized, rounded lesions attached to an intact bone surface; some lesions have been described as having a pedicle.

Treatment has been by local resection, but in a few recurrent lesions there has been ray resection. There have not been any metastases, and the lesions continue to be regarded as reactive.

(b) Pathology

Their histological composition is a mixture of cartilage and bone, the latter usually arising from the former, and sometimes fibrous tissue. The cartilage can be quite cellular, but without features of anaplasia.

13.8 CARTILAGE TUMOURS IN SOFT TISSUE

13.8.1 CHONDROMA

This category was established by Dahlin and Salvador (1974) and their experience has been added to by others (Chung and Enzinger, 1978; Humphreys *et al.*, 1986)

(a) Clinical features

The age range is the middle years.

(i)   Skeletal distribution

Digits of hands and feet; rarely trunk, head and neck, tongue.

Clinical presentation is as a painless mass. Treatment is local excision. There is some tendency to recurrence, but no metastases have been reported.

(b)   Pathology

(i)   Morbid anatomy

Circumscribed, encapsulated, lobulated, hyaline or myxoid cut surface. Calcification is common and may be evident by X-ray or on sectioning; sometimes it can be very abundant, obscuring the histological detail and raising the possibility of tumoral calcinosis.

(ii)   Histopathology

The tissue is usually hyaline cartilage of variable cellularity, which may be very pronounced and associated with a degree of pleomorphism and bi- or multinucleate forms. Mitoses are not seen. Since hyaline soft tissue chondrosarcomas are almost unknown (one reported case Steiner *et al.*, 1989) there should be little risk of making this diagnosis. However, when the tissue is myxoid there can be a problem with myxoid neoplasias, usually resolved by finding hyaline areas. Two additional features are the presence in some of osteoclasts at the periphery of lobules, and, very rarely, accumulation of lipid in the chondrocytes.

13.8.2   CHONDROSARCOMA

Chondrosarcomas composed of hyaline cartilage are excessively rare. Steiner *et al.* (1989) claim the first published case. This occurred 13 years after radical mastectomy and radiotherapy for carcinoma of the breast. More numerous, but not very common are mesenchymal and myxoid chondrosarcomas which constitute about 1–2% of soft tissue sarcomas (Fletcher and Krausz, 1988; Casadei *et al.*, 1991).

(a)   Mesenchymal chondrosarcoma (Figure 13.28)

This is the same as its counterpart in bone.

(i)   Clinical features

The age range is the second to eighth decade; mainly second to fourth.

Skeletal distribution Most common is the head and neck, but with a wide range of other sites.

Clinical presentation is the usual pattern of neoplasia.

(ii)   Pathology

Morbid anatomy The only distinctive feature is the presence of spotty mineralization in a proportion of cases, detectable by X-ray or other imaging.

Histopathology This is identical with the lesion in bone. As in bone the diagnosis depends in the first place on the identification of the islands of cartilage.

In the absence of the telltale chondroid tissue (including the possibility of inferring its presence on the basis of radiographically demonstrated mineral) the possibilities in the differential diagnosis are haemangiopericytoma (by reason of the vascular pattern), Ewing's sarcoma, synovial sarcoma (so-called monophasic type) and solid rhabdomyosarcoma. Swanson *et al.* (1990) noted that whereas ultrastructural studies indicate a similarity to fetal chondrogenic tissue, there was little information on the immunochemistry of this tumour. They studied nine tumours with antivimentin, Leu-7, antisynaptophysin, antidesmin, antimuscle specific actin, anti-cytokeratins (AE1/AE3, MAK6, CAM 5.2), anti-neurone-specific enolase, and anti-S100 protein (Table 13.10). Six samples of fetal cartilage were included in the study. On this basis a diagnosis of mesenchymal chondrosarcoma cannot be made immunochemically. But the results do not counter the premise that it is a chondrogenic neoplasm.

(b) Myxoid chondrosarcoma (Figure 13.36)

(i) Clinical features

The age range is middle age. The site is principally the limbs. The clinical presentation has no specific features.

Treatment is compartmental excision.

These tumours tend to recur locally and metastasize late. Five-year survival is about 50%.

(ii) Pathology

Morbid anatomy This is an encapsulated, lobulated tumour with a gelatinous cut surface.

Histopathology (Figure 13.36) The lobules have a cellular periphery, but are poorly cellular centrally. The cells have small, generally uniform, nuclei; at the periphery they have little cytoplasm; centrally the cytoplasm is more evident. Mitoses are rare. In some tumours the cells are arranged in cords, which led to the suggestion of chordoid sarcoma,

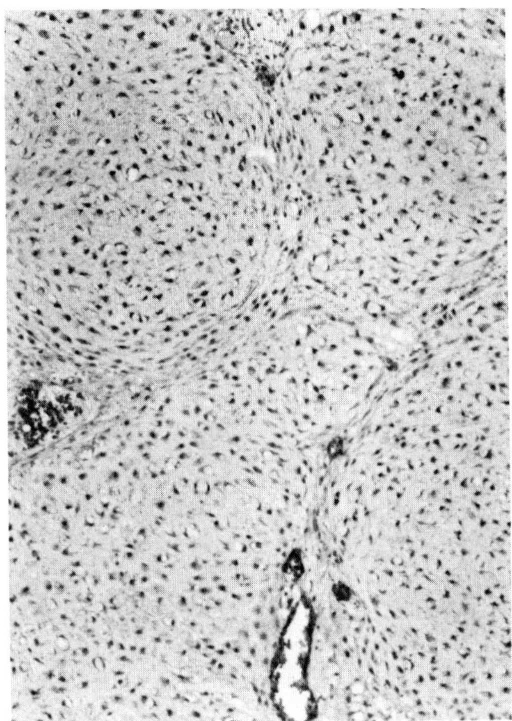

Figure 13.36 Myxoid chondrosarcoma. A very cellular, lobulated tumour. Blood vessels running in the septae are associated with mineral deposition. There is moderate pleomorphism, and a few double nuclei.

which has since been discounted. In some tumours there is formation of cartilage matrix.

If chondroid matrix is present the diagnosis is established. Otherwise it can be established by demonstrating chondroitin and keratan sulphates in the matrix by critical

Table 13.10 Comparison of the immunochemistry of mesenchymal chondrosarcoma cells with fetal chondrogenic tissue (Swanson *et al.*, 1990)

	VIM	S100	Leu-7	SNP	NSE	DES	ACT	Cker	EMA
Mesenchymal chondrosarcoma cells									
Small	9	0	6	0	4	0	0	0	0
Lacunar	9	6	6	0	7	0	0	0	0
Fetal cartilaginous cells									
Small	6	0	5	0	2	0	0	0	0
Lacunar	6	5	4	0	3	0	0	0	0

electrolyte concentration staining procedures (Fletcher and Krausz, 1988).

In the absence of clear cartilage differentiation the lesion is confused with other myxoid soft tissue tumours. A number of methods as shown below are utilized in the diagnosis:

Myxoid chondroma	site, histology
Myxoma	negative for
Myxoid liposarcoma	chondroitin/keratan
Myxoid MFH	sulphates
Myxoid neurilemmoma	glycogen negative

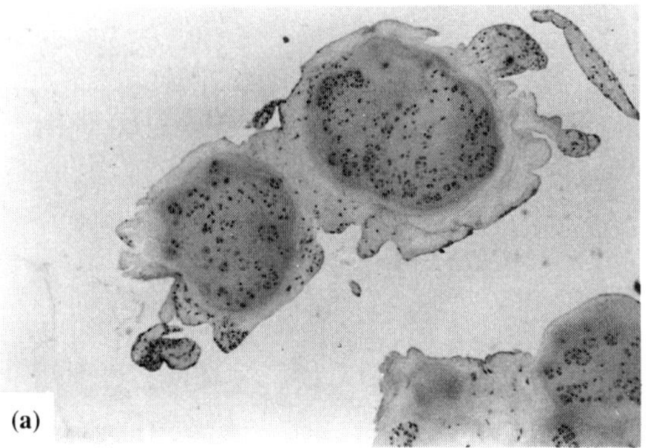

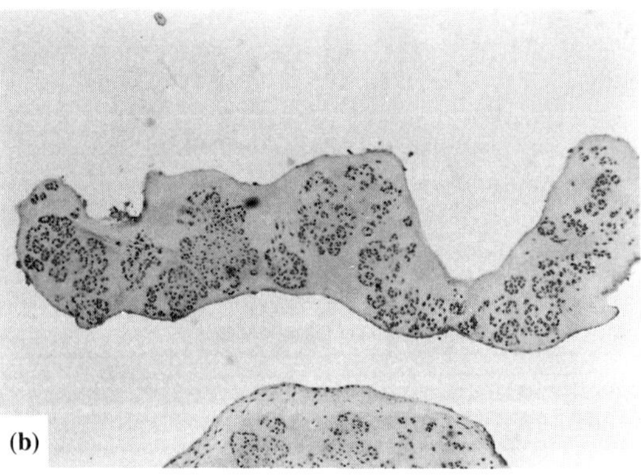

Figure 13.37 Synovial chondromatosis. (a) Photomicrograph of cartilage nodules in a synovial villus (the continuity with the synovial membrane is not complete in the plane of the section). (b) The joint also contained numerous detached cartilage nodules, one type of the so-called 'rice bodies'. The feature of the tissue is chondrocyte clusters in a hyaline matrix.

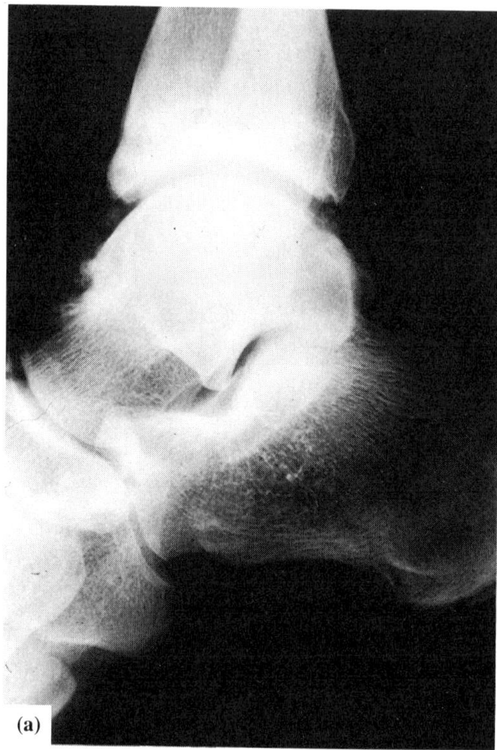

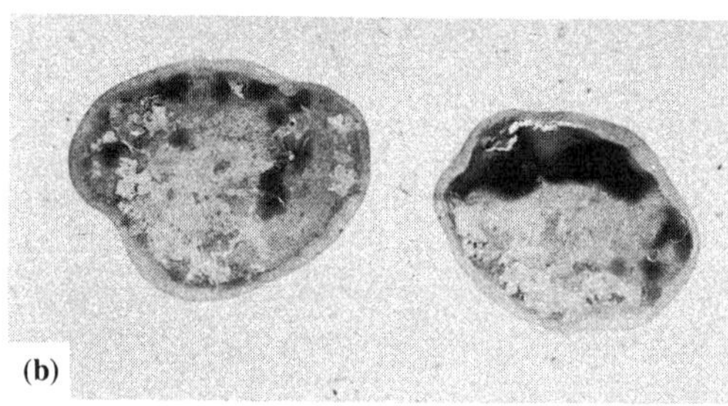

Figure 13.38 Male aged 46 years. Synovial chondromatosis. Presented with pain in ankle. (a) Radiograph showing small intra-articular mineralized bodies in the ankle joint. In some cases, the nodules remain attached and become ossified, in others, only mineralization of the cartilage takes place. (b) In this case, the joint contained unattached, partly calcified, cartilage nodules of approximately 1 cm diameter. Radiograph courtesy of Mr P.W. Skinner.

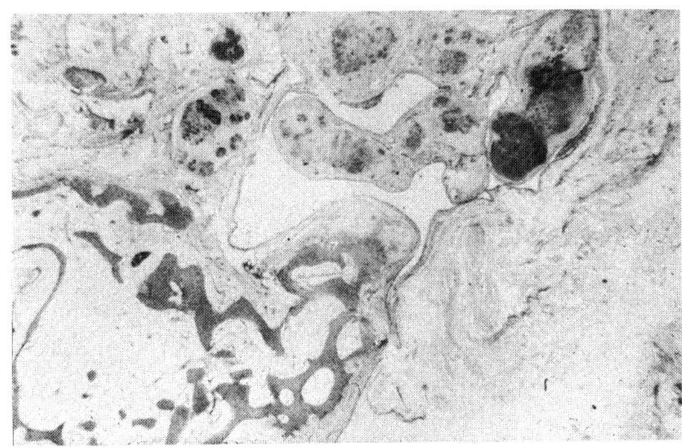

Figure 13.39 Adult male, knee joint. Synovial osteochondromatosis. The radiograph showed several large calcified bodies. The knee was explored and a portion of nodular synovium was removed. The section shows large and small synovial villi, in which there are small metaplastic cartilage nodules, and part of one large ossified cartilage nodule.

13.9   CARTILAGE TUMOURS IN JOINTS

13.9.1   BENIGN (FIGURES 13.37–13.39)

There are no true benign cartilage neoplasms of joints. There is however a metaplastic lesion of synovial membrane which gives rise to a few or many cartilage nodules. This is synovial (osteo)chondromatosis. In some cases the nodules vary around 1 cm in size, are located at individual sites, sometimes pedunculated, and undergo ossification. In others, the affected area is small, and this one focus produces numerous small (a few mm) cartilage nodules which come away and float free in the joint space. There is said to be an association with osteoarthritis; but, since loose bodies occur in that condition and may be incorporated in synovium, it is difficult to establish priority. The joint most usually affected is the knee. It is also known for chondrosarcoma to develop in an affected joint (Bertoni *et al.*, 1991).

13.9.2   MALIGNANT

Malignant cartilage tumour in joint has been reviewed by Bertoni *et al.* (1991). The study was of ten cases from the Mayo Clinic; four were in-patients and six were consultation cases. One case from each group had been previously reported in the literature, where ten cases have been described.

(a)   Clinical features

The age ranged from 25 to 70 years, with 15 cases between 30 and 58 years. The site of the tumours was 13 knees, four hips, two ankles and one elbow. When recorded the symptoms were pain and/or swelling. Treatment

Table 13.11 Comparison of synovial chondromatosis with chondrosarcoma in joint

	Benign	*Malignant*
Cells in small clusters	yes	no, or focal
Diffusely spread	no	yes
With minor atypia*	yes	yes
Crowded, round/spindle	no	yes
Mitosis	rare	may be present
Necrosis	no	may be present
Columniated†	no	yes
Myxoid foci	no	may be present
Edge of lesion	pushing and/or permeative (satellite)	pushing or permeative (satellite)
Bone infiltration	pushing border	marrow permeation

* nuclei hyperchromatic, plump, irregular, more than occasionally multiple.
† cells in single files or ribbons.

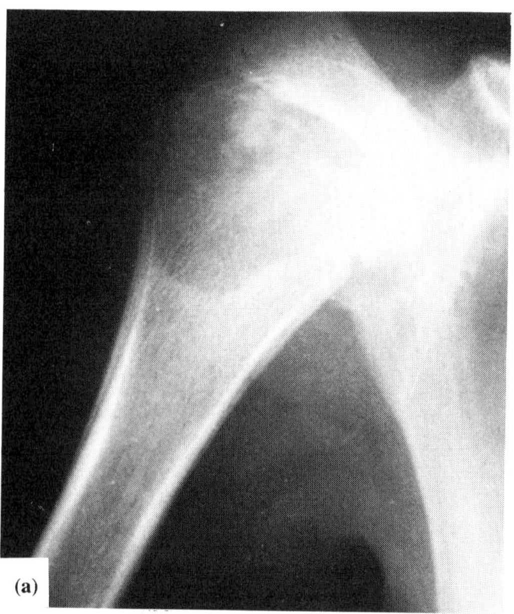

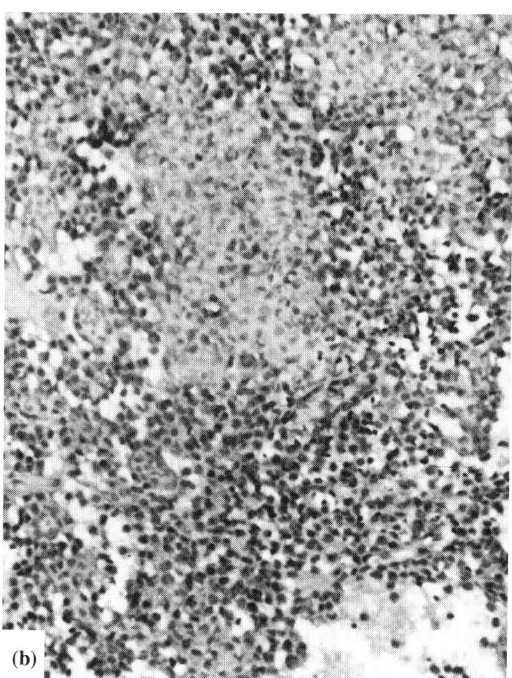

Figure 13.40 Male aged 8 years. (a) Benign chondroblastoma of proximal humerus. A large eccentric global osteolytic lesion centred on the epiphysis, but extending into the metaphysis is well demarcated with a narrow sclerotic transition zone. There is punctate mineralization in the upper portion. There is a periosteal reaction extended down the metaphysis. (b) Cellular tissue with chondroid foci.

is amputation and the prognosis is good.

(b)   Pathology

(i)   Morbid anatomy

Bertoni *et al.* (1991) found in the material available to them that, macroscopically, the synovium was bulky and contained nodules, some were free in the joint, but to distinguish between primary chondrosarcoma of synovium and chondrosarcoma secondary to synovial chondromatosis was not always possible.

(ii)   Histopathology

They considered, on histological grounds, that five cases had definite chondromatosis, three had suggestive but not diagnostic fea-

tures; in two the chondrosarcoma was judged to be primary. The 10 cases for which there was material were compared with 30 cases of synovial chondromatosis and the criteria found to be useful for differentiation are summarized in Table 13.11.

The diagnosis requires swelling of the joint as an indicator of tumour growth, the production of lobulated cartilage within the joint and histological features of malignancy.

Given convincing evidence of chondrosarcoma and no outside source there is little alternative.

13.10   BENIGN CHONDROID TUMOURS

13.10.1   BENIGN CHONDROBLASTOMA (FIGURE 13.40)

This is a rare benign neoplasm whose cells

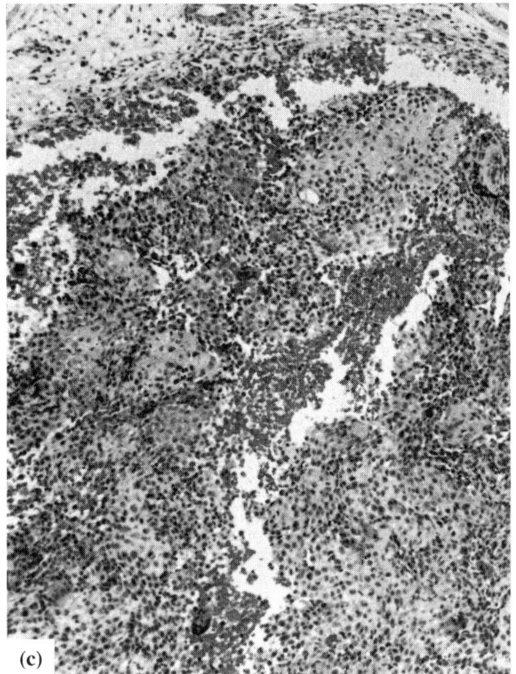

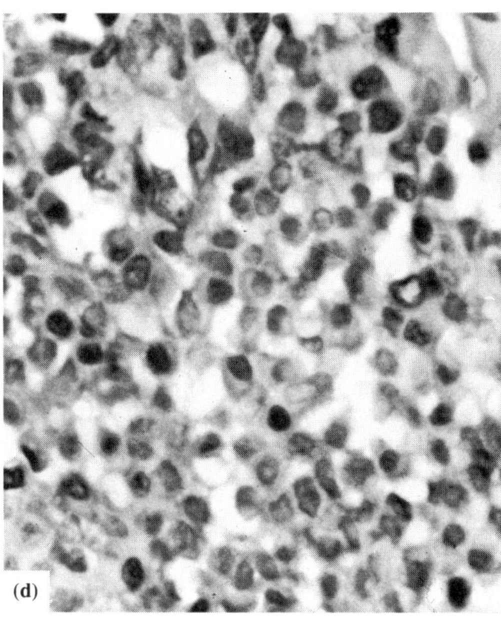

Figure 13.40 Male aged 8 years. Benign chondroblastoma of proximal humerus. (c) The cells are closely packed, except where they have produced matrix which separates them a little. Elsewhere the tissue appears looser because the cells are vacuolated. There are no osteoclasts nor foci of mineralization in this field. (d) There is some variability in nuclear staining and size. A multinucleated cell is present in one corner. Taken in isolation, this field would prompt consideration of 'round cell' tumour.

are identified as chondroblasts on the basis of the presence of foci of chondroid matrix in the tissue. They also have the ultrastructure associated with physeal cartilage cells (Levine and Bensch, 1972). Osteoclasts are a prominent feature. Some of these tumours and some chondromyxoid fibromas have structural features in common, suggesting a close relationship. Notwithstanding its benign character, patients die as a result of complications (Matsuno *et al.*, 1987), and cases with metastases have been reported (Kyriakos *et al.*, 1985). Collected cases are presented by Springfield *et al.* (1985) and Schajowicz and Gallardo (1970). Three cases of soft tissue chondroblastoma have been reported (Abdul-Karim *et al.*, 1985).

(a)   Clinical features

The vast majority occur in the second decade, with few beyond the age of 25 years. The upper age limit is about 60 years, but cases as young as 3 years and as old as 72 years have been reported (McBryde and Goldner, 1970; Wright and Sherman, 1964).

(i)   Skeletal distribution

- Jaws
- Skull   +
- Other flat bones
  - ribs   4
  - girdles
    - shoulder: scapula   +
    - pelvic   4

- Spine   +
- Long tubular   68
    - femur, tibia, humerus   65
    - fibula, radius, ulna   3
- Hands and feet   18
    - short tubular
        - metacarpals, metatarsals,
            - phalanges   +
        - cuboidal   14
        - carpals, tarsals

Note: + = recorded but < 1%

This is one of the tumours that was regarded as a form of giant cell tumour until recognized by Jaffe and Lichtenstein (Jaffe, 1958) as a distinct entity and given its present name. With rare exceptions this tumour occurs in the epiphysis. The exceptions are located in the skull and ribs, and very rarely in the metaphysis of a long bone. The symptoms are pain and disability, or swelling in the case of skull and rib lesions.

Curettage is the usual treatment, although in particularly large lesions local resection and even amputation have been employed.

The response to treatment is generally good, and recurrence is uncommon. Death can occur from complications (Matsuno *et al.*, 1987). Metastases are known, but have not all been fatal; Kyriakos *et al.* (1985) report a case and review the literature on atypical, aggressive and malignant chondroblastoma. They conclude that the incidence of these is so small that it should not influence conventional treatment.

(b)   Pathology

(i)   *Morbid anatomy* (Figure 13.40)

With rare exceptions the lesion is centred on the epiphysis (Sotelo-Avila *et al.*, 1986). Radiographs reveal a translucent lesion, usually (up to 60%, Mirra, 1989) with fine spotty calcification. It is often eccentric, and confined to the epiphysis. With growth it can cross the physis, and extend in the metaphysis. Demarcation is

good with a somewhat lobulated contour, and a narrow, sclerotic transition zone. Where it impinges on the endosteum the cortex is thinned and expanded. But there is no periosteal reaction, unless the lesion becomes greatly enlarged and causes considerable bone expansion. In the intact specimen the tissue is red, soft and gritty, sometimes contains lobules of cartilage, or is cystic. Necrosis of calcified foci may occur and be identified as yellow spots. Curetted material breaks up into small, soft and gritty pieces.

(ii)   *Histopathology* (Figure 13.40)

The stromal tissue is composed of closely arranged, discrete, polygonal cells of moderate, but variable size. Pleomorphism is not a feature, but occasional mitoses are not unexpected. There is a variable population of osteoclasts, and inconstant foci of chondroid matrix distributed through this tissue. The cytoplasm of the stromal cells, which is featureless in H & E paraffin sections, contains glycogen granules. The nuclei are variable in shape and may be indented or lobulated, and have a fine chromatin pattern. Ultramicroscopically they resemble cells of physeal cartilage. Reticulin fibres surround individual cells. A distinctive feature of the tissue is deposition of mineral in the reticulin creating foci likened to chicken wire. The cells in these foci may become necrotic, and more mineral precipitated. On occasion mineral is deposited in the chondroid foci. Together these account for the pattern of mineral found radiographically (about 60% cases) and histologically (about 75% cases; both estimates from Mirra, 1989). The proportion of matrix in chondroid foci is much less than in hyaline cartilage, nor are they precisely demarcated from the contiguous stroma. In some tumours there are hyaline or, more usually, chondromyxoid nodules. These do not mineralize. The latter are the same as those of chondromyxoid fibroma, and if, as sometimes occurs in lesions otherwise conforming to benign chondroblastoma, they are a predominant part of the tissue it becomes difficult to sustain the diagnosis of benign chondroblastoma over chondromyxoid fibroma. The number and size of the osteoclasts is variable throughout the tissue; substantial fields may be free of them, but nowhere are they the only cells. The tissue has a supporting network of blood vessels. Vascular channels may be prominent; haemorrhage sometimes occurs, and this may lead to collections of foamy histiocytes and cholesterol crystal clefts; cystic spaces are present in some tumours and may have the structure of aneurysmal bone cyst.

The following discussion presupposes biopsy. Fine needle aspiration is considered below. The typical morbid anatomy of the radiograph (demarcated epiphyseal lesion with punctate calcification) is of itself diagnostic. The discrete rounded cells, the chondroid matrix, calcified, with focal necrosis and the osteoclasts add, in their own right, successively to the strength of the diagnosis. Together the radiological and histological

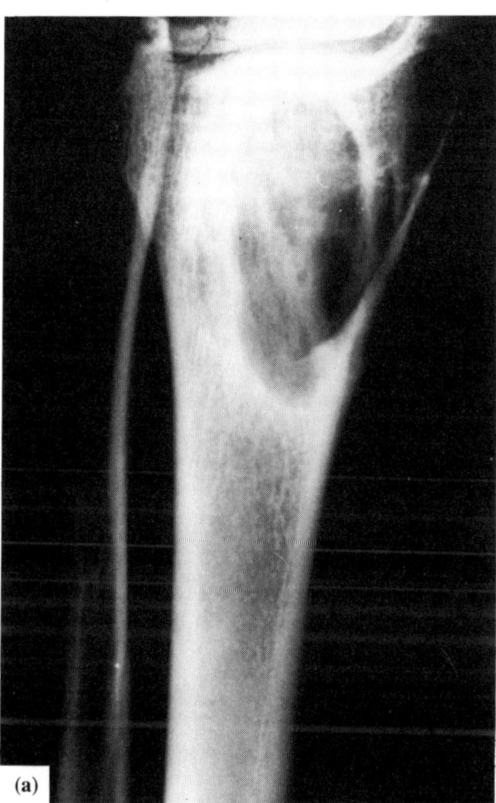

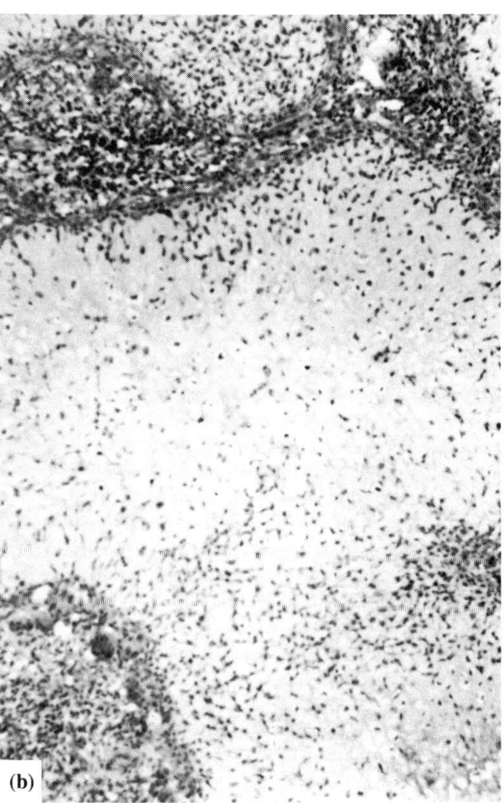

Figure 13.41 Female aged 12 years. Chondromyxoid fibroma. (a) An eccentric, ovoid, global osteolytic lesion of the upper tibial metaphysis. The transition zone is sclerotic. The tibia distal to the lesion is porotic. A small osteolytic focus at the level of the mid-point of the lesion may also be due to porosis, or may be an extension of the tumour. In the latter case there would be difficulty in complete curettage. The thin shell of cortical cover has been fractured. (b) The specific pattern of chondromyxoid fibroma: avascular lobules of chondro (centrally) myxoid (peripherally) tissue separated by bands of fibrovascular tissue, which can contain a range of ancillary cells and sometimes bone spicules (see text). In this section osteoclasts line the surfaces of the lobules.

evidence are incontrovertible. Lesions of the rib, where there is no epiphysis, or of small bones where the landmarks are obscured by the relative size of the lesion, lose one diagnostic feature, but the demarcation between lesion and bone remains.

The principal possibilities which might arise in the differential diagnosis are: giant cell tumour; clear cell chondrosarcoma; and chondromyxoid fibroma.

Focal calcification, matrix production (with or without calcification) and discrete cells with glycogen are features to refute the diagnosis of giant cell tumour. Mirra (1989) records a case in which he could not make a decision. The similarity to clear cell chondrosarcoma is cytological; the pattern of the matrix formations should serve to differentiate. When features of both chondroblastoma and chondromyxoid fibroma are present it is a matter of the weight of evidence for choosing between them (Dahlin, 1956).

(iii)   Cytology

Fine needle aspiration (FNA) findings in 12 lesions are reported by Fanning *et al.* (1990), and compared with the histological sections after curettage.

    FNA results were:
    BC certain   7
    BC suggestive   1
    BC on review   1
    Undiagnosable   2
    GCT   1
      (sections had both types of tissue)

The diagnostic features were separated chondroblasts, giving a pebbled appearance; randomly admixed osteoclasts; and chondroid matrix fragments. They conclude that the diagnostic hallmark is the cytology of the chondroblasts.

13.10.2 CHONDROMYXOID FIBROMA (FIGURE 13.41)

This arises with about half the frequency of benign chondroblastoma. It was established as an entity by Jaffe and Lichtenstein in 1948 (Jaffe, 1958). Reports in the literature to 1985 reached 400 (Kreicsberg *et al.*, 1985).

(a)   Clinical features

These tumours present mainly in the first three decades (75%). The range is 4–79 years (Mirra, 1989).

(i)   Skeletal distribution (from Mirra, 1989; 101 cases).

* Flat bones
    ribs   3
    girdles
      shoulder: scapula   1
      pelvic   9
* Spine, cervical   2
* Long tubular   62
    femur, tibia (37) humerus   45
    fibula (9), radius (4), ulna (4)   17
* Hands (3), feet (20)   23

Clinical presentation is with variable degrees of pain, swelling and disability, with a few cases found incidentally.

Curettage is frequently employed as treatment. However, the high recurrence rate (reported as between 12 and 25%) is an argument for block resection (Gherlinzoni *et al.*, 1983).

The propensity to recur has been discussed. Superimposed malignancy is a curiosity (Iwata and Coley, 1958; Gilmer *et al.*, 1963; Dahlin, 1978).

(b)   Pathology

(i)   Morbid anatomy (Figure 13.41)

The lesion is primarily metaphyseal, with a small proportion in the diaphysis. The cut surface shows lobules of firm pale tissue surrounded by darker material which is sometimes pigmented by haemosiderin.

This tissue replaces the normal bone to produce an osteolytic lesion; in larger bones it extends from the region of the physis into the metaphysis. In radiographs the outline is often lobulated and there may be satellite nodules, some at a considerable remove from the main mass. These are responsible for the high recurrence rate following curettage. The transition zone is narrow and sclerotic. Some lesions extend into the epiphysis.

(ii) Histopathology (Figure 13.41)

The basic structure of the tissue is lobules of chondromyxoid tissue separated by a fibrovascular stroma in which there may be a variety of other elements. Prominent among these, and the most constant are osteoclasts. They are generally located at or near to the borders of the lobules. The other components are macrophages containing haemosiderin and, on occasion, lipid; reactive bone and stromal cells of the chondroblast type. The latter may be so abundant as to be the major element of the lesion, presenting a problem in diagnosis complementary to the reverse situation in benign chondroblastoma (Dahlin, 1956). The structure of the lobules is a chondroid matrix in which the more centrally placed cells are rounded and in lacunae as in hyaline cartilage, but approaching the periphery they become stellate and then spindled, and the proportion of matrix to cells declines. There is a tendency for cells at the periphery of the lobules to be pleomorphic and hyperchromatic, sufficiently so to give rise to concern about malignancy. But mitoses, particularly abnormal ones, are not a feature.

The tissue pattern of this tumour is very distinctive when it is well developed. But there are cases where the myxoid element, the stellate cells and rather poorly formed matrix, are dominant with little clear lobulation, and myxoma becomes a diagnostic possibility. However, since myxomas are odontogenic and restricted to the jaws the problem is resolvable (Schajowicz, 1981).

Tumours with a poorly developed pattern may be mistaken for some form of chondrosarcoma. Differentiation is made on the basis of clinical and radiological findings as well as histology. The absence of cytological malignancy will be an important point.

REFERENCES

Abdul-Karim, F.W., Ayala, A.G. and Spujt, H.J. (1985) Case report 321. Diagnosis: extraosseous chondroblastoma in the subcutaneous tissues of the right shoulder. *Skeletal Radiol.*, **14**, 73–3.

Barnes, R. and Catto, M. (1966) Chondrosarcoma of bone. *J. Bone Joint Surg.*, **48B**, 729–64.

Bertoni, F., Boriani, S., Laus, M. *et al.* (1982) Periosteal chondrosarcoma and periosteal osteosarcoma. Two distinct entities. *J. Bone Joint Surg.*, **64B**, 370–6.

Bertoni, F., Unni, K.K., Beabout, J.W. *et al.* (1991) Chondrosarcoma of the synovium. *Cancer*, **67**, 155–62.

Bjornsson, J., Unni, K.K., Dahlin, D.C. *et al.* (1984) Clear cell chondrosarcoma of bone. Observations in 47 cases. *Am. J. Surg. Pathol.*, **8**, 223–30.

Bourgouin, P.M., Tampieri, D., Robitaille, Y. *et al.* (1992) Low grade myxoid chondrosarcoma of the base of the skull: CT, MR, histopathology. *J. Comput. Assist. Tomogr.*, **16**, 268–73.

Brooks, J.J., Trojanowski, J.Q. and LiVolsi, V.A. (1989) Chondroid chordoma: a low grade chondrosarcoma and its differential diagnosis. *Curr. Top. Pathol.*, **80**, 165–81.

Campanacci, M., Bertoni, F. and Laus, M. (1980) Clear cell chondrosarcoma. *Ital. J. Orthop. Traumatol.*, **6**, 365–72.

Casadei, R., Ricci, M., Ruggieri, P. *et al.* (1991) Chondrosarcoma of the soft tissues. Two different subgroups. *J. Bone Joint Surg.*, **73B**, 162–8.

Charpentier, Y., Forest, M., Postel, M. *et al.* (1979) Clear cell chondrosarcoma. A report of 5 cases including an ultrastructural study. *Cancer*, **44**, 622–9.

Chung, E.B. and Enzinger, F.M. (1978) Chondroma of soft parts. *Cancer*, **41**, 1414–24.

Dahlin, D.C. (1956) Chondromyxoid fibroma of bone with emphasis on its relationship to benign chondroblastoma of bone. *Cancer*, **9**, 195–203.

Dahlin, D.C. (1978) *Bone Tumors*, 3rd edn, Charles C. Thomas, Springfield, IL.

Dahlin, D.C. and Beabout, J.W. (1971) Dedifferentiation of low grade chondrosarcoma. *Cancer*, **28**, 461–6.

Dahlin, D.C. and Salvador, A.H. (1974). Cartilaginous tumours of the soft tissues of the hands and feet. *Mayo Clin. Proc.*, **49**, 721–6.

Dahlin, D.C. and Unni, K.K. (1988). *Bone Tumors;* 4th edn, Charles C. Thomas, Springfield, IL.

Delling, G. and Welkerling, H. (1992) Pathomorphology of malignant chondrogenic bone tumors – an analysis of 94 cases from the Hamburg Bone Tumor Registry (1974–1989). *Z. Orthop. Grenzgebeit*, **130**, 1–8.

DelSignore, J.L., Torre, B.A. and Miller, R.J. (1990) Extraskeletal chondrosarcoma of the hand. Case report and review of the literature. *Clin. Orthop.*, **254**, 147–52.

Dupree, W.B. and Enzinger, F.M. (1986) Fibroosseous pseudotumor of the digits. *Cancer*, **58**, 2103–9.

Fanning, C.V., Sneige, N.S., Carrasco, C.H. *et al.* (1990) Fine needle biopsy in benign chondroblastoma. *Cancer*, **65**, 1847–63.

Fletcher, C.D.M. and Krausz, T. (1988) Cartilaginous tumours of soft tissue. *Appl. Pathol.*, **6**, 208–20.

Garrington, G.E. and Collett, W.K. (1988) Chondrosarcoma. I. A selected literature review. *J. Oral Pathol.*, **17**, 1–11.

Garrison, R.C., Unni, K.K., McLeod, R.A. *et al.* (1982) Chondrosarcoma arising in osteochondroma. *Cancer*, **49**, 1890–7.

Gherlinzoni, F., Rock, M. and Picci, P. (1983) Chondromyxoid fibroma. The experience at the Instituto Ortopedica Rizzoli. *J. Bone Joint Surg.*, **65A**, 198–204.

Gilmer et al. (1963) *Atlas of Bone Tumors.* C.V. Mosby, St Louis, pp. 36–9.

Goldman, R.L. (1967) Mesenchymal chondrosarcoma, a rare malignant chondroid tumor usually primary in bone. Report of a case arising in extraskeletal soft tissue. *Cancer*, **20**, 1494–8.

Hoehn, J.G. and Coletta, C. (1992) Subungual exostosis of the fingers. *J. Hand Surg.*, **17**, 468–71.

Humphreys, S., Pambakian, H., McKee, P.H. *et al.* (1986). Soft tissue chondroma. *Histopathology*, **10**, 147–59.

Huvos, A.G., Rosen, G., Dabska, M. *et al.* (1983) Mesenchymal chondrosarcoma: a clinicopathologic analysis of 35 patients with emphasis on treatment. *Cancer*, **51**, 1230–7.

Iwata, S. and Coley, B.L. (1958) Report of six cases of chondromyxoid fibroma of bone. *Surg. Gynecol. Obstet.*, **101**, 571–6.

Jaffe, H.L. (1958) *Tumors and Tumorous Conditions of Bones and Joints.* Lea and Febiger, Philadelphia.

Kreicsberg, A., Lonnquist, P.A. and Willems, J. (1985) Chondromyxoid fibroma of bone. A review of the literature and a report on our own experience. *Acta Pathol. Microbiol. Scand.*, **93A**, 189–97.

Kyriakos, M., Land, V.T., Penning, L. *et al.* (1985) Metastatic chondroblastoma. Report of two cases and review of the literature. *Cancer*, **55**, 1770–89.

Levine, G.D. and Bensch, K.G. (1972) Chondroblastoma – the nature of the basic cell. A study by means of histochemistry, tissue culture, electron microscopy and autoradiography. *Cancer*, **29**, 1546–62.

Lewis, M.M., Kenan, S., Yabut, S.M. *et al.* (1990) Periosteal chondroma. A report of 10 cases and review of the literature. *Clin. Orthop.*, **256**, 185–92.

Lewis, R.J. and Ketchum, A.S. (1973) Maffuci's syndrome: functional and neoplastic significance. *J. Bone Joint Surg.*, **55A**, 1465–79.

Lichtenstein, L. and Bernstein, D. (1959) Unusual benign and malignant chondroid tumors of bone – a survey of some mesenchymal cartilage tumors and malignant chondroblastic tumors, including a few multicentric ones, as well as many atypical benign chondroblastomas and chondromyxoid fibromas. *Cancer*, **12**, 1142–5.

Liu, J., Hudkins, P.G., Swee, R.G. *et al.* (1987) Bone sarcomas associated with Ollier's disease. *Cancer*, **59**, 1376–85.

Matsuno, T., Hasegawa, I. and Masuda, T. (1987) Chondroblastoma arising in the tri-radiate cartilage. Report of two cases with review of the literature. *Skeletal Radiol.*, **16**, 216–22.

McBryde, A. and Goldner J.L. (1970) Chondroblastoma of bone. *Am. J. Surg.*, **36**, 94–108.

Milgram, J.W. (1983) The origins of osteochondromas and enchondromas. *Clin. Orthop.*, **174**, 264–84.

Mirra, J.M. (1989) *Bone Tumors.* Lea and Febiger, Philadelphia.

Mirra, J.M., Gold, R., Downs, J. *et al.* (1985) A new histologic approach to the differentiation of enchondroma from chondrosarcoma of the bones. A clinicopathologic analysis of 51 cases. *Clin. Orthop.*, **201**, 214–37.

Nelson, D.L., Abdul-Karim, F,W., Carter, J.R. *et al.*

(1990) Chondrosacoma of the small bones of the hand arising from enchondroma. *J. Hand Surg.*, **15**, 655–9.

Nojima, T., Unni, K.K., McLeod, R.A. *et al.* (1985) Periosteal chondroma and periosteal chondrosarcoma. *Am. J. Surg. Pathol.*, **9**, 666–77.

Nora, F., Dahlin, D.C. and Beabout, J.W. (1983) Bizarre parosteal osteochondromatous proliferations of hands and feet. *Am. J. Surg. Pathol.*, **7**, 245–50.

Norman, A. and Sissons, H.A. (1984) Radiographic hallmarks of peripheral chondrosarcoma. *Radiology*, **151**, 589–96.

Ollier, M. (1900) Dyschondroplasia. *Lyon. Med.*, **93**, 23–4.

Reid, R. (1991) New developments in the diagnosis of chondrosarcoma. *J. Pathol.*, **163**, 93–4.

Salvador, A.H., Beabout, J.W. and Dahlin, D.C. (1971) Mesenchymal chondrosarcoma – observations on 30 new cases. *Cancer*, **28**, 605–15.

Schajowicz, F. (1981) *Tumors and Tumorlike Lesions of Bone and Joints*. Springer, New York.

Schajowicz, F. and Gallardo, H. (1970) Epiphyseal chondroblastoma of bone. A clinico-pathologic study of sixty-nine cases. *J. Bone Joint Surg.*, **52B**, 205–26.

Schajowicz, F. and McGuire, M.H. (1989) Diagnostic difficulties in skeletal pathology. *Clin. Orthop.*, **240**, 281–310.

Schajowicz, F., Ackerman, L.W. and Sissons, H.A. (1972) Histologic typing of bone tumors. *International Classification of Tumors*. Vol. 6. World Health Organization, Geneva.

Sotelo-Avila, C., Sundaram, M., Kyriakos, M. *et al.* (1986) Case report 373. Diametaphyseal chondroblastoma of the upper portion of the left femur. *Skeletal Radiol.*, **15**, 387–90.

Springfield, D.S., Capanna, R., Gherlinzoni, F. *et al.* (1985) Chondroblastoma. A review of 70 cases. *J. Bone Joint Surg.*, **67A**, 748–55.

Spujt, H.J. and Dorfman, H.D. (1981) Florid reactive periostitis of the tubular bones of the hands and feet. A benign lesion which may simulate osteosarcoma. *Am. J. Surg. Pathol.*, **5**, 423–33.

Steiner, E., Barrabes, M.H., Lequang, M.L. *et al.* (1989) Chondrosarcoma of the soft parts of the thoracic wall. A propos of a case after surgery and irradiation of breast adenocarcinoma. *J. Gynecol. Obstet. Biol. Reprod.*, **18**, 496–9.

Swanson, P.E., Lillimoe, T.J., Manivel, J.C. *et al.* (1990) Mesenchymal chondrosarcoma. An immunohistochemical study. *Arch. Pathol. Lab. Med.*, **114**, 943–8.

Unni, K.K., Dahlin, D.C. and Beabout, J.W. (1976) Periosteal osteosarcoma. *Cancer*, **37**, 2476–85.

Unni, K.K., Dahlin, D.C., Beabout, J.W. *et al.* (1976) Chondrosarcoma clear-cell variant. A report of sixteen cases *J. Bone Joint Surg.*, **58A**, 676–83.

Wright, J.V. and Sherman, M.S. (1964) An unusual chondroblastoma. *J. Bone Joint Surg.*, **46A**, 597–600.

Young, C.L., Sim, F.H., Unni, K.K. *et al.* (1990) Chondrosarcoma of bone in children. *Cancer*, **66**, 1641–8.

Zillmer, D.A. and Dorfman, H.D. (1989) Chondromyxoid fibroma of bone: thirty-six cases with clinicopathologic correlation. *Hum. Pathol.*, **20**, 952–64.

NON-OSTEOBLASTIC, NON-CARTILAGINOUS NEOPLASMS

14

Jonathan R. Salisbury and Paul D. Byers

14.1 CHORDOMA

(a) Clinical features

Chordomas are rare slow-growing tumours that are malignant because of local invasion of bone and surrounding tissues. Chordomas represented 4% of malignant primary bone tumours reported from the Mayo Clinic, Minnesota (Dahlin and Unni, 1986) but this was almost certainly an overestimate as it included many referred patients. Chordomas accounted for 1% of the malignant tumours in Schajowicz's (1981) series.

Most chordomas occur in adults, with the peak in the decade 55–65 years, although cases do occur both in children (Horton *et al.*, 1990) and in old age. Tumours described as chordomas have even been reported at birth, e.g. Willis (1962) described a large coccygeal chordoma in a female infant who also had cervical spina bifida occulta, but these may represent examples of the split notochord syndrome. There is some evidence that spheno-occipital chordomas arise in a younger age group than do sacrococcygeal tumours and that they are more common in children (Wold and Laws, 1983; Dahlin and Unni, 1986). Males are affected about twice as frequently as females (Willis, 1962; Dahlin and Unni, 1986), the preponderance of males being greater in the sacral than in the cranial group.

The large majority of chordomas arise at the ends of the spinal column and so the two main locations are at the base of the skull, near the site of the sphenoid–occipital synchondrosis (over 30%), and in the sacrococcygeal region (over 50%). Sacral chordomas often attain great sizes. Occasional cases occur in the cervical, lumbar and thoracic vertebrae. This strict localization to the midline of the body is an important diagnostic sign.

(i)   Skeletal distribution (from Dahlin and Unni, 1986)

- Skull   37%
- Spine
    - cervical   6%
    - thoracic   3%
    - lumbar   3%
    - sacral   51%

The duration of symptoms before diagnosis is usually over 5 years. Metastasis by both lymphatic and venous systems does occur but is relatively uncommon. Some patients survive for many years (19 years in Stewart's case (1922)), even without modern treatments. The ultimate prognosis is poor except for those sacral chordomas where complete radical removal is possible. Some chordomas are radiosensitive and so radiotherapy can be employed with palliative benefit, especially for inoperable spheno-occipital chordomas.

(b) Pathology

(i) *Morbid anatomy*

Morbid anatomical examination of gross specimens shows that chordomas are soft and gelatinous with areas of haemorrhage (Figure 14.1).

(ii) *Histopathology*

Histological examination shows the tumours to be composed of rounded or polyhedral cells, arranged in lobules or trabeculae, and separated by variable amounts of extracellular mucins (Figure 14.2a). Some of the cells are very large and contain numerous intracytoplasmic vacuoles of varying sizes; these are known as 'physaliphorous' cells. Histochemistry has shown that some of these cytoplasmic vacuoles contain glycogen (Crawford, 1958). A second population of smaller, spindle-shaped cells are referred to as 'stel-late' cells and are thought to be the precursors of the physaliphorous cells. Anisonucleosis and intranuclear inclusions are prominent features in some cases (Finley *et al.*, 1986). Mitotic figures can be found but are rare, as might be expected in such a slow-growing tumour. Some chordomas contain a malignant spindle-cell component (Rone *et al.*, 1986); DNA flow cytometry shows these tumours are all aneuploid–multiploid, in contrast to 'usual' chordomas where about one-quarter of the tumours are aneuploid–multiploid (Hruban *et al.*, 1990b). Rare cases of sacral chordomas may have both high-grade malignant cartilaginous and spindle-cell components (Hruban *et al.*, 1990a).

The histopathological diagnosis of chordoma can be straightforward or it can be notoriously difficult. Included in the microscopic differential diagnosis are chondrosarcoma, metastatic carcinoma (Figure 14.2b), particularly from renal cell carcinoma, signet

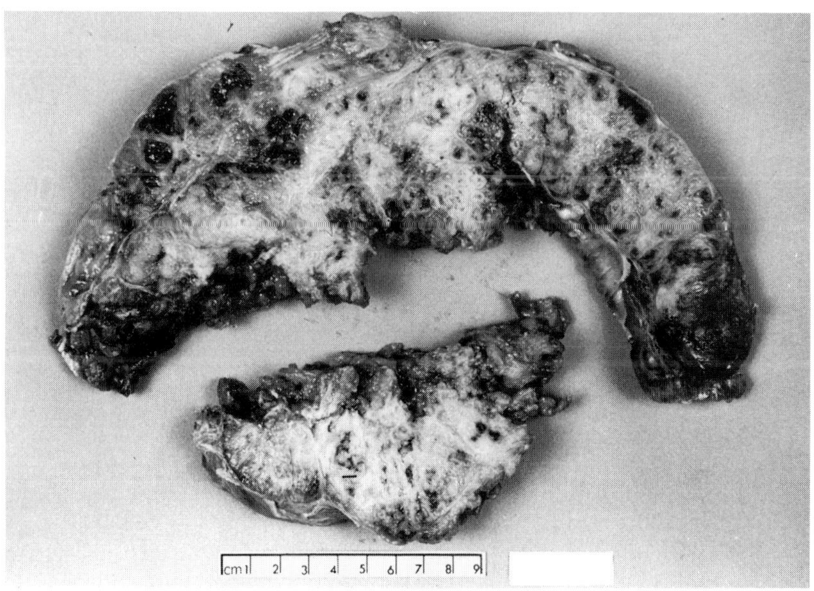

Figure 14.1 Female aged 64 years. Sacrococcygeal chordoma.

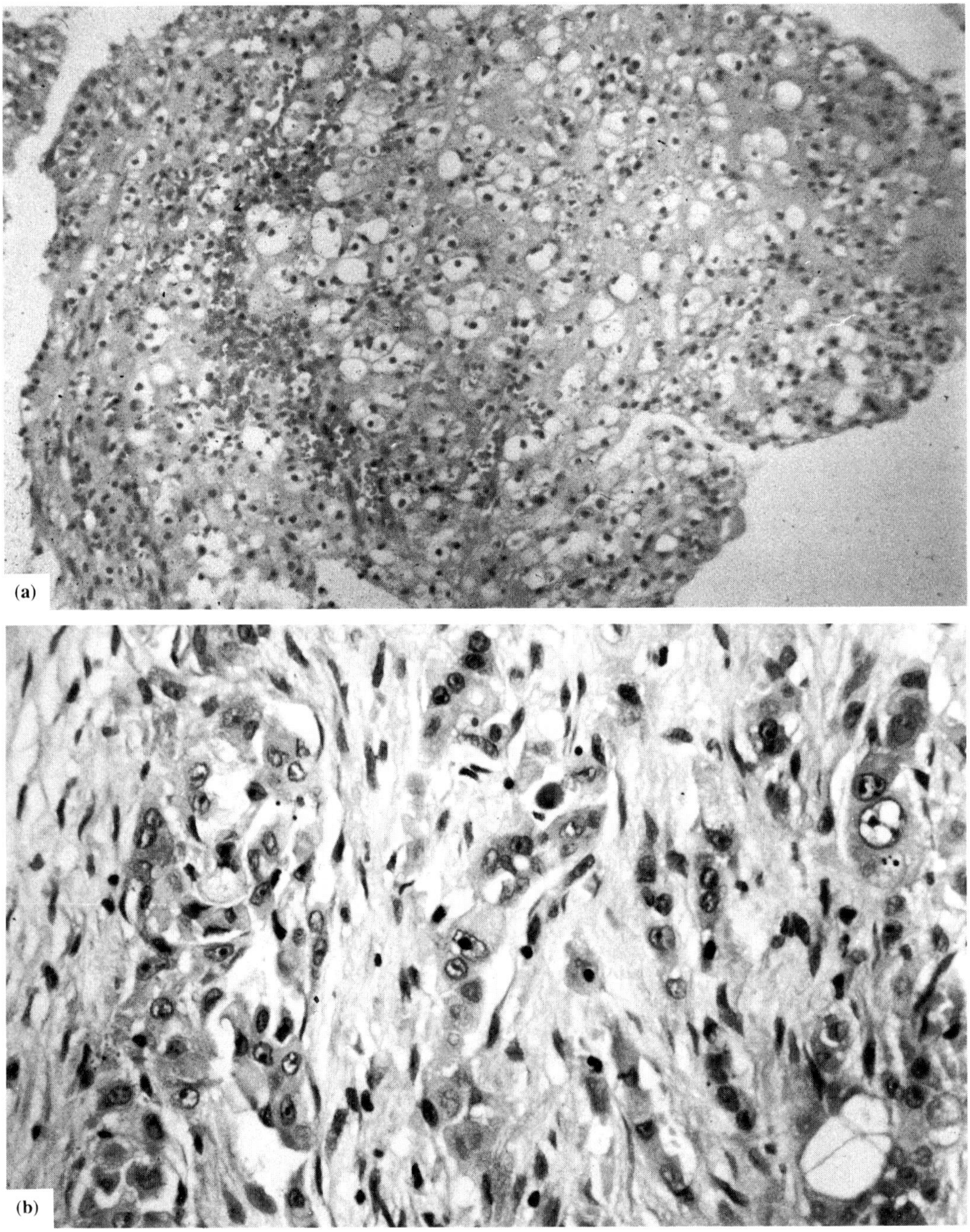

Figure 14.2 Photomicrographs of chordoma. (a) Section of tissue from sacral lesion with the usual pattern of chordoma; numerous physaliphorous cells supported by matrix. (b) The cells are arranged in clusters and trabeculae and show intra- and extracellular matrix production. Distinction from metastatic adenocarcinoma is clearly difficult and is dependent upon clinicoradiological information and S-100 protein immunoreactivity.

ring adenocarcinoma of rectum and myxo-papillary ependymoma. No straightforward histochemical stain is known to differentiate between chordoma and chondrosarcoma (Crawford, 1958; Kindblom and Angervall, 1975).

(iii) *Immunohistochemistry*

Immunohistochemistry shows that chordomas stain positively for cytokeratins and for epithelial membrane antigen as does human fetal notochord (Salisbury and Isaacson, 1985). They also stain positively for vimentin (Coindre *et al.*, 1986) and for S-100 protein (Nakamura *et al.*, 1983), as do chondrosarcomas (Salisbury and Isaacson, 1985), so these two antibodies cannot be used to distinguish between chordoma and chondrosarcoma. Most chordomas express α_1-antichymotrypsin (Meis and Giraldo, 1988), EGF (epithelial growth factor) receptor and *c-neu* oncogene product (Tamayama and Maruyama, 1990). Expression of neurofilaments (Coindre *et al.*, 1986; Maiorano *et al.*, 1992), CEA (carcinoembryonic antigen) and lysozyme is variable (Miettinen, 1984; Meis and Giraldo, 1988; Tamayama *et al.*, 1990). Chordomas are negative for AFP (alpha-fetoprotein) (Tamayama *et al.*, 1990), desmin, glial fibrillary acidic protein (Finley *et al.*, 1986) and for transferrin receptor (Tamayama and Maruyama, 1990). The spindle cells in those chordomas with malignant spindle-cell components show weak staining for cytokeratins and for epithelial membrane antigen (Hruban *et al.*, 1990b).

(iv) *Cytopathology*

Fine-needle aspiration biopsy of chordomas shows the presence of microtissue fragments, cells in a dissociate pattern and an abundant metachromatic extracellular matrix (Finley *et al.*, 1986).

(v) *Electron microscopy*

Ultrastructurally, peculiar mitochondrial–endoplasmic reticulum complexes have been described in chordomas (Erlandson, 1968) but they are not a consistent or a specific finding. Occasional desmosome-like junctions and abundant extracellular matrix, adherent to the tumour cells, are also seen (Finley *et al.*, 1986).

14.1.1 CHONDROID CHORDOMAS

A distinct group of predominantly spheno-occipital and upper cervical neoplasms, which are histologically composed of both typical chordomatous and cartilaginous tissue, are known as chondroid chordomas (Heffelfinger *et al.*, 1973). Rare cases of chondroid chordoma have been reported in the sacrococcygeal and lumbar regions (Chu, 1987; Wojno *et al.*, 1992). In the chondromatous areas neoplastic cells within lacunae are surrounded by stroma resembling cartilage. The tumours share ultrastructural features with both typical chordoma and chondrosarcoma (Valderrama *et al.*, 1983). Immunohistochemistry shows the same positivity for cytokeratins and epithelial membrane antigen as ordinary chordomas, even for those cells in the 'chondromatous' areas (Salisbury, 1987), although in the study by Meis and Giraldo (1988) there was a lack of epithelial marker positivity in two of three chondroid chordomas located at the base of the skull. The existence of chondroid chordoma as a separate entity is still controversial, some investigators claim it cannot be distinguished from cartilaginous tumours (Brooks *et al.*, 1987). Wojno *et al.* (1992) analysed 17 cases of cartilaginous neoplasms of the craniospinal axis by immunohistochemistry and showed that 14 had the expected morphology and immunophenotype of chondroid chordomas. It is important to distinguish between chondroid chordomas and chondrosarcomas of the skull base because of the better prognosis and survival associated with chondroid chordomas.

(a) Histogenesis

Chordomas are thought to arise from notochordal cells (Figures 14.3 and 14.4), not only because of their morphological similarity, but also because their distribution accords with that of notochord rests and ecchordoses. Postmortem studies of adult spinal columns have shown that a small percentage of adults have little, non-neoplastic masses of vestigial notochordal tissue, most frequently at the two ends of the axis, in the sphenooccipital or sacro-coccygeal areas (Willis, 1962). The upper end of the notochord in the embryo closely approaches the dural surface of the sphenoid, whereas more caudally, in the basiocciput, it lies close to or on the pharyngeal surface of the bone, and it may even

come into contact with the pharyngeal epithelium. Notochord vestiges may persist in both these situations, especially the former; if at autopsy the dura mater is stripped off the dorsum sellae, a tiny gelatinous bead of notochordal tissue embedded in the surface of the bone can be found in 4–5% of adult subjects. At the lower end of the spinal axis also, aberrant buds of the notochord have been noted on the anterior aspects of the sacral and coccygeal vertebrae (Horwitz, 1941). Aberrant chordal tissue has rarely been seen at other levels of the spine, but Musgrove (1891) reported it in the lumbar region of an adult.

Ecchordoses are soft, gelatinous pedunculated masses, usually only a few millimetres but sometimes more than 2 cm or more in diameter, with flat inner surfaces where they have lain against the brain-stem in the base of the skull. These ecchordoses

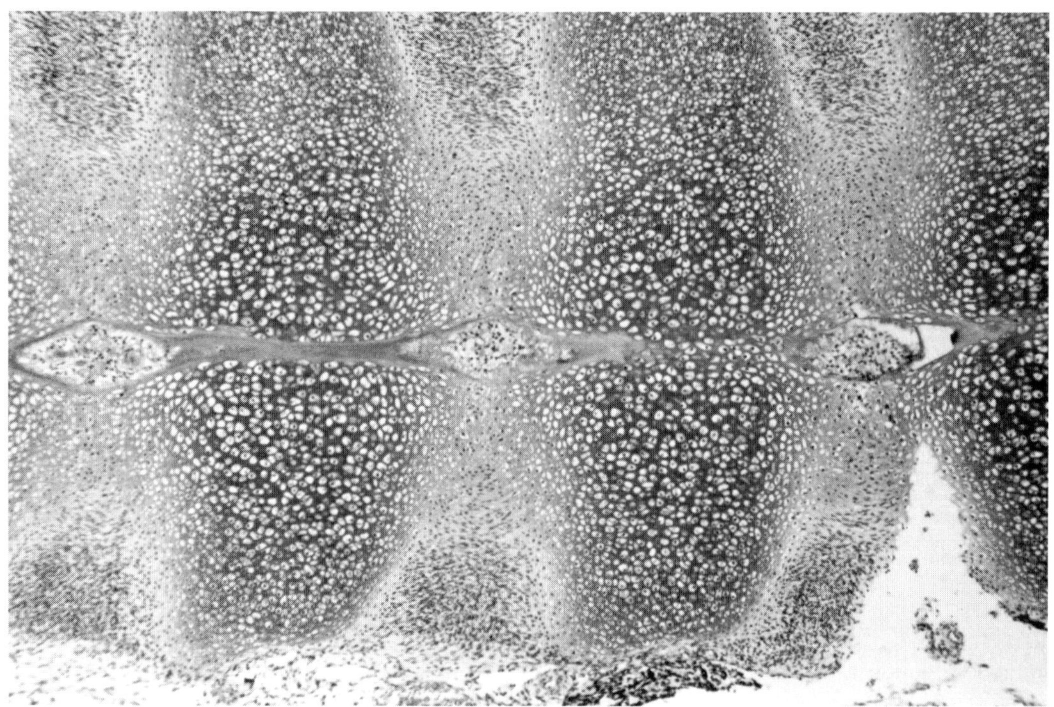

Figure 14.3 Longitudinal section of a human fetal spine at 6 weeks gestational age. Expansions of notochord are present at the site of the future intervertebral discs. These are surrounded by the notochordal sheath which also persists within the cartilaginous models of the future vertebral bodies.

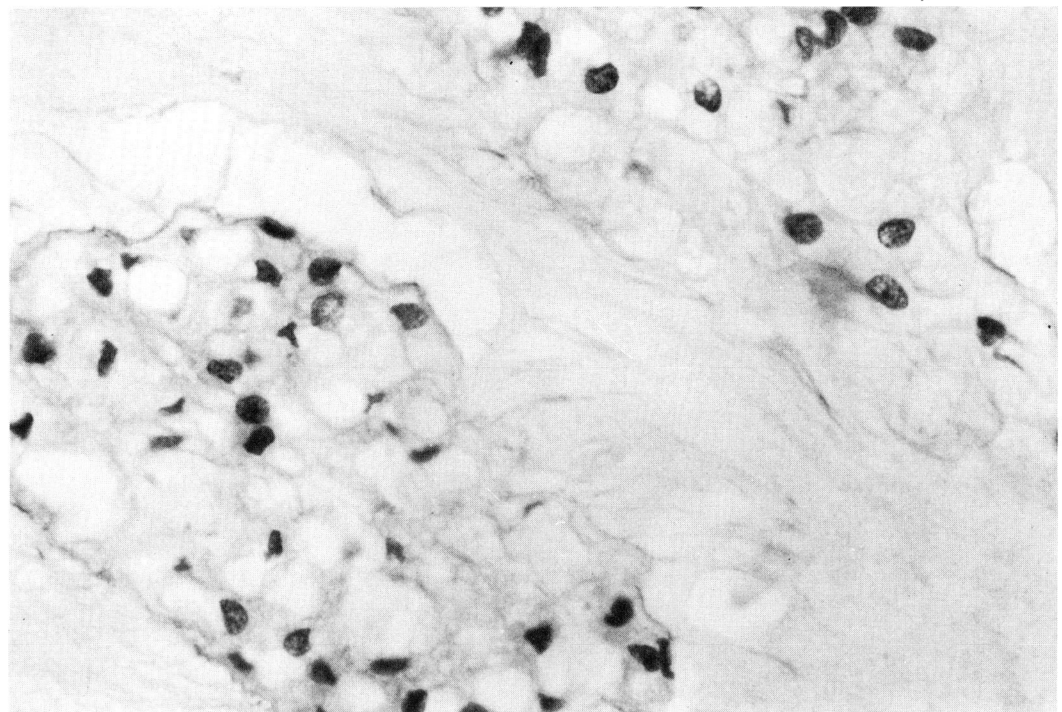

Figure 14.4 Notochordal tissue from a human fetal spine at 26 weeks gestational age shows a morphological resemblance to the cells of chordoma.

physaliphora were first noted by Luschka (1856) and Virchow (1857) who regarded them as cartilaginous and called them 'ecchondroses physaliphora'. They were soon shown by Muller (1858) to arise from notochord remains, an origin confirmed by Ribbert (1894). Their incidence has been variously reported as 2% (Ribbert, 1894), 1.1% (Stewart and Morin, 1926) and 0.5% (Willis, 1962). Typically, ecchordoses are connected by a pedicle, often a mere thread, mooring the mass loosely in the dorsum sellae. The pedicle traverses a small aperture in the dura mater and is often connected with a remnant of notochord in the bone (Willis, 1962).

That chordomas and notochords share the same immunohistochemical staining pattern (S-100 protein positive, low molecular weight cytokeratin positive, epithelial membrane antigen positive, vimentin positive)

adds support to the hypothesis that chordomas derive from notochordal vestiges (Nakamura *et al.*, 1983, Salisbury and Isaacson, 1985).

REFERENCES

Brooks, J.J., LiVolsi, V.A. and Jaffe, H.L. (1987) Does chondroid chordoma exist? *Acta Neuropathol.*, **72**, 229–35.

Chu, T.A. (1987) Chondroid chordoma of the sacrococcygeal region. *Arch. Pathol. Lab. Med.*, **111**, 861–4.

Coindre, J.-M., Rivel, J., Trojani, M. *et al.* (1986) Immunohistochemical study of chordomas. *J. Pathol.*, **150**, 61–3

Crawford, T. (1958) The staining reactions of chordoma. *J. Clin. Pathol.*, **1**, 110–3.

Dahlin, D.C. and Unni, K.K. (1986) Chordoma. In *Bone Tumors: General Aspects and Data on 8542 Cases*, 4th edn. Charles C Thomas, Springfield, IL, pp. 379–93.

Erlandson, R.A., Tandler, B., Lieberman, P.H. *et al.* (1968) Ultrastructure of human chordoma. *Cancer Res.*, **28**, 2115–25.

Finley, J.L., Silverman, J.F., Dabbs, D.J. *et al.* (1986) Chordoma: diagnosis by fine-needle aspiration biopsy with histologic, immunocytochemical, and ultrastructural confirmation. *Diagn. Cytopathol.*, **2**, 330–7.

Heffelfinger, M.J., Dahlin, D.C., MacCarty, C.S. *et al.* (1973) Chordomas and cartilaginous tumors at the skull base. *Cancer*, **32**, 410–20.

Horton, K.M., Levey, M.S., Owl-Smith, F.A. *et al.* (1990) Metastasizing chordoma in early childhood: report of a case at 1.5 T. *Magn. Reson. Imaging*, **7**, 689–91.

Horwitz, T. (1941) Chordal ectopia and its possible relation to chordoma. *Arch. Pathol.*, **31**, 354–62.

Hruban, R.H., May, M., Marcove, R.C. *et al.* (1990a) Lumbo-sacral chordoma with high-grade malignant cartilaginous and spindle cell component. *Am. J. Surg. Pathol.*, **14**, 384–9.

Hruban, R.H., Traganos, F., Reuter, V.E. *et al.* (1990b) Chordomas with malignant spindle cell components. A DNA flow cytometric and immunohistochemical study with histogenetic implications. *Am. J. Pathol.*, **137**, 435–47.

Kindblom, L.-G. and Angervall, L. (1975) Histochemical characterization of mucosubstances in bone and soft tissue tumors. *Cancer*, **36**, 985–94.

Luschka, H. (1856) Die altersveranderungen der zwischenwirbelknorpel. *Virchows Archiv.* [A], **9**, 311–27.

Maiorano, E., Rezulli, G., Favia, G. *et al.* (1992) Expression of intermediate filaments in chordomas. *Pathol. Res. Pract.*, **188**, 901–7.

Meis, J.M. and Giraldo, A.A. (1988) Chordoma. An immunohistochemical study of 20 cases. *Arch. Pathol. Lab. Med.*, **112**, 553–6.

Miettinen, M. (1984) Chordoma. Antibodies to epithelial membrane antigen and carcinoembryonic antigen in differential diagnosis. *Arch. Pathol. Lab. Med.*, **108**, 891–2.

Muller, H. (1858) Ueber das vorkommen von resten der chorda dorsalis bei menschen nach der gerbut und uber ihr verhaltnis zu den gallertgeschwulsten am clivus. *Z. Ration. Medic.*, **2**, 202–29.

Musgrove, J. (1891) Persistence of the notochord in the human subject. *J. Anat. Physiol.*, **25**, 386–9.

Nakamura, Y., Becker, L.E. and Marks, A. (1983) S-100 protein in human chordoma and human and rabbit notochord. *Arch. Pathol. Lab. Med.*, **107**, 118–20.

Ribbert, H. (1894) Uber die ecchondrosis physalifora sphenooccipitalis. *Zentralbl. Allg. Pathol.*, **5**, 457–61.

Rone, R., Ramzy, I. and Duncan, D. (1986) Anaplastic sacrococcygeal chordoma. Fine needle aspiration cytologic findings and embryologic considerations. *Acta Cytol.*, **30**, 183–8.

Salisbury, J.R. (1987) Demonstration of cytokeratins and an epithelial membrane antigen in chondroid chordoma. *J. Pathol.*, **153**, 37–40.

Salisbury, J.R. and Isaacson, P.G. (1985) Demonstration of cytokeratins and an epithelial membrane antigen in chordomas and in human fetal notochord. *Am. J. Surg. Pathol.*, **9**, 791–7.

Schajowicz, F. (1981) Other tumors 1. Chordoma. In *Tumors and Tumorlike Lesions of Bone and Joints*. Springer-Verlag, New York, pp. 377–83.

Stewart, M.J. (1922) Malignant sacrococcygeal chordoma. *J. Pathol. Bacteriol.*, **25**, 40–62.

Stewart, M.J. and Morin, J.E. (1926) Chordoma: a review, with report of a new sacrococcygeal case. *J. Pathol. Bacteriol.*, **29**, 41–60.

Tamayama, C. and Maruyama, K. (1990) Expression of EGF receptor and c-neu oncogene product in chordomas. *Gan No Rinsho*, **36**, 773–6.

Tamayama, C., Miyauchi, M. and Maruyama, K. (1990) Expression of embryonal and differentiational proteins in chordomas and in the notochord. *Gan No Rinsho*, **36**, 7–12.

Valderrama, E., Kahn, L.B., Lipper, S. *et al.* (1983) Chondroid chordoma: electron-microscopic study of two cases. *Am. J. Surg. Pathol.*, **7**, 161–70.

Virchow, R. (1857) Untersuchungen uber die entwicklungen des schadelgrundes im gesunden und krankhaften zustande und uber den einfluss derselben auf schadelform, gesichtsbildung und gehirnban. G. Reiner, Berlin, p. 47.

Willis, R.A. (1962) *The Borderland of Embryology and Pathology*. Butterworths, London, pp. 2–5, 9–10, 19–29, 37, 299–301.

Wojno, K.J., Hruban, R.H., Garin-Chesa, P. *et al.* (1992) Chondroid chordomas and low-grade chondrosarcomas of the craniospinal axis: an immunohistochemical analysis of 17 cases. *Am. J. Surg. Pathol.*, **16**, 1144–52.

Wold, L.E. and Laws, E.R. Jr (1983) Cranial chordomas in children and young adults. *J. Neurosurg.*, **59**, 1043–7.

14.2   GIANT CELL TUMOUR

Synonym: Osteoclastoma

(a)   Clinical features

This uncommon tumour can show a range of biological behaviour from completely benign to a tumour that produces pulmonary metastases, even though the tumour appears cytologically benign (Vanel *et al.*, 1983). The large majority of giant cell tumours are benign, but often locally aggressive, tumours with a distinct tendency toward local recurrence. Malignant transformation is comparatively rare: for example, 28 out 407 cases reported by Dahlin (1985) developed malignant change histologically (7%). Only seven of these tumours (less than 2% of all cases) had not had radiotherapy included in the treatment of the primary tumour. Giant cell tumours represented 5% of all primary bone tumours (21% of the benign tumours) in the Mayo Clinic series (Dahlin and Unni, 1986).

Most giant cell tumours occur in young adults, with the peak in the decade 20–30 years, although there is a wide age distribution and cases have occurred in 4-year-olds and in 75-year-olds. Approximately 2% of giant cell tumours occur in the skeletally immature. In contrast to most bone tumours, there is a female preponderance, 56.4% in the Mayo series (Dahlin and Unni, 1986); a female:male ratio of 1.5:1 in Schajowicz's (1981) series.

(i)   Skeletal distribution (from Schajowicz, 1981 and Dahlin and Unni, 1986)

- Skull   1%
- Other flat bones
    Ribs
    Girdles   5%
- Spine
    Cervical   1%
    Thoracic   1%
    Lumbar   1%
    Sacral   5%
- Long tubular bones
    Femur   28%
    Tibia   29%
    Humerus   7%
    Fibula, radius, ulna   16%
- Hands and feet   4%

Most giant cell tumours are epiphyseal tumours which extend to the articular surface. Occasionally, they are limited to the metaphysis (Dahlin, 1985). In only 2% of patients are they adjacent to an open growth plate (Campanacci *et al.*, 1987). Giant cell tumours sometimes invade the articular space or involve the ligaments or synovial membrane. Extension to an adjacent bone through the joint space can occur in 5% of cases (Campanacci *et al.*, 1987).

A few cases of giant cell tumours are known to have developed in association with Paget's disease (Dahlin, 1985; Pazzaglia *et al.*, 1988; Carles *et al.*, 1989). Rare cases are multicentric (Dahlin, 1985; Bottke and Hankin, 1989; Wiemann *et al.*, 1990); clearly, hyperparathyroidism must be excluded. Multicentric tumours may affect contiguous bones or involve distant and unrelated bones. Whether multicentric giant cell tumours arise independently, arise by multifocal origin or represent haematogenous metastases, is unclear. Some multicentric cases behave in a more aggressive manner. Experience at the Mayo Clinic has shown that when the small bones of the hand are involved, giant cell tumours are more likely to be multicentric, and to recur (two-thirds) than other giant-cell-bearing lesions of bone of the hands (Dahlin, 1987).

Prognosis for giant cell tumour must be guarded as the recurrence rate after curettage is between 25% and 50% (25% for long bone tumours). About 90% of recurrences occur within three years of surgery (Campanacci *et al.*, 1987). Recurrence may be in the soft tissues. Treatment depends on tumour size and site (Eckardt and Grogan, 1986). Most giant cell tumours are curetted and bone grafted but it is usual to remove expendable bones such as fibula. A number of physical methods have been employed to reduce the local recurrence rate including thermal cautery, cryosurgery with liquid nitrogen, phenol instillation, the use of methylmethacrylate and, experimentally, a CO_2 laser beam (Kenan *et al.*, 1988). Radiotherapy is used to treat those giant cell tumours of the spine and sacrum that are not amenable to complete surgical resection. Sarcomas, usually malignant fibrous histiocytomas, have followed in up to 10% of patients treated primarily by curettage and radiotherapy. These radiation-induced or secondary malignant giant cell tumours have a much worse prognosis than those giant cell tumours with dedifferentiation occurring *de novo*.

(ii)   Radiology

The radiologic appearances of giant cell tumour (Figure 14.5) include: (1) well-defined (geographic) margins, occasionally with a delicate sclerotic rim, (2) prominent trabeculations, (3) 'expanded' bone contour, (4) frequent extension to the subchondral plate, and (5) absence of internal mineralization (Aoki *et al.*, 1989). Giant cell tumours all show increased uptake on bone scanning but bone scans often overestimate the limits of bone involvement and fail to detect soft tissue extension (Levine *et al.*, 1984). CT or conventional tomography are more useful in planning surgical margins. Fluid–fluid levels can be demonstrated within some giant cell tumours by CT and NMR (Buetow *et al.*, 1990).

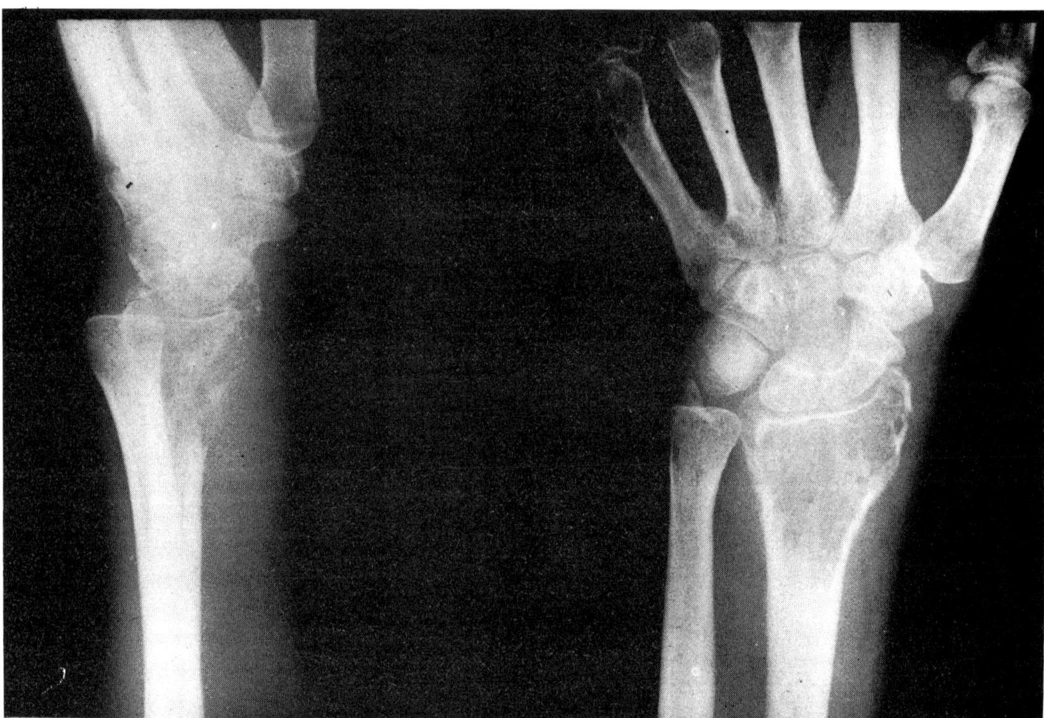

Figure 14.5 Radiograph of giant cell tumour. An osteolytic lesion involving the distal end of the radius of an adult. There is expansion of the cortex. There is no periosteal reaction. As in the majority of these tumours, the lesional tissue extends up to the articular cartilage.

(b) Pathology

(i) *Morbid anatomy*

Morbid anatomical examination of gross specimens shows that giant cell tumours are soft, red to grey and friable (Figures 14.6 and 14.7). Small areas of fibrosis, cystic change or necrosis may be present. Large areas of cystic degeneration can resemble aneurysmal bone cysts.

(ii) *Histopathology*

Histological examination of giant cell tumours shows two obvious cell populations – small mononuclear stromal cells and osteoclast giant cells (Figure 14.8). The stromal cells have poorly defined cytoplasm and may have rounded, oval or spindle-shaped nuclei. They are the proliferating cells and mitotic figures may be quite numerous. There is usually no production of intercellular material but collagen (Figure 14.9) or osteoid can be produced after interference, e.g. fracture or unsuccessful treatment. The osteoclasts are usually numerous and evenly distributed throughout the tumour tissue but occasional tumours contain rather large fields of mononuclear stromal cells devoid of multinucleated giant cells (Figure 14.10).

The main histopathological differential diagnosis is the 'brown tumour' of hyperparathyroidism (Figure 14.7b) and hyperparathyroidism should always be excluded by biochemical investigation before a diagnosis of giant cell tumour is made. Osteoclast-rich osteosarcoma may also need to be excluded; these tumours are nearly always metaphyseal and occur in a younger age group.

Histological examination of sections from tumours that subsequently recurred, and from those that did not, shows no observable cytological differences between the primary tumours (Komiya *et al.*, 1986). However, there is evidence that certain features best demonstrated on macrosections, such as cortical and subchondral invasion, capsular and reactive bony zone infiltration, 'digital'

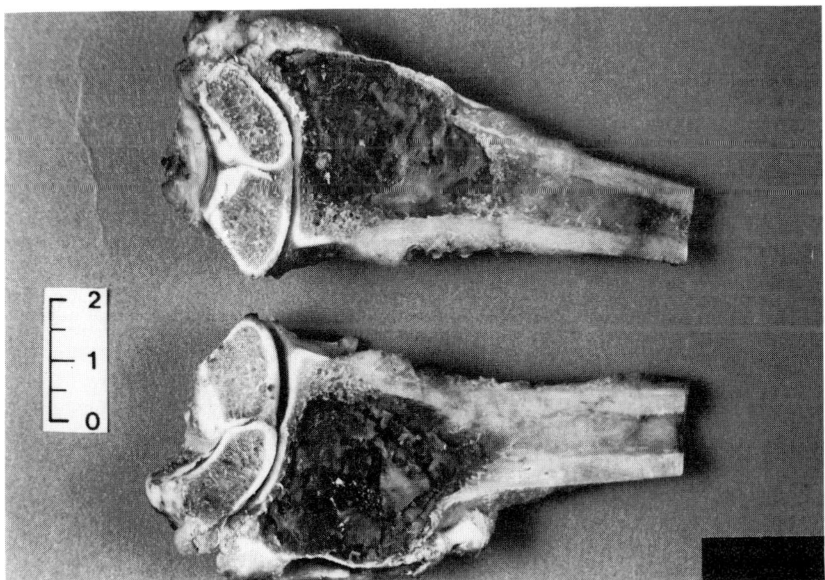

Figure 14.6 Male aged 24 years. Giant cell tumour of the radius.

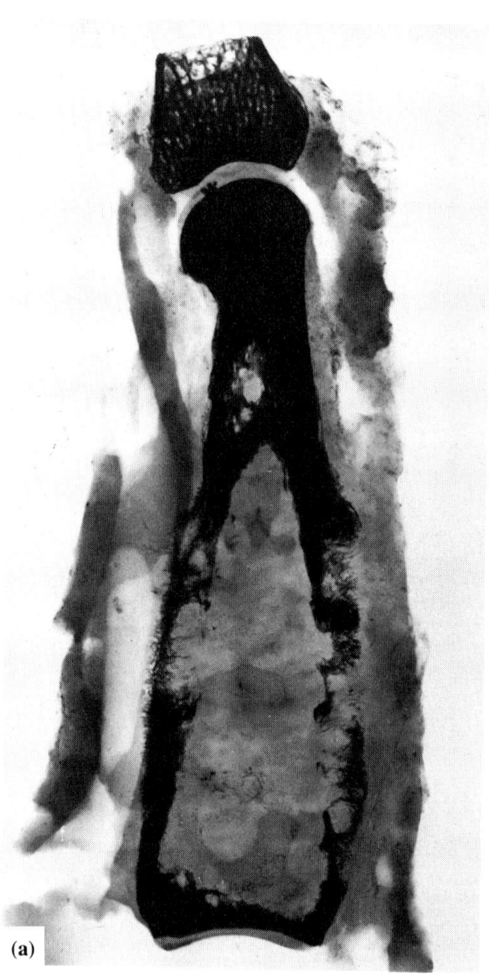

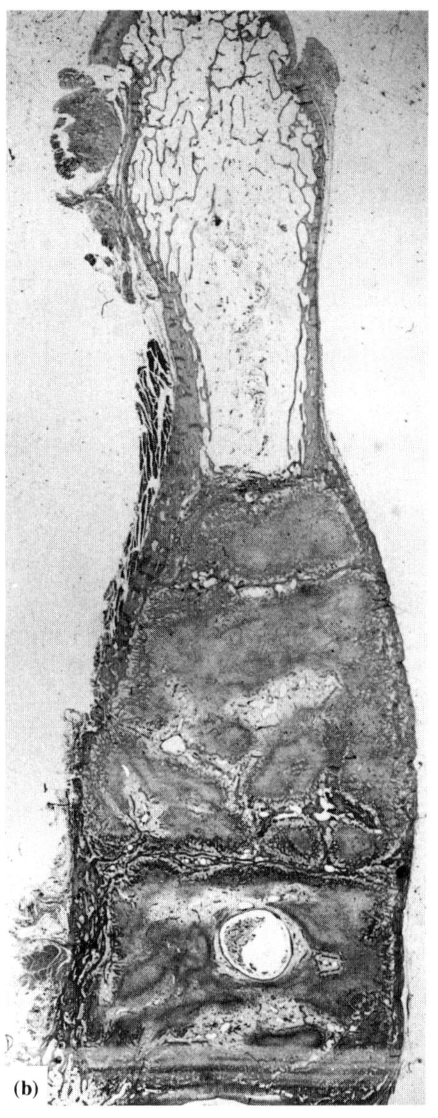

Figure 14.7 (a) Fine detail radiograph of a giant cell tumour of the metacarpal. The proximal part of the metacarpal is expanded and eroded. (b) Photomicrograph of a 'brown tumour' of hyperparathyroidism in a metacarpal. The location and expansion are similar to (a). The distinctive feature of 'brown tumour' is its nodularity but the distal portion of this tumour is more uniform and would present greater diagnostic difficulty which might have to be resolved biochemically. Note the periosteal resorption at the distal articular margin.

extension of the tumour, and neovascularity, correlate well with the aggressiveness found on staging studies (Present *et al.*, 1986).

(iii) Immunohistochemistry

Immunohistochemical studies show that stromal cells stain positively for vimentin but

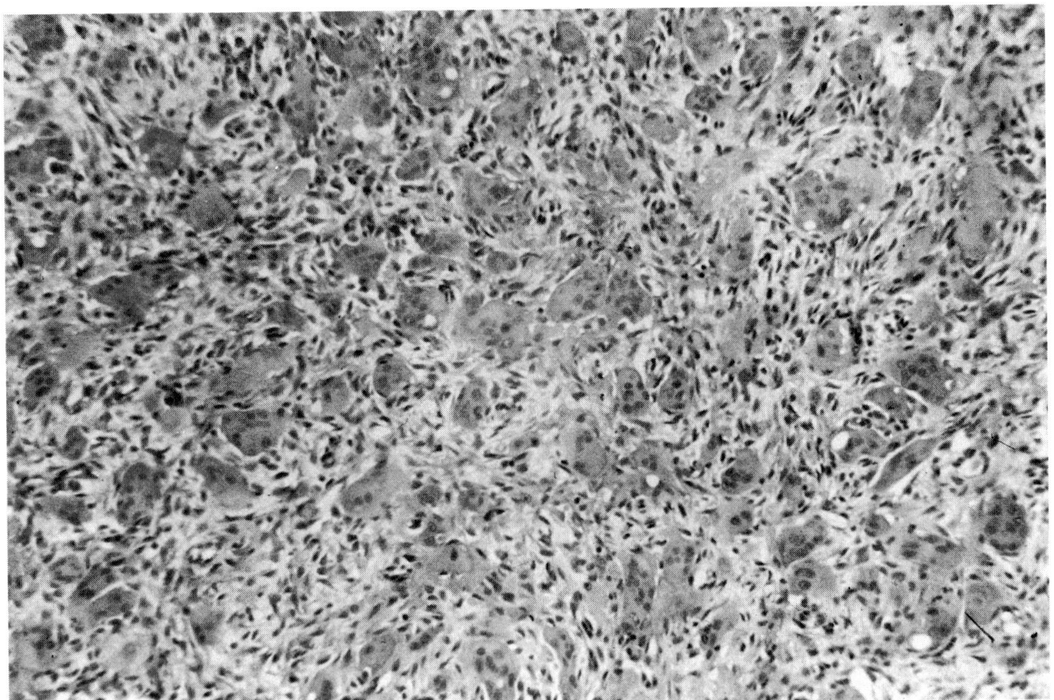

Figure 14.8 Giant cell tumour of bone showing a mononuclear spindle-celled stroma which contains numerous osteoclasts.

negatively for alpha-antichymotrypsin, CD11b, CD35, CD45, epithelial membrane antigen, factor VIII-related antigen, HLA-Dr, lysozyme and mononuclear phagocyte-markers (Brecher *et al.*, 1986). There is one report that some stromal cells react positively with S-100 protein (Liu *et al.*, 1989). The multinucleate osteoclastic giant cells in giant cell tumours stain for α1-antitrypsin (Ling *et al.*, 1986), CD45 (Aqel *et al.*, 1988), CD68 (EBM11) (Athanasou *et al.*, 1985; Brecher *et al.*, 1986), with 25-F-9, an antibody against mature tissue macrophages (Roessner *et al.*, 1987) and with MB1 (Chilosi *et al.*, 1988), and weakly with UCHM1 and KB90 (Brecher *et al.*, 1986). They do not react with the majority of antibodies specific for myeloid cells or HLA-Dr (Aqel *et al.*, 1988). The interrelationship of the multinucleate giant cells and the stromal cells has also been investigated immunohistochemically by staining for Ia and monocyte–macrophage lineage antigens (Ling *et al.*, 1988). Immunocytochemical studies have also shown that the osteoclasts within giant cell tumours possess receptors for calcitonin (Goldring *et al.*, 1987) and produce an integrin complex that is absent in cells of the monocyte–macrophage lineage (Zambonin-Zallone *et al.*, 1989).

(iv) Cytogenetics

Many giant cell tumours show random chromosomal abnormalities when analysed cytogenetically, although some show clonal abnormalities. An unusual anomaly, telomeric fusion, is the most striking random chromosomal abnormality described (Bridge *et al.*, 1990). A case of 12;19 translocation has also been reported (Noguera *et al.*, 1989). Interestingly, chromosomal abnormalities are almost always present in those tumours

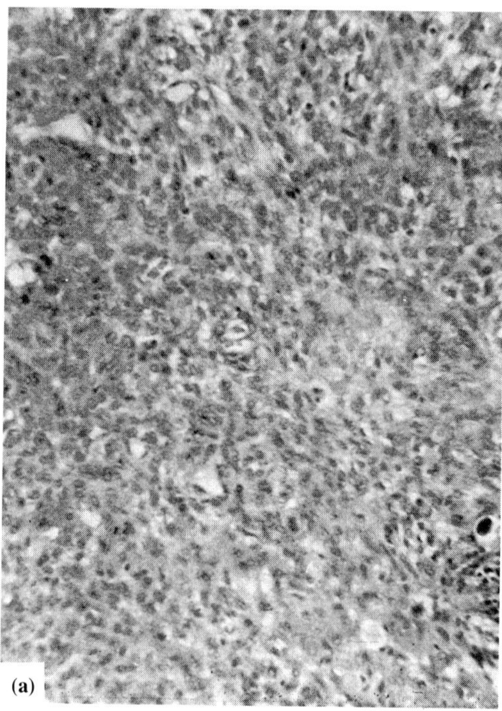 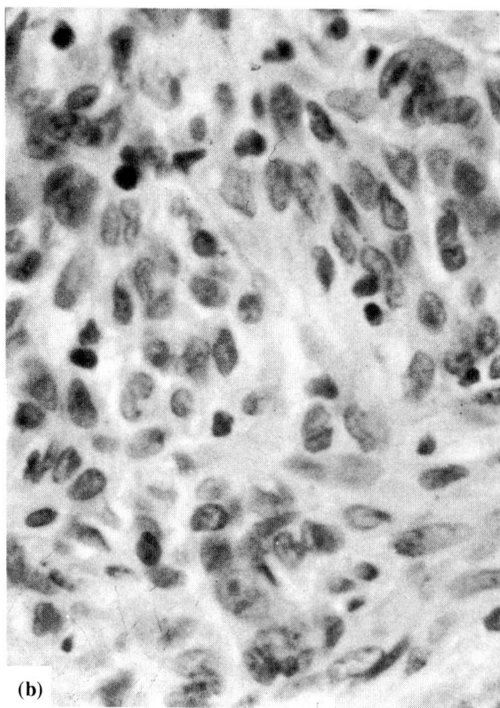

Figure 14.9 (a, b) A giant cell tumour of bone in which there were fields that did not contain osteoclasts. The stroma is composed of cells with round and oval nuclei. This tissue is not diagnostic of giant cell tumour.

which are locally aggressive, recurrent or metastatic, and are rare in those that behave in an innocent fashion (Bridge *et al.*, 1990). This suggests that cytogenetic analysis may be a worthwhile means of predicting the biological behaviour of these tumours.

(v) Histogenesis

Despite the descriptive names applied to this tumour (giant cell tumour, osteoclastoma), the multinucleated giant cells are osteoclasts (Athanasou *et al.*, 1985), and can be seen as a reactive population in other tumours (Flanagan and Chambers, 1989), and not the neoplastic population. An intriguing, although difficult to understand, finding is that, in continuous *in vitro* culture, two seemingly distinct populations of multinucleated giant cells are observed (Zhou, 1990). One population is short-lived (2–3 weeks) whereas the other maintains growth and formation. The small mononuclear stromal cells between the osteoclasts are the neoplastic clone and can be shown to be the proliferating cells by epi-illumination cytofluorometry, tissue culture (Goldring *et al.*, 1987), autoradiography, electron microscopy or immunohistochemical studies using antibodies against Ki-67 or proliferation-associated nuclear antigen (Roessner *et al.*, 1987, 1989). Presumably they secrete cytokine(s) that act as an attractant for the osteoclast precursors and/or cause the precursors to fuse into multinucleated giant cells. The older idea that the multinucleated giant cells were formed by fusion of the neoplastic stromal cells has been largely disproved (Aqel *et al.*, 1988) and there is now substantial evi-

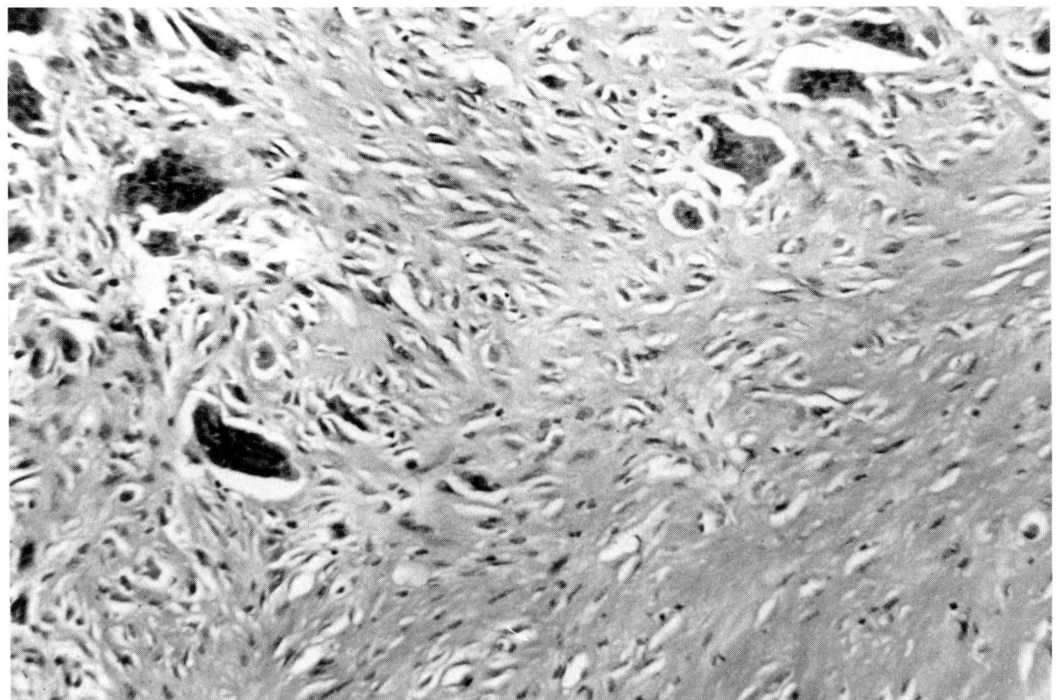

Figure 14.10 An illustration of the extensive stromal fibrosis that can occur in giant cell tumour of bone. Seen in isolation, such a field would not be diagnostic.

dence that osteoclasts are part of the mononuclear phagocyte system and are formed by fusion of macrophage-like precursors derived ultimately from stem cells in the bone marrow. Mononuclear macrophages are present in all giant cell tumours although their numbers vary considerably. They can be distinguished from the mononuclear stromal cells by immunohistochemical staining (Roessner *et al.*, 1987; Aqel *et al.*, 1988; Liu *et al.*, 1989) and by their ability to form rosettes. Small numbers of T and B lymphocytes can also be identified in some tumours (Aqel *et al.*, 1988). The origin of the neoplastic stromal cells is unknown but it is speculated that they are derived from a connective tissue stromal cell or other primitive mesenchymal bone cell.

REFERENCES

Aoki, J., Moser, R.P. Jr and Vinh, T.N. (1989) Giant cell tumor of the scapula. A review of 13 cases. *Skeletal Radiol.*, **18**, 427–34.

Aqel, N.M., Pringle, J.A. and Horton, M.A. (1988) Cellular heterogeneity of giant cell tumour of bone (osteoclastoma). An immunohistochemical study of 16 cases. *Histopathology*, **13**, 675–85.

Athanasou, N.A., Bliss, E., Gatter, K.C. *et al.* (1985) An immunohistological study of giant-cell tumour of bone: evidence for an osteoclast origin of the giant cells. *J. Pathol.*, **147**, 153–8.

Bottke, C.A. and Hankin, F.M. (1989) Bilateral giant cell tumour of the distal radius: a case report. *J. Hand Surg.*, **14B**, 338–40.

Brecher, M.E., Franklin, W.A. and Simon, M.A. (1986) Immunohistochemical study of mononuclear phagocyte antigens in giant cell tumor of bone. *Am. J. Pathol.*, **125**, 252–7.

Bridge, J.A., Neff, J.R., Bhatia, P.S. *et al.* (1990) Cytogenetic findings and biologic behaviour of giant cell tumors of bone. *Cancer*, **65**, 2697–703.

Buetow, P.C., Newman, S. and Kransdorf, M.J. (1990) Giant-cell tumor of the tibia in a child presenting as an expansile mass with fluid–fluid levels on MR. *Magn. Reson. Imaging*, **8**, 341–4.

Campanacci, M., Baldini, N., Boriani, S. *et al.*

(1987) Giant-cell tumor of bone. *J. Bone Joint Surg.*, **69A**, 106–14.

Carles, D., Rivel, J., Devars, F. *et al.* (1989) Giant cell tumors developing in Paget's disease. Presentation of two cases with an ultrastructural study. *Ann. Pathol.*, **9**, 47–53.

Chilosi, M., Gilioli, E., Lestani, M. *et al.* (1988) Immunohistochemical characterization of osteoclasts and osteoclast-like cells with monoclonal antibody MB1 on paraffin-embedded tissues. *J. Pathol.*, **156**, 251–4.

Dahlin, D.C. (1985) Caldwell Lecture. Giant cell tumor of bone: highlights of 407 cases. *Am. J. Roentgenol.*, **144**, 955–60.

Dahlin, D.C. (1987) Giant-cell-bearing lesions of bone of the hands. *Hand Clin.*, **3**, 291–7.

Dahlin, D.C. and Unni, K.K. (1986) Giant cell tumor (osteoclastoma). In *Bone Tumors: General Aspects and Data on 8542 cases*, 4th edn. Charles C Thomas, Springfield, IL, pp. 119–40.

Eckardt, J.J. and Grogan, T.J. (1986) Giant cell tumor of bone. *Clin. Orthop.*, **204**, 45–58.

Flanagan, A.M. and Chambers, T.J. (1989) Osteoclasts are present in the giant cell variant of malignant fibrous histiocytoma. *J. Pathol.*, **159**, 53–7.

Goldring, S.R., Roelke, M.S., Petrison, K.K. *et al.* (1987) Human giant cell tumors of bone: identification and characterization of cell types. *J. Clin. Invest.*, **79**, 483–91.

Kenan, S., Kirby, E.J., Buchalter, J. *et al.* (1988) The potential role of the laser in marginal sterilization of giant cell tumor following curettage. *Bull. Hosp. Jt. Dis. Orthop. Inst.*, **48**, 93–101.

Komiya, S., Inoue, A., Nakashima, A. *et al.* (1986) Prognostic factors in giant cell tumor of bone. A modified histological grading system useful as a guide to prognosis. *Arch. Orthop. Trauma Surg.*, **105**, 67–72.

Levine, E., De Smet, A.A., Neff, J.R. *et al.* (1984) Scintigraphic evaluation of giant cell tumor of bone. *Am. J. Roentgenol.*, **143**, 343–8.

Ling, L., Klein, M.J., Sissons, H.A. *et al.* (1986) Lysozyme and alpha 1-antitrypsin in giant-cell tumor of bone and in other lesions that contain giant cells. *Arch. Pathol. Lab. Med.*, **110**, 713–8.

Ling, L., Klein, M.J., Sissons, H.A. *et al.* (1988) Expression of Ia and monocyte–macrophage lineage antigens in giant cell tumor of bone and related lesions. *Arch. Pathol. Lab. Med.*, **112**, 65–9.

Liu, T.C., Ji, Z.M. and Wang, L.T. (1989) Giant cell tumors of bone. An immunohistochemical study. *Pathol. Res. Prac.*, **185**, 448–53.

Noguera, R., Llombart-Bosch, A., Lopez-Gines, C. *et al.* (1989) Giant-cell tumor of bone, stage II, displaying translocation t(12;19) (q13;q13). *Virchows Arch. A*, **415**, 377–82.

Pazzaglia, U.E., Barbieri, D. and Ceciliani, L. (1988) An epiphyseal giant cell tumor associated with early Paget's disease. A case report. *Clin. Orthop.*, **234**, 217–20.

Present, D., Bertoni, F., Hudson, T. *et al.* (1986) The correlation between the radiologic staging studies and histopathologic findings in aggressive stage 3 giant cell tumor of bone. *Cancer*, **57**, 237–44.

Roessner, A., Vassallo, J., Vollmer, E. *et al.* (1987) Biological characterization of human bone tumors. X. The proliferation behaviour of macrophages as compared to fibroblastic cells in malignant fibrous histiocytoma and giant cell tumor of bone. *J. Cancer Res. Clin. Oncol.*, **113**, 559–62.

Roessner, A., Vollmer, E., Zwadlo, G. *et al.* (1989) The cytogenesis of macrophages and osteoclast-like giant cells in bone tumors with special emphasis on the so-called fibrohistiocytic tumors. *Curr. Top. Pathol.*, **80**, 205–27.

Schajowicz, F. (1981) Giant-cell tumor (Osteoclastoma). In *Tumors and Tumorlike Lesions of Bone and Joints*. Springer-Verlag, New York, pp. 205–42.

Vanel, D., Contesso, G., Rebibo, G. *et al.* (1983) Benign giant cell tumours of bone with pulmonary metastases and favourable prognosis. Report on two cases and review of the literature. *Skeletal Radiol.*, **10**, 221–6.

Wiemann, B., Albert, H., Knolle, H. *et al.* (1990) Bilateral primary giant cell tumor (osteoclastoma) of the ribs. *Z. Erkr. Atmungsorgane*, **174**, 155–60.

Zambonin-Zallone, A., Teti, A., Grano, M. *et al.* (1989) Immunocytochemical distribution of extracellular matrix receptors in human osteoclasts: a beta 3 integrin is colocalized with vinculin and talin in the podosomes of osteoclastoma giant cells. *Exp. Cell Res.*, **182**, 645–52.

Zhou, L. (1990) Multinucleated giant cells in cultured giant cell tumor of bone. *Chung Hua Wai Ko Tsa Chih*, **27**, 689–91.

14.3 ROUND CELL NEOPLASMS

14.3.1 EWING'S TUMOUR

(a) Clinical features

Ewing's tumour is an uncommon neoplasm which represents about 10% of all malignant primary bone tumours. It was first described by Ewing in 1921. The large majority of cases occur in patients between 7 and 30 years old, predominantly 10–15 years old (Kissane *et al.*, 1983). Very few cases are known to have arisen in infants less than 2 years old. Ewing's tumour is commoner in males than females. It is predominantly a disease of Caucasians and is rare in non-whites.

(i)   Skeletal distribution (from Schajowicz, 1981 and Dahlin and Unni, 1986)

- Jaws   0.5%
- Skull   1%
- Other flat bones
    Ribs   7%
    Girdles
        Shoulder: clavicle, scapula,
        sternum   7%
        Pelvis: ilium, pubis, sacrum   20%
- Spine: cervical, thoracic, lumbar   4%
- Long tubular
    Femur, tibia, humerus   46%
    Fibula, radius, ulna   10%
- Hands and feet
    Short tubular
        Metacarpals, metatarsals,
        phalanges   1%
    Cuboidal
        Carpals, tarsals   2%

As can be seen, most Ewing's tumours arise in the extremities. They are uncommon in the distal extremities (Chen *et al.*, 1983; Shirley *et al.*, 1985), for example, there are only 20 cases of Ewing's tumour of the hand in the literature (Euler *et al.*, 1990) and they are very rare in the feet (Wu, 1989). Approximately 4% of primary Ewing's tumours arise

in the bones of the head and neck (Siegal *et al.*, 1987). Involvement of the jaws by Ewing's tumour is also uncommon; when it occurs it may mimic an inflammatory pericoronitis (McGlumphy *et al.*, 1987).

There are no known preceding factors for Ewing's tumour. Single case reports exist of Ewing's tumour following bilateral retinoblastoma (Schifter *et al.*, 1983) and developing in a lesion of fibrous dysplasia (Roth *et al.*, 1985).

A mass or swelling, high ESR and low-grade fever are common presenting features, although the length of the preoperative symptoms does not seem to alter prognosis. The clinical features which do have prognostic significance are the size of the tumour at presentation (whether measured by tumour volume (Gobel *et al.*, 1987) or by maximum diameter (Hayes *et al.*, 1989)), the peripheral blood white cell count (Hayes *et al.*, 1989), the presence of metastatic disease, elevation of the erythrocyte sedimentation rate and location of the tumour in the pelvis (Kissane *et al.*, 1983; Wilkins *et al.*, 1986). In addition, patients who undergo complete surgical excision of the primary tumour have a better survival rate (74% at 5 years) than those who do not (34% at 5 years) (Wilkins *et al.*, 1986). The 3-year disease-free survival rate (Kaplan–Meier life table analysis) is 78% for tumours with a volume less than 100 ml compared to 17% for tumours greater than 100 ml (Gobel *et al.*, 1987). The Kaplan–Meier estimate of disease-free survival at 3 years is 82% for those with tumours less than 8 cm in maximum diameter and 64% for those with tumours greater than 8 cm in maximum diameter (Hayes *et al.*, 1989). A high white blood cell count predicts worse disease-free survival (Hayes *et al.*, 1989). The site of the primary tumour is generally of no prognostic value (Gobel *et al.*, 1987; Hayes *et al.*, 1989), although larger tumours are primarily located in central and proximal extremity sites. The serum lactase dehydrogenase (LDH) level at presentation has no prognostic significance, but the LDH level at recurrence may be significantly higher than the follow-up LDH level of those without recurrence (Farley *et al.*, 1987). Prognosis of head and neck Ewing's tumours is significantly better than Ewing's tumours overall (Siegal *et al.*, 1987). The prognosis of periosteal Ewing's tumours may be more favourable than that of the central type (Kolar *et al.*, 1989).

All patients, even those with apparently localized tumours, are treated with cytotoxic chemotherapy on the assumption that subclinical metastases are already present. Before the introduction of chemotherapy, Ewing's tumour had a 10% 5-year survival. Now, treated by chemotherapy in combination with radiotherapy and/or surgical resection, some centres are estimating 5-year survival for all patients at 80% (Hayes *et al.*, 1989). About one-third of tumours recur locally 6 months to 10 years after radiotherapy, therefore primary tumours are resected if possible. Almost all local recurrences occur in patients with tumours greater than 8 cm in diameter (Hayes *et al.*, 1989). Metastases are usually to the lungs and skeletal system; central nervous system involvement is rare (Yu *et al.*, 1990). Pulmonary metastases may be successfully treated with radiotherapy.

Occasional cases of Ewing's tumour present in the soft tissues. These were first described by Angervall and Enzinger in 1975 (see Auge and Pusel (1990) for review). These extraskeletal Ewing's tumour patients range in age from 5 to 14 years (average age 10.3 years) and have a male to female ratio of 1:3. The same treatment rules as for skeletal Ewing's tumour apply to extraskeletal Ewing's tumours.

(ii) Radiology

The classical radiographic appearance shows a tumour with 'onion-skinning' and Codman's triangles but these are not specific features. About 40% of cases show diffuse

sclerosis, usually combined with areas of lysis and/or a periosteal reaction. Some tumours show erosion of bone from the outside, secondary to soft tissue extension. Rare tumours originate in a periosteal location and intact endosteal cortical surfaces with a tumour-free medullary cavity can be demonstrated by CT or MRI (Kolar *et al.*, 1989).

(b) Pathology

(i) Morbid anatomy

Macroscopically, at surgery, some Ewing's tumours resemble pus; most are more solid.

(ii) Histopathology

Histological examination shows small tumour cells in large clumps (Figure 14.11). The dominant histological pattern may be diffuse, filigree (an organoid pattern consisting of bicellular tumour strands separated by filmy vascular stroma) or 'endothelial-like'. There is usually little reticulin. Cytologically, Ewing's tumour cells are uniform, oval cells without prominent nuclear chromatin clumping and with inconspicuous nucleoli. Necrotic tumour and layers of new bone formation lead to the 'onion-skinning'. The diffuse sclerosis seen radiologically is related to dead bone (Shirley *et al.*, 1985). Viable cells survive between radionecrotic bone after radiotherapy and are responsible for recurrence. Radiotherapy can also lead to variation in the size and shape of the Ewing's cells. Most tumours are periodic acid–Schiff (PAS) positive but not all (section 14.3.2). Only two histological features have any prognostic significance, the presence of necrosis and the presence of a filigree pattern; both are of poor prognostic value (Kissane *et al.*, 1983; Llombart Bosch *et al.*, 1986).

The histological differential diagnosis is between embryonal rhabdomyosarcoma

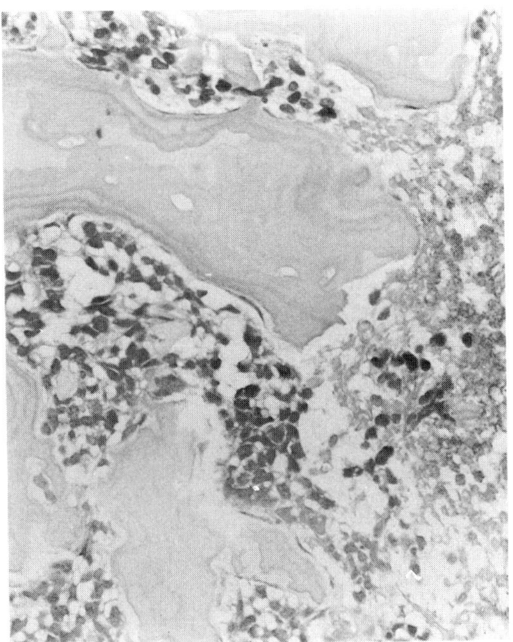

Figure 14.11 Ewing's sarcoma. Section of secondary spongiosa from the pubic ramus (note the cores of cartilage in the trabeculae), in which the marrow is replaced by viable and necrotic small round cell tumour. The cytological feature of malignancy here is the hyperchromatic nuclei; uniformity of the cells is also indicative of neoplasia in this context.

invading bone, acute leukaemia or extranodal lymphoma, metastatic neuroblastoma or medulloblastoma, small cell osteosarcoma, mesenchymal chondrosarcoma, Askin tumours of bone and soft tissues, and primitive neuroectodermal tumour of bone.

(iii) Immunohistochemistry

Immunohistochemistry using avidin–biotin immunoperoxidase techniques shows positivity for CD57 (Leu 7) (Pinto *et al.*, 1989), MB2 (Kahn and Thorner, 1989), neuroblastoma cell surface antigen (NBCA), neurofilaments, neurone cell surface antigen (NCSA), neurone-specific enolase (Ushigome *et al.*, 1989) and vimentin in the majority of tumours. Occasional cases show positive staining for S-100 protein (Ushigome *et al.*, 1989). Ewing's tumours are negative for α_1-antitrypsin, α_1-antichymotrypsin, factor VIII-related antigen, immunoglobulin heavy and light chains and myoglobin (Navas-Palacios *et al.*, 1984). Extraskeletal Ewing's tumours possess the same immunohistochemical profile as osseous Ewing's tumours (Ushigome *et al.*, 1989).

(iv) Cytopathology

Fine-needle aspiration of Ewing's tumours produces very cellular smears of relatively small, round to oval, uniform tumour cells (Dahl *et al.*, 1986). Glycogen deposits appear as punched-out clear spaces in the cytoplasm (Akhtar *et al.*, 1985). Two cell types can be distinguished. There is a predominance of lighter 'principal' or 'chief' cells which are interspersed with darker, smaller 'dark' cells (Dahl *et al.*, 1986).

(v) Electron microscopy

Electron microscopy of skeletal Ewing's tumours shows round cells with oval nuclei, smooth nuclear membranes and abundant euchromatin. There are scanty cytoplasmic organelles, abundant glycogen, occasional lipid vacuoles and primitive intercellular junctions (Navas-Palacios *et al.*, 1984). There are no cell processes or other evidence of neural differentiation.

(vi) Cytogenetics

Cytogenetic analysis of Ewing's tumours shows a specific and consistent reciprocal translocation between chromosomes 11 and 22 (t(11;22) (q24;q12)) (Turc-Carel *et al.*, 1984; Aurias *et al.*, 1984; Whang-Peng *et al.*, 1986; Callen *et al.*, 1987). Extraskeletal Ewing's tumours (Whang-Peng *et al.*, 1986), peripheral neuroepithelioma (Whang-Peng *et al.*, 1984) and Askin tumours (De Chadarevian *et al.*, 1984; Whang-Peng *et al.*, 1986) all show the same translocation. Ewing's tumours have also been reported in patients with Down's syndrome (trisomy 21) (Bridge *et al.*, 1990). In contrast with their high malignancy, Ewing's tumours show an unexpectedly low proportion of DNA aneuploid stemlines (Mellin *et al.*, 1989).

(vii) Histogenesis

The cell of origin of Ewing's tumour is debatable. Undifferentiated mesenchymal cells in the bone marrow have long been proposed as a possible candidate (Melnick, 1933; Jaffe, 1958; Llombart-Bosch *et al.*, 1978, 1982; Navas-Palacios *et al.*, 1984; Moll *et al.*, 1987) but the experimental work of Cavazzana *et al.*, (1987) provides fairly convincing evidence for a neural histogenesis. Triche and Cavazzana (1988) have suggested that Ewing's tumour, Askin tumour and primitive neuroectodermal tumour (PNET) of bone can all be considered as non-neuroblastomatous neural tumours of bone that vary in the extent of their neural differentiation, which is an interesting and worthwhile concept. Ewing's tumour lacks neural differentiation *in vivo* whereas Askin tumour and PNET of bone show limited neural differentiation, the degree of which can vary from tumour to tumour. Cell lines established from Ewing's tumour show evidence of neural differentiation *in vitro*; immunophenotypically, in their hormone sensitivity (van Valen *et al.*, 1988), and, after treatment with cyclic AMP or TPA (phorbol 12-myristate 13-acetate), morphologically and ultrastructurally (Cavazzana *et al.*, 1987). All tumours in the 'Ewing's group' show *c-myc* expression.

REFERENCES

Akhtar, M., Ali, M.A. and Sabbah, R. (1985) Aspiration cytology of Ewing's sarcoma. Light and electron microscopic correlations. *Cancer*, **56**, 2051–60.

Auge, B. and Pusel, J. (1990) Extra-skeletal Ewing's sarcoma. A case report with detailed review of the literature. *Arch. Anat. Cytol. Pathol.*, **38**, 65–71.

Aurias, A., Rimbaut, C., Buffe, D. *et al.* (1984) Translocation involving chromosome 22 in Ewing's sarcoma: a cytogenetic study of four fresh tumors. *Cancer Genet. Cytogenet.*, **12**, 21–5.

Bridge, J.A., Neff, J.R., Borek, D.A. *et al.* (1990) Primary skeletal Ewing's sarcoma in Down's syndrome. *Cancer Genet. Cytogenet.*, **47**, 61–8.

Callen, D.F., Smith, R.D. and Bourne, A.J. (1987) Chromosomal analysis in Ewing's sarcoma. *Pathology*, **19**, 64–6.

Cavazzana, A.O., Miser, J.S., Jefferson, J. *et al.* (1987) Experimental evidence for a neural origin of Ewing's sarcoma of bone. *Am. J. Pathol.*, **127**, 507–18.

Chen, K.T., McGann, P.D. and Flam, M.S. (1983) Ewing's sarcoma of the phalangeal bone. *J. Surg. Oncol.*, **22**, 92–4.

Dahl, I., Akerman, M. and Angervall, L. (1986) Ewing's sarcoma of bone. A correlative cytological and histological study of 14 cases. *Acta Pathol. Microbiol. Immunol. Scand. A*, **94**, 363–9.

Dahlin, D.C. and Unni, K.K. (1986) Ewing's tumor. In *Bone Tumors: General Aspects and Data on 8542 Cases*, 4th edn, Charles C Thomas, Springfield, IL, pp. 322–36.

De Chadarevian, J.-P., Vekemans, M. and Seemayer, T. (1984) Reciprocal translocation in small-cell sarcomas (Letter). *N. Engl. J. Med.*, **311**, 1702.

Euler, E., Wilhelm, K., Permanetter, W. *et al.* (1990) Ewing's sarcoma of the hand: localization and treatment. *J. Hand. Surg.*, **15A**, 659–62.

Ewing, J. (1921) Diffuse endothelioma of bone. *Proc. New York Pathol. Soc.*, **21**, 17–24.

Farley, F.A., Healey, J.H., Caparros-Sison, B. *et al.* (1987) Lactase dehydrogenase as a tumor marker for recurrent disease in Ewing's sarcoma. *Cancer*, **59**, 1245–8.

Gobel, V., Jurgens, H., Etspuler, G. *et al.* (1987) Prognostic significance of tumor volume in localized Ewing's sarcoma of bone in children and adolescents. *J. Cancer Res. Clin. Oncol.*, **113**, 187–91.

Hayes, F.A., Thompson, E.I., Meyer, W.H. *et al.* (1989) Therapy for localized Ewing's sarcoma of bone. *J. Clin. Oncol.*, **7**, 208–13.

Jaffe, H.L. (1958) *Tumors and Tumorous Conditions*

of the Bones and Joints. Lea and Febiger, Philadelphia, pp. 350–1.

Kahn, H.J. and Thorner, P.S. (1989) Monoclonal antibody MB2: a potential marker for Ewing's sarcoma and primitive neuroectodermal tumor. *Pediatr. Pathol.,* **9**, 153–62.

Kissane, J.M., Askin, F.B., Foulkes, M. *et al.* (1983) Ewing's sarcoma of bone: clinicopathologic aspects of 303 cases from the Intergroup Ewing's Sarcoma Study. *Human. Pathol.,* **14**, 773–9.

Kolar, J., Zidkova, H., Matejovsky, Z. *et al.* (1989) Periosteal Ewing's sarcoma. *ROFO,* **150**, 179–82.

Llombart-Bosch, A., Blache, R. and Peydro-Olaya, A. (1978) Ultrastructural study of 23 cases of Ewing's sarcoma: typical and atypical forms. *Cancer,* **41**, 1362–73.

Llombart-Bosch, A., Blache, R. and Peydro-Olaya, A. (1982) Round-cell sarcomas of bone and their differential diagnosis (with particular emphasis on Ewing's sarcoma and reticulosarcoma): a study of 233 tumors with optical and electron microscopic techniques. *Pathol. Annu.,* **17**, 113–45.

Llombart-Bosch, A., Contesso, G., Henry-Amar, M. *et al.* (1986) Histopathological predictive factors in Ewing's sarcoma of bone and clinicopathological correlations. A retrospective study of 261 cases. *Virchows Arch. A,* **409**, 627–40.

McGlumphy, E.A., Zysset, M.K. and Montgomery, M.T. (1987) Ewing's sarcoma metastatic to the gingiva. *J. Oral Maxillofac. Surg.,* **45**, 444–7.

Mellin, W., Dierschauer, W., Hiddemann, W. *et al.* (1989) Flow cytometric DNA analysis of bone tumors. *Curr. Top. Pathol.,* **80**, 115–52.

Melnick, P.J. (1933) Histogenesis of Ewing's sarcoma with post-mortem of a case. *Am. J. Cancer,* **19**, 353–63.

Moll, R., Lee, I., Gould, V.E. *et al.* (1987) Immunocytochemical analysis of Ewing's tumors. Patterns of expression of intermediate filaments and desmosomal proteins indicate cell type heterogeneity and pluripotential differentiation. *Am. J. Pathol.,* **127**, 288–304.

Navas-Palacios, J.J., Aparicio-Duque, R. and Valdes, M.D. (1984) On the histogenesis of Ewing's sarcoma. An ultrastructural, immunohistochemical, and cytochemical study. *Cancer,* **53**, 1882–901.

Pinto, A., Grant, L.H., Hayes, F.A. *et al.* (1989) Immunohistochemical expression of neuron-specific enolase and Leu 7 in Ewing's sarcoma of bone. *Cancer,* **64**, 1266–73.

Roth, A., Touzet, P. and Rigault, P. (1985) Association of Ewing's sarcoma with fibrous dysplasia of the tibia. Apropos of a case report. *Rev. Chir. Orthop.,* **71**, 133–7.

Schajowicz, F. (1981) Marrow tumors. In *Tumors and Tumorlike Lesions of Bone and Joints.* Springer-Verlag, New York, pp. 244–67.

Schifter, S., Vendelbe, L., Jensen, O.M. *et al.* (1983) Ewing's tumor following bilateral retinoblastoma. A case report. *Cancer,* **51**, 1746–9.

Shirley, S.K., Askin, F.B., Gilula, L.A. *et al.* (1985) Ewing's sarcoma in bones of the hands and feet: a clinicopathologic study and review of the literature. *J. Clin. Oncol.,* **3**, 686–97.

Siegal, G.P., Oliver, W.R., Reinus, W.R. *et al.* (1987) Primary Ewing's sarcoma involving the bones of the head and neck. *Cancer,* **60**, 2829–40.

Triche, T.J. and Cavazzana, A. (1988) Round cell tumors of bone. In *Bone Tumors* (ed. K.K. Unni), Churchill Livingstone, New York, pp. 199–223.

Turc-Carel, C., Philip, I., Berger, M. -P. *et al.* (1984) Chromosome study of Ewing's sarcoma (ES) cell lines. Consistency of a reciprocal translocation t(11;22) (q24;q12). *Cancer Genet. Cytogenet.,* **12**, 1–9.

Ushigome, S., Shimoda, T., Takaki, K. *et al.* (1989) Immunocytochemical and ultrastructural studies of the histogenesis of Ewing's sarcoma and putatively related tumors. *Cancer,* **64**, 52–62.

Van Valen, F., Proir, R., Wechsler, W. *et al.* (1988) Immunocytochemical and biochemical studies of an Ewing sarcoma cell line: evidence for neural differentiation in vitro. *Klin. Padiatr.,* **200**, 256–70.

Whang-Peng, J., Triche, T.J., Knutsen, T. *et al.* (1984) Chromosome translocation in peripheral neuroepithelioma. *N. Engl. J. Med.,* **311**, 584–5.

Whang-Peng, J., Triche, T.J., Knutsen, T. *et al.* (1986) Cytogenetic characterization of selected small round cell tumors of childhood. *Cancer Genet. Cytogenet.,* **21**, 185–208.

Wilkins, R.M., Pritchard, D.J., Burgert, E.O. Jr *et al.* (1986) Ewing's sarcoma of bone. Experience with 140 patients. *Cancer,* **58**, 2551–5.

Wu, K.K. (1989) Ewing's sarcoma of the foot. *J. Foot Surg.,* **28**, 166–70.

Yu, L., Craver, R., Baliga, M. *et al.* (1990) Isolated CNS involvement in Ewing's sarcoma. *Med. Paediatr. Oncol.,* **18**, 354–8.

14.3.2 ATYPICAL EWING'S TUMOUR

(a) Clinical features

Atypical Ewing's tumours are rare tumours that have the same clinical features as classical Ewing's tumours (Llombart-Bosch *et al.*, 1978). The 'atypical' refers to their histological appearance. This histological variant is apparently without prognostic significance. Its importance lies in providing a link between classical Ewing's tumour and primitive neuroectodermal tumour of bone.

(b) Pathology

Atypical Ewing's tumours are defined histologically as those sarcomas which, although very similar to Ewing's tumour, contain rosettes and are periodic acid–Schiff negative. The rosette formation is a prominent feature but they also have obvious extracellular stroma (compared with the virtual absence of stroma in classical Ewing's tumour) and may be formed of more pleomorphic or larger cells than those found in classical Ewing's tumour. Immunohistochemistry using avidin–biotin techniques shows positivity for CD57 (Leu 7), neurone-specific enolase and vimentin. Electron microscopy shows cells with poorly formed or absent cell processes and no true dense core granules although variably sized, pleomorphic neurosecretory granules may be seen.

REFERENCE

Llombart-Bosch, A., Blache, R. and Peydro-Olaya, A. (1978) Ultrastructural study of 23 cases of Ewing's sarcoma: typical and atypical forms. *Cancer*, **41**, 1362–73.

14.3.3 PRIMITIVE NEUROECTODERMAL TUMOUR OF BONE

(a) Clinical features

Primitive neuroectodermal tumours (PNETs) are rare bone neoplasms with clinical features similar to Ewing's tumour of bone. The patients range in age from 3 to 34 years but most are 13–17 years of age. The tumour is commoner in females and male:female ratios of between 4:5 and 3:11 have been reported (Llombart-Bosch *et al.*, 1988).

(i) Skeletal distribution

Tumours predominantly involve the limbs, especially legs, and humerus, pelvis and scapula in that order of frequency. Involvement is both diaphyseal and metaphyseal.

Fever is the commonest systemic symptom. Up to a third of patients present with a fracture, and about one-half have metastases at presentation. Metastasis is often to other bones. Prognosis is poor; death occurs on average 8 months following diagnosis if metastases are present initially, and 36 months after the diagnosis otherwise (Rousselin *et al.*, 1989).

(ii) Radiology

Radiologically, PNETs of bone appear similar to Ewing's tumours. They are aggressive, poorly demarcated tumours, with cortical destruction, periosteal reaction and soft tissue invasion (Rousselin *et al.*, 1989).

(b) Pathology

(i) Histopathology

Histologically, PNET of bone shows a lobular growth pattern and possesses rosette-like structures mimicking Homer–Wright rosettes (Jaffe *et al.*, 1984) (Figure 14.12), as seen in neuroectodermic neoplasms (neuroblastoma, peripheral neuroepithelioma). Some tumours contain pseudoalveolar spaces (Steiner *et al.*, 1988) and there may be a fibrillary background (Llombart-Bosch *et al.*, 1988). The proliferating cells are small and round with variable amounts of glycogen from sparse to abundant. Tumours that recur after treatment may show the histological features of pleomorphic neuroblastoma (Llombart-Bosch *et al.*, 1987). There are case reports of PNETs of bone showing melanocytic features, confirmed by electron microscopy (Young and Gonzalez-Crussi, 1985).

The differential diagnosis from Ewing's tumour by light microscopy alone can be extremely difficult. A diagnosis of PNET can be made when at least one of the following are recognized: (1) definite neurofibrils, (2) differentiation to ganglion cells, or (3) ultrastructural evidence of a neurogenic origin (e.g. neurosecretory granules or cell processes with microtubules. The presence or

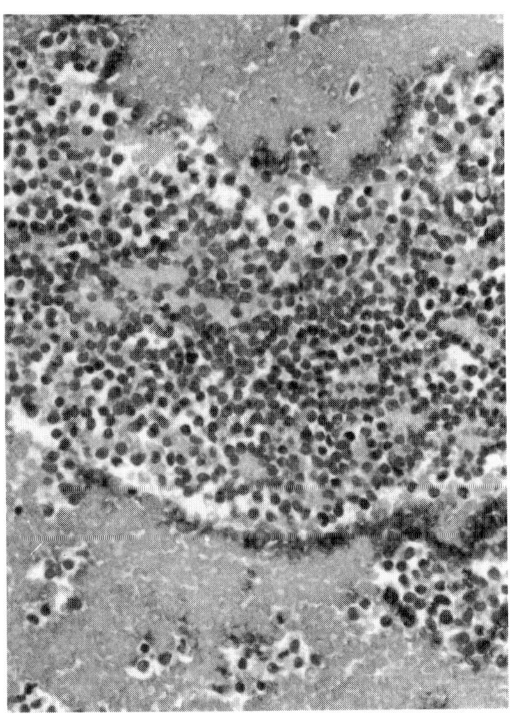

Figure 14.12 Male aged 5 years. A peripheral neuroectodermal tumour from the femoral diaphysis. Necrotic tumour tissue encloses viable malignant round cell tumour. Some of the tumour cells surround amorphous material, not readily distinguished from necrosis, but the pattern suggests rosettes, confirmable by electron microscopy. The diagnosis can also be supported by immunoreactivity for neurone-specific enolase.

absence of rosette-like structures of tumour cells and abundant glycogen in tumour cells is not conclusive.

(ii) Immunohistochemistry

Immunohistochemistry using avidin–biotin peroxidase techniques shows PNETs of bone are positive for β_2-microglobulin, CD57 (Leu 7), chromogranin, MB2, neuroblastoma cell surface antigen (NBCA), neurofilaments, neuron cell surface antigen (NCSA), neurone-specific enolase, *n-myc* oncogene product, synaptophysin and vimentin (Jaffe *et al.*, 1984; Kawaguchi and Koike, 1986; Llombart-Bosch *et al.*, 1987, 1988; Kahn and Thorner, 1989; Tsuneyoshi *et al.*, 1989; Ushigome *et al.*, 1989). Rare cases demonstrate positivity for S-100 protein (Steiner *et al.*, 1988; Ushigome *et al.*, 1989).

(iii) Electron microscopy

Electron microscopy shows small round tumour cells with a dense chromatin pattern and abundant glycogen. Neurites of irregular calibre, synaptic-like buttons, microtubules and intermediate filaments are present (Jaffe *et al.*, 1984; Llombart-Bosch *et al.*, 1987). Dense core granules are seen, albeit that they may include rather variably sized and pleomorphic forms (Llombart-Bosch *et al.*, 1988; Steiner *et al.*, 1988). Basement membrane-like condensations may surround the cells (Llombart-Bosch *et al.*, 1987). Scanning electron microscopy of one case confirmed the presence of rosette-like figures and cell elongations with short dendritic projections (Llombart-Bosch *et al.*, 1987).

(iv) Histogenesis

The relationship between PNETs of bone and Askin tumours (section 14.3.4) was recognized by the original authors (Jaffe *et al.*, 1984). More recent speculation has focused on the possibility that Ewing's sarcoma and

PNET are closely related histogenetically, without directly answering the question of histiogenesis (Dehner, 1993). Tumours histologically identical to PNETs of bone also occur in the soft tissues (peripheral neuroepithelioma of soft tissue). Cell lines established from PNETs of bone show evidence of neural differentiation (Jaffe *et al.*, 1984; Isayama *et al.*, 1990).

REFERENCES

Dehner, L.P. (1993) Primitive neuroectodermal tumor and Ewing's sarcoma. *Am. J. Surg. Pathol.*, **17**, 1–13.

Isayama, T., Iwasaki, H., Kikuchi, M. *et al.* (1990) Neuroectodermal tumor of bone. Evidence for neural differentiation in a cultured cell line. *Cancer*, **65**, 1771–81.

Jaffe, R., Santamaria, M., Yunis, E.J. *et al.* (1984) The neuroectodermal tumor of bone. *Am. J. Surg. Pathol.*, **8**, 885–98.

Kahn, H.J. and Thorner, P.S. (1989) Monoclonal antibody MB2: a potential marker for Ewing's sarcoma and primitive neuroectodermal tumor. *Pediatr. Pathol.*, **9**, 153–62.

Kawaguchi, K. and Koike, M. (1986) Neuron-specific enolase and Leu-7 immunoreactive small round-cell neoplasm. The relationship to Ewing's sarcoma in bone and soft tissue. *Am. J. Clin. Pathol.*, **86**, 79–83.

Llombart-Bosch, A., Lacombe, M.J., Contesso, G. *et al.* (1987) Small round blue cell sarcoma of bone mimicking atypical Ewing's sarcoma with neuroectodermal features. An analysis of five cases with immunohistochemical and electron microscopic support. *Cancer*, **60**, 1570–82.

Llombart-Bosch, A., Lacombe, M.J., Peydro-Olaya, A. *et al.* (1988) Malignant peripheral neuroectodermal tumours of bone other than Askin's neoplasm: characterization of 14 new cases with immunohistochemistry and electron microscopy. *Virchows Arch. A*, **412**, 421–30.

Rousselin, B., Vanel, D., Terrier-Lacombe, M.J. *et al.* (1989) Clinical and radiologic analysis of 13 cases of primary neuroectodermal tumors of bone. *Skeletal Radiol.*, **18**, 115–20.

Steiner, C.G., Graham, S. and Lewis, M.M. (1988) Malignant round cell tumour of bone with neural differentiation (neuroectodermal tumor). *Ultrastruct. Pathol.*, **12**, 505–12.

Tsuneyoshi, M., Yokoyama, R., Hashimoto, H. *et al.* (1989) Comparative study of neuroectodermal tumor and Ewing's sarcoma of bone. Histopathologic, immunohistochemical and ultrastructural features. *Acta Pathol. Jpn.*, **39**, 573–81.

Ushigome, S., Shimoda, T., Takaki, K. *et al.* (1989) Immunocytochemical and ultrastructural studies of the histogenesis of Ewing's sarcoma and putatively related tumors. *Cancer*, **64**, 52–62.

Young, S. and Gonzalez-Crussi, F. (1985) Melanocytic neuroectodermal tumor of the foot. Report of a case with multicentric origin. *Am. J. Clin. Pathol.*, **84**, 371–8.

14.3.4 ASKIN TUMOUR

Synonym: Malignant small cell tumour of the thoracopulmonary region in childhood

(a) Clinical features

Askin tumours (malignant small cell tumours of the thoracopulmonary region in childhood) are rare tumours of children and young adults (Askin *et al.*, 1979). Whether Askin tumours arise in bone or soft tissue is unclear; nevertheless, almost all show rib involvement. Many authorities believe that Askin tumours are primary soft tissue tumours arising in the chest wall which involve rib secondarily.

Askin tumours usually present with a chest wall mass, or pain, or both. The patients may be dyspnoeic and have a fever (Askin *et al.*, 1979). Metastases occur most commonly to bone, lung and other structures in the chest (Askin *et al.*, 1979; Miser *et al.*, 1985).

(i) Radiology

Radiologically, Askin tumours present most commonly (70%) as pleural disease. A chest wall soft tissue mass is seen in approximately 50%. A peripheral intrapulmonary mass which is associated with pleural disease, is seen in approximately 25%, and radiologically apparent rib involvement in under 50%. Apparent pulmonary involvement by Askin tumours is caused by the tumour masses growing into the pleural space and compressing adjacent lung. Tumour spread in the hilum or mediastinum, calcification within the soft tissue mass, or a paraspinal soft tissue mass as the sole presenting feature, are rarer manifestations (Askin *et al.*, 1979; Fink *et al.*, 1985, 1992).

(b) Pathology

(i) Histopathology

Histologically, Askin tumours are rare true round cell sarcomas of bone that may or may not contain glycogen as determined by the periodic acid–Schiff stain with and without diastase (Askin *et al.*, 1979; Linnoila *et al.*, 1986). Immunocytochemically, Askin tumours always stain positively for neurone-specific enolase and vimentin but may be either positive or negative for neurofilaments. They are negative for CD45, CD57 (unlike Ewing's tumour (Pinto *et al.*, 1989)), and for desmin and cytokeratins. Electron microscopy shows minimal neural differentiation with clusters of variably sized dense core granules. Neurites or definitive cell processes are absent.

An unusual case of a neurone-specific enolase positive, but otherwise completely undifferentiated, round cell tumour originating in rib was reported by Haas *et al.* (1987) that showed a unique karyotype 45, XY, -21, t(11;22) (q23;q11), del(22)t(21;22) (q11.2;p11).

REFERENCES

Askin, F.B., Rosai, J., Sibley, R.K. *et al.* (1979) Malignant small cell tumor of the thoracopulmonary region in childhood. A distinctive clinicopathologic entity of uncertain histogenesis. *Cancer*, **43**, 2438–51.

Fink, I.J., Kurtz, D.W., Cazenave, L. *et al.* (1985) Malignant thoracopulmonary small cell ('Askin') tumor. *Am. J. Roentgenol* **145**, 517–20.

Fink, M., Salisbury, J.R. and Gishen, P. (1992) Askin tumours: three case histories and a review of the literature. *Eur. J. Radiol.*, **14**, 178–80.

Haas, O.A., Chott, A., Ladenstein, R. *et al.* (1987) Poorly differentiated, neuron-specific enolase positive round cell tumor with two translocations t(11;22) and t(21;22). *Cancer*, **60**, 2219–23.

Linnoila, R.J., Tsokos, M., Triche, T.J. *et al.* (1986) Evidence for neural origin and PAS positive variants of the malignant small cell tumor of thoracopulmonary region ('Askin tumour'). *Am. J. Surg. Pathol.*, **10**, 124–33.

Miser, J.S. and Pizzo, P.A. (1985) Soft tissue sarcomas in childhood. *Pediatr. Clin. North Am.*, **32**, 779–800.

Pinto, A., Grant, L.H., Hayes, F.A. *et al.* (1989) Immunohistochemical expression of neuron-specific enolase and Leu 7 in Ewing's sarcoma of bone. *Cancer*, **64**, 1266–73.

14.3.5   PRIMARY MALIGNANT LYMPHOMA OF BONE

Synonyms:
>   Lymphosarcoma of bone
>   Reticulosarcoma of bone
>   Parker–Jackson reticulosarcoma

(a)   Clinical features

At the beginning, a distinction needs to be made between those lymphomas which appear to arise primarily within bones and the skeletal involvement that is seen in disseminated malignant lymphomas that have arisen primarily in lymph nodes (secondary involvement of bone). Primary malignant lymphomas of bone are rare bone tumours that occur between 2 and 86 years of age, mean age 46 years (Ostrowski *et al.*, 1986). They are infrequent tumours in children (Howat *et al.*, 1987). Of children with non-Hodgkin's lymphoma 2.8% present with a bone primary, usually in the femur (Furman *et al.*, 1989). There is a male predominance with male:female ratio in adults of 1.6:1 (Ostrowski *et al.*, 1986).

(i) Skeletal distribution (from Schajowicz, 1981 and Dahlin and Unni, 1986)

- Jaws   5%
- Skull   5%
- Other flat bones
    Ribs   7%
    Girdles
        Shoulder: clavicle, scapula,
        sternum   9%
        Pelvis: ilium, pubis, sacrum   20%
- Spine: cervical, thoracic, lumbar   10%
- Long tubular
    Femur, tibia, humerus   34%
    Fibula, radius, ulna   2%
- Hands and feet
    Short tubular
        Metacarpals, metatarsals,
        phalanges   0.5%
    Cuboidal
        Carpals, tarsals   1%

Rare case reports document parosteal involvement (Smith, 1984).

Patients often have little in the way of systemic symptoms, although there may be local pain or an associated soft tissue swelling or mass (Ostrowski *et al.*, 1986). Pathological fractures are relatively frequent and are thought to be related to the permeative growth pattern. Exceptional case reports document malignant lymphomas which have developed secondarily to chronic osteomyelitis or have arisen within a congenital neurofibroma of bone and soft tissue (Radi *et al.*, 1988).

The biological behaviour of primary malignant lymphomas of bone is unpredictable and the long-term prognosis should be guarded. Most respond quite well to radiotherapy alone. For multifocal osseous disease and simultaneous osseous and nodal or soft tissue involvement, radiotherapy plus cytotoxic chemotherapy is the usual course of treatment.

More than 50% of cases at presentation fall into the category of disseminated skeletal lesions. The clinical features may simulate multiple myeloma or metastatic carcinoma with disseminated osteolytic lesions and hypercalcaemia (Rossi *et al.*, 1987; Plaza *et al.*, 1989). Some of the disseminated skeletal lesions seem to be multicentric malignant bone lymphomas rather than secondary involvement although this can obviously be a difficult diagnosis to establish. These multicentric cases have a worse prognosis than the single tumours. Magnetic resonance imaging may reveal other foci of disease undetected by routine staging studies (Salter *et al.*, 1989). The distinction between primary and secondary lymphoma is important prognostically. Patients with primary lymphomas of bone have a 66% 3-year, 44% 5-year and 34% 10-year survival whereas patients with secondary lymphoma of bone have a 23% 5-year and 18% 10-year survival. In some sites, however, it becomes almost impossible to know whether the lymphoma is a primary bone tumour or represents secondary involvement – this is particularly true for malignant lymphomas along the spine and from the maxillary sinus. Involvement of the bony cavities of the face is uncommon. Two distinct clinicopathological entities are recognized: orbital non-Hodgkin's lymphomas which are generally stage 1, of low or intermediate histological grade and carry a good prognosis; and nasosinusal non-Hodgkin's lymphomas which are often locally advanced, associated with other disease sites, of intermediate or high histological grade and which carry a poor prognosis (Demard *et al.*, 1989).

No convincing cases of Hodgkin's disease primarily arising in bone exist; all osseous cases are believed to represent secondary involvement.

(ii) Radiology

Primary malignant lymphomas of bone appear radiologically as destructive lesions but often have small areas of sclerosis within (Figures 14.13 and 14.14). Permeative destruction is the usual finding but some cases have sclerotic or lytic borders or show layered periosteal reactions or eccentric cortical destruction. The radiographic pattern of bone involvement does not have prognostic significance (Clayton *et al.*, 1987; Franczyk *et al.*, 1989). There may or may not be a soft tissue extension which can even lead to ulceration of the overlying skin.

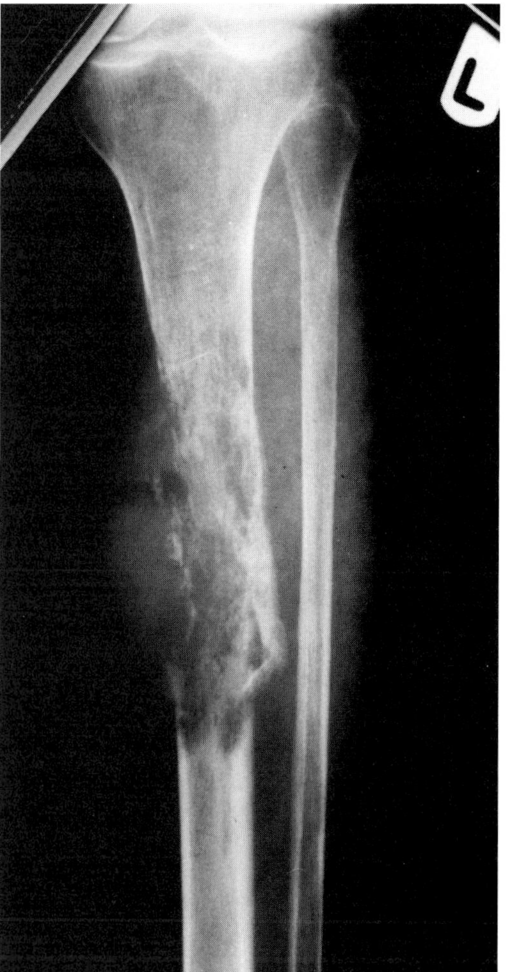

Figure 14.14 Female aged 79 years. Radiograph of a primary B cell non-Hodgkin's lymphoma. Pathological fracture through a large lytic area with permeative margins in the left tibial diaphysis. In addition, there is an extensive soft tissue swelling. Radiograph courtesy of Mr P.W. Skinner.

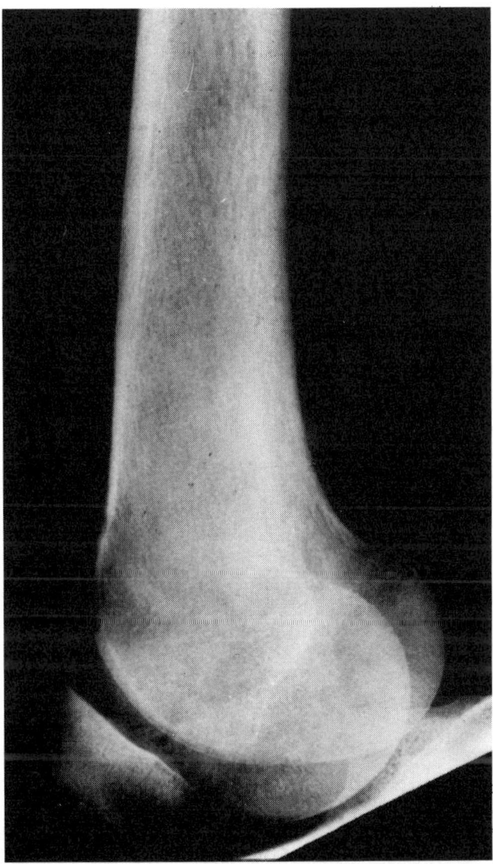

Figure 14.13 Radiograph of a primary non-Hodgkin's lymphoma. The distal end of the femur shows permeative destruction of the bone with complete destruction of the bone at the anterior metaphyseal surface and on the posterior aspect of a condyle. The shaft shows loss of density and a minimal periosteal reaction.

(b) Pathology

(i) *Histopathology*

Histological examination shows a small round cell tumour (Figure 14.15) that typically penetrates among bone trabeculae and marrow fat. A reticular framework separates the tumour cells and can be accentuated by a reticulin stain. All tumours are associated with fibrosis: 45% have delicate reticulin fibrosis, 33% have fibrous bands, 21% have hyalinized dense fibrosis and <1% have bony sclerosis with osteoid (Ostrowski *et al.*, 1986). The sclerotic process seen radiologically is reflected by appositional new bone formation. The tumour cells are usually pleomorphic with round to irregularly shaped, sometimes folded, nuclei. The nuclei possess finely distributed heterochromatin and one or two prominent, but small to medium-sized, nucleoli. The cytoplasm is scanty to moderate and slightly basophilic. A periodic acid–Schiff stain for glycogen is classically negative (Price and Ross, 1972) but variations from the usual pattern include tumours with clear cells and clustering that can simulate carcinoma, spindle-celled

forms (Kluin *et al.*, 1984) and tumours where clustering of cells gives rise to 'alveolar' formations (Ostrowski *et al.*, 1986). Mucin stains are always negative in lymphomas.

Most primary lymphomas of bone are large cell lymphomas of high-grade malignancy; they are often difficult to classify further. When further classification is attempted, then most are classed as centroblastic lymphomas of polymorphic subtype (Kiel classification) (Falini *et al.*, 1988; Radaszkiewicz and Hansmann, 1988) with some examples of immunoblastic lymphoma and of lymphoblastic lymphoma (Clayton *et al.*, 1987; Vassallo *et al.*, 1987; Vassallo *et al.*, 1988). There is also an unusually high incidence of tumours with large-cleaved or multilobated cells in primary bone lymphomas (Clayton *et al.*, 1987; Vassallo *et al.*, 1988; Pettit *et al.*, 1990)

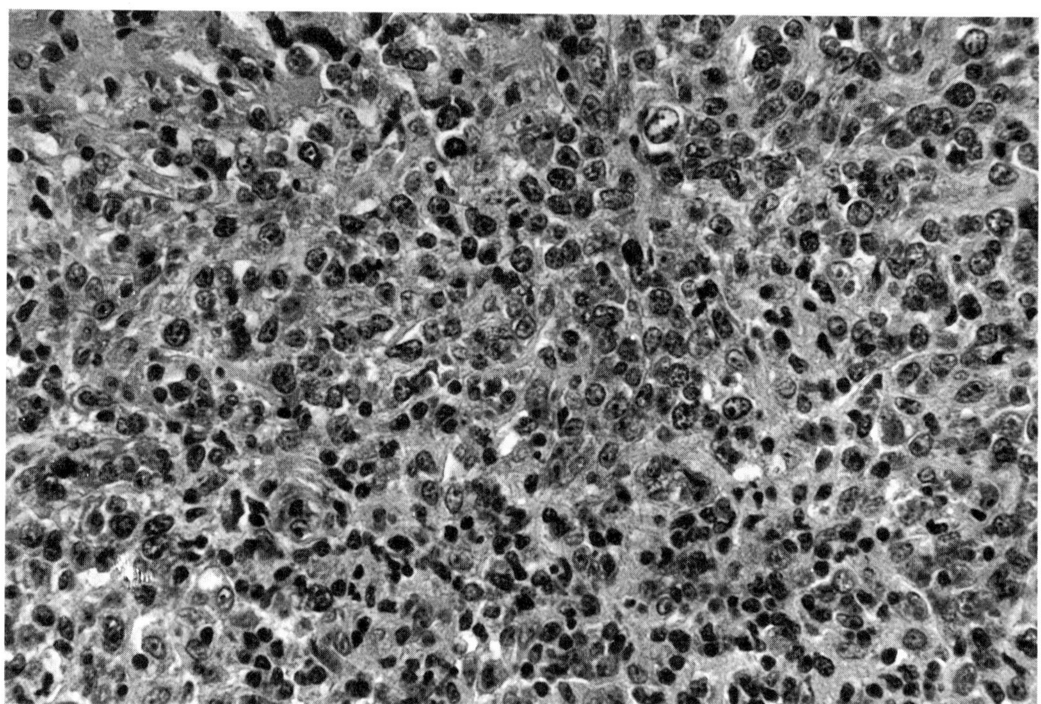

Figure 14.15 Female aged 27 years. Primary B cell non-Hodgkin's lymphoma in the ilium. The larger cells are the neoplastic cells; there is also a reactive population of small lymphocytes.

compared with their rarity as nodal lymphomas. Primary osseous malignant lymphomas of low-grade malignancy (lymphocytic, centroblastic/centrocytic and centrocytic subtypes) are uncommon (Clayton *et al.*, 1987; Vassallo *et al.*, 1987).

The histological differential diagnosis of malignant lymphoma of bone is with other small round cell sarcomas of bone, Langerhans cell histiocytosis, osteomyelitis (Ostrowski *et al.*, 1986), granulocytic sarcoma, malignant fibrous histiocytoma (Kluin *et al.*, 1984) and small cell anaplastic carcinoma.

One report has suggested that stage and histological pattern significantly correlate with long-term survival among large cell lymphomas (Clayton *et al.*, 1987). The opinion of other authorities, however, is that none of the lymph node-based classifications of lymphoma (Kiel, Working Formulation, etc.) seems to have any relationship to prognosis when applied to primary bone lymphomas and that staging alone remains the most important prognostic indicator (Ostrowski *et al.*, 1986). The Mayo Clinic group, for example, separates malignant lymphoma of bone into four major groups based on the stage of the disease (Ostrowski *et al.*, 1986):

1. Primary lymphoma of bone (lymphoma presenting in an osseous site with no evidence of disease elsewhere for at least 6 months after diagnosis)
2. Multifocal osseous disease (lymphoma in two or more osseous sites only, without evidence of soft tissue or nodal involvement, also for at least 6 months after diagnosis)
3. Lymphoma of bone and nodal or soft tissue (or both) disease presenting simultaneously (or these lesions developed within 6 months)
4. Lymphoma of bone diagnosed at least 6 months after an original diagnosis of nodal or soft tissue (or both) disease

(ii) Immunohistochemistry

Immunohistochemical studies of primary osseous lymphomas are scarce when compared with studies of lymphomas at other sites. They show that the large majority of primary bone lymphomas are of B cell lineage (Vassallo *et al.*, 1987; Falini *et al.*, 1988). The tumours are positive for CD19, CD20, CD22 and CD45 and possess monotypic immunoglobulins, often IgG kappa which suggests a post-germinal centre stage of differentiation. Like nodal lymphomas, some primary B cell lymphomas of bone contain an abundant reactive T lymphocyte population (Fiche *et al.*, 1990). Rare primary T cell malignant lymphomas of bone do occur; some of these contain 'Reed-Sternberg-like' cells. Occasional cases of primary B cell bone lymphomas also contain giant cells similar to Reed-Sternberg cells (Radaszkiewicz and Hansmann, 1988). Some anaplastic large cell Ki-1 lymphomas have also presented in bone (Chan *et al.*, 1989).

REFERENCES

Chan, J.K., Ng, C.S., Hui, P.K. *et al.* (1989) Anaplastic large cell Ki-1 lymphoma. Delineation of two morphological types. *Histopathology*, **15**, 11–34.

Clayton, F., Butler, J.J., Ayala, A.G. *et al.* (1987) Non-Hodgkin's lymphoma in bone. Pathologic and radiologic features with clinical correlates. *Cancer*, **60**, 2494–501.

Dahlin, D.C. and Unni, K.K. (1986) Malignant lymphoma of bone (reticulum cell sarcoma). In *Bone Tumors: General Aspects and Data on 8542 Cases*, 4th edn. Charles C Thomas, Springfield, IL, pp. 208–26.

Demard, F., Santini, J., Ettore, F. *et al.* (1989) Malignant non-Hodgkin's lymphoma of the bony cavity of the face. Apropos of 17 cases. *Rev. Laryngol. Otol. Rhinol.*, **110**, 191–5.

Falini, B., Binazzi, R., Pileri, S. *et al.* (1988) Large cell lymphoma of bone. A report of three cases of B-cell origin. *Histopathology*, **12**, 177–90.

Fiche, M., Le Tourneau, A., Audouin, J. *et al.* (1990) A case of primary osseous malignant immunoblastic B-cell lymphoma with intracytoplasmic mu lambda immunoglobulin inclusions. *Histopathology*, **16**, 167–72.

Franczyk, J., Samuels, T., Rubenstein, J. *et al.* (1989) Skeletal lymphoma. *Can. Assoc. Radiol. J.*, **40**, 75–9.

Furman, W.L., Fitch, S., Hustu, H.O. *et al.* (1989) Primary lymphoma of bone in children. *J. Clin. Oncol.*, **7**, 1275–80.

Howat, A.J., Thomas, H., Waters, K.D. *et al.* (1987) Malignant lymphoma of bone in children. *Cancer*, **59**, 335–9.

Kluin, P.M., Slootweg, P.J., Schuurman, H.J. *et al.* (1984) Primary B-cell malignant lymphoma of the maxilla with a sarcomatous pattern and multilobated nuclei. *Cancer*, **54**, 1598–605.

Ostrowski, M.L., Unni, K.K., Banks, P.M. *et al.* (1986) Malignant lymphoma of bone. *Cancer*, **58**, 2646–55.

Pettit, C.K., Zukerberg, L.R., Gray, M.H. *et al.* (1990) Primary lymphoma of bone. A B-cell neoplasm with a high frequency of multilobated cells. *Am. J. Surg. Pathol.*, **14**, 329–34.

Plaza, V., Urbano-Ispizua, A., Paz, M.A. *et al.* (1989) High-degree malignancy non-Hodgkin's lymphoma simulating a disseminated carcinoma. Presentation of 2 cases. *Med. Clin.*, **92**, 344–6.

Price, C.H.G. and Ross, F.G.M. (1972) *Bone, Certain Aspects of Neoplasia*. Butterworth, London.

Radaszkiewicz, T. and Hansmann, M.L. (1988) Primary high-grade malignant lymphomas of bone. *Virchows Arch. A*, **413**, 269–74.

Radi, M.J., Foucar, E., Palmer, C.H. *et al.* (1988) Malignant lymphoma arising in a large congenital neurofibroma of the head and neck. Report of a case. *Cancer*, **61**, 1667–73.

Rossi, J.F., Bataille, R., Chappard, D. (1987) B cell malignancies presenting with unusual bone involvement and mimicking multiple myeloma. *Am. J. Med.*, **83**, 10–16.

Salter, M., Sollaccio, R.J., Bernreuter, W.K. *et al.* (1989) Primary lymphoma of bone: the use of MRI in pretreatment evaluation. *Am. J. Clin. Oncol.*, **12**, 101–5.

Schajowicz, F. (1981) Marrow tumors. In: *Tumors and Tumorlike Lesions of Bone and Joints*. Springer-Verlag, New York, pp. 267–80.

Smith, R.G. (1984) Parosteal lymphoblastic lymphoma. A human counterpart of Abelson virus-induced lymphosarcoma of mice. *Cancer*, **54**, 471–6.

Vassallo, J., Roessner, A., Vollmer, E. *et al.* (1987) Malignant lymphomas with primary bone manifestation. *Pathol. Res. Pract.*, **182**, 381–9.

Vassallo, J., Assuncao, M.C. and Machado, J.C. (1988) Primitive malignant lymphomas of bone. Study of 14 cases. *Ann. Pathol.*, **8**, 44–8.

14.3.6 MULTIPLE MYELOMA AND SOLITARY PLASMACYTOMA

(a) Clinical features

These tumours of malignant plasma cells occur mainly between 45 and 90 years of age. Their site distribution is that of the red marrow and most are derived therefore from the central axial skeleton.

(i) Skeletal distribution (from Dahlin and Unni, 1986)

- Jaws   2%
- Skull   8%
- Other flat bones

Ribs	16%
Girdles	
Shoulder: clavicle, scapula, sternum	8%
Pelvis: ilium, pubis, sacrum	15%

- Spine: cervical, thoracic, lumbar   33%
- Long tubular

Femur, tibia, humerus	15%
Fibula, radius, ulna	0.5%

Very rare cases are known to have occurred secondary to chronic osteomyelitis. Most cases of multiple myeloma are dead within 2 years.

(ii) Radiology

Radiographs show myelomas to be destructive lesions affecting almost any bones (Figures 14.16 and 14.17a); the skull appearance may be particularly characteristic, so-called 'pepper-pot' skull. The number of osteolytic lesions correlates with the differentiation of the malignant plasma cells (Hokamp and Grundmann, 1983). Sometimes myelomas are sclerosing tumours – these seem to be more indolent variants. Non-secretory multiple myeloma usually has a high tumour cell mass and multiple areas of bone destruction (Cavo *et al.*, 1985).

(b) Pathology

(i) Morbid anatomy

Macroscopically, multiple myelomas are usually soft mushy tumours but they are sometimes meaty like a lymphoma.

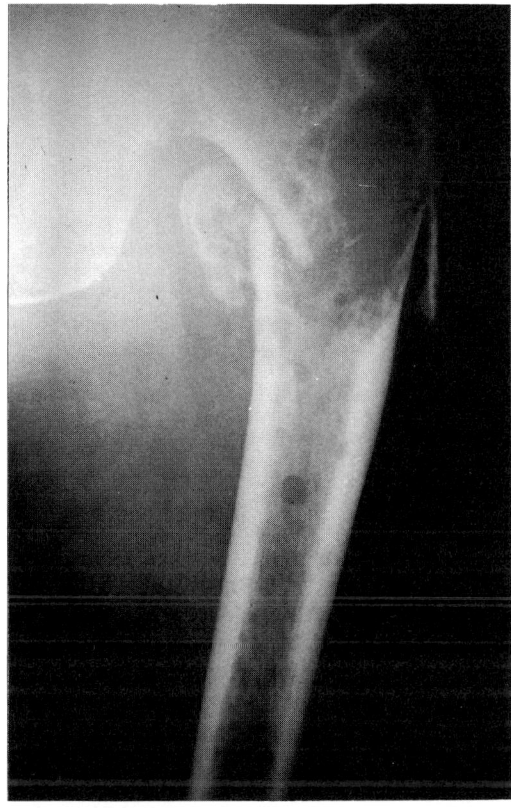

Figure 14.16 Male aged 60 years with multiple myeloma. There are small and large lesions in the femur. The former are round, clear-cut with no sclerotic margin. The large lesion in the metaphysis which extends into the greater trochanter, has expanded the bone, and has led to extensive cortical erosion and pathological fracture. The fracture occurred a fortnight or more before this radiograph as evidenced by the callus on the medial aspect of the femur.

(ii) Histopathology

Histologically, multiple myeloma is formed from pure sheets of plasma cells (Figure 14.17b). Immature variants show nuclear pleomorphism but still have eccentrically positioned nuclei. Myelomatous bone shows increased areas of bone resorption when compared with normal controls, the number of osteoclasts is significantly increased in zones invaded by myeloma cells, and osteoblastic activity is reduced (Charhon *et al.*, 1984). Rare 'clear cell' myelomas occur where the tumour cells contain cytoplasmic vacuoles (Chen *et al.*, 1985). Some cases show extensive amyloid deposits (Figure 14.17c), sometimes with a surrounding foreign body-type giant cell reaction. Sometimes solid amyloid deposits are found in bones ('amyloid tumours' or 'amyloidomas') – these are really multiple myeloma (Lai *et al.*, 1984; Le Loet *et al.*, 1986; Kruse and Sander, 1987).

The histological differential diagnosis of plasma cell infiltrates in bone is (1) ordinary multiple myeloma, (2) solitary myeloma or 'plasmacytoma' of bone, (3) 'plasma cell granuloma' of bone – chronic osteomyelitis with many plasma cells. Plasmacytosis may also be seen in benign monoclonal gammopathies and accompanying HIV changes in the bone marrow. Normal bone marrow contains plasma cells that can constitute up to 10% of the cells present. More than 10% of all cells present being plasma cells is pathological. Bone marrow examination is useful in the differential diagnosis of the plasma cell dyscrasias but has limitations because of the overlapping clinical and morphological features of these disorders and because of problems due to random marrow sampling (Buss *et al.*, 1988). The final diagnosis usually requires a synthesis of clinical, radiological and laboratory findings.

14.3.7 SOLITARY PLASMACYTOMA OF BONE

Solitary plasmacytomas of bone can occur in almost any bone, even in the foot (Sprinkle *et al.*, 1988). Ribs and spine are common sites

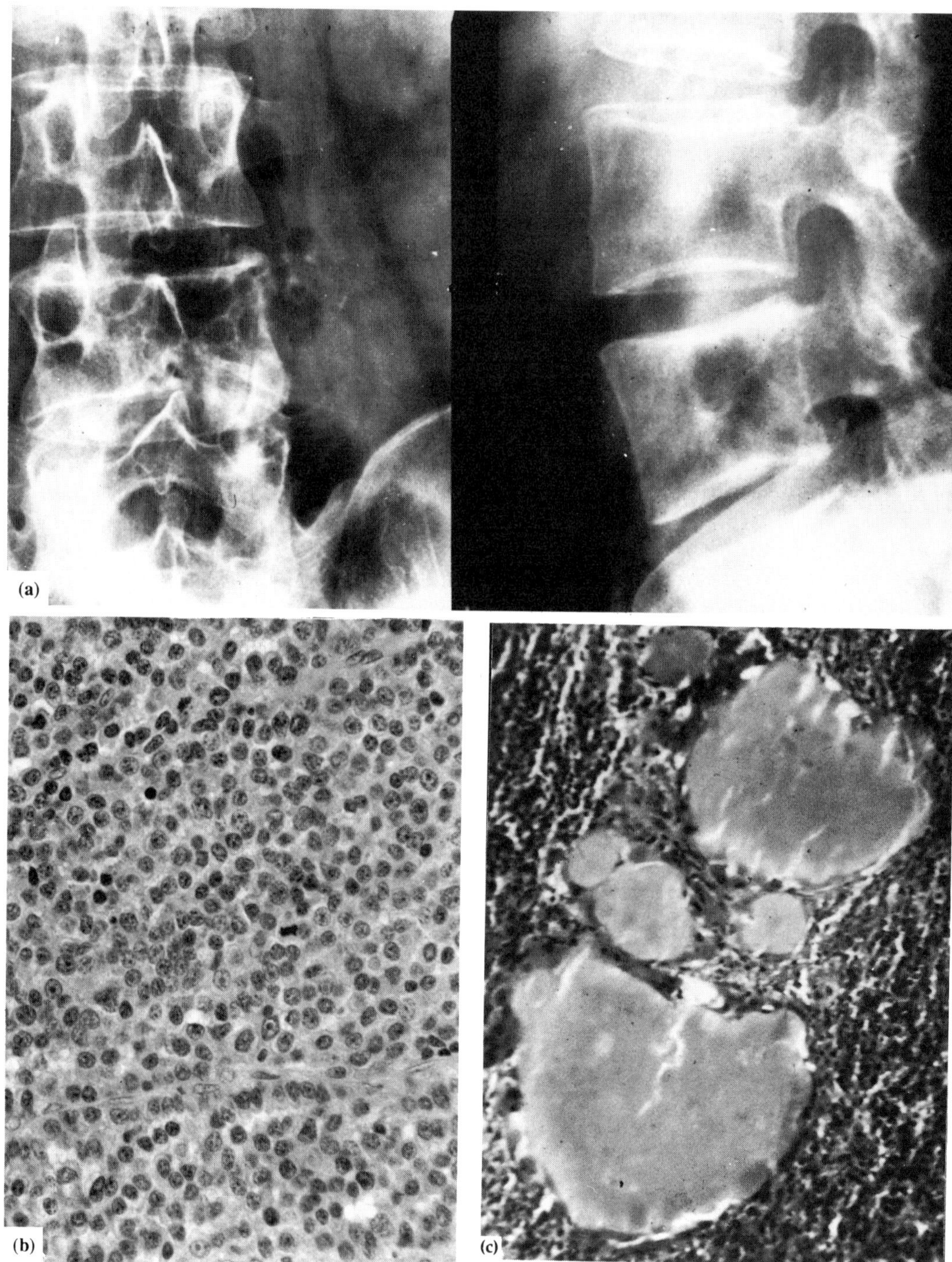

Figure 14.17 (a) Male aged 59 years. Investigation of low back pain revealed an osteolytic lesion in L4 vertebra. The lesion is well-demarcated with minimal bony reaction, characteristic of myeloma. (b) Medium power photomicrograph of myeloma. (c) Amorphous deposits of amyloid within the tumour.

(Wollersheim *et al.*, 1984). There are no known preceding factors; there is one case report of a solitary plasmacytoma of bone occurring in a patient with Hodgkin's disease (Gherlinzoni *et al.*, 1986). Solitary plasmacytomas of bone are best treated primarily by radiotherapy (Greenberg *et al.*, 1987). Radical surgical resections appear to be unwarranted. Solitary plasmacytomas of bone have a 5-year survival greater than 50%. Death resulting from progression of solitary plasmacytoma of bone to multiple myeloma occurs in between 36% and 50% of patients; prognosis and progression-free survival is much better for non-osseous extramedullary plasmacytomas (Kayrouz *et al.*, 1983; Knowling *et al.*, 1983). The histological parameters of nuclear immaturity and prominent nucleoli seem to be the best indicators of which patients will develop multiple myeloma (Meis *et al.*, 1987).

REFERENCES

Buss, D.H., Prichard, R.W. and Cooper, M.R. (1988) Plasma cell dyscrasias. *Hematol. Oncol. Clin. North Am.*, **2**, 603–15.

Cavo, M., Galieni, P., Gobbi, M. *et al.* (1985) Nonsecretory multiple myeloma. Presenting findings, clinical course and prognosis. *Acta Haematol.*, **74**, 27–30.

Charhon, S.A., Valentin-Opran, A., Edouard, C. *et al.* (1984) Myelomatous bone. Histomorphometric study and therapeutic effects. *Rev. Rhumat. Mul. Osteouartic.*, **51**, 657–62.

Chen, K.T., Ma, C.K., Nelson, J.W. *et al.* (1985) Clear cell myeloma. *Am. J. Surg. Pathol.*, **9**, 149–54.

Dahlin, D.C. and Unni, K.K. (1986) Myeloma. In *Bone Tumors: General Aspects and Data on 8542 Cases*, 4th edn, Charles C Thomas, Springfield, IL, pp. 193–207.

Gherlinzoni, F., Cavo, M., Pileri, S. *et al.* (1986) Solitary plasmacytoma of bone in a case of Hodgkin's disease. *Acta Haematol.*, **76**, 178–80.

Greenberg, P., Parker, R.G., Fu, Y.S. *et al.* (1987) The treatment of solitary plasmacytoma of bone and extramedullary plasmacytoma. *Am. J. Clin. Oncol.*, **10**, 199–204.

Hokamp, H.G. and Grundmann, E. (1983) Histological grading and staging of plasmacytomas. *J. Cancer Res. Clin. Oncol.*, **105**, 197–8.

Kayrouz, T., Jose, B., Chu, A.M. *et al.* (1983) Solitary plasmacytoma. *J. Surg. Oncol.*, **24**, 46–8.

Knowling, M.A., Harwood, A.R. and Bergsagel, D.E. (1983) Comparison of extramedullary plasmacytomas with solitary and multiple plasma cell tumors of bone. *J. Clin. Oncol.*, **1**, 255–62.

Kruse, C. and Sander, P. (1987) Amyloid tumor of bone. *Zentralbl. Allg. Pathol.*, **133**, 3–6.

Lai, K.N., Chan, K.W., Siu, D.L. *et al.* (1984) Pathologic hip fractures secondary to amyloidoma. Case report and review of the literature. *Am. J. Med.*, **77**, 937–43.

Le Leot, X., Ducastelle, T., Cambon, C. *et al.* (1986) Amyloid pseudotumor disclosing non-secretory myeloma. Ultrastructural demonstration of the role of histiocytes in intratumoral amyloidogenesis. *Ann. Med. Int.*, **137**, 123–8.

Meis, J.M., Butler, J.J., Osborne, B.M. *et al.* (1987) Solitary plasmacytomas of bone and extramedullary plasmacytomas. A clinicopathologic and immunohistochemical study. *Cancer*, **59**, 1475–85.

Schajowicz, F. (1981) Marrow tumors. In *Tumors and Tumorlike Lesions of Bone and Joints*. Springer-Verlag, New York, pp. 281–98.

Sprinkle, R.L., Santangelo, L. and De Ugarte, R. (1988) Solitary plasmacytoma of bone in the calcaneus. *J. Am. Podiatr. Med. Assoc.*, **78**, 636–42.

Wollersheim, H.C., Holdrinet, R.S. and Haanen, C. (1984) Clinical course and survival in 16 patients with localized plasmacytoma. *Scand. J. Haematol.*, **32**, 423–8.

14.3.8 LEUKAEMIA INCLUDING GRANULOCYTIC SARCOMA

(a) Clinical features

Solitary skeletal lesions can be the initial manifestations of a number of systemic haematological diseases (Kittel *et al.*, 1984; Akber *et al.*, 1988). Osteolytic bone lesions are a well-recognized occurrence in hairy cell leukaemia (Arkel *et al.*, 1984; Bastien *et al.*, 1984; Huaux *et al.*, 1984) and can be associated with widespread or localized demineralization with a predilection for the femoral head and neck (Herold *et al.*, 1988).

Osteolytic bone lesions can, rarely, be the presenting feature of chronic lymphocytic leukaemia (Hekselman *et al.*, 1988). Most granulocytic sarcomas are localized to bone (Cassi *et al.*, 1984), usually associated with subperiosteal bony structures. The most common sites are the skull, paranasal sinuses, sternum, ribs, vertebrae and pelvis. Granulocytic sarcoma may pursue an indolent clinical course or be associated with highly destructive skeletal disease (Welch *et al.*, 1986). Occasionally long-term survivors of acute lymphoblastic leukaemia re-present with isolated bone relapse (Wong *et al.*, 1983).

Bone lesions of leukaemia usually present with localized and persistent pain.

(i) Radiology

Radiography may show osteolytic bone lesions (Figure 14.18a). Magnetic resonance imaging can be helpful in evaluating the extent of marrow infiltration and will also demonstrate foci of involvement in bones that appear normal on plain films (Herold *et al.*, 1988).

(b) Pathology

(i) Histopathology

Histologically, leukaemias and granulocytic sarcomas are composed of a relatively uniform population of immature cells (Figure 14.18b). Eosinophil or myeloid precursors may be present in granulocytic sarcoma and suggest the diagnosis. The chloroacetate stain can be very helpful in establishing the diagnosis. Other enzyme cytochemical stains (not applicable to paraffin sections) show the tumour cells are positive for myeloperoxidase and negative for non-specific esterase (Welch *et al.*, 1986). Immunocytochemical studies of granulocytic sarcoma show the tumour cells are positive for CD11b, CD15 and lysozyme and are negative for B and T

lymphocyte markers and for HLA-Dr (Welch *et al.*, 1986). Electron microscopy of granulocytic sarcoma may show cells with the ultrastructural features of promyelocytes (Welch *et al.*, 1986). Cytogenetic analysis shows the cells are clonal (Welch *et al.*, 1986).

REFERENCES

Akber, J., Gallagher, M.T., Mathew, L. *et al.* (1988) Destructive skeletal lesions as the primary initial manifestation of acute childhood leukemia. *Am. J. Pediatr. Hematol. Oncol.*, **10**, 258–60.

Arkel, Y.S., Lake–Lewin, D., Savopoulos, A.A. *et al.* (1984) Bone lesions in hairy cell leukemia. A case report and response of bone pain to steroids. *Cancer*, **53**, 2401–3.

Bastien, P., Huaux, J.P., Noel, H. *et al.* (1984) Tricholeukocyte leukemia complicated by osteolytic lesions. *Rev. Rhumat. Mal. Osteoartic.*, **51**, 287–8.

Cassi, E., Tosi, A., De'Paoli, A. *et al.* (1984) Granulocytic sarcoma without evidence of acute leukemia. 2 cases with unusual localization (uterus and breast) and 1 case with bone localization. *Haematol. Pavia*, **69**, 464–96.

Hekselman, I., Kitai, E. and Hallel, T. (1988) Chronic lymphocytic leukemia presenting with osteolytic ankle lesions. *Harefuah*, **115**, 369–70.

Herold, C.J., Wittich, G.R., Schwarzinger, I. *et al.* (1988) Skeletal involvement in hairy cell leukaemia. *Skeletal Radiol.*, **17**, 171–5.

Huaux, J.P., Noel, H., Bastien, P. (1984) Bony lesions in hairy cell leukemia. Various therapeutic considerations apropos of a case report. *Acta Clin. Belg.*, **39**, 339–51.

Kittel, G., Roessner, A., Vollmer, E. *et al.* (1984) Solitary skeletal lesions as the initial manifestation of systemic hematologic diseases. A contribution to the differential pathologic diagnosis of malignant bone tumors. *Pathologe*, **5**, 143–7.

Welch, P., Grossi, C., Carroll, A. *et al.* (1986) Granulocytic sarcoma with an indolent course and destructive skeletal disease. Tumor characterization with immunologic markers, electron microscopy, cytochemistry, and cytogenetic studies. *Cancer*, **57**, 1005–10.

Wong, K.Y., Benton, C., Gelfand, M.J. *et al.* (1983) Isolated bone relapse in long-term survivors of acute lymphoblastic leukaemia. *J. Pediatr.*, **102**, 92–4.

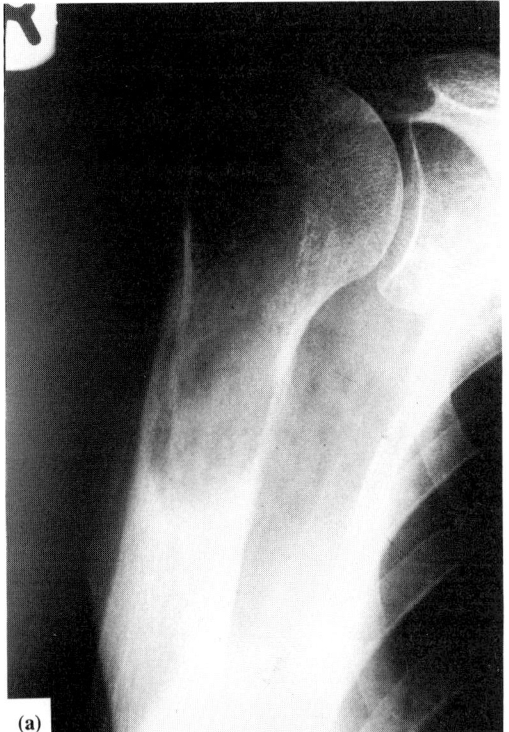

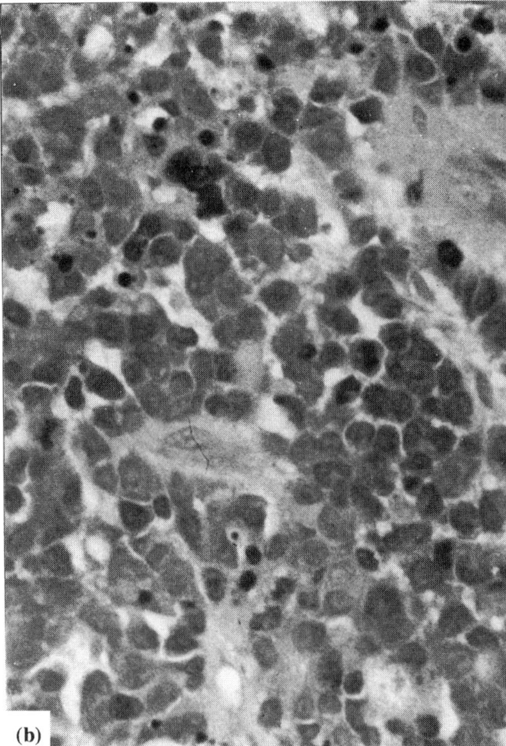

Figure 14.18 Female aged 60 years. Long history of chronic granulocytic leukaemia. Presented with pain in the upper arm and radiograph (a) showed permeative destruction affecting the proximal end of the humerus with total lysis of a large part of the lateral metaphyseal–epiphyseal region and periosteal reaction more distally. (b) Needle biopsy showed cells with the cytology of myeloblasts with fine nuclear chromatin and 2–4 nucleoli. The appearance was that of a granulocytic sarcoma or chloroma; such masses may represent the initial manifestation of blast crisis of chronic granulocytic leukaemia. Radiograph courtesy of Dr G.J. Mufti.

14.3.9 MASTOCYTOSIS

(a) Clinical features

Mastocytosis characteristically affects the skin but the skeleton is the second most involved site in adults (Lennert and Parwaresch, 1979; Brunning *et al.*, 1983). Both localized and generalized osteoclastic and osteoblastic lesions may be present (systemic mastocytosis) and can cause bone pain. The course of systemic mastocytosis is progressive and the ultimate prognosis is poor.

(b) Pathology

Histologically, the bone marrow space is infiltrated by clumps of round-to-oval mast cells with clear or granular cytoplasm and rounded nuclei (Figure 14.19). Eosinophils may encircle and be admixed with the mast cell collections. Metachromatic stains such as Giemsa, toluidine blue or polychrome methylene blue are best for demonstrating the mast cell granules. Monoclonal antibodies specific for mast cells have also been described (Rimmer *et al.*, 1984).

REFERENCES

Brunning, R.D., McKenna, R.W., Rosai, J. *et al.* (1983) Systemic mastocytosis. Extracutaneous manifestations. *Am. J. Surg. Pathol.*, **7**, 425–38.
Lennert, K. and Parwaresch, M.R. (1979) Mast cells and mast cell neoplasia. A review. *Histopathology*, **3**, 349–65.
Rimmer, E.F., Turberville, C. and Horton M. (1984) Human mast cells detected by monclonal antibodies. *J. Clin. Pathol.*, **37**, 1249–55.

14.4 SPINDLE-CELLED TUMOURS

14.4.1 BENIGN FIBROUS HISTIOCYTOMA

(a) Clinical features

Benign fibrous histiocytoma is a very rare lesion, e.g. there were only 10 examples in the series of 8542 bone tumours reported by Dahlin and Unni (1986). All patients were adults, with ages ranging from 17 to 60 years. Benign fibrous histiocytoma should be distinguished from non-ossifying fibroma because it occurs in a different age range, involves different sites and has different radiological features.

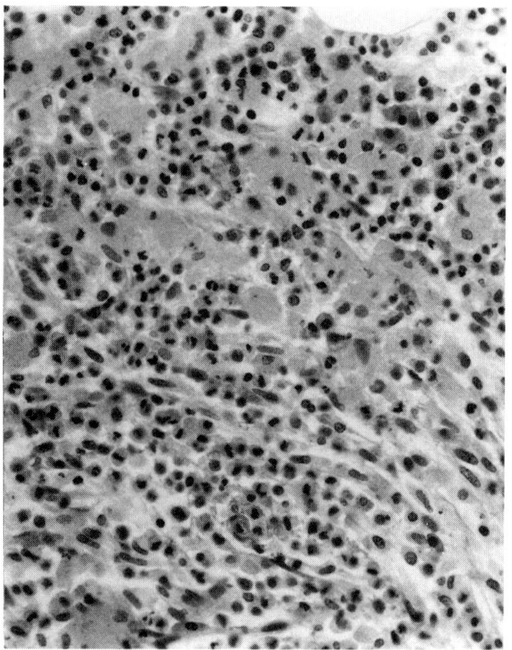

Figure 14.19 Female aged 45 years. Systemic mastocytosis. Section shows a mixture of mast cells and eosinophils. The mast cells have abundant cytoplasm and round-to-oval nuclei. In addition to the small, bilobed eosinophils, there is a scattering of plasma cells.

(i) Skeletal distribution

Benign fibrous histiocytomas are commonest in the long tubular bones and the pelvis (Dahlin and Unni, 1986). Other sites are spine and the short tubular bones of the hand. Rare cases occur in unusual sites such as rib (Friedman *et al.*, 1989).

Benign fibrous histiocytomas present with a high frequency of pain and sometimes with pathological fractures. Radiologically, benign fibrous histiocytomas of bone are lytic lesions.

(b) Pathology

Histologically, benign fibrous histiocytomas of bone are composed of a mixture of cells with either fibroblastic or histiocytic features

and have a similar appearance to the much commoner benign fibrous histiocytomas found in soft tissues. They are identical histologically to non-ossifying fibromas of childhood. Occasional cases appear myxoid histologically (Marcove *et al.*, 1989). The histological picture of benign fibrous histiocytoma can be seen in foci in other lesions of bone (giant cell tumour, aneurysmal bone cyst, fibrous dysplasia) where these areas are secondary reactive tissue (Bertoni *et al.*, 1986).

REFERENCES

Bertoni, F., Calderoni, P., Bacchini, P. *et al.* (1986) Benign fibrous histiocytoma of bone. *J. Bone Joint Surg.*, **68A**, 1225–30.
Dahlin, D.C. and Unni, K.K. (1986) Benign and

atypical fibrous histiocytoma. In *Bone Tumors: General Aspects and Data on 8542 Cases*, 4th edn. Charles C Thomas, Springfield, IL, pp. 141–8.

Friedman, L., Patel, M., Lew, E. *et al.* (1989) Benign histiocytic fibroma of rib with CT correlation. *Can. Assoc. Radiol. J.*, **40**, 114–16.

Marcove, R.C., Lindeque, B.G. and Huvos, A.G. (1989) Fibromyxoma of bone. *Surg. Gynecol. Obstet.*, **169**, 115–18.

14.4.2 NON-OSSIFYING FIBROMA

Synonyms:
    Metaphyseal fibrous cortical defect
    Fibroxanthoma

(a) Clinical features

Non-ossifying fibromas are common lesions. Most are situated at characteristic sites on the circumference of the metaphysis of long tubular bones.

(i) *Skeletal distribution* (from Schajowicz, 1981 and Dahlin and Unni, 1986)

- Jaws   0.5%
- Skull   1%
- Other flat bones
    Ribs   1%
    Girdles
        Shoulder: clavicle, scapula,
        sternum   <0.5%
        Pelvis: ilium, pubis, sacrum   1.5%
- Spine: cervical, thoracic, lumbar
- Long tubular
    Femur, tibia, humerus   90%
    Fibula, radius, ulna   4%
- Hands and feet
    Short tubular
        Metacarpals, metatarsals,
        phalanges   1%
    Cuboidal
        Carpals, tarsals   <0.5%

Multiple non-ossifying fibromas of bone sometimes occur (The Jaffe–Campanacci syndrome) (Peuchmaur *et al.*, 1985; Moser *et al.*, 1987; Blau *et al.*, 1988). They may be more common than previously suspected as at least 8% of the 900 patients with non-ossifying fibromas re-evaluated by Moser *et al.* (1987) had multiple skeletal non-ossifying fibromas. Some cases of the Jaffe–Campanacci syndrome occur in association with von Recklinghausen neurofibromatosis (Erlemann *et al.*, 1987; Steinmetz *et al.*, 1988); 5% of patients with multiple skeletal non-ossifying fibromas had coexistent neurofibromatosis in the series of Moser *et al.* (1987).

(ii) *Radiology*

Radiologically, non-ossifying fibromas show a characteristic course over time rather than a typical single appearance (Figure 14.20). The radiological findings therefore allow conclusions to be made about the age of a non-ossifying fibroma (Ritschl *et al.*, 1988). Moser *et al.* (1987) noted four radiographic patterns in their study of multiple non-ossifying fibromas:

1. Clustered lesions – usually about the knee.
2. Non-clustered lesions – in opposite ends of long bones.
3. Coalescent lesions – several lesions coalescing over time.
4. Emergent lesions – lesions appearing in previously unaffected bone.

(b) Pathology

(i) *Histopathology*

Histologically, non-ossifying fibromas are characterized by a proliferation of spindle cells (Figure 14.21), disposed either randomly or in a storiform pattern, and with numerous scattered multinucleated giant cells. Haemosiderin pigment may be present. The multiple lesions are histologically indistinguishable from their solitary counterparts (Moser *et al.*, 1987). Electron microscopy

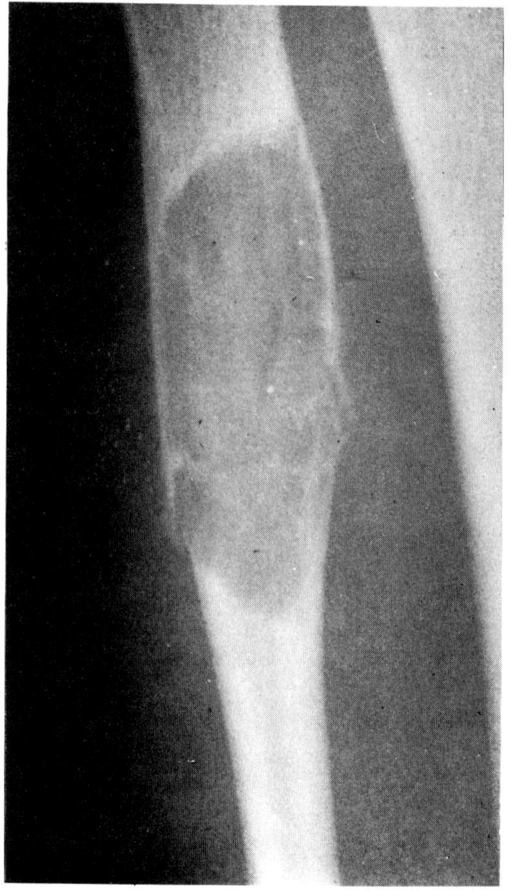

Figure 14.20 Female aged 12 years. Non-ossifying fibroma. A pathological fracture through a central osteolytic lesion of the fibular diaphysis. Endosteal erosion has exceeded periosteal apposition resulting in slight expansion of the bone but thinning of the cortex. The lesion is demarcated from the cancellous space by a thin sclerotic border.

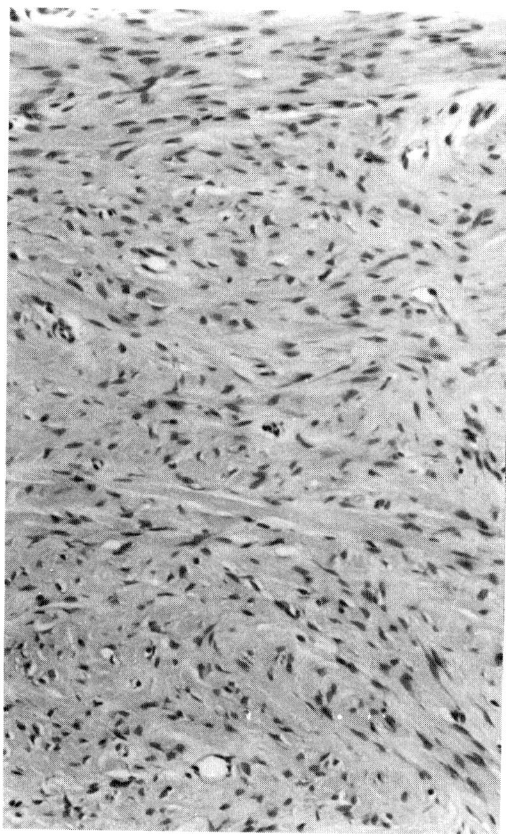

Figure 14.21 Non-ossifying fibroma. Irregularly arranged fascicles of spindle cells. The cells appear cytologically benign. These tumours may also contain histiocytes and these contain lipid or haemosiderin.

shows the spindle cells have features of both fibroblasts and myofibroblasts (Peuchmaur *et al.*, 1985).

(ii) Histogenesis

The pathogenesis of metaphyseal fibrous defect is thought to be related to the insertion of a tendon or ligament into the peri-

chondrium of the epiphyseal growth plate (Ritschl *et al.*, 1988, 1990).

REFERENCES

Blau, R.A., Zwick, D.L. and Westphal, R.A. (1988) Multiple non-ossifying fibromas. A case report. *J. Bone Joint Surg.*, **70A**, 299–304.

Dahlin, D.C. and Unni, K.K. (1986) Metaphyseal fibrous defect (fibroma, nonosteogenic fibroma), myxoma, cortical 'desmoid', fibromatosis and 'xanthoma'. In *Bone Tumors: General Aspects and Data on 8542 Cases*, 4th edn. Charles C Thomas, Springfield, IL, pp. 149–66.

Erlemann, R., Fischedick, A.R., Edel, G. *et al.*

(1987) Neurofibromatosis and multiple nonossifying bone fibromas. *ROFO* **147**, 20–4.

Moser, R.P. Jr, Sweet, D.E., Haseman, D.B. *et al.* (1987) Multiple skeletal fibroxanthomas: radiologic–pathologic correlation of 72 cases. *Skeletal Radiol.*, **16**, 353–9.

Peuchmaur, M., Forest, M., Tomeno, B. *et al.* (1985) Multifocal nonosteogenic fibroma: report of a case with ultrastructural findings. *Hum. Pathol.*, **16**, 751–3.

Ritschl, P., Karnel, F. and Hajek, P. (1988) Fibrous metaphyseal defects – determination of their origin and natural history using a radiomorphological study. *Skeletal Radiol.*, **17**, 8–15.

Ritschl, P., Lintner, F., Pechmann, U. *et al.* (1990) Fibrous metaphyseal defect. *Int. Orthop.*, **14**, 205–11.

Schajowicz, F. (1981) Tumorlike lesions. In *Tumors and Tumor-like Lesions of Bone and Joints.* Springer-Verlag, New York, pp. 449–63.

Steinmetz, J.C., Pilon, V.A. and Lee, J.K. (1988) Jaffe–Campanacci syndrome. *J. Pediatr. Orthop.*, **8**, 602–4.

14.4.3 DESMOPLASTIC FIBROMA AND CHILDHOOD FIBROMATOSES

(a) Clinical features

Desmoplastic fibroma is a rare tumour; only 127 cases are reported in the literature. It usually grows in a locally aggressive manner. The majority of these tumours (about 75%) occur in young adults less than 30 years old.

(i) *Skeletal distribution*

Usually in the metaphysis or metadiaphyseal region of a long bone. Other sites such as the scapula and os calcis can be involved (Bertoni *et al.*, 1984). Rare cases occur in rib (Butters *et al.*, 1985).

Desmoplastic fibroma can present with dull pain. Very rarely, desmoplastic fibroma arises in fibrous dysplasia (West *et al.*, 1983; Bridge *et al.*, 1989). Treatment is en bloc resection as curettage leads to recurrence. The case report of Graudal (1984) lists 78 references dealing with desmoplastic fibroma. Radiography characteristically shows desmoplastic fibroma as a centrally located and well-demarcated osteolytic lesion. A trabeculated 'soap-bubble' appearance is common (Bertoni *et al.*, 1984).

(b) Pathology

(i) *Histopathology*

Histologically, desmoplastic fibroma is identical with both fibromatosis and desmoid tumour of the soft tissues. It contains areas with abundant collagen fibres and densely packed areas composed of fibroblasts and myofibroblasts (Meerbach, 1987). The collagen fibres may have an amyanthoid appearance. Myofilaments have been detected by electron microscopy in the myofibroblasts.

Desmoplastic fibroma is not synonymous with fibromatosis. No case of fibromatosis arising *de novo* in adult bone has ever been reported.

Cytogenetic analysis of a case of desmoplastic fibroma has shown non-random karyotypic abnormalities, namely a primary abnormal clone trisomic for both chromosomes 3 and 5 and two subclones, one trisomic for chromosome 3 and one trisomic for chromosome 5 (Bridge *et al.*, 1989).

14.4.4 INFANTILE MYOFIBROMATOSIS

Synonym: Congenital fibromatosis

Infantile myofibromatosis is a very rare disease which may be solitary or multiple and can involve skin, soft tissues and internal organs (Stout, 1954; Enzinger and Weiss, 1988). Some cases show multiple bone involvement (Chan *et al.*, 1989) or involve bone secondarily (Ortega-Martos *et al.*, 1986). The lesion(s) are usually noted at birth or within the first few months of life. The multiple bone lesions can be very numerous, e.g. the case of Heiple *et al.* (1972) had more than 100 skeletal lesions. Those cases where only the bones are involved (Lluch *et al.*, 1985) usually heal spontaneously with time. If soft tissues, liver or other organs are also involved then there is a very poor prognosis.

Radiological examination shows the bone lesions of infantile myofibromatosis are circumscribed and osteolytic. There is marginal sclerosis and usually no penetration of the cortex (Enzinger and Weiss, 1988). Histologically, infantile myofibromatosis appears as bland, spindle-celled fibrous tissue; both fibroblasts and smooth muscle-like cells may be present. The bone nodules are usually poorly delineated compared with those found in skin and subcutis.

14.4.5 JUVENILE HYALINE FIBROMATOSIS

Juvenile hyaline fibromatosis (fibromatosis hyalinica multiplex) is an extremely rare, autosomal recessive disease that usually appears two or more years after birth. The lesions are commonest in skin, subcutis and gums (Murray, 1873; Enzinger and Weiss, 1988). Bone involvement can occur producing punched-out osteolytic lesions (Remberger *et al.*, 1985). Light microscopy reveals cords of fibroblasts associated with deposits of hyaline ground substance, shown immunohistochemically to be collagen types I and III (Remberger *et al.*, 1985).

REFERENCES

Bertoni, F., Calderoni, P., Bacchini, P. *et al.* (1984) Desmoplastic fibroma of bone. A report of six cases. *J. Bone Joint Surg.*, **66B**, 265–8.

Bridge, J.A., Rosenthal, H., Sanger, W.G. *et al.* (1989) Desmoplastic fibroma arising in fibrous dysplasia. Chromosomal analysis and review of the literature. *Clin. Orthop.*, **247**, 272–

Butters, M., Hamann, H. and Mohr, W. (1985) Desmoplastic fibroma of the rib. *Thorac. Cardiovasc. Surg.*, **33**, 317–8.

Chan, Y.F., Lau, J.H. and Tong, C.Y. (1989) Congenital generalized fibromatosis with predominant osseous involvement in a Chinese newborn. *J. Pediatr. Orthop.*, **9**, 64–8.

Enzinger, F.M. and Weiss, S.W. (1988) Fibrous proliferations of infancy and childhood. In *Soft Tissue Tumors*, 2nd edn. C.V. Mosby, St Louis, pp. 171–81.

Graudal, N. (1984) Desmoplastic fibroma of bone. Case report and literature review. *Acta Orthop. Scand.*, **55**, 215–9.

Heiple, K.G., Perrin, E. and Aikawa, M. (1972) Congenital generalized fibromatosis. A case limited to osseous lesions. *J. Bone Joint Surg.*, **54A**, 663–9.

Lluch, M.D., Gonzalez-Hachero, J., Campora, R. *et al.* (1985) Congenital fibromatosis of exclusively bone localization. *An. Esp. Pediatr.*, **23**, 609–11.

Meerbach, W. (1987) Desmoplastic fibroma as a rare bone tumor. *Zentralbl. Allg. Pathol.*, **133**, 243–8.

Murray, J. (1873) On three peculiar cases of molluscum fibrosum in children. *Med. Chir. Trans.*, **38**, 235.

Ortega-Martos, L., Fernandez-Ortiz, B., Martinez de Victoria, J.M. *et al.* (1986) Congenital generalized fibromatosis. Presentation of a case and review of the literature. *An. Esp. Pediatr.*, **25**, 96–100.

Remberger, K., Krieg, T., Kunze, D. *et al.* (1985) Fibromatosis hyalinica multiplex (juvenile hyalin fibromatosis). Light microscopic, electron microscopic, immunohistochemical, and biochemical findings. *Cancer*, **56**, 614–24.

Stout, A.P. (1954) Juvenile fibromatoses. *Cancer*, **7**, 953.

West, R., Huvos, A.G. and Lane, J.M. (1983) Desmoplastic fibroma of bone arising in fibrous dysplasia. *Am. J. Clin. Pathol.*, **79**, 630–3.

14.4.6 BENIGN NEURAL TUMOURS OF BONE

Synonyms:
  Neurilemmoma
  Schwannoma

(a) Clinical features

Primary benign neural tumours of bone are very rare and examples in the literature are limited (de la Monte *et al.*, 1984). There is a high frequency of mandibular involvement in the reported cases. Benign neural tumours of bone appear radiologically as osteolytic lesions. Soft tissue extension is common.

(b) Pathology

Reported cases of intraosseous schwannomas have shown similar histological features to schwannomas of the soft tissues (Enzinger and Weiss, 1988). Some cases have been fairly cellular and the Antoni type A and B patterns have been subtle (de la Monte *et al.*, 1984). Rare cases show the light microscopic and ultrastructural features characteristic of melanotic schwannoma (Myers *et al.*, 1990).

14.4.7 'NEUROFIBROMATOSIS OF BONE'

Neurofibromatosis is an hamartomatous malformation that most commonly involves skin and the nervous system. It is inherited as an autosomal dominant trait with varying (usually high) degrees of penetrance. The gene for NF1 is located on chromosome 17 (Barker *et al.*, 1987). Clinically, the disease can be subdivided into a peripheral form and a central form (Enzinger and Weiss, 1988).

Skeletal changes in neurofibromatosis occur in 40–50% of patients with peripheral neurofibromatosis (Hunt and Pugh, 1961) but are not seen in those with the central form of the disease. Many lesions are ero sive defects secondary to soft tissue tumours. Scoliosis, often severe and angular, is the commonest primary abnormality (Allibone *et al.*, 1960; Scott, 1965; Zorab and Edwards, 1972). Congenital bowing of the long bones with pseudarthrosis (especially of the tibia), localized gigantism, intrathoracic meningocoele, vertebral scalloping, unilateral orbital malformations and intraosseous cystic lesions are also seen (Hunt and Pugh, 1961).

It was suggested that the scoliosis was a destructive and/or regenerative phenomenon secondary to a 'neurofibroma' of a periosteal nerve (Brooks and Lehman, 1924)

but no histological biopsy or autopsy investigations of the scoliosis of neurofibromatosis has ever confirmed this and there is no histological abnormality of the vertebral bodies (Moe, quoted by Zorab and Edwards, 1972). Clinical examination of the nervous system to the trunk in patients with scoliosis is also entirely normal (Zorab and Edwards, 1972). Pseudarthroses are occasionally surgically excised but show only fibrosis and other reparative changes. The fibrous tissue can appear rather 'neural' histologically with wavy nuclei in the spindle cells but immunohistochemical staining for S-100 protein is negative. Biopsy of bones involved by localized gigantism shows only sclerotic 'reactive' bone. These findings all lend weight to the hypothesis that the neurofibromatosis gene is producing its skeletal effects by affecting bone modelling, remodelling and turnover rather than by the production of 'neurofibromatous' tissue in bone.

The intraosseous cystic lesions have the histological appearance of non-ossifying fibromas. They are composed of fascicles of fibroblasts arranged in short intersecting fascicles (sometimes in a storiform pattern) with scattered osteoclasts. A single case report exists of an intraosseous 'neurofibroma' in a patient with neurofibromatosis (Kaufman *et al.*, 1984). The tumour had been originally diagnosed as a desmoplastic fibroma. Given the well-recognized association between neurofibromatosis and non-ossifying fibroma (the Jaffe–Campanacci syndrome, see 14.4.2), a non-ossifying fibroma was probably the correct diagnosis. No convincing case reports of true neurofibromas of bone exist. 'Neurofibromatosis of bone' is, nonetheless, probably the best term to describe the bone changes seen in individuals with neurofibromastosis. Neurofibromatosis can, then, be thought of as a generalized mesenchymal hamartomatous syndrome, rather than a purely neurocutaneous syndrome.

REFERENCES

Allibone, E.C., Illingworth, R.S. and Wright, T. (1960) Neurofibromatosis (von Recklinghausen's disease) of the vertebral column. *Arch. Dis. Child.*, **35**, 153–8.

Barker, D., Wright, E., Nguyen, K. *et al.* (1987) Gene for von Recklinghausen neurofibromatosis is in the pericentromeric region of chromosome 17. *Science*, **236**, 1100–2.

Brooks, B. and Lehman, E.P. (1924) The bone changes in Recklinghausen's neurofibromatosis. *Surg. Gynecol. Obstet.*, **38**, 587.

de la Monte, S.M., Dorfman, H.D., Chandra, R. *et al.* (1984) Intraosseous schwannoma: histologic features, ultrastructure, and review of the literature. *Hum. Pathol.*, **15**, 551–8.

Enzinger, F.M. and Weiss, S.W. (1988) Benign tumors of peripheral nerves. In *Soft Tissue Tumors*, 2nd edn. C.V. Mosby, St Louis, pp. 725–35.

Hunt, J.C. and Pugh, D.G. (1961) Skeletal lesions in neurofibromatosis. *Radiology*, **76**, 1–20.

Kaufman, A., Sherman, F.C., Black, W. *et al.* (1984) Osseous destruction by neurofibroma diagnosed in infancy as 'desmoplastic fibroma'. *J. Pediatr. Orthop.*, **4**, 239–42.

Myers, J.L., Bernreuter, W. and Dunham, W. (1990) Melanotic schwannoma. Clinicopathologic, immunohistochemical, and ultrastructural features of a rare primary bone tumor. *Am. J. Clin. Pathol.*, **93**, 424–9.

Scott, J.C. (1965) Scoliosis and neurofibromatosis. *J. Bone Joint Surg.*, **47B**, 240–6.

Zorab, P. and Edwards, H. (1972) Spinal deformity in neurofibromatosis [letter]. *Lancet*, **ii**, 823.

14.4.8 HAEMANGIOPERICYTOMA

(a) Clinical features

Primary intraosseous haemangiopericytomas are very rare tumours. Most are described as single case reports (Vathana, 1984). Some of the neoplasms associated with tumour-induced osteomalacia or rickets have been haemangiopericytomas of bone (McClure and Smith, 1987; Nuovo *et al.*, 1989). A single case has been reported of an extrarenal juxtaglomerular cell tumour in the terminal phalanx of the thumb (Chen and

Chang, 1987) that was shown by electron microscopy to contain renin granules and trapezoid crystalloids. The light microscopic appearance had some features of haemangiopericytoma.

(b) Pathology

Primary haemangiopericytomas of bone have the same histological features as their counterparts described in the soft tissues (Enzinger and Weiss, 1988). They are composed of plump, short, spindle cells, typically surrounding staghorn-shaped vessels.

REFERENCES

Chen, W.-S. and Chang, J.-W. (1987) Extrarenal juxtaglomerular cell tumor in bone. Report of a case with review of the literature. *Chin. Med. J.*, **100**, 78–82.

Enzinger, F.M. and Weiss, S.W. (1988) Hemangiopericytoma. In *Soft Tissue Tumors*, 2nd edn. C.V. Mosby, St Louis, pp. 596–613.

McClure, J. and Smith, P.S. (1987) Oncogenic osteomalacia. *J. Clin. Pathol.*, **40**, 446–53.

Nuovo, M.A., Dorfman, H.D., Sun, C.C. *et al.* (1989) Tumor-induced osteomalacia and rickets. *Am. J. Surg. Pathol.*, **13**, 588–99.

Vathana, P. (1984) Primary hemangiopericytoma of bone in the hand: a case report. *J. Hand Surg.*, **9A**, 761–4.

14.4.9 MALIGNANT FIBROUS HISTIOCYTOMA INCLUDING FIBROSARCOMA

(a) Clinical features

Malignant fibrous histiocytoma is a rare bone tumour, about ten times less frequent than osteosarcoma (Huvos *et al.*, 1985). It represented only 0.8% of the 6514 primary bone tumours described from the Mayo Clinic (Dahlin and Unni, 1986) but others report an incidence of between 4 and 8%. The age range is large, between 7 and 80 years, but the tumour is most common in middle age with a mean of 40.5 years (Huvos *et al.*, 1985).

(i)   Skeletal distribution (from Schajowicz, 1981 and Dahlin and Unni, 1986)

* Jaws   5%
* Skull   5%
* Other flat bones
    Ribs   2%
    Girdles
        Shoulder: clavicle, scapula,
        sternum   3%
        Pelvis: ilium, pubis, sacrum   16%
* Spine: cervical, thoracic, lumbar   8%
* Long tubular
    Femur, tibia, humerus   55%
    Fibula, radius, ulna   5%
* Hands and feet
    Short tubular
        Metacarpals, metatarsals,
        phalanges   1%
    Cuboidal
        Carpals, tarsals   1%

The appendicular skeleton is the commonest site of involvement. About 60% of tumours involve the long bones, most frequently the metaphyseal area, but there is a wide skeletal distribution with the other cases at a variety of sites (Destouet *et al.*, 1980; Hankin *et al.*, 1987; Duck *et al.*, 1989; Grieco *et al.*, 1989).

Most malignant fibrous histiocytomas of bone (72%) arise without any obvious predisposing factors (Huvos *et al.*, 1985) but a moderate number are associated with previous radiotherapy (Vanel *et al.*, 1983; Huvos *et al.*, 1985, 1986), Paget's disease (Huvos *et al.*, 1985) or bone infarcts (Furey *et al.*, 1960; Heselson *et al.*, 1983; Frierson *et al.*, 1987), usually multiple infarcts (Mirra *et al.*, 1974). Most of the cases of malignant fibrous histiocytomas arising in bone infarcts have been in males although occasional examples occur in females (Abdelwahab *et al.*, 1988). It has been suggested that high levels of platelet-derived growth factor (PDGF) may be involved in tumour induction in these sarcomas appearing on bone infarcts. Where previous radiotherapy is a factor, it may have been given for a giant cell tumour or other benign bone lesion or for non-osseous disease. The mean radiation dose in these patients was 6000 rads, and the latent period between irradiation and the appearance of the bone sarcoma ranged from 4 to 47 years, mean 16.5 years (Huvos *et al.*, 1986). Very occasionally, malignant fibrous histiocytomas arise in patients with neurofibromatosis (and can be shown immunohistochemically to be negative with neural and Schwannian markers) (Ducatman *et al.*, 1983), in giant cell tumours (Meis *et al.*, 1989), enchondromata (Sanerkin and Woods, 1979), osteochondromatosis (Voutsinas, 1988), bone lipomas (Milgram, 1990), ameloblastic or desmoblastic fibromas, secondarily to chronic osteomyelitis (Kirshbaum, 1949) and after orthopaedic implants (Bago-Granell *et al.*, 1984; Troop *et al.*, 1990). A very rare autosomal dominant bone dysplasia, diaphyseal medullary stenosis, commonly terminates in malignant fibrous histiocytoma (Hardcastle *et al.*, 1986). Occasional multicentric, or multiple and familial, cases of malignant fibrous histiocytoma of bone are reported (Castillo *et al.*, 1987; Finci *et al.*, 1990).

The 5-year survival overall is about 35% (Capanna *et al.*, 1984) for high-grade tumours and 80% for low-grade tumours (Bertoni *et al.*, 1984), but reported survival times vary widely from a mean of 19 months (Spanier *et al.*, 1975), through 53% 5-year survival (Huvos *et al.*, 1985) to 67% 5-year survival (Huvos, 1976). Features which determine prognosis are the age of the patient (older patients do worse), whether the tumour is primary *de novo* or a secondary sarcoma (secondary tumours do worse) (Huvos *et al.*, 1985), the maximal tumour size and the duration of disease. Metastases from malignant fibrous histiocytoma of bone nearly always go to the lungs. The optimal treatment for malignant fibrous histiocytomas of bone is cytotoxic chemotherapy (Urban *et al.*, 1983; Weiner *et al.*, 1983) followed by surgical excision and, for long bone tumours, prosthetic replacement. Malignant fibrous histiocytoma responds at least as frequently as osteosarcoma to chemotherapy.

'Dedifferentiated' low-grade chondrosarcomas often have the appearance of high-grade malignant fibrous histiocytomas (Dahlin and Beabout, 1971) as do 'dedifferentiated' areas within some liposarcomas, chordomas (Halpern *et al.*, 1984), and well differentiated intraosseous and parosteal osteosarcomas. The presence of these high-grade malignant components generally portends a more ominous prognosis.

(ii)   Radiology

Radiologically, malignant fibrous histiocytomas are usually clearly malignant tumours (Feldman and Norman, 1972), often with a moth-eaten pattern of bone destruction and a wide zone of transition. Low-grade tumours have generally well-defined margins and a 'soap-bubble' appearance. High-grade tumours appear permeative and more aggressive (Bertoni *et al.*, 1984). 'Benign' bone is present within the tumour in a small number of cases, and may be related to fracture. Taconis and Mulder (1984) studied 102 cases of spindle-celled sarcoma of bone, initially all classified as fibrosarcoma, about 50% of which were subsequently reclassified as malignant fibrous histiocytomas on review. However, both tumour groups had the same clinical picture, radiological appearance and survival. Radiographic signs which suggest a longer survival are eccentric location, geographic bone destruction (rather than moth-eaten or permeative) and cortical destruction involving less than half the bone circumference (Taconis and Mulder, 1984). Some malignant fibrous histiocytomas contain fluid–fluid levels indicative of prior haemorrhage (Tsai *et al.*, 1990) and some are cold on technetium bone scans (Sanders *et al.*, 1990).

(b)   Pathology

(i)   Morbid anatomy

Macroscopically, malignant fibrous histiocytomas often look yellowish because of the fat content.

(ii)   Histopathology

Histologically, the majority of osseous malignant fibrous histiocytomas have the appearance of the pleomorphic–storiform type of malignant fibrous histiocytoma of soft tissues (Enzinger and Weiss, 1988) (Figure 14.22a), but their degree of differentiation ranges from anaplastic to extremely well differentiated. Pleomorphic refers to the presence of bizarre polynuclear tumour giant cells although the nuclei of the spindle cells also display anaplasia (Figure 14.22b). Storiform is derived from 'storia' = 'matting' and describes the arrangement of the interlacing bundles of collagen fibres – rather like a cartwheel pattern. Mitotic figures are numerous and include atypical forms. Distinctive morphological changes occur in bone during invasion by malignant fibrous histiocytoma, dependent upon the extent of tumour invasion (Gruber *et al.*, 1987). Changes affect bone formation but not resorption, and osteoblast number and activity are significantly altered. The changes are local in nature and probably reflect osteoblast response to local tumour factor(s). Foci of rounded cells with foamy or vacuolated cytoplasm (histiocyte-like) are present within malignant fibrous histiocytomas and led, in part, to the rather unsatisfactory name by which these tumours are now known. True macrophage cells are present in these tumours as a reactive transit population, as in most other neoplasms (Wood and Gollahon, 1977). Double-labelling immunohistochemical techniques using antibodies against mature tissue macrophages and Ki-67 or proliferation-associated nuclear antigen have shown that it is only the fibroblast-like cells, which do not react with the macrophage-specific antibodies, that express Ki-67 or proliferation-associated nuclear antigen (Roessner *et al.*, 1987, 1989). Some cases of malignant fibrous histiocytoma of bone appear myxoid (Frassica *et al.*, 1988), histologically rather like the myxoid type of malignant fibrous histiocytoma described in the soft tissues (Enzinger and Weiss, 1988), about 8% are giant cell-rich variants (Huvos *et al.*, 1985), and some can be positively 'small cell' in appearance. Survival is not dependent on the histological subtype of the tumour, but is strongly influenced by the histological grade of malignancy (Huvos *et al.*, 1985). Some low-grade malignant fibrous histiocytomas 'dedifferentiate' into high-grade malignant fibrous histiocytomas with the passage of time. Osteoid is present in some tumours which can lead to a rather sterile argument as to whether they should be considered as malignant fibrous histiocytomas or as osteosarcomas. The metastases from malignant fibrous histiocytomas can certainly appear histologically as pure osteosarcomas.

(iii) Immunohistochemistry

The main use of immunohistochemistry in the diagnosis of malignant fibrous histiocytomas is to exclude other possibilities such as metastases, smooth muscle neoplasms or S-100 positive tumours. The exclusion of metastatic carcinoma is made more difficult by a report of cytokeratin expression by a post-irradiation malignant fibrous histiocytoma of the sacrum (Weiss *et al.*, 1988). Cytokeratin expression by malignant fibrous histiocytoma of the soft tissues, presumably due to uncontrolled or poorly regulated gene expression, is well recognized (Dawson *et al.*, 1987; Hirose *et al.*, 1989; Miettinen and Soini, 1989). Some sarcomatoid forms of metastatic renal cell carcinoma can look just like malig-

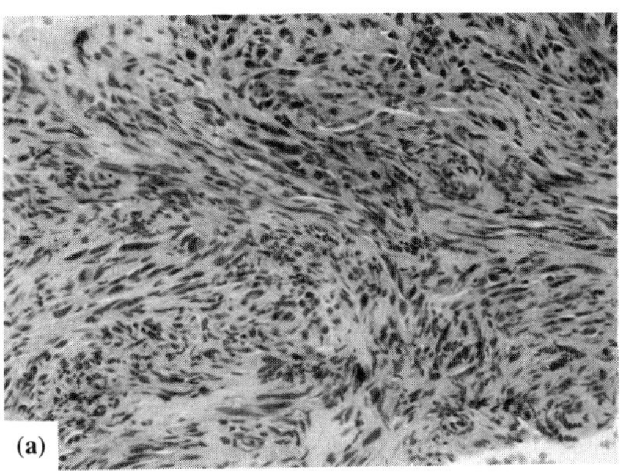

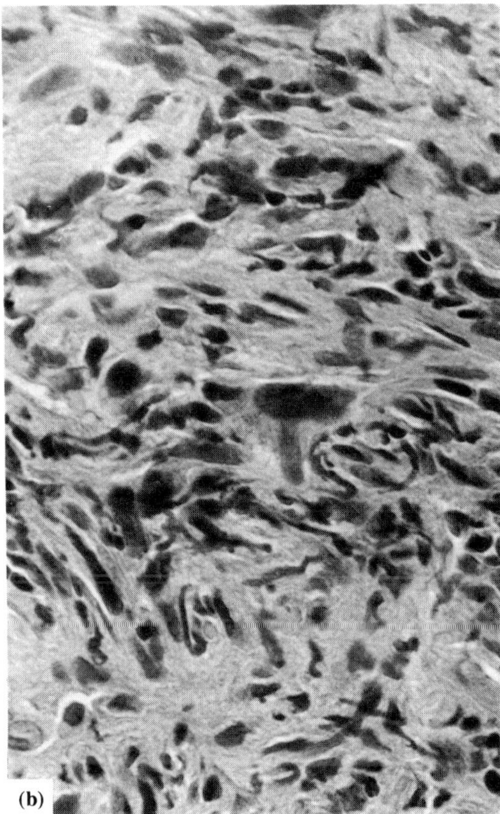

Figure 14.22 Malignant fibrous histiocytoma from a thoracic vertebra. (a) Pleomorphic hyperchromatic spindle cells in fascicles arranged in a storiform pattern. (b) Cytological features: variable nuclear size with some tumour giant cells, most nuclei are hyperchromatic.

nant fibrous histiocytoma in areas, therefore it is always necessary to hunt around the sections for clear cells. The tumour cells of malignant fibrous histiocytomas are positive for vimentin and with the 'anti-muscle antigen' – antibody HHF 35 (Martorell *et al.*, 1989). Some recent studies have suggested that malignant fibrous histiocytomas express HLA-Dr whereas histologically similar pleomorphic malignant neoplasms do not, but others have not confirmed this (Swanson and Wick, 1990).

(iv)   Electron microscopy

Ultrastructural examination shows fibroblasts and myofibroblasts are the main tumour cells (Martorell *et al.*, 1989).

(v)   Cytogenetics

Numerical and structural chromosomal abnormalities, including ring chromosomes, dicentric chromosomes and telomeric associations, are present in the tumour cells (Mandahl *et al.*, 1988; Bridge *et al.*, 1990). Chromosomal rearrangements are also found (Bridge *et al.*, 1990).

(vi)   Histogenesis

The cell of origin of malignant fibrous histiocytoma of bone is unknown. It has been speculated to be a primitive mesenchymal stem cell; alternatively 'malignant fibrous histiocytoma' may be a morphological endstage for a number of anaplastic neoplasms. There are doubts about the whole concept of pleomorphic malignant fibrous histiocytoma as a diagnosis for undifferentiated soft tissue tumours (Salisbury, 1989); similar misgivings have not yet been voiced about malignant fibrous histiocytoma of bone but it may just be a matter of time.

REFERENCES

Abdelwahab, I.F., Hermann, G., Lewis, M.M. *et al.* (1988) Transformation of an idiopathic bone infarct into malignant fibrous histiocytoma in a female. A case report. *Bull. Hosp. Jt Dis. Orthop. Inst.*, **48**, 197–203.

Bago-Granell, J., Aguirre-Canyadell, M., Nardi, J. *et al.* (1984) Malignant fibrous histiocytoma of bone at the site of a total hip arthroplasty. A case report. *J. Bone Joint Surg.*, **66B**, 38–40.

Bertoni, F., Capanna, R., Calderoni, P. *et al.* (1984) Primary central (medullary) fibrosarcoma of bone. *Semin. Diagn. Pathol.*, **1**, 185–98.

Bridge, J.A., Sanger, W.G., Neff, J.R. *et al.* (1990) Cytogenetic findings in a primary malignant fibrous histiocytoma of bone and the lung metastasis. *Pathology*, **22**, 16–9.

Capanna, R., Bertoni, F., Baochini, P. *et al.* (1984) Malignant fibrous histiocytoma of bone. The experience at the Rizzoli Institute: report of 30 cases. *Cancer*, **54**, 177–87.

Castillo, M., Tehranzadeh, J., Becerra, J. *et al.* (1987) Case report 408: malignant fibrous histiocytoma of innominate bones and femur (multicentric). *Skeletal Radiol.*, **16**, 74–7.

Dahlin, D.C. and Beabout, J.W. (1971) Dedifferentiation of low-grade chondrosarcomas. *Cancer*, **28**, 461–6.

Dahlin, D.C. and Unni, K.K. (1986) Malignant (fibrous) histiocytoma. In *Bone Tumors*, 4th edn. Charles C Thomas, Springfield, IL, pp. 357–65.

Dawson, C.W., Fisher, C. and Gatter, K.C. (1987) An immunohistochemical study of differentiation in malignant fibrous histiocytoma. *Histopathology*, **11**, 375–83.

Destouet, J.M., Kyriakos, M. and Gilula, L.A. (1980) Fibrous histiocytoma (fibroxanthoma) of a cervical vertebra. A report with a review of the literature. *Skeletal Radiol.*, **5**, 241–6.

Dock, W., Hajek, P., Wittich, G. *et al.* (1989) Primary malignant fibrous histiocytoma of the metacarpal bone: a new localization. *Br. J. Radiol.*, **62**, 940–2.

Ducatman, B.S., Scheithauer, B.W. and Dahlin, D.C. (1983) Malignant bone tumors associated with neurofibromatosis. *Mayo Clin. Proc.*, **58**, 578–82.

Enzinger, F.M. and Weiss, S.W. (1988) Malignant fibrous histiocytoma. In *Soft Tissue Tumors*, 2nd edn. C.V. Mosby, St Louis, pp. 273–300.

Feldman, F. and Norman, D. (1972) Intra- and extraosseous malignant histiocytoma (malignant fibrous xanthoma). *Radiology*, **104**, 497–508.

Finci, R., Gunhan, O., Ucmakli, E. *et al.* (1990) Multiple and familial malignant fibrous histiocytoma of bone. A report of two cases. *J. Bone Joint Surg.*, **72A**, 295–8.

Frassica, F.J., Sim, F.H. and Wold, L.E. (1988) Case report 462: Grade 2 myxoid fibrosarcoma of femur. *Skeletal Radiol.*, **17**, 77–80.

Frierson, H.F. Jr, Fechner, R.E., Stallings, R.G. *et al.* (1987) Malignant fibrous histiocytoma in bone infarct. Association with sickle cell trait and alcohol abuse. *Cancer*, **59**, 496–500.

Furey, J., Ferrer-Torells, M. and Reagan, J.W. (1960) Fibrosarcoma arising at the site of bone infarcts. A report of two cases. *J. Bone Joint Surg.*, **42A**, 802–10.

Grieco, A., Caputo, S., Silvestri, E. *et al.* (1989) Malignant fibrous histiocytoma of sternum: an unusual cause of fever of undetermined origin. *Postgrad. Med. J.*, **65**, 929–31.

Gruber, H.E., Marshall, G.J., Moore, T.M. *et al.* (1987) Alteration in osteoblast cell number and cell activity in the presence of invading malignant fibrous histiocytoma. *Cancer*, **59**, 755–60.

Halpern, J., Kopolovic, J. and Catane, R. (1984) Malignant fibrous histiocytoma developing in irradiated sacral chordoma. *Cancer*, **53**, 2661–2.

Hankin, F.M., Hankin, R.C. and Louis, D.S. (1987) Malignant fibrous histiocytoma involving a digit. *J. Hand Surg.*, **12A**, 83–6.

Hardcastle, P., Nade, S. and Arnold, W. (1986) Hereditary bone dysplasia with malignant change. Report of three families. *J. Bone Joint Surg.*, **68A**, 1079–89.

Heselson, N.G., Price, S.K., Mills, E.E. *et al.* (1983) Two malignant fibrous histiocytomas in bone infarcts. Case report. *J. Bone Joint Surg.*, **65A**, 1166–71.

Hirose, T., Kudo, E., Hasegawa, T. *et al.* (1989) Expression of intermediate filaments in malignant fibrous histiocytomas. *Hum. Pathol.*, **20**, 871–7.

Huvos, A.G. (1976) Primary malignant fibrous histiocytoma of bone: clinicopathological study of 18 patients. *N. Y. State J. Med.*, **76**, 552–9.

Huvos, A.G., Heilweil, M. and Bretsky, S.S. (1985) The pathology of malignant fibrous histiocytoma of bone. A study of 130 patients. *Am. J. Surg. Pathol.*, **9**, 853–71.

Huvos, A.G., Woodard, H.Q. and Heilweil, M. (1986) Postradiation malignant fibrous histiocytoma of bone. A clinicopathologic study of 20 patients. *Am. J. Surg. Pathol.*, **10**, 9–18.

Kirshbaum, J.D. (1949) Fibrosarcoma of the tibia following chronic osteomyelitis. Report of a case. *J. Bone Joint Surg.*, **31A**, 413–16.

Mandahl, N., Heim, S., Arheden, K. *et al.* (1988) Rings, dicentrics, and telomeric associations in histiocytomas. *Cancer Genet. Cytogenet.*, **30**, 23–33.

Martorell, M., Calabuig, C., Peydro-Olaya, A. *et al.* (1989) Fibroblast and myofibroblast participation in malignant fibrous histiocytoma (MFH) of bone. Ultrastructural study of eight cases with immunohistochemical support. *Pathol. Res. Pract.*, **184**, 582–90.

Meis, J.M., Dorfman, H.D., Nathanson, S.D. *et al.* (1989) Primary malignant giant cell tumor of bone: 'Dedifferentiated' giant cell tumor. *Mod. Pathol.*, **2**, 541–5.

Miettinen, M. and Soini, Y. (1989) Malignant fibrous histiocytoma. Heterogeneous patterns of intermediate filament proteins by immunohistochemistry. *Arch. Pathol. Lab. Med.*, **113**, 1363–6.

Milgram, J.W. (1990) Malignant transformation in bone lipomas. *Skeletal Radiol.*, **19**, 347–52.

Mirra, J.M., Bullough, P.G., Marcove, R.C. *et al.* (1974) Malignant fibrous histiocytoma and osteosarcoma in association with bone infarcts. Report of four cases, two in caisson workers. *J. Bone Joint Surg.*, **56A**, 932–40.

Roessner, A., Vassallo, J., Vollmer, E. *et al.* (1987) Biological characterization of human bone tumors. X. The proliferation behaviour of macrophages as compared to fibroblastic cells in malignant fibrous histiocytoma and giant cell tumor of bone. *J. Cancer Res. Clin. Oncol.*, **113**, 559–62.

Roessner, A., Vollmer, E., Zwadlo, G. *et al.* (1989) The cytogenesis of macrophages and osteoclast-like giant cells in bone tumors with special emphasis on the so-called fibrohistiocytic tumors. *Curr. Top. Pathol.*, **80**, 205–27.

Salisbury, J.R. (1989) Malignant fibrous histiocytoma [leading article]. *Postgrad. Med. J.*, **65**, 872–4.

Sanders, T.G., Wilf, L.H. and Northup, H.M. (1990) Malignant fibrous histiocytoma: Etiology for a cold defect on technetium-99m-methylene diphosphonate bone scan. *J. Nucl. Med.*, **31**, 1104–5.

Sanerkin, N.G. and Woods, C.G. (1979) Fibrosarcomata and malignant fibrous histiocytoma arising in relation to enchondromata. *J. Bone Joint Surg.*, **61B**, 366–72.

Schajowicz, F. (1981) Other connective tissue

tumors. In *Tumors and Tumorlike Lesions of Bone and Joints*. Springer-Verlag, New York, pp. 342–59.

Spanier, S.S., Enneking, W.F. and Enriquez, P. (1975) Primary malignant fibrous histiocytoma of bone. *Cancer*, **36**, 2084–98.

Swanson, P.E. and Wick, M.R. (1990) HLA-Dr (Ia-like) reactivity in tumors of bone and soft tissue: an immunohistochemical comparison of monoclonal antibodies LN3 and LK8D3 in routinely processed specimens. *Mod. Pathol.*, **3**, 113–9.

Taconis, W.K. and Mulder, J.D. (1984) Fibrosarcoma and malignant fibrous histiocytoma of long bones: Radiographic features and grading. *Skeletal Radiol.*, **11**, 237–45.

Troop, J.K., Mallory, T.H., Fisher, D.A. *et al.* (1990) Malignant fibrous histiocytoma after total hip arthroplasty. A case report. *Clin. Orthop.*, **253**, 297–300.

Tsai, J.C., Dalinka, M.K., Fallon, M.D. *et al.* (1990) Fluid–fluid level: a nonspecific finding in tumors of bone and soft tissue. *Radiology*, **175**, 779–82.

Urban, C., Rosen, G., Huvos, A.G. *et al.* (1983) Chemotherapy of malignant fibrous histiocytoma of bone. A report of five cases. *Cancer*, **51**, 795–802.

Vanel, D., Hagy, C., Rebibo, G. *et al.* (1983) Study of thrre radio-induced malignant fibrohistiocytomas of bone. *Skeletal Radiol.*, **9**, 174–8.

Voutsinas, S.A. (1988) Spindle-cell sarcoma in patients who have osteochondromatosis. A report of two cases [letter]. *J. Bone Joint Surg.*, **70A**, 1430.

Weiner, M., Sedlis, M., Johnston, A.D. *et al.* (1983) Adjuvant chemotherapy of malignant fibrous histiocytoma of bone. *Cancer*, **51**, 25–9.

Weiss, S.W., Bratthauer, G.L. and Morris, P.A. (1988) Post-irradiation malignant fibrous histiocytoma expressing cytokeratin: implications for immunodiagnosis of sarcomas. *Am. J. Surg. Pathol.*, **12**, 554–7.

Wold, L.E. (1988) Fibrohistiocytic tumors of bone. In *Bone Tumors* (ed. K.K. Unni), Churchill Livingstone, New York, pp. 183–97.

Wood, G.W. and Gollahon, K.A. (1977) Detection and quantitation of macrophage infiltration into primary human tumors with the use of cell-surface markers. *J. Natl. Cancer Inst.*, **59**, 1081–7.

14.4.10 INFANTILE FIBROSARCOMA OF BONE

(a) Clinical features

Infantile fibrosarcoma is an exceptionally rare bone tumour (Bernado *et al.*, 1987); most examples of this tumour arise in the soft tissues (Chung and Enzinger, 1976). Infantile fibrosarcoma of bone is a rapidly growing neoplasm that, if allowed, attains a large size within a few months. Treatment may have to be amputation.

(b) Pathology

Macroscopically, infantile fibrosarcoma is a poorly circumscribed tumour that may extensively infiltrate adjacent soft tissues. Microscopically, infantile fibrosarcoma is a highly cellular neoplasm composed of immature-appearing spindle-shaped cells. Ultrastructural examination shows mesenchymal cells with fibroblastic and histiocytic differentiation.

REFERENCES

Bernado, L., Admella, C., Lucaya, J. *et al.* (1987) Infantile fibrosarcoma of femur. *Pediatr. Pathol.*, **7**, 201–17.

Chung, E.B. and Enzinger, F.M. (1976) Infantile fibrosarcoma. *Cancer*, **38**, 729–39.

14.4.11 LEIOMYOSARCOMA

(a) Clinical features

Primary leiomyosarcoma of bone is a very rare tumour with only 43 cases reported in the literature (Evans and Sanerkin, 1965; Angervall *et al.*, 1980; von Hochstetter *et al.*, 1984; Berlin *et al.*, 1987; Eady *et al.*, 1987). Primary leiomyosarcomas of bone are very rare compared with secondary deposits of leiomyosarcoma in bone. With most leiomyosarcomas in bone, eventually a primary tumour is discovered elsewhere, especially in women where most are secondaries from uterine leiomyosarcomas (Fornasier and Paley, 1983).

(i)   *Skeletal distribution*

Most tumours are found around the knee (lower femur, upper tibia) or in the jaws and facial bones. Rare cases occur at other sites (Eady *et al.*, 1987; Marymont and Clanton, 1990).

Presenting features are a dull ache or pain, the presence of a mass and pathological fracture. Metastases mostly occur in the lungs and in other bones. The likelihood of metastases from primary leiomyosarcomas of bone is the same as from malignant fibrous histiocytoma of bone. Adequate treatment of primary leiomyosarcoma of bone requires surgical ablation with the goals being those for any malignant tumour of bone – eradication of the tumour with preservation of as much function as is possible (Young *et al.*, 1988).

(ii)   *Radiology*

Radiologically, primary leiomyosarcomas of bone appear as malignant tumours with permeative destruction of bone. The tumours may grow out of the bone and diffusely infiltrate the surrounding soft tissues.

(b)   **Pathology**

(i)   *Histopathology*

Histologically, leiomyosarcomas of bone are tumours composed of fascicles of spindle cells with hyperchromatic and pleomorphic 'cigar-shaped' nuclei. There may be areas of necrosis or of palisading. Mitotic figures are frequent. A leiomyosarcomatous component can be produced by some dedifferentiated chondrosarcomas (Munk *et al.*, 1988).

(ii)   *Immunohistochemistry*

Immunohistochemistry shows positivity for muscle-specific actin, vimentin and desmin, although poorly differentiated areas in these tumours are often desmin negative. It is important to take multiple sections and use the most well-differentiated areas for immunohistochemical studies. Antibodies to myoglobin are always negative. Electron microscopy shows numerous intermediate filaments and also thin filaments with dense bodies which are the myofilaments (Trojani *et al.*, 1983).

(iii)   *Histogenesis*

Histogenesis is speculative; primary leiomyosarcomas of bone may originate from the smooth muscle of vascular walls within bone but this is unproven.

REFERENCES

Angervall, L., Berlin, O., Kindblom, L.-G. *et al.* (1980) Primary leiomyosarcoma of bone. A study of five cases. *Cancer*, **46**, 1270–9.

Berlin, O., Angervall, L., Kindblom, L.-G. *et al.* (1987) Primary leiomyosarcoma of bone. A clinical, radiographic, pathologic-anatomic, and prognostic study of 16 cases. *Skeletal Radiol.*, **16**, 364–76.

Eady, J.L., McKinney, J.D. and McDonald, E.C. (1987) Primary leiomyosarcoma of bone. A case report and review of the literature. *J. Bone Joint Surg.*, **69A**, 287–9.

Evans, D.M.D. and Sanerkin, N.G. (1965) Primary leiomyosarcoma of bone. *J. Pathol. Bacteriol.*, **90**, 348–50.

Fornasier, V.L. and Paley, D. (1983) Leiomyosarcoma of bone: primary or secondary? A case report and review of the literature. *Skeletal Radiol.*, **10**, 147–53.

Marymont, J.V. and Clanton, T.O. (1990) Leiomyosarcoma of the os calcis. *Foot Ankle*, **10**, 239–42.

Munk, P.L., Connell, D.G. and Quenville, N.F. (1988) Dedifferentiated chondrosarcoma of bone with leiomyosarcomatous mesenchymal component: a case report. *Can. Assoc. Radiol. J.*, **39**, 218–20.

Trojani, M., Coquet, M., Peres, P. *et al.* (1983) Primary leiomyosarcoma of bone. A case with ultrastructural study. Review of the literature. *Semin. Hopit. Paris*, **59**, 1179–83.

von Hochstetter, A.R., Eberle, H. and Ruttner, J.R. (1984) Primary leiomyosarcoma of extragnathic bones. Case report and review of literature. *Cancer*, **53**, 2194–200.

Young, C.L., Wold, L.E., McLeod, R.A. *et al.* (1988) Primary leiomyosarcoma of bone. *Orthopedics*, **11**, 615–8.

14.4.12   LEIOMYOMA OF BONE

Exceptional cases of true primary leiomyomas of bone occur. They are among the rarest of all bone tumours.

14.4.13   GLOMUS TUMOUR OF BONE

(a)   Clinical features

Primary intraosseous glomus tumours are very rare tumours (Bergstrand, 1937; Lattes and Bull, 1948; Bog *et al.*, 1983; Sunderraj *et al.*, 1989).

(i)   *Skeletal distribution*

Almost all glomus tumours of bone have occurred in the phalanges (Bjorkengren *et al.*, 1986), but there are solitary examples of cases in a metacarpal bone (Serra *et al.*, 1985) and in the ulna (Rozmaryn *et al.*, 1987).

Intraosseous glomus tumours present with progressive pain and swelling. One case has been in association with neurofibromatosis (Siegel, 1967). Excision of intraosseous glomus tumours is followed by complete relief of symptoms. Bone curettage, with or without grafting, also affords relief.

(b)   Pathology

Glomus tumours are benign vascular tumours composed of round to oval uniform cells associated with vascular structures. Those glomus tumours that have been reported in bones appear histologically identical to their counterparts described in the soft tissues (Enzinger and Weiss, 1988). They arise from the glomus apparatus which is an arteriovenous anastomosis commonest in the nail beds but which may be sometimes be found in bone. Glomus cells appear closely related to smooth muscle cells when studied ultrastructurally (Venkatachalam and Greally, 1969).

REFERENCES

Bergstrand, H. (1937) Multiple glomic tumors. *Am. J. Cancer*, **29**, 470.

Bjorkengren, A.G., Resnick, D., Haghighi, P. *et al.* (1986) Intraosseous glomus tumor. Report of case and review of literature. *Am. J. Radiol.*, **147**, 739–41.

Bog, J., Lessel, W. and Dominok, G.W. (1983) Intraosseous glomus tumors. *Zentralbl. Chir.*, **108**, 1155–7.

Enzinger, F.M. and Weiss, S.W. (1988) Glomus tumor. In *Soft Tissue Tumors*, 2nd edn. C.V. Mosby, St Louis, pp. 581–95.

Lattes, R. and Bull, D.A. (1948) Case of glomus tumor with primary involvement of bone. *Ann. Surg.*, **127**, 187–91.

Rozmaryn, L.M., Sadler, A.H. and Dorfman, H.D. (1987) Intraosseous glomus tumour in the ulna. A case report. *Clin. Orthop.*, **220**, 126–9.

Serra, J.M., Muirragui, A. and Tadjalli, H. (1985) Glomus tumor of the metacarpophalangeal joint: a case report. *J. Hand Surg.*, **10**, 142–3.

Siegel, M.M. (1967) Intraosseous glomus tumor. *Am. J. Orthop.*, **9**, 68–9.

Sunderraj, S., Al-Khalifa, A.A., Pal, A.K. *et al.* (1989) Primary intra-osseous glomus tumour. *Histopathology*, **14**, 532–6.

Venkatachalam, M.A. and Greally, J.G. (1969) Fine structure of glomus tumor: similarity of glomus cells to smooth muscle. *Cancer*, **23**, 1176–84.

14.5   VACUOLATED OR CLEAR CELLED NEOPLASMS

14.5.1   LIPOMA

(a)   Clinical features

Primary lipomas of bone are very rare bone tumours that are usually identified as an incidental radiographic finding. Their incidence has been estimated at 1 in 1000 primary bone tumours (Leeson *et al.*, 1983).

(i) Skeletal distribution

Lipomas occur most often in the metaphysis of long bones. There is a single case report of involvement of the ilium (Buckley and Burkus, 1988). Many bone lipomas are parosteal (periosteal) in location (Demos *et al.*, 1984; Krajewska *et al.*, 1988) rather than intraosseous; they occur on major long bones and metacarpal shafts (Schajowicz, 1981). Rare cases with definite intraosseous origin show significant extension into the soft tissues (Buckley and Burkus, 1988). Circumscribed foci of fatty marrow are not uncommon in the vertebral bodies but they are not true lipomas.

Very rare cases with multiple intraosseous sites have also been described (Milgram, 1988). The prognosis is generally excellent so conservative treatment is mandatory. Many intraosseous lipomas appear to undergo spontaneous involution, so that surgical excision becomes unnecessary.

(ii) Radiology

Radiology of intraosseous lipomas shows sharply defined 'cystic' lesions with dense central sclerosis and fat-equivalent CT values (Ramos *et al.*, 1985; Schumacher *et al.*, 1988). Parosteal lipomas appear as round or ovoid, well-delimited soft tissue masses adjacent to bone. They show a central bone density because of spicular, radiating, reactive, periosteal bone formation (Schajowicz, 1981).

(b) Pathology

(i) Histopathology

Histologically, bone lipomas are composed of mature fat-cells (Figure 14.23) like the much commoner subcutaneous lipomas.

Some intraosseous lipomas undergo focal infarction (Gero and Kahn, 1988) and Milgram (1988) has proposed subdividing intraosseous lipomas into three groups depending on this degree of involution:

1. Solid tumours of viable lipocytes.
2. Transitional cases with partial fat necrosis and focal calcification but also regions with viable lipocytes.
3. Late cases in which the fat-cells have died with variable degree of cyst formation, calcification and reactive new bone formation.

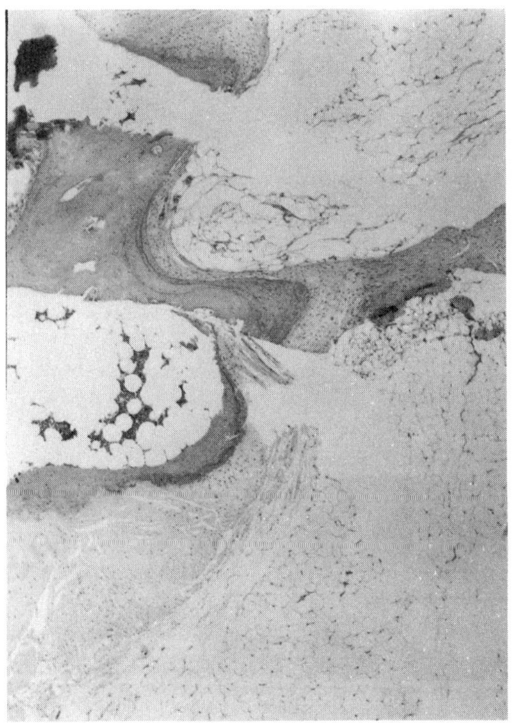

Figure 14.23 Female aged 71 years. Parosteal lipoma. Presented with swelling over the tibial shaft. Radiograph was normal but the CT showed a soft tissue mass, with the attributes of fat, applied to the bone. The section shows benign adipose tissue resting on fibrous tissue (from which septae arise), attached to bone. It is not clear whether the fibrous tissue is periosteum or tumour capsule or both.

REFERENCES

Buckley, S.L. and Burkus, J.K. (1988) Intraosseous lipoma of the ilium. A case report. *Clin. Orthop.*, **228**, 297–301.

Demos, T.C., Bruno, E., Armin, A. *et al.* (1984) Parosteal lipoma with enlarging osteochondroma. *Am. J. Roentgenol.* **143**, 365–6.

Gero, M.J. and Kahn, L.B. (1988) Case report 498: Intraosseous lipoma of the distal end of the fibula with focal infarction. *Skeletal Radiol.*, **17**, 443–6.

Krajewska, I., Vernon-Roberts, B. and Sorby-Adams, G. (1988) Parosteal (periosteal) lipoma. *Pathology*, **20**, 179–83.

Leeson, M.C., Kay, D. and Smith, B.S. (1983) Intraosseous lipoma. *Clin. Orthop.*, **181**, 186–90.

Milgram, J.W. (1988) Intraosseous lipomas. A clinicopathologic study of 66 cases. *Clin. Orthop.*, **231**, 277–302.

Ramos, A., Castello, J., Sartoris, D.J. *et al.* (1985) Osseous lipoma: CT appearance. *Radiology*, **157**, 615–19.

Schajowicz, F. (1981) Other connective tissue tumors. In *Tumors and Tumorlike Lesions of Bone and Joints*. Springer-Verlag, New York, pp. 341–2.

Schumacher, K.A., Reuther, G. and Friedrich, J.M. (1988) Radiological diagnosis of intraosseous lipomas. *ROFO*, **149**, 286–8.

14.5.2 EPITHELIOID HAEMANGIOENDOTHELIOMA

(a) Clinical features

Epithelioid haemangioendothelioma is a rare, borderline malignant, tumour. It is the prototype of a group of vascular tumours characterized by an epithelioid or histiocytoid endothelial cell (Weiss *et al.*, 1986).

Not infrequently, epithelioid haemangioendotheliomas present as multiple bony lesions or as multiple soft tissue and bony lesions. Rarely tumours are periosteal (Hirose *et al.*, 1987). Some tumours have occurred at the site of a prosthesis (van der List *et al.*, 1988); others have been associated with hypercalciuria (Cortet *et al.*, 1990).

Some patients present with pain. The clinical course is characteristically prolonged.

(i) Radiology

Radiologically, epithelioid haemangioendotheliomas appear as osteolytic lesions without reactive new bone formation (Maruyama *et al.*, 1985).

(b) Pathology

(i) Histopathology

Histologically, epithelioid haemangioendotheliomas show epithelioid tumour cells with frequent intracytoplasmic vacuoles arranged in small nests or cords in hyalinized stroma.

(ii) Immunohistochemistry

Immunohistochemical studies show the tumour cells are positive for cytokeratins, the endothelial markers factor VIII-related antigen (FVIII-RAg) and *Ulex europaeus* agglutinin I, HLA-Dr and vimentin (Maruyama *et al.*, 1985; Hirose *et al.*, 1987). Coexpression of cytokeratin and FVIII-RAg has been demonstrated in the same tumour cells by means of step sections (van Haelst *et al.*, 1990).

(iii) Electron microscopy

Ultrastructural examination supports an endothelial origin for the epithelioid tumour cells by demonstrating the presence of Weibel–Palade bodies. An unusual case has been reported where the tumour cells contained leptomeric fibrils (often noted in normal skeletal muscle cells) and crystalline filamentous aggregates (Hirose *et al.*, 1987).

REFERENCES

Cortet, B., Houvenagel, E., Creusy, C. *et al.* (1990) A case of hemangioendothelioma of the rib associated with hypercalciuria. *Rev. Rhum. Mal. Osteoartic.*, **57**, 185–7.

Hirose, T., Sano, T., Shinomiya, S. *et al.* (1987) Periosteal epithelioid hemangioendothelioma with leptomeric fibrils. *Ultrastruct. Pathol.*, **11**, 405–10.

Maruyama, N., Kumagai, Y., Ishida, Y. *et al.* (1985) Epithelioid hemangioendothelioma of the bone tissue. *Virchows Arch. A*, **407**, 159–65.

van der List, J.J., van Horn, J.R., Slooff, T.J. (1988) Malignant epithelioid hemangioendothelioma at the site of a hip prosthesis. *Acta Orthop. Scand.*, **59**, 328–30.

Van Haelst, U.J., Pruszczynski, M., ten Cate, L.N. *et al.* (1990) Ultrastructural and immunohistochemical study of epithelioid hemangioendothelioma of bone: coexpression of epithelial and endothelial markers. *Ultrastruct. Pathol.*, **14**, 141–9.

Weiss, S.W., Ishak, K.G., Dail, D.H. *et al.* (1986) Epithelioid hemangioendothelioma and related lesions. *Semin. Diagn. Pathol.*, **3**, 259–87.

14.5.3 LIPOSARCOMA

(a) Clinical features

Primary liposarcomas of bone are very rare bone tumours (Torok *et al.*, 1983). Only 35 cases were reported in the 50-year period from 1930 to 1980 (see Catto and Stevens, 1963; Goldman, 1964; Schwartz *et al.*, 1970 for good examples).

(i) Skeletal distribution (from Catto and Stevens, 1963 and Schwartz *et al.*, 1970 but based on a small number of cases because of the rarity of the neoplasm)

- Flat bones
  - Ribs
  - Girdles
    - Shoulder: clavicle, scapula, sternum
    - Pelvis: ilium, pubis, sacrum   8%
- Long tubular
  - Femur, tibia, humerus   58%
  - Fibula, radius, ulna   25%
- Hands and feet
  - Short tubular
    - Metacarpals, metatarsals, phalanges   8%
  - Cuboidal
    - Carpals, tarsals

Very rare cases are thought to arise from pre-existing simple bone cysts (Johnson *et al.*, 1962), non-ossifying fibroma (Retz, 1961) and bone lipomas (Milgram, 1990). Soft tissue liposarcomas sometimes produce skeletal metastasis that may mimic primary liposarcoma of bone. Liposarcomas arising in the soft tissues adjacent to bone seldom infiltrate the bone.

(ii) Radiology

Radiology shows that primary liposarcomas of bone are ill-defined, expanding, lytic lesions which usually show cortical erosion and may be associated with an overlying soft tissue swelling.

(b) Pathology

(i) Histopathology

Histologically, primary liposarcomas of bone infiltrate the marrow spaces without greatly destroying the spongy bone (Catto and Stevens, 1963). The tumours are lobulated, cellular and well vascularized. The neoplastic cells have pleomorphic nuclei with coarse chromatin and prominent nucleoli. Mitoses are numerous and scattered multinucleated tumour giant cells are sometimes seen. Occasional areas in some tumours may be composed largely of non-vacuolated spindle cells (Goldman, 1964). Rare cases of liposarcoma mixed with another component have been reported, e.g. osteoliposarcoma (Ross and Hadfield, 1968) and liposarcoma with osteosarcomatous foci (Downey *et al.*, 1982).

(ii) Histochemistry

Intracytoplasmic fat-globules are present, and can be demonstrated by Oil red O and Sudan stains in frozen sections. Some cells contain a single large globule and an eccentric nucleus, others contain multiple globules indenting the nucleus (lipoblasts). Alcian blue staining for acid mucins is also positive.

REFERENCES

Catto, M. and Stevens, J. (1963) Liposarcoma of bone. *J. Pathol. Bacteriol.*, **86**, 248–53.

Downey, E.F. Jr, Worsham, G.F. and Brower, A.C. (1982) Liposarcoma of bone with osteosarcomatous foci: case report and review of the literature. *Skeletal Radiol.*, **8**, 47–50.

Goldman, R.L. (1964) Primary liposarcoma of bone. Report of a case. *Am. J. Clin. Pathol.*, **42**, 503–8.

Johnson, L.C., Vetter, H. and Putschar, W.J.G. (1962) Sarcomas arising in bone cysts. *Virchows Arch. A*, **335**, 428–51.

Milgram, J.W. (1990) Malignant transformation in bone lipomas. *Skeletal Radiol.*, **19**, 347–52.

Retz, L.D. Jr (1961) Primary liposarcoma of bone. Report of a case and review of the literature. *J. Bone Joint Surg.*, **43A**, 123–9.

Ross, C.F. and Hadfield, G. (1968) Primary osteo-liposarcoma of bone (malignant mesenchymoma). Report of a case. *J. Bone Joint Surg.*, **50B**, 639–43.

Schwartz, A., Shuster, M. and Becker, S.M. (1970) Liposarcoma of bone. Report of a case and review of the literature. *J. Bone Joint Surg.*, **52A**, 171–7.

Torok, G., Meller, Y. and Maor, E. (1983) Primary liposarcoma of bone. Case report and review of the literature. *Bull. Hosp. Jt Dis. Orthop. Inst.*, **43**, 28–37.

14.6 NEOPLASMS WITH SPACES

14.6.1 ANGIOMA AND VARIANTS

Synonyms:
Haemangioma
Lymphangioma

(a) Clinical features

Angiomas are common bone lesions. Rare angiomas occur at uncommon sites (Warman and Myssiorek, 1989; Boker *et al.*, 1990). Exceptionally rare angiomas are subperiosteal (Kenan *et al.*, 1988). Angiomas may be single or multiple and may remain stable or

increase in size. An adjacent soft tissue mass may be present (Ortega *et al.*, 1986).

(i)   Skeletal distribution for solitary angiomas (from Dahlin and Unni, 1986)

- Jaws   5%
- Skull   50%
- Other flat bones
  - Ribs   2.5%
  - Girdles
    - Shoulder: clavicle, scapula, sternum   1%
    - Pelvis: ilium, pubis, sacrum   2.5%
- Spine: cervical, thoracic, lumbar   25%
- Long tubular
  - Femur, tibia, humerus   11%
  - Fibula, radius, ulna   1%

Subperiosteal angiomas are most commonly located in the midshaft of a long tubular bone (Kenan *et al.*, 1988).

The commonest clinical features of angiomas are swelling and pain or tenderness. Malignant transformation has not been reported unless radiotherapy has been used.

The treatment of subperiosteal angiomas is marginal excision; local recurrences have not been reported after such treatment (Kenan *et al.*, 1988).

A variant of angioma is known as histiocytoid haemangioma. This disease, or spectrum of diseases, has a characteristic histological feature, namely distinctive histiocytoid endothelial cells. Most of the tumours are cutaneous but extracutaneous sites can include bone (Ose *et al.*, 1983; Dannaker *et al.*, 1989). Some osseous cases have had lesions at multiple sites (Cone *et al.*, 1983). Radiotherapy results in clinical improvement.

'Vanishing bone disease', 'disappearing bone disease', Gorham's disease and the Gorham–Stout syndrome are all synonyms for the very rare skeletal haemangiomatosis which can be diffuse or focal (Rebaud *et al.*, 1985; Krzok and Flossel, 1988). Some cases of

Gorham's disease have been caused by diffuse lymphangiomatosis (Brown *et al.*, 1986). Generalized bony lymphangiomatosis may also be associated with cystic hygroma (Bowman *et al.*, 1984).

Three further, very rare, angioma variants sometimes occur in bones. Haemangioblastoma is predominantly a tumour of the cerebellum but has been recorded as a solitary vertebral tumour (Stevens *et al.*, 1983). Cystic angiomatosis (Johnsen *et al.*, 1984), can involve multiple bones without visceral involvement and be associated with pancytopenia and coagulation disorders (Guisasola *et al.*, 1988). Myxoid angioblastomatosis is also usually multicentric and is characterized by slowly progressive, multiple lytic bone defects (Mirra and Kameda, 1985).

Disseminated cat-scratch disease in patients with AIDS can produce multiple angiomatous nodules within long bones (Koehler *et al.*, 1988).

(ii) Radiology

Radiologically, angiomas show an expanded cortex and bone destruction with irregular trabeculation (Ortega *et al.*, 1986). Subperiosteal angiomas appear as shallow cup-shaped depressions surrounded by cortical thickening (Kenan *et al.*, 1988).

(b) Pathology

(i) Histopathology

Histologically, angiomas are formed of anastomosing vessels within the marrow space. In most cases, the vessels are blood vessels (haemangiomas) but in some they are of lymphatic origin (lymphangiomas).

Histological examination of cases of histiocytoid haemangioma shows a proliferation of histiocytoid endothelial cells with a variable inflammatory response. The histiocytoid endothelial cells possess intracytoplasmic vacuoles and associated vascular lumen formation (Dannaker *et al.*, 1989).

Histologically, capillary haemangioblastoma shows numerous compressed capillaries and larger endothelium-lined vascular spaces. The blood vessels are separated by polygonal cells with small, round nuclei and abundant, foamy cytoplasm (Stevens *et al.*, 1983). Myxoid angioblastomatosis shows capillary-like cellular tubes with occasional red blood cells within cytoplasmic lumina. Immunohistochemical staining is positive for Factor VIII-related antigen. Electron microscopy shows the cells contain Weibel–Palade bodies, numerous pinocytic vesicles, prominent microvilli, elaborate intercellular contacts, desmosomes and arrays of fine intracytoplasmic filaments (Mirra and Kameda, 1985).

The angiomatous nodules seen in disseminated cat-scratch disease in AIDS patients can be demonstrated to contain numerous clumps of bacteria by Warthin–Starry staining or electron microscopy, and the bacteria can be stained with antisera raised against the cat-scratch disease bacillus (Koehler *et al.*, 1988).

REFERENCES

Boker, S.M., Cullen, G.M., Swank, M. *et al.* (1990) Case report 593: haemangioma of sternum. *Skeletal Radiol.*, **19**, 77–8.

Bowman, C.A., Wittee, M.H., Wittee, C.L. *et al.* (1984) Cystic hygroma reconsidered: hamartoma or neoplasm? Primary culture of an endothelial cell line from a massive cervicomediastinal cystic hygroma with bony lymphangiomatosis. *Lymphology*, **17**, 15–22.

Brown, L.R., Reiman, H.M., Rosenow, E.C. *et al.* (1986) Intrathoracic lymphangioma. *Mayo Clin. Proc.*, **61**, 882–92.

Cone, R.O., Hudkins, P., Nguyen, V. *et al.* (1983) Histiocytoid hemangioma of bone: a benign lesion which may mimic angiosarcoma. Report of a case and review of the literature. *Skeletal Radiol.*, **10**, 165–9.

Dahlin, D.C. and Unni, K.K. (1986) Benign vascular tumors. In *Bone Tumors*, 4th edn. Charles C Thomas, Springfield, IL, pp. 167–80.

Dannaker, C., Piacquadio, D., Willoughby, C.B. *et al.* (1989) Histiocytoid hemangioma: a disease spectrum. Report of a case with simultaneous cutaneous and bone involvement limited to one extremity. *J. Am. Acad. Dermatol.*, **21**, 404–9.

Guisasola, F.J., Gonzalez, H., del Real, M. *et al.* (1988) Cystic angiomatosis of bone with hematologic involvement. Report of a case. *An. Esp. Pediatr.*, **28**, 455–8.

Johnsen, A., Rotne, H., Berner, J. *et al.* (1984) Cystic angiomatosis of bone. *Ugeskr. Laeger*, **146**, 3035–40.

Kenan, S., Bonar, S., Jones, C. *et al.* (1988) Subperiosteal hemangioma. A case report and review of the literature. *Clin. Orthop.*, **232**, 279–83.

Koehler, J.E., Le Boit, P.E., Egbert, B.M. *et al.* (1988) Cutaneous vascular lesions and disseminated cat-scratch disease in patients with the acquired immunodeficiency syndrome (AIDS) and AIDS-related complex. *Ann. Intern. Med.*, **109**, 449–55.

Krzok, G. and Flossel, C. (1988) Gorham–Stout syndrome and diffuse skeletal hemangiomatosis. *Beitr. Orthop. Traumatol.*, **35**, 219–25.

Mirra, J.M. and Kameda, N. (1985) Myxoid angioblastomatosis of bones. A case report of a rare, multifocal entity with light, ultramicroscopic, and immunopathologic correlation. *Am. J. Surg. Pathol.*, **9**, 450–8.

Ortega, W., Mahboubi, S., Dalinka, M.K. *et al.* (1986) Computed tomography of rib hemangiomas. *J. Comput. Assist. Tomogr.*, **10**, 945–7.

Ose, D., Vollmer, R., Shelburne, J. *et al.* (1983) Histiocytoid hemangioma of the skin and scapula. A case report with electron microscopy and immunohistochemistry. *Cancer*, **51**, 1656–62.

Rebaud, P., Larbre, F., Pracros, J.P. *et al.* (1985) Bone angiomatoses in children. Apropos of 3 personal cases. *Pediatrie*, **40**, 613–22.

Stevens, J., Love, S., Davis, C. *et al.* (1983) Case report. Capillary haemangioblastoma of bone resembling a vertebral haemangioma. *Br. J. Radiol.*, **56**, 571–5.

Warman, S. and Myssiorek, D. (1989) Hemangioma of the zygomatic bone. *Ann. Otol. Rhinol. Laryngol.*, **98**, 655–8.

14.6.2 ANGIOSARCOMA

Synonyms:
  Haemangiosarcoma
  Haemangioendothelial sarcoma (Dorf-
man *et al.*, 1971)
Grades II and III haemangioendothelioma (Unni *et al.*, 1971)

(a) Clinical features

Angiosarcoma is a rare bone tumour with a variable history. Most cases are rapidly progressive. As in other vascular tumours, multifocal bone lesions can occur. Occasional examples are believed to arise in chronic osteomyelitis (Bacchini *et al.*, 1984). The prognosis is ominous and most cases are dead within two years with metastases to lungs and other bones.

(b) Pathology

Radiology shows a malignant tumour with extensive cortical erosion and destruction and wide penetration into soft tissues (Schajowicz, 1981). Histologically, angiosarcoma of bone is characterized by the formation of vascular channels, lined by one or more layers of atypical endothelial cells, often of immature appearance, and accompanied by solid masses of poorly differentiated or anaplastic tissue.

REFERENCES

Bacchini, F., Calderoni, P., Gherlinzoni, F. *et al.* (1984) Angiosarcoma in chronic osteomyelitis. *Ital. J. Orthop. Traumatol.*, **10**, 393–8.

Dorfman, H.D., Steiner, G.C. and Jaffe, H.L. (1971) Vascular tumors of bone. *Hum. Pathol.*, **2**, 349–76.

Schajowicz, F. (1981) Vascular tumors. In *Tumors and Tumorlike Lesions of Bone and Joints*. Springer-Verlag, New York, pp. 329–31.

Unni, K.K., Ivins, J.C., Beabout, J.W. *et al.* (1971) Hemangioma, hemangiopericytoma and hemangioendothelioma (angiosarcoma) of bone. *Cancer*, **27**, 1403–14.

14.7 EPITHELIAL NEOPLASMS

14.7.1 METASTASES

(a) Clinical features

Secondary deposits are very common in

bones, particularly in the older age groups. Most secondary deposits are metastatic carcinomas but osseous metastases from malignant melanomas, sarcomas, carcinoid tumours, germ cell tumours (Collis and Eckert, 1985) and even gliomas (Campbell *et al.*, 1984; Spencer *et al.*, 1984; Strom and Lie, 1988; Myers *et al.*, 1990) are all seen occasionally.

(i)   Skeletal distribution

In some cases the site of the deposits may suggest a likely primary. Prostatic adenocarcinoma frequently metastasizes to the male lumbar spine, and bone metastases from carcinoma of the rectum occur predominantly in the lumbar spine and pelvis (Talbot *et al.*, 1989). Skeletal metastases from follicular carcinoma of the thyroid have a predilection for the shoulder girdle, sternum, skull and iliac bone (Nagamine *et al.*, 1985). Skeletal metastases are relatively rare below the knee.

At presentation, secondary deposits may be multiple, which aids their recognition, or single. Individual deposits may come to attention because of pain, swelling or a pathological fracture. If the patient is known to have a primary tumour, secondary deposits in bones do not usually present a diagnostic problem. Difficulties can occur when a secondary deposit is the first indication that a particular patient has a malignancy.

Carcinomas sometimes metastasize to bones involved with Paget's disease (Agha *et al.*, 1976; Kelemen, 1977; Powell, 1983), possibly related to the hypervascularity (Kalinowski and Goodwin, 1981); it has been suggested that this occurs more commonly than is recognized (Nicholas *et al.*, 1987). Metastatic deposits are described very rarely in joints (Newton *et al.*, 1984) and, exceptionally, metastatic carcinoma can be the cause of an arthritis (Philipson *et al.*, 1983; Garcia-Morteo *et al.*, 1987).

(ii)   Radiology

Radiologically, most secondary deposits are lytic lesions but some are usually sclerotic, e.g secondaries from prostatic adenocarcinoma. The bone in osteosclerotic metastases of prostatic origin often shows co-existing osteomalacia, thought due to an inability to satisfy the high calcium demand of the new bone induced by the prostatic cells (Charhon *et al.* 1983). Unusual examples of secondary deposits mimic other bone lesions (Ghandur-Mnaymneh *et al.*, 1984).

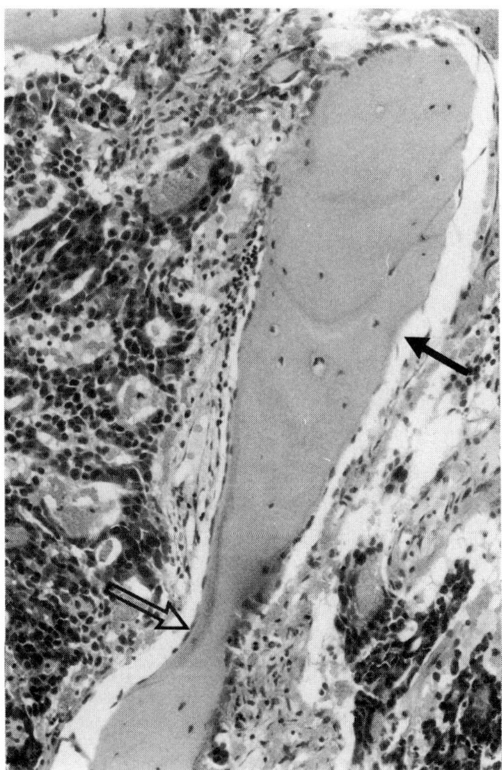

Figure 14.24 Male aged 70 years. Metastatic prostatic adenocarcinoma. The marrow space is infiltrated by sheets of cells in an acinar arrangement. These are separated from the bone by a thin layer of fibrous tissue. The bone surface shows both resorption (black arrow) and formation (open arrow). There are two reversal lines above.

(b)   Pathology

(i)   Histopathology

Histopathological examination of a secondary deposit, in a patient with a known primary, may be warranted to confirm the diagnosis before treatment. Examination of a metastasis where the primary is not known may give a clue as to the site of the primary tumour, e.g. metastatic squamous carcinoma suggests a primary bronchial carcinoma. Many secondary deposits, however, are metastatic adenocarcinoma (Figures 14.24 and 14.25). The histological appearance may suggest the site of the primary tumour. Alternatively, immunohistochemical demonstration of cell lineage-specific products such as prostatic-specific antigen or thyroglobulin in

the cells of the metastasis may confirm their origin. In some cases all that can be drawn up is a list of suggestions and so it is worthwhile knowing which carcinomas commonly metastasize to bone. In adults these are, in order of frequency, with their approximate percentage of all epithelial metastases (Schmid *et al.*, 1983):

1.   Prostatic adenocarcinoma (54%)
2.   Breast adenocarcinoma (27%)
3.   Gastric adenocarcinoma (19%)
4.   Lung carcinoma [all types] (8%)
5.   Follicular carcinoma of the thyroid
6.   Renal cell carcinoma
7.   Colonic adenocarcinoma

Metastatic carcinoma in adults may appear as a spindle-cell carcinoma and it is always

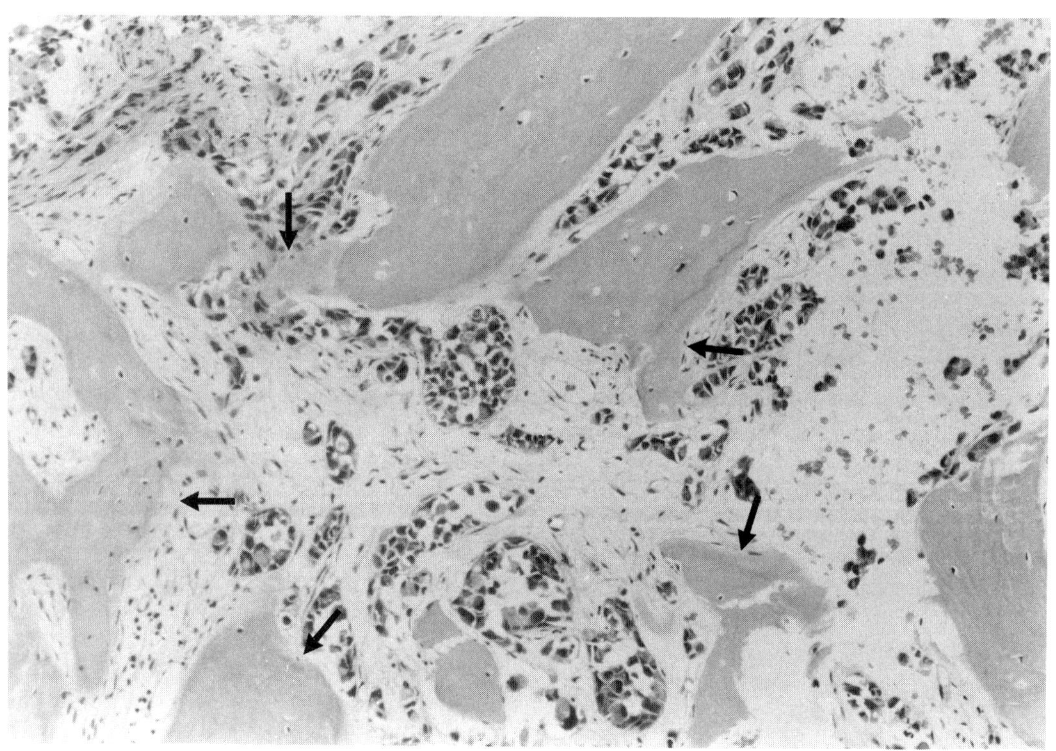

Figure 14.25 Female aged 60 years. Metastatic breast adenocarcinoma. Clusters of epithelial cells, some acinar formations, in a fibrous stroma. The bone shows many empty osteocyte lacunae, this could be age-related. There is reactive bone formation at several surfaces (arrows).

worthwhile performing cytokeratin immuno-histochemical stains on every malignant spindle-celled tumour arising in the adult skeleton.

For some tumours such as prostatic adeno-carcinoma, the growth rate of the osseous secondary deposits is considerably greater than that of the primary tumour. Cell culture studies have suggested that novel mitogenic factors, produced by bone marrow stromal cells, account for this preferential growth of metastases in bone (Chackal *et al.*, 1989). All primary tumours are composed of heterog-enous subpopulations of neoplastic cells whereas only specific subpopulations have metastatic potential. There is some evidence, for prostatic adenocarcinoma, that evaluation of the p21 protein of the *ras* oncogene family may be useful as a predictor for metastatic potential to bone (Fan, 1988). In newly diag-nosed patients with prostatic adenocarci-noma, measurement of the serum concentration of prostatic specific antigen can be used as a predictor for bone metastases (Oesterling *et al.*, 1993), and is cheaper than bone scanning.

(ii)   Secondary deposits in children

In children, neuroblastoma is the commonest skeletal metastasis (Figure 14.26) (Eggerath *et al.*, 1983). Detection of metastatic neuroblas-toma in the bone marrow is more successful by trephine biopsy than by aspiration (Mac-Manus, 1983) and can be enhanced by using indirect immunofluorescence with the monoclonal antibody UJ13A (Rogers *et al.*, 1989). Rare cases of neuroblastoma in adults can present as primary bone tumours (Mackay and Ordonez, 1987). Some child-hood tumours have a particular propensity to metastasize to bone, e.g. bone metastasizing renal tumour of childhood (BMRTC) (also known as clear cell sarcoma of the kidney) (Gonzalez-Crussi and Baum, 1983; Lamego and Zerbini, 1983; Schmidt *et al.*, 1985; Sleight and Lock, 1986). Macroscopically,

BMRTC appears as a soft white tumour with areas of necrosis. Histologically, it is formed of groups of clear cells separated by a striking pattern of capillaries, well demonstrated by a reticulin stain. BMRTC is usually treated with chemotherapy. Interestingly, BMRTC is able to invade native collagen gels, because of an absence of fibronectin, whereas Wilm's tumour and mesoblastic nephroma are not (Kumar *et al.*, 1984).

About 30% of stage IV childhood rhab-domyosarcomas have bone metastases at diagnosis. The histology is frequently alveo-lar and bone involvement is a poor prognos-

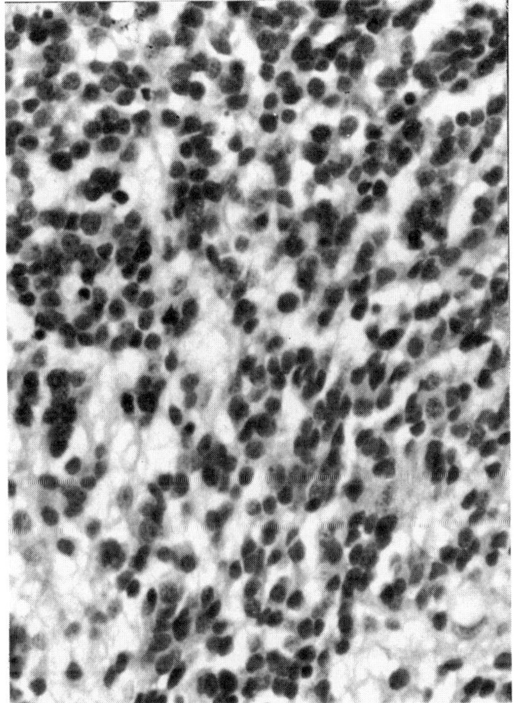

Figure 14.26 Female aged 10 years, known to have neuroblastoma. Returned with pain and swelling of upper forearm and an osteolytic lesion of the radius indicative of malignant neoplasia. The photomicrograph shows uniform malignant round cells which were immunoreactive for S-100 protein. The diagnosis is dependent on clinical and biochemical data, which were already known at the time of this presentation.

tic sign (Ruymann *et al.*, 1984). Initial widespread disease without a clinically apparent primary rhabdomyosarcoma is a rare presentation (Almanaseer *et al.*, 1984). Of the childhood primary intracranial tumours, medulloblastoma is the tumour associated most frequently with extracranial metastases, and the majority of these are bone or bone marrow metastases (Campbell *et al.*, 1984).

REFERENCES

Agha, F.P., Norman, A., Hirschl, S. *et al.* (1976) Paget's disease co-existent with metastatic carcinoma. *N. Y. State J. Med.*, **76**, 734–5.

Almanaseer, I.Y., Trujillo, Y.P., Taxy, J.B. *et al.* (1984) Systemic rhabdomyosarcoma with diffuse bone marrow involvement. Case report of an unusual presentation. *Am. J. Clin. Pathol.*, **82**, 345–53.

Campbell, A.N., Chan, H.S., Becker, L.E. *et al.* (1984) Extracranial metastases in childhood primary intracranial tumors. A report of 21 cases and review of the literature. *Cancer*, **53**, 974–81.

Chackal, R.M., Niemeyer, C., Moore, M. *et al.* (1989) Stimulation of human prostatic carcinoma cell growth by factors present in human bone marrow. *J. Clin. Invest.*, **84**, 43–50.

Charhon, S.A., Chapuy, M.C., Delvin, E.E. *et al.* (1983) Histomorphometric analysis of sclerotic bone metastases from prostatic carcinoma: special reference to osteomalacia. *Cancer*, **51**, 918–24.

Collins, C.H. and Eckert, H. (1985) Seminoma of testis with bone involvement: a report of three cases. *Clin. Radiol.*, **36**, 467–8.

Eggerath, A., Porsigchl, M. and Mortono, R. (1983) Typical skeletal changes in metastatic neuroblastoma. *ROFO*, **139**, 534–9.

Fan, K. (1988) Heterogeneous subpopulations of human prostatic adenocarcinoma cells: potential usefulness of p21 protein as a predictor for bone metastasis. *J. Urol.*, **139**, 318–22.

Garcia-Morteo, D., Lema, B., Maldonado-Cocco, J.A. *et al.* (1987) Carcinomatous arthritis of the elbow caused by metastatic breast carcinoma. *Clin. Rheumatol.*, **6**, 273–5.

Ghandur-Mnaymneh, L., Broder, L.E. and Mnaymneh, W.A. (1984) Lobular carcinoma of the breast metastatic to bone with unusual clinical, radiologic, and pathologic features mimicking osteopoikilosis. *Cancer*, **53**, 1801–3.

Gonzalez-Crussi, F. and Baum, E.S. (1983) Renal sarcomas of childhood. A clinicopathologic and ultrastructural study. *Cancer*, **51**, 898–912.

Kalinowski, D.T. and Goodwin, C.A. (1981) Metastatic disease developing in Paget's disease of bone in the distal end of the femur. *Skeletal Radiol.*, **7**, 229–31.

Kelemen, G. (1977) Temporal bone showing otosclerosis, Paget's disease and adenocarcinoma. *Ann. Otol. Rhinol. Laryngol.*, **86**, 381–5.

Kumar, S., Marsden, H.B. and Calabuig, M.C. (1984) Childhood kidney tumours: in vitro studies and natural history. *Virchows Arch. A*, **405**, 95–111.

Lamego, C.M. and Zerbini, M.C. (1983) Bone-metastasizing primary renal tumors in children. *Radiology*, **147**, 449–54.

MacKay, B. and Ordonez, N.G. (1987) Adult neuroblastoma of bone: a case report. *Ultrastruct. Pathol.*, **11**, 455–64.

MacManus, M. (1983) The diagnosis and staging of neuroblastoma. *Clin. Radiol.*, **34**, 523–7.

Myers, T., Egelhoff, J. and Myers, M. (1990) Glioblastoma multiforme presenting as osteoblastic metastatic disease: case report and review of the literature. *Am. J. Neuroradiol.*, **11**, 802–3.

Nagamine, Y., Suzuki, J., Katakura, R. *et al.* (1985) Skull metastasis of thyroid carcinoma. Study of 12 cases. *J. Neurosurg.*, **63**, 526–31.

Newton, P., Freemont, A.J., Noble, J. *et al.* (1984) Secondary malignant synovitis: report of three cases and review of the literature. *Q. J. Med.*, **53**, 135–43.

Nicholas, J.J., Srodes, C.H., Herbert, D. *et al.* (1987) Metastatic cancer in Paget's disease of bone. A case report. *Orthopedics*, **10**, 725–9.

Oesterling, J.E., Martin, S.K., Bergstralh, E.J. *et al.* (1993) The use of prostate-specific antigen in staging patients with newly diagnosed prostatic cancer. *J. Am. Med. Assoc.*, **269**, 57–60.

Philipson, J.D., Birkhead, R. and Phillips, P.E. (1983) Arthritis of the elbow caused by metastatic bronchogenic carcinoma. *Clin. Exp. Rheumatol.*, **1**, 165–9.

Powell, N. (1983) Metastatic carcinoma in association with Paget's disease of bone. *Br. J. Radiol.*, **56**, 582–5.

Rogers, D.W., Treleaven, J.G., Kemshead, J.T. *et al.* (1989) Monoclonal antibodies for detecting bone marrow invasion by neuroblastoma. *J. Clin. Pathol.*, **42**, 422–6.

Ruymann, F.B., Newton, W.A. Jr, Ragab, A.H. *et al.* (1984) Bone marrow metastases at diagnosis in children and adolescents with rhabdomyosarcoma. A report from the intergroup rhabdomyosarcoma study. *Cancer*, **53**, 368–73.

Schmid, C., Marocolo, D., Tombesi, V. *et al.* (1983) Bone marrow biopsy in the staging of malignant epithelial tumors. *Appl. Pathol.*, **1**, 343–7.

Schmidt, D., Harms, D., Evers, K.G. *et al.* (1985) Bone metastasizing renal tumor (clear cell sarcoma) of childhood with epithelioid elements. *Cancer*, **56**, 609–13.

Sleight, G. and Lock, M.M. (1986) Clear cell sarcoma of the kidney: a renal tumor of childhood that metastasizes to bone [clinical conference]. *Am. J. Roentgenol.*, **146**, 64–6.

Spencer, C.D., Weiss, R.B., Van Eys, J. *et al.* (1984) Medulloblastoma metastatic to the marrow. Report of four cases and review of the literature. *J. Neurooncol.*, **2**, 223–35.

Strom, E.H. and Lie, B. (1988) Metastasizing glioma. *Tidsskr. Nor. Laegeforen*, **108**, 2490.

Talbot, R.W., Irvine, B., Jass, J.R. *et al.* (1989) Bone metastases in carcinoma of the rectum: a clinical and pathological review. *Eur. J. Surg. Oncol.*, **15**, 449–52.

14.7.2 ADAMANTINOMA

(a) Clinical features

Adamantinomas are rare epithelial bone tumours. The name 'adamantinoma' was given to this neoplasm because of its histological resemblance to the common adamantinoma (ameloblastoma) of the jaw. These tumours occur from childhood to late adult life with the median age being in the early thirties (Dahlin and Unni, 1986). There is a slight male predominance.

(i) Skeletal distribution

Adamantinomas usually arise in the anterior midshaft of the tibia. They are rare in other long bones, e.g. fibula (Henneking *et al.*, 1984; Sowa and Dorfman, 1986). There is one report of a primary rib tumour (Plump *et al.*, 1986).

Adamantinomas are slowly growing, expansile tumours that eventually cause thinning or destruction of the overlying cortical bone. Pain is the commonest presenting feature. Treatment should be by *en bloc* resection (Braud *et al.*, 1987). Curettage is almost always followed by recurrence. Metastasis to the lungs occurs in a small number of cases and can be diagnosed by brush cytology (Tabei *et al.*, 1988).

Tumours histologically identical to adamantinoma can arise primarily in the pretibial soft tissues (Mills and Rosai, 1985).

(ii) Radiology

Radiologically, the most common appearance of an adamantinoma is that of multiple, sharply circumscribed, radiolucent defects of different sizes, with sclerotic bone between, above and below the lucent zones (Dahlin and Unni, 1986). Typically, one of the lytic areas, usually in the midshaft, is the largest and most destructive, actually destroying the cortex. Rarely, adamantinomas present as large, multiloculated cystic areas with a soap-bubble appearance.

(b) Pathology

(i) Histopathology

Histologically, adamantinomas are formed of palisading nests of small cells with either prominent nucleoli or spindle-shaped hyperchromatic nuclei, the so-called spindle-cell type. Exclusively spindle-celled forms of adamantinoma occur but, even in these, immunohistochemical stains demonstrate tiny islands of cytokeratin-positive cells. Rarer cases have a more 'vascular' appearance (Muretto and Raspugli, 1985). Diagnosis can be made by fine-needle aspiration cytology (Hales and Ferrell, 1988).

Immunohistochemistry shows the tumour cells stain positively for CEA and cytokeratins and negatively for Factor VIII-related antigen (Eisenstein and Pitcock, 1984; Mori *et al.*, 1984; Perez-Atayde *et al.* 1985). Ultrastructurally, adamantinomas have tonofilaments, desmosomes, hemidesmosomes, gap junctions, microvillous-like projections and basement membranes (Eisenstein and Pitcock, 1984; Mori *et al.*, 1984; Perez-Atayde *et al.*, 1985).

(ii) Histogenesis

Histogenesis is problematic. The immunohistochemical and electron microscopic findings demonstrate that the differentiation of the tumour cells is epithelial and an enzyme histochemical study has suggested eccrine features (Eisenstein and Pitcock, 1984). Because most adamantinomas occur in bones near a cutaneous surface, traumatic implantation has been postulated as the cause but seems unlikely. 'Congenital rests of epithelium', another suggested origin, remain undemonstrated. The problem with these suggestions is that the differentiation shown by tumour cells is not necessary a guide to the likely cell of origin. The relationship between adamantinoma and cortical osteofibrous dysplasia remains unclear (Sweet *et al.*, 1992).

REFERENCES

Braud, P., Tomeno, B., Courpied, J.P. *et al.* (1987) A peculiar tumor. Adamantinoma of the long bones. Apropos of 7 consecutive cases followed up after resection. *Rev. Chir. Orthop.*, **73**, 3–13.

Dahlin, D.C. and Unni, K.K. (1986) 'Adamantinoma' of long bones. In *Bone Tumors*, 4th edn. Charles C Thomas, Springfield, IL, pp. 346–56.

Eisenstein, W. and Pitcock, J.A. (1984) Adamantinoma of the tibia. An eccrine carcinoma. *Arch. Pathol. Lab. Med.*, **108**, 246–50.

Hales, M.S. and Ferrell, L.D. (1988) Fine-needle aspiration biopsy of tibial adamantinoma: a case report. *Diag. Cytopathol.*, **4**, 67–70.

Henneking, K., Rehm, K.E. and Schulz, A. (1984) Adamantinoma of the long tubular bones. Case report of a fibular tumor. *Chirurgie*, **55**, 407–10.

Mills, S.E. and Rosai, J. (1985) Adamantinoma of the pretibial soft tissue. Clinicopathologic features, differential diagnosis, and possible relationship to intraosseous disease. *Am. J. Clin. Pathol.*, **83**, 108–14.

Mori, H., Yamamoto, S., Hiramatsu, K. *et al.* (1984)

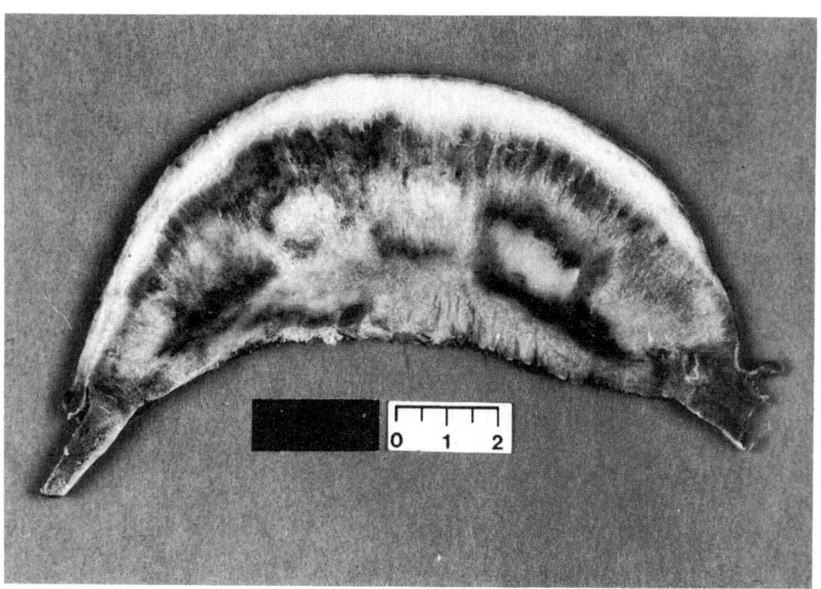

Figure 14.27 Female aged 21 years. Skull infiltrated by endotheliomatous meningioma.

Adamantinoma of tibia. Ultrastructural and immunohistochemic study with reference to histogenesis. *Clin. Orthop.*, **190**, 299–310.

Muretto, P. and Raspugli, P. (1985) 'Angioblastic' adamantinoma of tibia. An immunohistochemical study. *Tumori*, **71**, 387–90.

Perez-Atayde, A.R., Kozakewich, H.P. and Vawter, G.F. (1985) Adamantinoma of the tibia. An ultrastructural and immunohistochemical study. *Cancer*, **55**, 1015–23.

Plump, D., Haponik, E.F., Katz, R.S. *et al.* (1986) Primary adamantinoma of rib: thoracic manifestations of a rare bone tumor. *South. Med. J.*, **79**, 352–5.

Sowa, D. T. and Dorfman, H.D. (1986) Unusual localization of adamantinoma of long bones. Report of a case of isolated fibular involvement. *J. Bone Joint Surg.*, **68A**, 293–6.

Sweet, D.E., Vinh, T.N. and Devaney, K. (1992) Cortical osteofibrous dysplasia of long bone and its relationship to adamantinoma. A clinicopathologic study of 30 cases. *Am. J. Surg. Pathol.*, **16**, 282–90.

Tabei, S.Z., Abdollahi, B. and Nili, F. (1988) Diagnosis of metastatic adamantinoma of the tibia by pulmonary brushing cytology. *Acta Cytol.*, **32**, 579–81.

14.7.3 MENINGIOMA

(a) Clinical features

Meningiomas are neoplasms arising from and composed of meningothelial (arachnoid) cells. The large majority occur in the meninges of adults but some extend into, or occur primarily in, the bones of the skull (Figure 14.27). Extension of meningeal meningiomas into the dura mater, major sinuses and skull is a feature inherent to these neoplasms and not a sign of malignancy (Rosai, 1989).

(b) Pathology

The histopathology of those meningiomas primary to the skull bones or which secondarily extend into the skull bone is no different from that of meningeal meningiomas generally, and general texts should be consulted for a description of the variety of histological patterns (Rosai, 1989).

REFERENCE

Rosai, J. (1989) Neuromuscular system. In *Ackerman's Surgical Pathology*, Vol. 2. C.V. Mosby, St Louis. pp. 1743–9.

NON-NEOPLASTIC LESIONS THAT MAY MIMIC BONE TUMOURS

Jonathan R. Salisbury and Paul D. Byers

15.1 SIMPLE BONE CYST

(a) Clinical features

Simple bone cysts are common developmental abnormalities that occur at the ends of long bones. Most cases present during the first two decades of life (Dahlin and Unni, 1986).

(i) Skeletal distribution (from Schajowicz, 1981)

- Flat bones
  Ribs
  Girdles
      Shoulder: clavicle, scapula,
      sternum   0.5%
      Pelvis: ilium, pubis, sacrum   2%
- Spine: cervical, thoracic, lumbar
- Long tubular
  Femur, tibia, humerus   84%
  Fibula, radius, ulna   5%
- Hands and feet
  Short tubular
      Metacarpals, metatarsals,
      phalanges   2%
  Cuboidal
      Carpals, tarsals   5%

The lesions in the long tubular bones occur in the upper part of the diaphysis of the humerus, the diaphysis of the femur, or the proximal part of the diaphysis of the tibia, in that order of frequency (Dahlin and Unni, 1986). Some patients present with local pain or swelling but most present with pathological fracture. Treatment is curettage and bone grafting, injection of methylprednisolone acetate (Scaglietti *et al.*, 1979) or drilling multiple holes into the cyst.

(ii) Radiology

Radiology of a simple bone cyst (Figure 15.1a) shows a lucency in the medullary portion of the shaft and abutting the epiphyseal plate. Typically, the involved bone shows only slight expansion, which does not exceed that of the epiphyseal plate (Dahlin and Unni, 1986). The cortex is eroded and thinned but is intact unless pathological fracture has occurred. Some simple bone cysts contain fluid–fluid levels indicative of prior haemorrhage (Tsai *et al.*, 1990).

(b) Pathology

(i) Histopathology

Histologically, curettings from simple bone cysts are often very unsatisfactory. There is usually just a delicate fibrous lining. Thicker areas, if present, may show fibrous tissue with small numbers of scattered osteoclasts, chronic inflammatory cells and haemosiderin granules. Cysts which have fractured may contain callus (Figure 15.1b).

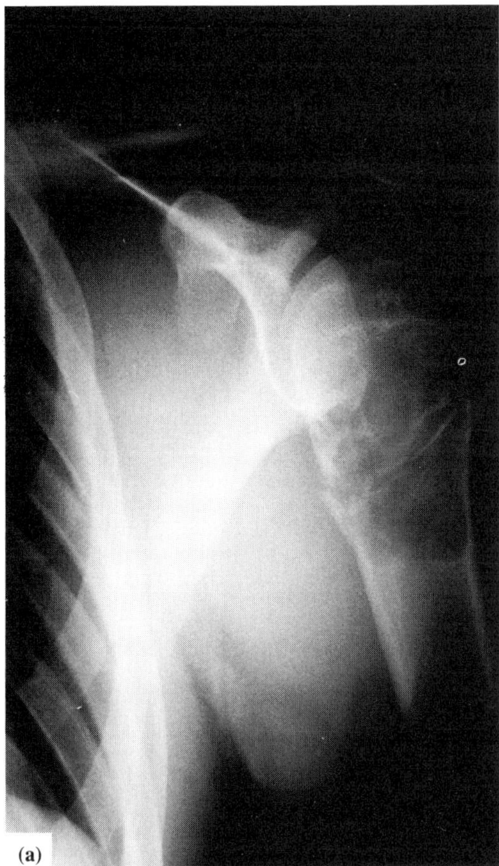

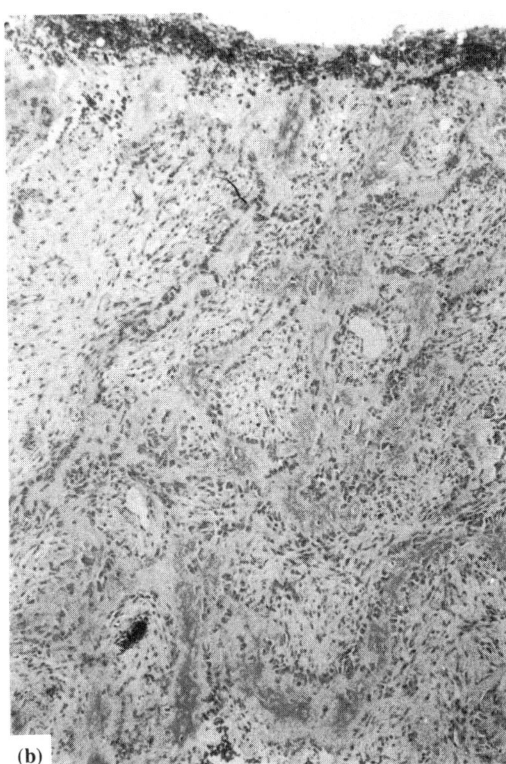

Figure 15.1 Male aged 19 years. Simple bone cyst. (a) A well-demarcated osteolytic lesion is present in the left humeral metaphysis. Unequal endosteal resorption has thinned the cortex and created a pseudoloculated appearance. There is a transverse fracture through the mid-region of the lesion. Following a needle biopsy, the lesion was injected with contrast medium which established that the cavity was a unilocular cyst. Methylprednisolone was then injected for treatment. (b) Section of needle biopsy showing fracture callus with the typical uniformly spaced trabeculae with a single layer of osteoblasts and intervening granulation tissue. The lining of these cysts is usually so thin that it is seldom obtained. Radiograph courtesy of Mr J.E. Nixon.

(ii) Histogenesis

Theories of pathogenesis abound and range from a disturbance in growth at the epiphyseal plate (Dahlin and Unni, 1986) to vascular obstruction in foci of fibrous tissue (non-ossifying fibromas) in areas of rapid bone remodelling (Broder, 1968).

REFERENCES

Broder, H.M. (1968) Possible precursor of unicameral bone cysts. *J. Bone Joint Surg.*, **50A**, 503–7.

Dahlin, D.C. and Unni, K.K. (1986) Conditions that commonly simulate primary neoplasms of bone. In *Bone Tumors*, 4th edn, Charles C Thomas, Springfield, Illinois, pp. 440–2.

Scaglietti, O., Marchetti, P.G. and Bartolozzi, P. (1979) The effects of methylprednisolone acetate in the treatment of bone cysts: results of three years follow-up. *J. Bone Joint Surg.*, **61B**, 200–4.

Schajowicz, F. (1981) Tumorlike lesions. In *Tumors and Tumorlike Lesions of Bone and Joints.* Springer-Verlag, New York, pp. 417–24.

Tsai, J.C., Dalinka, M.K., Fallon, M.D. *et al.* (1990) Fluid–fluid level: a nonspecific finding in tumors of bone and soft tissue. *Radiology*, **175**, 779–82.

15.2 ANEURYSMAL BONE CYST

(a) Clinical features

The usual aneurysmal bone cyst is a rapidly growing blood-filled cystic mass at the end of a long bone in a patient of 20 years or younger. About 77% of the patients in Dahlin and Unni's (1986) series were less than 20 years old. There is a slight female predominance. Aneurysmal bone cysts are uncommon bone lesions.

(i) Skeletal distribution (from Schajowicz, 1981 and Dahlin and Unni, 1986)

- Jaws   3%
- Skull   2%
- Other flat bones
  - Ribs   3%
  - Girdles
    - Shoulder: clavicle, scapula, sternum   4%
    - Pelvis: ilium, pubis, sacrum   10%
- Spine: cervical, thoracic, lumbar   14%
- Long tubular
  - Femur, tibia, humerus   37%
  - Fibula, radius, ulna   11%
- Hands and feet
  - Short tubular
    - Metacarpals, metatarsals, phalanges   9%
  - Cuboidal
    - Carpals, tarsals   4%

Aneurysmal bone cysts may occur as periosteal/cortical lesions and it can then be difficult to distinguish these from myositis ossificans with aneurysmal bone cyst-like areas. Most cases of aneurysmal bone cyst present with pain and swelling. Vertebral cysts can produce spinal cord compression. At least one-third of aneurysmal bone cysts are secondary to other bone lesions particularly giant cell tumour, chondroblastoma, chondromyxoid fibroma and fibrous dysplasia. Rare cases are not cystic but have sufficient similarity to aneurysmal bone cysts to justify the term 'solid aneurysmal bone cyst'.

Surgical removal of the entire lesion, or as much as possible, with bone grafting if necessary, is the best treatment. Recurrences sometimes occur, up to 33% for aneurysmal bone cysts of the bones of the hand in Dahlin's (1987) experience, but recurrence is rarer at other sites. Some cases of osteosarcomas have been described arising in aneurysmal bone cysts after radiotherapy. Apart from this, aneurysmal bone cysts never become malignant.

(ii) Radiology

Radiologically, aneurysmal bone cysts have a characteristic appearance (Figure 15.2) with a well-circumscribed and eccentric zone of rarefaction associated with an obvious soft tissue extension. Up to 25% of aneurysmal bone cysts can look very aggressive radiologically. Some aneurysmal bone cysts contain fluid–fluid levels indicative of prior haemorrhage (Tsai *et al.*, 1990). CT scanning may demonstrate a 'layering effect' of the blood within the cyst, rather like a haematocrit, but this is not a specific finding and can also be seen in telangiectatic osteosarcomas and in 'secondary' aneurysmal bone cysts.

(b) Pathology

(i) Histopathology

Histologically, aneurysmal bone cysts are composed of large cavernous spaces, often filled with blood, separated by thin septae

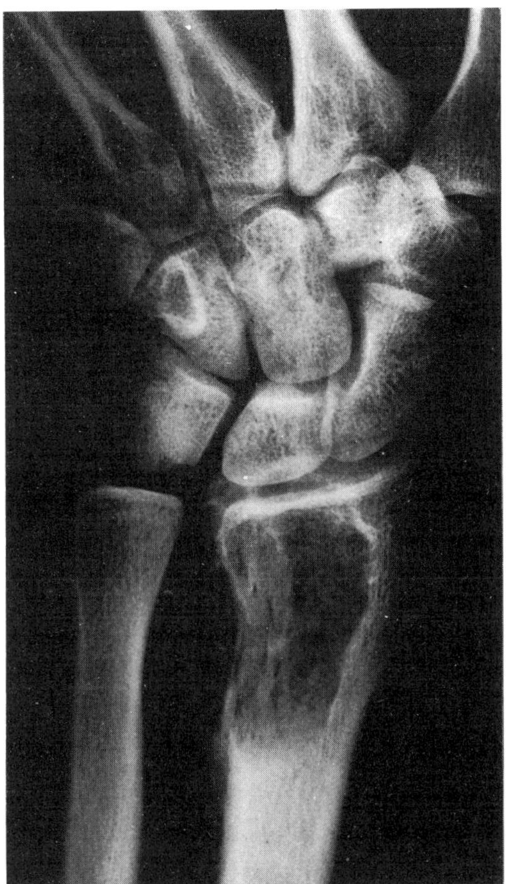

Figure 15.2 Young adult male. An osteolytic lesion in the distal end of the radius, extending to the articular surface, has expanded the bone. The cortex on the ulnar side has been completely eroded and the bulging periosteum can be faintly discerned. This 'aneurysmal' swelling was the basis for the naming of the lesion. On exploration there was a blood-filled multiloculated lesion with delicate septae.

of fibrovascular tissue containing immature bone and histiocytes (Figure 15.3). Osteoclasts are often present in large numbers. Electron microscopic and immunohistochemical studies show the walls of the cystic cavities are covered by a single layer of flattened fibroblast-like cells and that there are no endothelium, basement membranes or pericytes (Alles and Schulz, 1986;

Vollmer *et al.*, 1987). Some aneurysmal bone cysts may have areas with small or no spaces and thick trabeculae or solid tissue (section 15.2.1).

(ii) Histogenesis

The histogenesis of aneurysmal bone cyst is unknown. The idea of a vascular origin, although superficially attractive, seems unlikely in view of the ultrastructural findings and the lack of enzyme histochemical and immunohistochemical endothelial markers in the lining cells of the cyst wall (Vollmer *et al.*, 1987).

15.2.1 'SOLID' VARIANT OF ANEURYSMAL BONE CYST

Solid aneurysmal bone cysts occur mostly in children, often in the spine. By imaging techniques, they are shown to be predominantly soft tissue masses but with involvement of underlying bone. Grossly, solid aneurysmal bone cysts are not multicystic but appear red and granular. Histologically, there is a loose arrangement of the tissues (like nodular fasciitis), many osteoclasts and much bone formation (Sanerkin *et al.*, 1983; Edel *et al.*, 1992). The bone pattern is reactive, i.e. interconnecting trabeculae, poorly mineralized, many osteoblasts and osteoclasts (like heterotopic ossification) The main histological differential diagnoses are giant cell tumour and low-grade osteosarcoma. Unni (1992) has pointed out that giant cell tumours often lack the fibrogenic quality and bone formation seen in solid aneurysmal bone cyst. In the vertebral column, precise location is important – if the lesion is in the body, it is a giant cell tumour, if it is in the posterior elements, it is an aneurysmal bone cyst. Solid aneurysmal bone cysts appear much more cellular and mitotically active than low-grade osteosarcoma. The pattern of bone formation is also different – the bone in low-grade osteosarcoma lacks the osteoblastic rimming

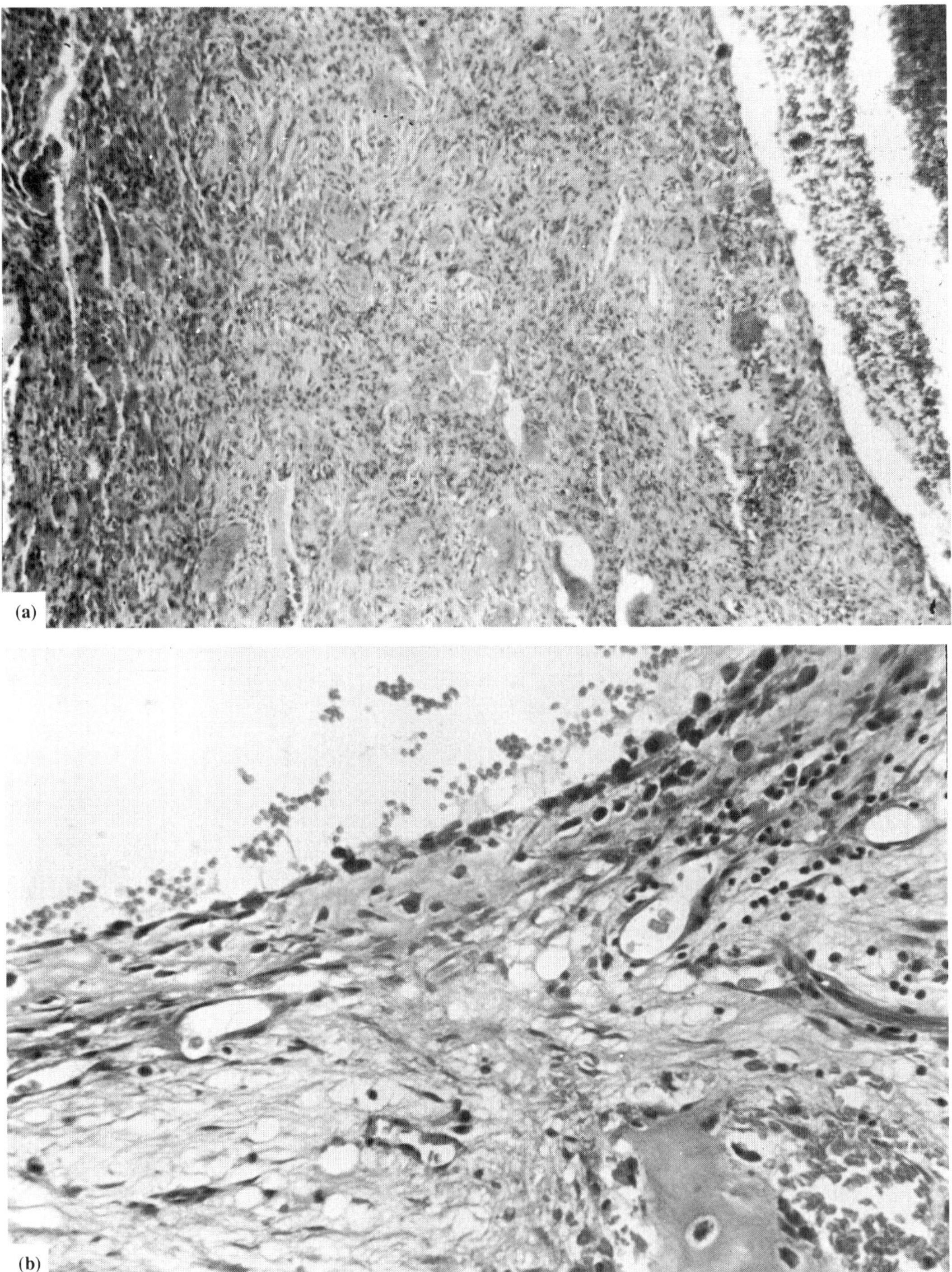

Figure 15.3 Photomicrographs of aneurysmal bone cysts. (a) The more substantial portion of a septum with ill-defined lining cells on the surfaces of a fibrovascular tissue containing scattered osteoclasts and delicate bone trabeculae. (b) A higher power view showing the lining cells, the delicate woven bone spicules and poorly cellular fibrovascular stroma.

seen in aneurysmal bone cyst (Unni, 1992).

REFERENCES

Alles, J.U. and Schulz, A. (1986) Immunocytochemical markers (endothelial and histiocytic) and ultrastructure of primary aneurysmal bone cyst. *Hum. Pathol.*, **17**, 39–45.

Dahlin, D.C. (1987) Giant-cell-bearing lesions of bone of the hands. *Hand Clin.*, **3**, 291–7.

Dahlin, D.C. and Unni, K.K. (1986) Conditions that commonly simulate primary neoplasms of bone. In *Bone Tumors*, 4th edn, Charles C. Thomas, Springfield, IL, pp. 420–30.

Edel, G., Roessner, A., Blasius, S. *et al.* (1992) 'Solid' variant of aneurysmal bone cyst. *Pathol. Res. Pract.*, **188**, 791–6.

Sanerkin, N.G., Mott, M.G. and Roylance, J. (1983) An unusual intraosseous lesion with fibroblastic, osteoclastic, osteoblastic, aneurysmal and fibromyxoid elements. 'Solid' variant of aneurysmal bone cyst. *Cancer*, **51**, 2278–86.

Schajowicz, F. (1981) Tumorlike lesions. In *Tumors and Tumorlike Lesions of Bone and Joints.* Springer-Verlag, New York, pp. 424–39.

Tsai, J.C., Dalinka, M.K., Fallon, M.D. *et al.* (1990) Fluid–fluid level: a nonspecific finding in tumors of bone and soft tissue. *Radiology*, **175**, 779–82.

Unni, K.K. (1992) 'Solid' variant of aneurysmal bone cyst. Letter to the case. *Pathol. Res. Pract.*, **188**, 796–7.

Vollmer, E., Roessner, A., Lipecki, K.H. *et al.* (1987) Biologic characterization of human bone tumors. VI. The aneurysmal bone cyst: an enzyme histochemical, electron microscopical, and immunohistochemical study. *Virchows Arch. B*, **53**, 58–65.

15.3 GANGLION OF BONE

Synonyms:
   Ganglion cyst of bone
   Intraosseous ganglion
   Periosteal ganglion

(a)   Clinical features

Ganglions are filled with a mucoid, glairy fluid (Figure 15.4). There is no association with degenerative changes in nearby joints (Dahlin and Unni, 1986).

(i)   Skeletal distribution

Ganglions occur most often in the epiphysis or metaphysis of a long bone. Very rarely, they develop in a diaphyseal location (Menendez *et al.*, 1988).

(b)   Pathology

Histologically, ganglions of bone have a thick fibrous wall and appear similar to ganglions of tendon sheath. It has been suggested that they may represent mucoid degeneration of periosteal tissue, or collections in synovial spaces in unusual locations, but neither of these explanations would seem entirely satisfactory.

REFERENCES

Dahlin, D.C. and Unni, K.K. (1986) Conditions that commonly simulate primary neoplasms of bone. In *Bone Tumors*, 4th edn, Charles C. Thomas, Springfield, IL, p. 442.

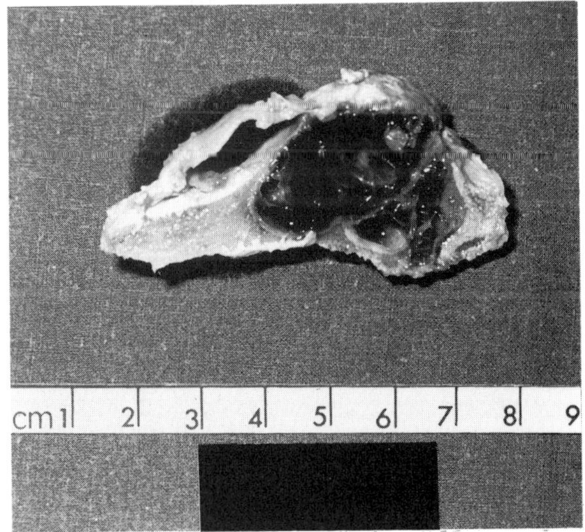

Figure 15.4 Female aged 21 years. Intraosseous ganglion of the proximal fibula.

Menendez, L.R., Chandler, D.R., Moore, T.M. *et al.* (1988) Diaphyseal intraosseous ganglion. *Clin. Orthop.*, **227**, 310–12.

15.4   EPIDERMOID CYST OF BONE

(a)   Clinical features

Epidermoid cysts are very rare bone lesions that occur exclusively in the terminal phalanges (Byers *et al.*, 1966) and skull (Roth, 1964; Dahlin and Unni, 1986). Squamous epithelium-lined cysts in the jaws are common but unrelated, as are the squamous epithelium-lined cysts sometimes seen in temporal bone following middle ear infection. Epidermoid cysts in the skull are developmental in origin, whereas those in the phalanges are believed due to traumatic implantation of epidermis.

(i)   Radiology

Epidermoid cysts expand the bone they are in and produce very sharply defined rarified defects surrounded by a thin layer of sclerotic bone (Dahlin and Unni, 1986).

(b)   Pathology

Histologically, the cysts are filled with masses of keratin flakes. A well-keratinized stratified squamous epithelium lines at least part of the cyst.

REFERENCES

Byers, P.D., Mantle, J. and Salm, R. (1966) Epidermal cysts of phalanges. *J. Bone Joint Surg.*, **48B**, 577–81.

Dahlin, D.C. and Unni, K.K. (1986) Conditions that commonly simulate primary neoplasms of bone. In *Bone Tumors*, 4th edn, Charles C. Thomas, Springfield, IL, pp. 443–4.

Roth, S.I. (1964) Squamous cysts involving the skull and distal phalanges. *J. Bone Joint Surg.*, **46B**, 1442–50.

15.5   GIANT CELL REPARATIVE GRANULOMA

(a)   Clinical features

Giant cell reparative granulomas are rare lesions. The mean age of the patients is 25 years, but the lesions are not uncommon in children under 10 years. There is a slight female predilection.

(i)   Skeletal distribution

Giant cell reparative granulomas occur predominantly in the jaws, skull and facial bones, but also in the small bones of the hands and feet (Herrmann and Goth, 1983; Caskey *et al.*, 1985; Lingg *et al.*, 1985; Merkow *et al.*, 1985; Picci *et al.*, 1986; Wold *et al.*, 1986; Dwyer *et al.*, 1989). Four cases (of varying credibility) of giant cell reparative granulomas were reported at sites other than jaws, hands and feet for the 5-year period 1985–1989. These sites were temporal bone (Lin and Huang, 1989), pituitary fossa (Siqueira *et al.*, 1989), humerus (Thomas *et al.*, 1988) and thoracic vertebra (Inoue *et al.*, 1986). A further case in a long bone (distal femur) has subsequently been reported (Hermann *et al.*, 1990) but the patient had been treated with systemic chemotherapy for a T cell lymphoma.

Isolated case reports of multicentric giant cell reparative granulomas exist (Robinson *et al.*, 1989). Clinical presentation is usually with localized pain or swelling. There are no known preceding factors. Upchurch *et al.* (1983) reported an apparent familial or geographic clustering of giant cell reparative granulomas occurring in jaws affected by Paget's disease. The treatment of giant cell reparative granuloma is thorough removal of the diseased tissues and grafting of autologous bone (Merkow *et al.*, 1985). For all sites overall, one-third to one-fifth of giant cell reparative granulomas recur; lesions in children seem to have a higher rate of recurrence compared to adults (Auclair *et al.*, 1988). Giant cell reparative granulomas of the bones of the hand also have a slightly higher recurrence rate of 39% (Dahlin, 1987).

(ii)   Radiology

Radiologically, giant cell reparative granulomas are lucent, expansile bone defects (Merkow *et al.*, 1985), which can perforate the cortex.

(b)   Pathology

Histologically, giant cell reparative granulomas show a spindle-celled fibroblastic stroma with scattered osteoclasts and areas of osteoid formation around foci of haemorrhage (Merkow *et al.*, 1985). The histological differential diagnosis is with giant cell tumour of bone and aneurysmal bone cyst. There are no histological differences between the recurrent and non-recurrent giant cell reparative granulomas that are useful in predicting the likelihood of recurrence (Auclair *et al.*, 1988). Pathogenesis is unclear; a reaction to trauma or a local disturbance of growth and/or development are possibilities.

REFERENCES

Auclair, P.L., Cuenin, P., Kratochvil, F.J. *et al.* (1988) A clinical and histomorphologic comparison of the central giant cell granuloma and giant cell tumor. *Oral Surg. Oral Med. Oral Pathol.*, **66**, 197–208.

Caskey, P.M., Wolf, M.D. and Fechner, R.E. (1985) Multicentric giant cell reparative granuloma of the small bones of the hand. A case report and review of the literature. *Clin. Orthop.*, **193**, 199–205.

Dahlin, D.C. (1987) Giant-cell-bearing lesions of bone of the hands. *Hand Clin.*, **3**, 291–7.

Dwyer, R.T., Bilous, A.M., Nade, S. *et al.* (1989) Giant cell reaction in a phalangeal bone. *Aust. N. Z. J. Surg.*, **59**, 586–9.

Hermann, G., Abdelwahab, I.F., Klein, M.J. *et al.* (1990) Giant cell reparative granuloma of the distal end of right femur. *Skeletal Radiol.*, **19**, 367–9.

Herrmann, H.J. and Goth, D. (1983) Giant cell reaction of short tubular bones. *Handchir. Mikrochir. Plast. Chir.*, **15**, 86–91.

Inoue, H., Tsuneyoshi, M., Enjoji, M. *et al.* (1986) Giant-cell reparative granuloma of the thoracic vertebra. *Acta Pathol. Jpn*, **36**, 745–50.

Lin, C.L. and Huang, T.S. (1989) Giant cell reparative granuloma in temporal bone – report of a case. *Chang Keng I Hsueh*, **12**, 62–6.

Lingg, G., Roessner, A., Fiedler, V. *et al.* (1985) Reparative giant-cell granuloma of the extremities. *ROFO* **142**, 185–8.

Merkow, R.L., Bansal, M. and Inglis, A.E. (1985) Giant cell reparative granuloma in the hand: report of three cases and review of the litera-

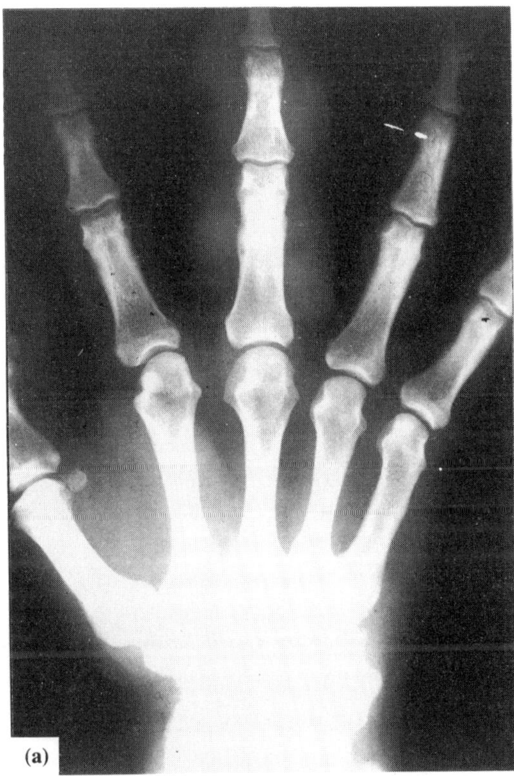

Figure 15.5 Male aged 40 years. Pigmented villonodular synovitis. (a) Radiograph of right hand showing soft tissue swelling around the middle finger. The finger was amputated because function could not be restored by excision of the lesion. Radiography courtesy of Mr P.W. Skinner.

ture. *J. Hand Surg.*, **10A**, 733–9.

Picci, P., Baldini, N., Sudanese, A. *et al.* (1986) Giant cell reparative granuloma and other giant cell lesions of the bones of the hands and feet. *Skeletal Radiol.*, **15**, 415–21.

Robinson, D., Hendel, D., Halperin, N. *et al.* (1989) Multicentric giant-cell reparative granuloma. A case in the foot. *Acta Orthop. Scand.*, **60**, 232–4.

Siqueira, E,. Tsung, J.S., Al-Kawi, M.Z. *et al.* (1989) Case report: idiopathic giant cell granuloma of the hypophysis: an unusual case of hypopituitarism. *Surg. Neurol.*, **32**, 68–71.

Thomas, I.H., Chow, C.W. and Cole, W.G. (1988) Giant cell reparative granuloma of the humerus. *J. Pediatr. Orthop.*, **8**, 596–8.

Upchurch, K.S., Simon, L.S., Schiller, A.L. *et al.* (1983) Giant cell reparative granuloma of Paget's disease of bone: a unique clinical entity. *Ann. Intern. Med.*, **98**, 35–40.

Wold, L.E., Dobyns, J.H., Swee, R.G. *et al.* (1986) Giant cell reaction (giant cell reparative granuloma) of the small bones of the hands and feet. *Am. J. Surg. Pathol.*, **10**, 491–6.

15.6 CHERUBISM

This rare heritable disorder was first described by Jones in 1933. Its incidence may be judged from the 10 cases seen between 1968 and 1984 at the Institute of Stomatology and Maxillo-facial Surgery in Paris (Chomette *et al.*, 1988). It is an autosomal dominant with variable expression and penetrance. It is usually detected in early childhood. The mandible is primarily affected, but maxillary involvement also occurs and this may extend to the orbital floor. The disease is bilateral, causing swelling of the affected bones: the mandibular enlargement gives rise to cherubic facies. Radiologically the lesions are radiolucent, with a multilocular appearance, well-defined without marginal or periosteal reactive bone. The condition has adverse effects on dentition, some teeth not developing and others being lost. The usual course is for the lesions to resolve after puberty. There is reason therefore not to interfere. But a

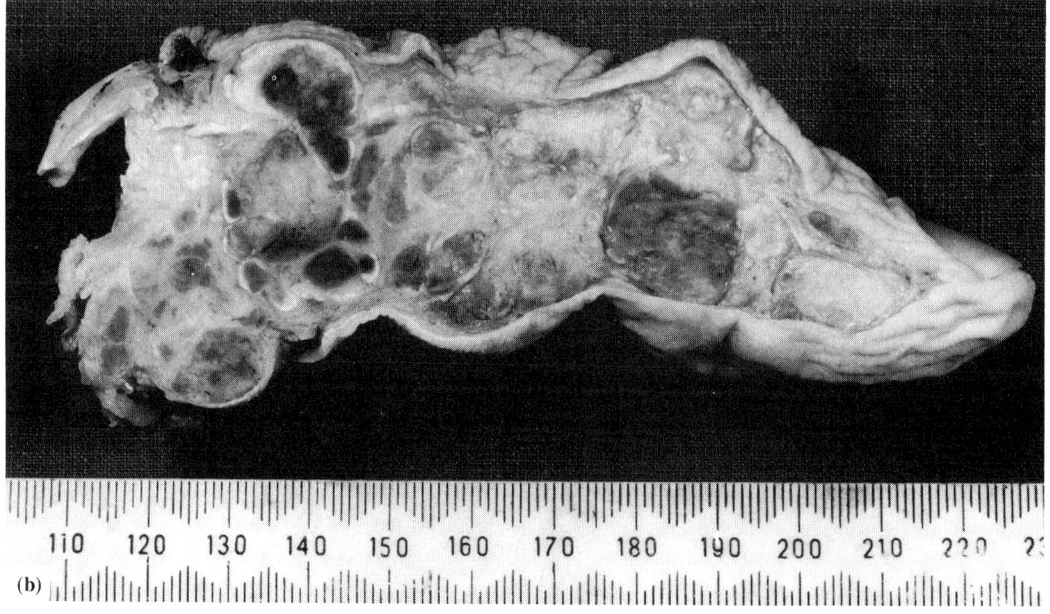

Figure 15.5 Male aged 40 years. Pigmented villonodular synovitis. (b) Longitudinal section of amputated right middle finger showing nodules of pigmented villonodular synovitis replacing most of the soft tissues. Specimen photograph courtesy of Dr W.L. Brander.

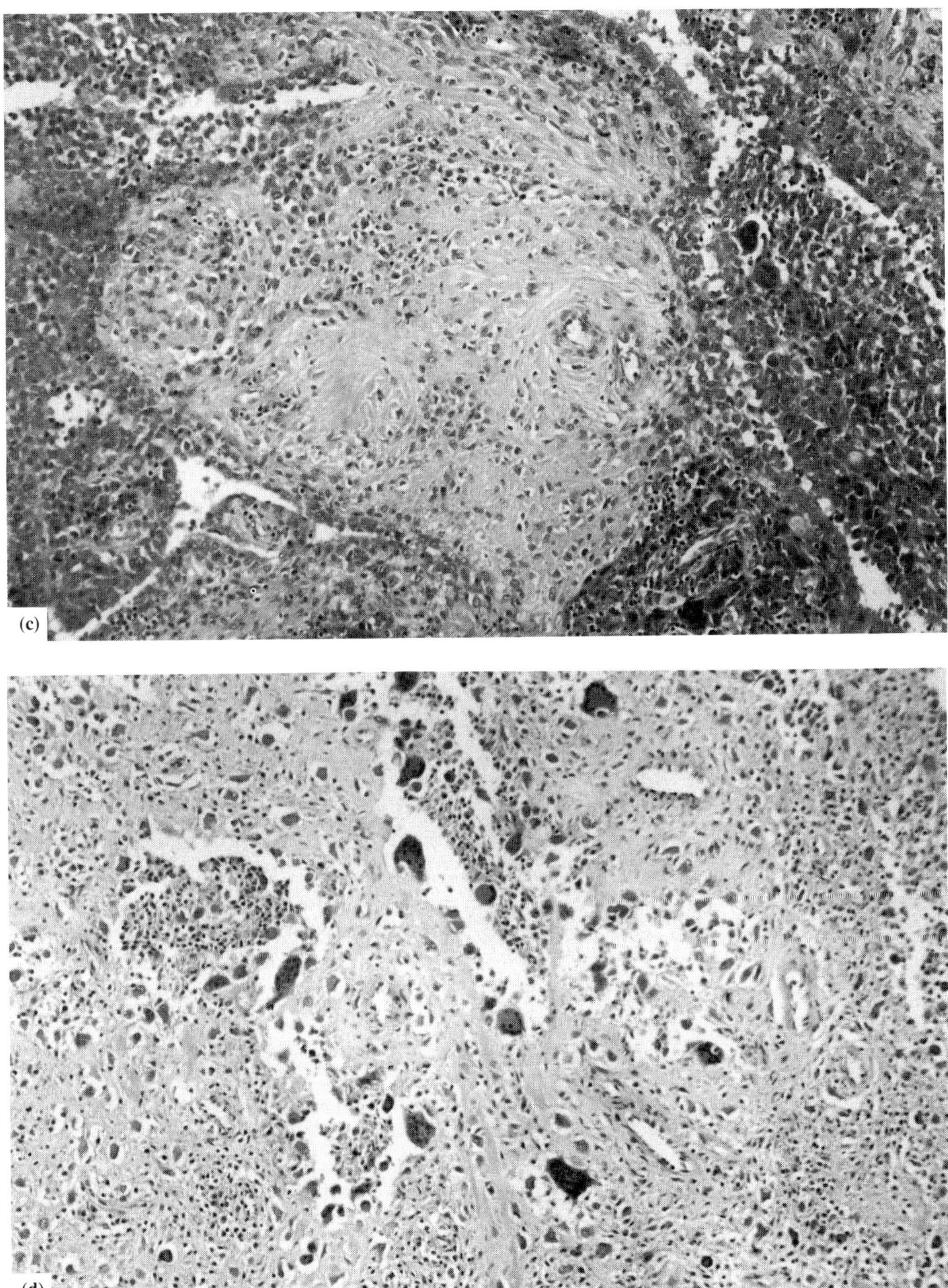

Figure 15.5 Male aged 40 years. Pigmented villonodular synovitis. (c) and (d) The variegated pattern of pigmented villonodular synovitis. This ranges from highly cellular, enlarged synovial villi with prominent lining cells and scattered osteoclasts to densely collagenous sheets and nodules containing large and small round cells and osteoclasts. In the dense tissue, osteoclasts and many of the cells are located in tissue spaces. The haemosiderin and lipid component, responsible for the light and dark areas in the gross specimen, can be made apparent by appropriate special stains.

variety of indications call for removal of tissue, and the pathology has been well established. There was a period, however, when the significance of the tissue was disputed and some classified the condition as fibrous dysplasia (Anderson and McClendon, 1962; McClendon *et al.*, 1962). But it now seems to be generally agreed that this is not fibrous dysplasia.

The tissue has the structure of fibro-vascular tissue with interspersed osteo-clasts, and is not distinguishable from giant cell reparative granuloma histol-ogically. At the purely histological level giant cell tumour and brown tumour of hyperparathyroidism might come in for consideration, but symmetry of lesions and normal serum chemistry are a neces-sary accompaniment to a diagnosis of cherubism.

REFERENCES

Anderson, D.E. and McClendon, J.L. (1962) Cherubism. Hereditary fibrous dysplasia of the jaws. I. Genetic considerations. *Oral Surg.*, **15**, suppl 2, 5–16.

Chomette, G., Auriol, M., Guilbert, F. *et al.* (1988) Cherubism: histo-enzymological and ultra-structural study. *Int. J. Oral Maxillofac. Surg.*, **17**, 219–23.

Jones, W.A. (1933) Familial multilocular cystic disease of the jaws. *Am. J. Cancer*, **17**, 946–50.

Khalifa, M.C. and Ibrahim, R.A. (1988) Cherubism. *J. Laryngol. Otol.*, **102**, 568–70.

McClendon, J.L., Anderson, D.E. and Cornelius, E.A. (1962) Cherubism. Hereditary fibrous dys-plasia of the jaws. II Pathologic considerations. *Oral Surg.*, **15**, suppl 2, 17–42.

15.7 PIGMENTED VILLONODULAR SYNOVITIS

Synonyms:
Xanthofibroma
Xanthoma of joint

(a) Clinical features

Pigmented villonodular synovitis is an uncommon lesion (Byers *et al.*, 1986) that tends to occur in young adults.

(i) Skeletal distribution

The knee joint is the commonest site. Ankle, hip, shoulder and elbow joints are also fre-quently affected, but almost any joint can be involved (Figure 15.5a,b).

Usually only a single joint is affected. Treatment is excision but complete removal may not be possible because of the diffuse nature of the process. Local recurrences are not uncommon and seem related to the adequacy of the primary procedure. Radio-therapy can be considered for treating recur-rences.

(b) Pathology

Histologically, pigmented villonodular synovitis is formed of proliferating masses of synovial tissue which form papillary projections and nodules (Figure 13.32c, d). The papillary projections are formed of foamy macrophages and haemosiderin-containing phagocytes whereas the nod-ules show variable patterns ranging from cellular to fibrotic hyaline areas. The pig-mented tissue contains abundant lipid, spaces, variable numbers of osteoclasts and a variable lymphocyte and plasma cell infil-trate. The main differential diagnosis is with repeated intra-articular haemorrhage, e.g. in haemophilia.

Pigmented villonodular synovitis can be accompanied by degenerative changes in the juxta-articular bone which produce 'cysts', particularly for lesions in the hip joint; histo-logically these 'cysts' are filled with myxoid material. Other cyst-like juxta-articular lesions result from erosion and penetration of the pigmented villonodular synovitis lesions into bone. Both these processes can be mistaken for a primary disease of bone (Dahlin and Unni, 1986).

REFERENCES

Byers, P.D., Cotton, R.E., Deacon, O.W. *et al* (1986) The diagnosis and treatment of pigmented villonodular synovitis. *J. Bone Joint Surg.*, **50B**, 290–305.

Dahlin, D.C. and Unni, K.K. (1986) Conditions that commonly simulate primary neoplasms of bone. In: *Bone Tumors*, 4th edn, Charles C Thomas, Springfield, II, p. 448.

15.8 LANGERHANS CELL HISTIOCYTOSIS

Synonyms:
  Histiocytosis X
  Eosinophilic granuloma
  Hand–Schuller–Christian disease
  Letterer–Siwe disease

(a) Clinical features

Langerhans cell histiocytosis is a complex and poorly understood entity (Osband, 1987). The term 'histiocytosis X' was originally used by Lichtenstein (1953) to describe this pathological entity. The disease is an extremely heterogeneous clinical disorder and includes infants with disseminated disease, fatal if untreated (Letterer–Siwe disease) (Donat *et al.*, 1986) as well as adults with solitary bony lesions (eosinophilic granuloma) (Makley and Carter, 1986) (Figures 15.6 and 15.7). Langerhans cell histiocytosis in childhood can present as early as 1 month of age (Matus-Ridley *et al.*, 1983).

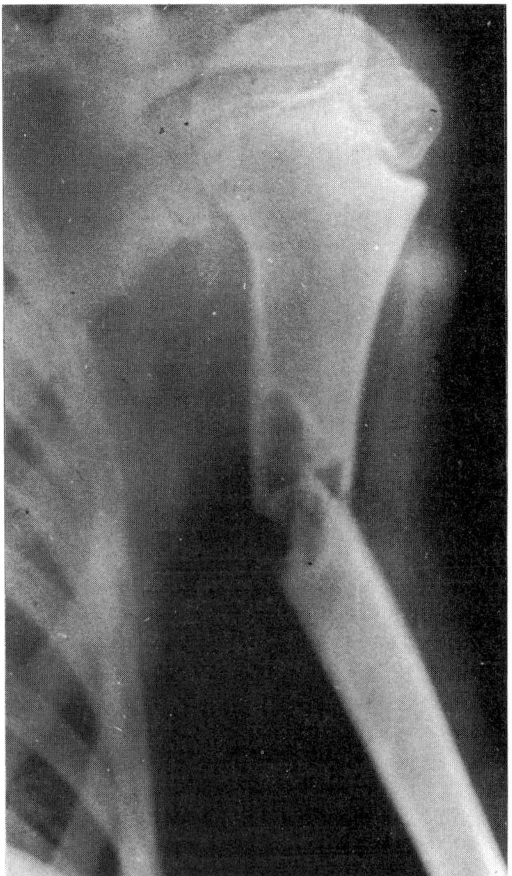

Figure 15.6 Male aged 9 years presented with pathological fracture through a benign loculated osteolytic lesion of the humerus with a well-developed sclerotic margin. The cortex has been thinned but there has been no periosteal reaction. Histology showed Langerhans cell histiocytosis.

(i) Skeletal distribution for solitary eosinophilic granulomas (from Schajowicz, 1981)

- Jaws   5%
- Skull   18%
- Other flat bones
    Ribs   9%
    Girdles
      Shoulder: clavicle, scapula,
      sternum   11%
      Pelvis: ilium, pubis, sacrum   10%
- Spine: cervical, thoracic, lumbar   8%
- Long tubular
    Femur, tibia, humerus   26%
    Fibula, radius, ulna   5%
- Hands and feet
    Short tubular
      Metacarpals, metatarsals, phalanges
    Cuboidal
      Carpals, tarsals   1.5%

Approximately two-thirds of cases of Langerhans cell histiocytosis have con-

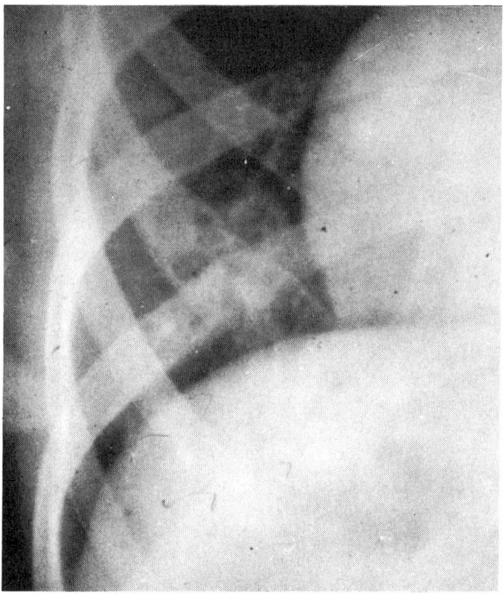

Figure 15.7 Female aged 24 years, incidental observation in a mass radiographic survey. A rib has been expanded by a well-demarcated, loculated lesion established as Langerhans cell histiocytosis histologically.

comitant or sequential osteolytic bone lesions. Abnormal liver function tests or a depressed peripheral blood count at presentation are ominous prognostic signs (Matus-Ridley *et al.*, 1983). Various treatment regimes including the use of surgery, steroids, cytotoxic chemotherapy and radiotherapy have all been used with success. Patients with localized Langerhans cell histiocytosis involving bone (eosinophilic granuloma) can be cured with surgery alone or with radiotherapy (Matus-Ridley *et al.*, 1983). By comparison, nearly one-half of patients with multifocal Langerhans cell histiocytosis (Hand–Schuller–Christian disease) develop recurrences; nevertheless, these patients have a favourable long-term outlook and do not usually require chemotherapy. Patients who have disseminated disease (Letterer–Siwe disease) generally fail to respond to treatment and die.

(b) Pathology

(i) *Histopathology*

Histologically, the cells of Langerhans cell histiocytosis show deeply folded nuclei with finely dispersed chromatin and small, inconspicuous nucleoli (Figure 15.8). The cytoplasm is abundant and eosinophilic or slightly vacuolated. Multinucleated giant cell forms and phagocytosis, including erthyrophagocytosis, may be present. Mitotic figures are usually absent and there is no nuclear atypia. An infiltrate of eosinophils usually accompanies the Langerhans cells and may be scanty or the predominant cell present.

Morphologically, Langerhans cells closely resemble the interdigitating reticulum cell of the T-dependent areas of lymph nodes (Wright and Isaacson, 1983). They can be distinguished from these cells only by the demonstration of Langerhans (Birbeck) granules by electron microscopy.

The Writing Group of the Histiocyte Society (1987) has described criteria reflecting confidence levels in diagnosis which should be used in reporting cases of Langerhans cell histiocytosis.

(ii) *Criteria of the Writing Group of the Histiocyte Society (1987) for the diagnosis of Langerhans cell histiocytosis (formerly histiocytosis X)*

1. Presumptive diagnosis: study of conventionally stained biopsy material with findings that are 'consistent' with those defined in the literature.

2. Diagnosis: an increased degree of diagnostic confidence with presumptive diagnosis plus presence of two or more features: positive stain for ATPase, S-100 protein, alpha mannosidase or peanut lectin.

3. Definitive diagnosis: requires the demonstration of Birbeck granules by elec-

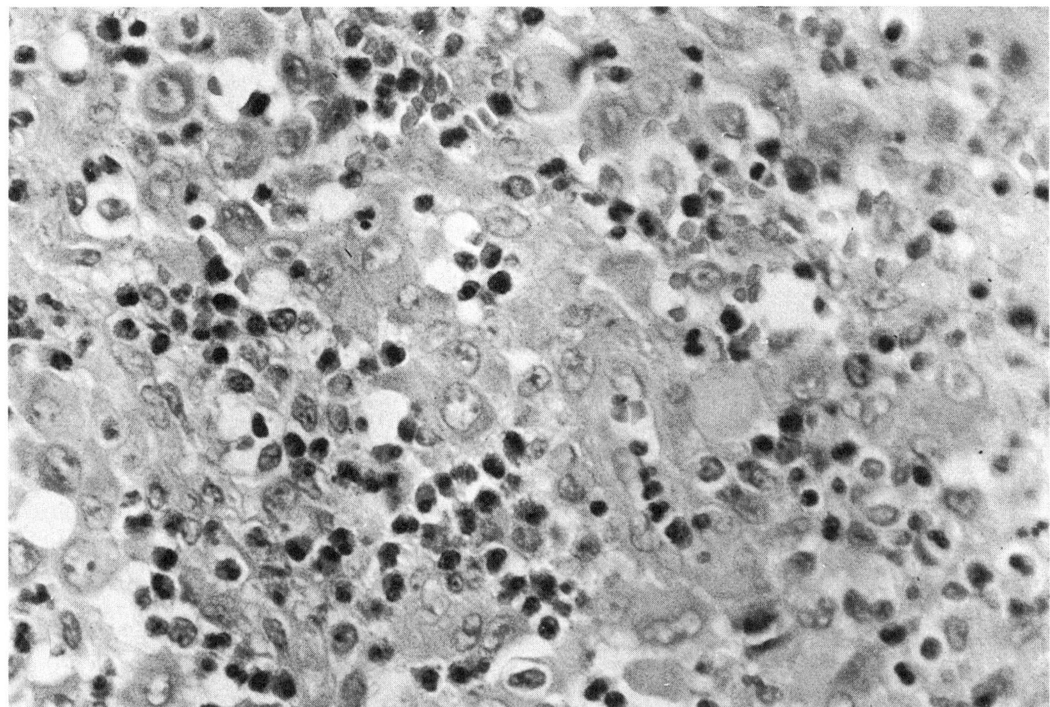

Figure 15.8 Langerhans cell histiocytosis. There is an admixture of large cells with abundant cytoplasm and vesicular nuclei, and eosinophils. Given the age of the patient and the benign radiographic appearance, these histological findings establish a presumptive diagnosis of Langerhans cell histiocytosis (see text for further diagnostic procedures).

tron microscopy or CD1 antigenic determinants (T6 positivity) on cryostat sections in the context of presumptive diagnosis or diagnosis.

(iii) Histogenesis

The Langerhans cell has been identified as the pathognomonic cell in the lesions of Langerhans cell histiocytosis and proliferates in this disease. It is unclear whether these Langerhans cells are truly normal Langerhans cells, responding appropriately to immune system signals, or if they are an abnormal variant, possibly even neoplastic (Osband, 1987). Most authors favour the position that the disease represents a non-neoplastic proliferation of Langerhans cells

(Nezelof *et al.*, 1973; Wright and Isaacson, 1983). Langerhans cells are derived from bone marrow monocytes (Katz *et al.*, 1979) which might account for the frequent occurrence of bone lesions in Langerhans cell histiocytosis.

REFERENCES

Donat, J., Fernandez-Delgado, R., Fernandez, L. *et al.* (1986) Histiocytosis X: localized and disseminated forms. Apropos of 13 cases. *An. Esp. Pediatr.*, **25**, 190–4.

Katz, S.I., Tamaki, K. and Sachs, D.H. (1979) Epidermal Langerhans cells are derived from cells originating in the bone marrow. *Nature*, **282**, 324–6.

Lichtenstein, L. (1953) Histiocytosis X: integration of eosinophilic granuloma of bone, 'Letterer-

Siwe disease' and 'Schuller–Christian disease' as related manifestations of a single nosologic entity. *Arch. Pathol.*, **56**, 84–102.

Makley, J.T. and Carter, J.R. (1986) Eosinophilic granuloma of bone. *Clin. Orthop.*, **204**, 37–44.

Matus-Ridley, M., Raney, R.B., Thawerani, H. *et al.* (1983) Histiocytosis X in children: patterns of disease and results of treatment. *Med. Pediatr. Oncol.*, **11**, 99–105.

Nezelof, C., Bassel, F. and Rousseau, M.F. (1973) Histiocytosis X: histogenetic arguments for a Langerhans cell origin. *Biomedicine*, **18**, 365–71.

Osband, M.E. (1987) Histiocytosis X. Langerhans' cell histiocytosis. *Hematol. Oncol. Clin. North Am.*, **1**, 737–51.

Schajowicz, F. (1981) Tumorlike lesions. In *Tumors and Tumorlike Lesion of Bone and Joints*. Springer-Verlag, New York, pp. 464–78.

Wright, D.H. and Isaacson, P.G. (1983) Lymphadenopathy simulating malignant lymphoma. In *Biopsy Pathology of the Lymphoreticular System*. Chapman & Hall, London, pp. 54–9.

Writing Group of the Histiocyte Society (1987) Histiocytosis syndromes in childhood. *Lancet*, **i**, 208–9.

15.9 SINUS HISTIOCYTOSIS WITH MASSIVE LYMPHADENOPATHY

Synonym: Rosai–Dorfman disease

(a) Clinical features

Sinus histiocytosis with massive lymphadenopathy (SHML) is a rare idiopathic condition that may involve bone (Walker *et al.* 1981; Foucar *et al.*, 1990). Usually the disease presents in lymph nodes or in non-osseous extranodal sites. Nine out of 33 patients with SHML involvement of bone had no evidence of lymphadenopathy (Foucar *et al.*, 1990). In some cases bone disease may represent extension from lesions growing in adjacent tissues. Unni (1988) described a lesion in the sacrum. Hamels *et al.* (1985) reported a case with greater cellular atypia than is usually seen in non-osseous sites but with benign evolution.

Radiology shows SHML in bone as well-circumscribed osteolytic lesions, sometimes multiple. Any part of a bone can be involved (Foucar *et al.*, 1990).

(b) Pathology

(i) Histopathology

Histologically, SHML shows a proliferation of a morphologically defined histiocyte subpopulation admixed with other haematolymphoid cells (Foucar *et al.*, 1990). Immunophenotyping shows that the SHML cells are true, functionally active macrophages and are not part of the family of dendritic cells (Eisen *et al.*, 1990).

REFERENCES

Eisen, R.N., Buckley, P.J. and Rosai, J. (1990) Immunophenotypic characterization of sinus histiocytosis with massive lymphadenopathy (Rosai–Dorfman disease). *Semin. Diagn. Pathol.*, **7**, 74–82.

Foucar, E., Rosai, J. and Dorfman, R. (1990) Sinus histiocytosis with massive lymphadenopathy (Rosai–Dorfman disease): Review of the entity. *Semin. Diagn. Pathol.*, **7**, 19–73.

Hamels, J., Fiasse, L. and Thiery, J. (1985) Atypical lymphohistiocytic bone tumour (osseous variant of Rosai–Dorfman disease?). *Virchows Arch. A*, **408**, 183–9.

Unni, K.K. (1988) Case report 457. Sinus histiocytosis with massive lymphadenopathy (Rosai–Dorfman disease) presenting as lesion in the sacrum. *Skeletal Radiol.*, **17**, 129–32.

Walker, P.D., Rosai, J. and Dorfman, R. (1981) The osseous manifestations of sinus histiocytosis with massive lymphadenopathy. *Am. J. Clin. Pathol.*, **75**, 131–9.

15.10 FIBROCARTILAGINOUS MESENCHYMOMA OF INFANCY

(a) Clinical features

Fibrocartilaginous mesenchymoma of infancy is a rare hamartomatous developmental malformation. It is found exclusively in newborns and the very young. The mesenchymoma always involves the chest wall although whether it arises from ribs or merely distorts them is not clear. Surgical excision can be very difficult because of the lesion's size but all patients with long-term follow-up survive free of disease (Dahlin and Unni, 1986).

(b) Pathology

Fibrocartilaginous mesenchymoma of infancy, as its name suggests, is composed largely of sheets of actively proliferating fibroblastic cells, without nuclear anaplasia, and islands of proliferating cartilage. These show maturation to well-formed bone trabeculae. Areas resembling aneurysmal bone cyst with large cavernous spaces occur not uncommonly (Moghal, 1990).

REFERENCES

Dahlin, D.C. and Unni, K.K. (1986) Conditions that commonly simulate primary neoplasms of bone. In *Bone Tumors*, 4th edn. Charles C Thomas, Springfield, IL, pp. 471–3.

Moghal, N. (1990) Vascular and cartilaginous hamartoma (mesenchymoma) of the ribs in infancy. *J. Pak. Med. Assoc.*, **40**, 114–15.

PART FOUR

The Cellular Biology of Bone

Paul D. Byers

Bone is a tissue, an organ (Figure 16.1) and an organ system. Different considerations come into play at each of these levels. They range from molecular to physical. To relate these in an integrated system requires theoretical formulations and empirical observations. The latter serves both to test and to construct the hypotheses. The hypotheses indicate the choice of empirical observation. It is possible gradually to elaborate a progressively more comprehensive structure with an increasing truth content (Magee, 1975), although the final goal may never be reached.

Frost has formulated an extended hypothesis concerning the operative and control mechanisms of the skeleton in the terms of an intermediary organization of the skeleton (Frost, 1983, 1986). Even the sketchiest acquaintance with this aids in recognizing the activities that are likely to take place in the skeleton at various times and circumstances; an understanding which can be used for explanation or prediction.

The core of his hypothesis is an hierarchical organization, each level making available to the one above some contribution essential to the latter's action. Central to this are three tissue levels, which he collectively calls the intermediary organization of the skeleton. For each of these three he has derived operating rules from clinical and laboratory studies extending over many years. The levels listed in descending order are (the abbreviation used to get around the rather lengthy nomenclature is a subscripted L (for level)):

The body – L_{is} (intact subject)
The integrated musculoskeletal system – L_{sk}
The skeletal organs – L_o
Three tissue levels – L_3, L_2, L_1
    units of the musculoskeletal system
    the organized tissue of those units
    the elemental tissues of the system

Cells – L_c
Organelles – L_{org}
Molecular activity – L_m

Some details about these are necessary to form a mental image of what they stand for.

The integrated musculoskeletal system is a reference to the articulated skeleton, with its joints, neuromuscular apparatus and neural and vascular supply.

Skeletal organs are the individual bones, intact joints, musculotendinous complexes, and other unitary complex structures.

The three tissue levels have been designated upper, middle and lower IO (intermediary organization).

1. Upper IO – L_3 – the complete structural units of the organs; e.g. joint capsule and synovium, articular cartilage, epiphysis, physis, metaphysis, the individual bone envelopes, etc. The term envelope has been used by Frost, and adopted widely, as a reference to the various bone surfaces, where the action of most bone cells take place. These surfaces (envelopes) are periosteal, osteonal, endocortical, trabecular.

2. Middle IO – L_2 – the tissues of L_3 units; e.g. capsular tissue, synovium, articular cartilage, growth cartilage, primary

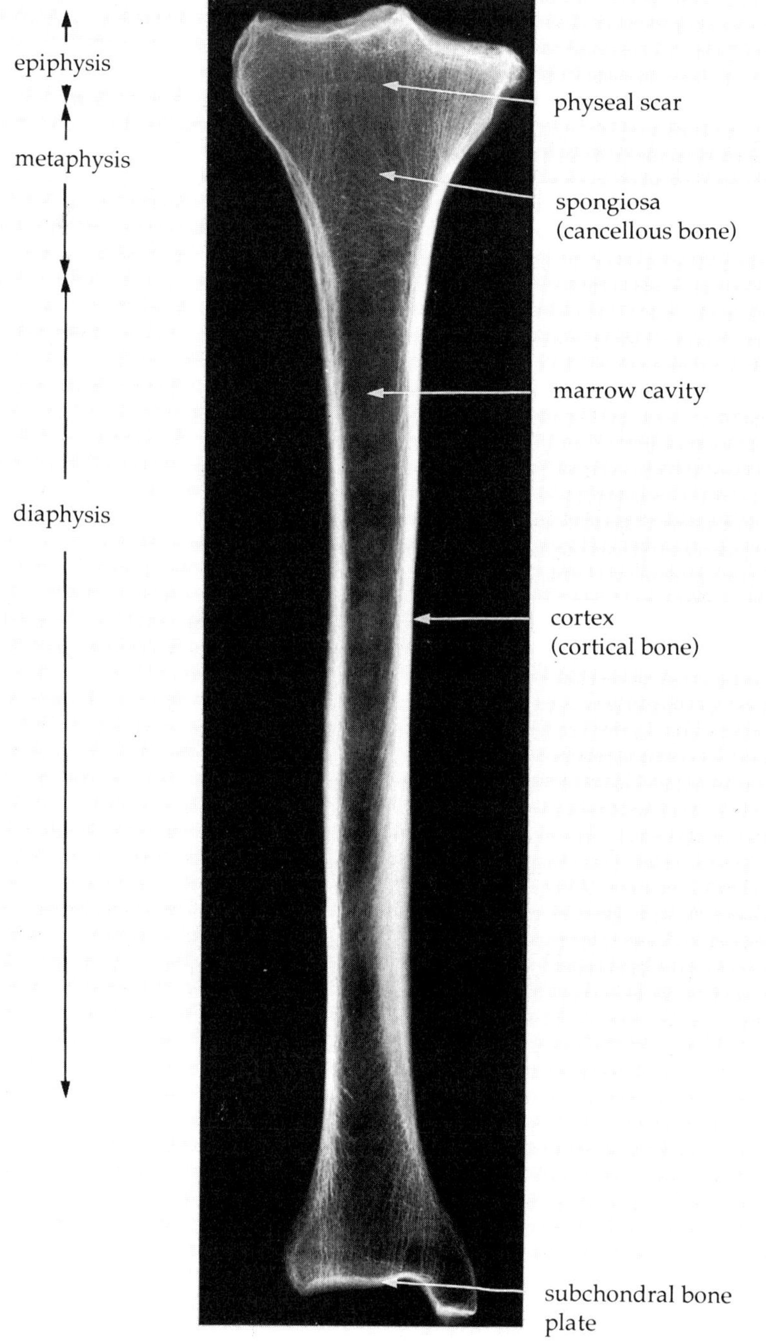

Figure 16.1 The anatomical regions of a mature bone.

spongiosa, secondary spongiosa, trabecular bone, compact bone, fibrocartilage of particular entities, collagenous tissue of the entities it forms, etc.

3. Lower IO – L_1 – lamellar bone, woven bone, hyaline cartilage, elastic cartilage, fibrocartilage, fibrous tissue, synovial tissue, etc.

Cells refers to the cells of the skeletal system, as discussed in following chapters.

Organelles are the membrane-bound compartments of the cell (Table 16.1), segregating various functions. This compartmentalization allows many thousands of different chemical reactions to be carried out simultaneously.

Molecules are the chemical entities of cells and tissues as shown in Table 16.2. In a mammalian cell the protein is in the order of 10^{10} molecules of 10 000 different kinds.

The overall concept is that at each level there are rules which determine the activities therein; these activities are independent of those in the level above, but dependent on the contribution from the level below. Controls are extrinsic, either systemic or local, or intrinsic. The hypothesis as it now stands elaborates these points for the three levels of the intermediary organization. All its detail requires a book on its own, and exceeds what is useful for present purposes. But there are some points which are of value to present here, and others which will find a place in other parts of this book. Elements of the scheme have been published in the periodical press recently, and are listed below.

It is obvious, although not something which immediately springs to mind, that this system, hierarchical in organization, is so in terms of scales of size and of time. Thus the lowest level incorporates the smallest physical entities which operate over the shortest distances and do so in the shortest time. As one moves up through the system larger and larger units of structure are encountered whose formation, modification or action takes place over progressively longer times. These time/domains are an important feature of aspects of the hypothesis and will be referred to in other sections.

Mow *et al.* (1992) also discuss hierarchical systems and advance cartilage and joints as a paradigm for hierarchical materials and structures.

Embryology is much concerned at present with the first few levels of this system, an interest which finds expression in the exploration of self-assembly of smaller into larger molecular structures, and of the latter into organelles and other component structures of the cell. Such activities lie outside the strict limits of concern to histopathology. Nevertheless they do feed upwards, where, under the appropriate stimuli, the histogenesis of tissues and their subsequent morphogenesis is a function of the first IO level. The formation of tissue necessarily involves growth and the organization of its products. This latter process can be termed micromodelling,

Table 16.1 Relative volumes of major intracellular compartments in a typical liver cell

Compartment	% cell volume	Number/cell
Cytosol	54	1
Mitochondria	22	1700
Rough ER cisternae	9	1
Smooth ER cisternae + Golgi cisternae	6	
Nucleus	6	1
Peroxisomes	1	400
Lysosomes	1	300
Endosomes	1	200

Table 16.2 The approximate chemical composition of a bacterial cell

	% total cell weight
Water	70
Inorganic ions	1
Miscellaneous small metabolites	3
Proteins	18
RNA	1.1
DNA	0.25
Phospholipids	3
Other lipids	2
Polysaccharides	2

and is responsible for the collagen organization, disposition of cells and other matrical components of connective tissues, e.g. cartilage, woven and lamellar bone, tendon, and so on. But there is a need for a higher level of the organization of growth, as exemplified by the physis where addition at the margins of new vertically oriented clones is required to increase the diameter. Or, in the case of bone, the provision of additional packets of bone in the remodelling activity (qv). These activities are postulated to be a function of the second IO level. Both these levels of growth respond to stimuli, extrinsic or intrinsic to the tissue, by altering the rate and duration of their action, or even ceasing temporarily.

Given normal physiology and genetics, the most potent stimulus to these L_2 tissues is from physical activity. The hypothesis elaborates principles of skeletal adaptation to mechanical usage (macromodelling, generally abbreviated to modelling) to account for observations of skeletal alteration during growth under normal and abnormal conditions. There are rules for bone, cartilage and fibrous tissues, in descending order of elaboration.

(Macro) modelling is presented as an activity primarily found during growth; it is, to a great degree, conditional on growth, and is responsible for the final shape of the bones and joints, and dimensions of ligaments and tendons. However, some vestiges of its activity remain in all three tissues of the adult skeleton. The system that alters bone tissue in the adult is remodelling. This is also present during growth, but then primarily as a means of substitution of one tissue for another during the conversion of the primary spongiosa to its secondary state.

The (macro) modelling and remodelling components of the hypothesis as applied to bone have found the widest critical acceptance and come to form an underlying tenet of histomorphometry. They are the result of the controlled activity of osteoclasts and osteoblasts. In modelling each of these two types of bone cells, osteoclasts and osteoblasts, act over a large surface, removing or forming relatively large volumes of bone. The control of where and for how long they act contributes to the shape and architecture of the region. By working on opposite surfaces of a structure, such as the endosteal (osteoclasts) and periosteal (osteoblasts) of diaphyseal cortex, they enlarge it, literally moving the cortex relative to a fixed point. This movement led to the use of the term 'drift' with respect to them, a word, in general use, which conveys the act of driving or that which is driven (*Concise Oxford English Dictionary*). Thus, one speaks of a resorption drift, a formation drift, and, collectively, a modelling drift. Whereas modelling is devoted in the main to shaping the skeleton, is active mainly in the growth period and has a less apparent unit structure, remodelling is active throughout life, has a well delineated format, and serves to modify skeletal shape, architecture, bone volume and to repair microdamage. The functional unit of remodelling is the Basic Multicellular Unit (BMU). Working on a bone surface, osteoclasts remove a small amount of bone; they are followed by osteoblasts which fill the excavation with osteoid that is mineralized to become bone. The operation of this simple process in terms of the sites and numbers that are activated, rates and volumes of bone removal and osteoid formation and mineralization, determines many features of the skeleton. As multicellular units, combining the activity of both osteoclasts and osteoblasts, they are regarded as an entity belonging to the second level IO. Further details of these and their contribution to the understanding of bone physiology and pathology are given in the chapters on bone growth, bone reactions, and metabolic bone disease.

REFERENCES AND FURTHER READING

Frost, H.M. (1983) The skeletal intermediary organisation. *J. Metab. Bone Dis.*, **4**, 281–90.

Frost, H.M. (1986) *The Intermediary Organisation of the Skeleton.* 2 volumes. CRC Press, Boca Raton, FL.

Frost, H.M. (1989) Some ABCs of skeletal pathophysiology. Introduction to the series. *Calcif. Tissue Int.*, **45**, 1–3.

Frost, H.M. (1989) General mediator properties. *Calcif. Tissue Int.*, **45**, 68–70.

Frost, H.M. (1989) Bone balance and the delta B.BMU. *Calcif. Tissue Int.*, **45**, 131–3.

Frost, H.M. (1989) The transient/steady state distinction. *Calcif. Tissue Int.*, **45**, 134–6.

Frost, H.M. (1991) Microdamage physiology. *Calcif. Tissue Int.*, **49**, 229–31.

Frost, H.M. (1991) The growth/modelling/remodelling distinction. *Calcif. Tissue Int.*, **49**, 301–2

Frost, H.M.(1991) Tissue mechanisms controlling bone mass. *Calcif. Tissue Int.*, **49**, 303–4.

Frost, H.M. (1992) The trivial physiologic/pathologic distinction. *Calcif. Tissue* Int., **50**, 105–6.

Frost, H.M. (1990) Skeletal structural adaptations to mechanical usage (SATMU). Redefining Wolff's Law: the bone modelling problem. *Anat. Rec.*, **226**, 403–13; 414–22.

Frost, H.M. (1990) The hyaline cartilage modelling problem. *Anat. Rec.*, **226**, 423–32.

Frost, H.M. (1990) Mechanical influences on intact fibrous tissue. *Anat. Rec.*, **226**, 433–9.

Magee, B. (1975) *Popper.* Fontana Modern Masters (ed. F. Kermode), Fontana/Collins.

Mow, V.C., Ratcliffe, A. and Poole, A.R. (1992) Cartilage and diarthrodial joints as paradigms for hierarchical materials and structures. *Biomaterials*, **13**, 67–97.

ASPECTS OF THE EMBRYOLOGY OF THE SKELETAL SYSTEM

Paul D. Byers

The early decades of this century saw the virtual completion of the morphological description of embryogenesis, and its last few decades are witnessing the initiation and advance of the understanding of the underlying control mechanisms as a result of the growth of cellular and molecular biology (Alberts *et al.*, 1989). Even though very far from complete, the knowledge already gained brings embryogenesis within the compass of practical imagination. A comprehensive discussion is beyond the scope of this book but a few comments will serve as a reminder or as an introduction to some of these mechanisms. Illustrations of the development of the musculoskeletal system are provided to have at hand in connection with any consideration of skeletal dysplasias. The possibility of such a request is increased by the growing demand for information about birth defects, both in general and with respect to individual cases, for purposes of genetic counselling. In any case, the paucity of histopathological information about most of these conditions behoves pathologists to collect data whenever possible. Information on this point is described in Chapter 5. Because the appearance of the face is often a consideration in the classification of these disorders it is helpful to know something of its development, which is also described.

Cells have the ability to respond to intra-cellular and intercellular messages in electronic, ionic, molecular or macromolecular form. This necessitates a complexity of organization for receiving sorting and routing the messages. In essence this is dependent on chemical stratification (inorganic and organic; lipid, carbohydrate and protein) and membrane compartmentalization. This stratification is already present in the oocyte through the differential distribution of the contents of the cytosol, so that, from the beginning, division results in difference, leading to asymmetry – head and tail, back and front – an essential requirement for positional information. The nature of the contact between cells is also a determining factor in the transmission of messages: tight and gap junctions preclude and permit diffusion between cells; chemical pumps rapidly move small molecules and ions in and out; receptors select from the array of large messenger molecules in their environment.

Chemical control and management is basically through the agency of proteins, whose manufacture is the function of genes in the form of DNA. Since all the cells of an individual derive from one cell, and since there is no evidence that any of the genetic component of cells is lost during development, the differences between cells must ultimately rest on various controls of gene expression. For example, the folding of the long DNA molecule to expose only a predetermined, limited segment for the manufacture of a specified protein, and the transmission of this pattern of DNA folding to daughter cells would ensure that they performed the same function as the parent – a property spoken of as cell memory, a necessary requirement for the establishment and stability of tissues. It is evident from experiment that many cells in the developing embryo, often at a very early stage, experience an event, which is 'remembered', that will ultimately result in their progeny assuming a particular role – they have been determined. The mechanism of determination is not clear, nor what takes place when the cell finally differentiates, that is, performs what it has been determined to do. In the hypothetical instance cited here that would be manifest by the folding of the DNA and the production of the specified protein. If there were no mechanism for undoing this folded pattern then the cells would be at an end-stage differentiation. Otherwise they might revert to some other role on demand. Differentiation is not always determined; uncommitted cells differentiate in response to local demands, and may afterwards revert to their original state.

Notwithstanding the simplistic nature of the foregoing, it serves to make the point that the growth and development of the embryo is a phenomenon ultimately explicable in molecular biological terms. It is possible to explore the complexities of the systems of controls and responses, or to enquire into the

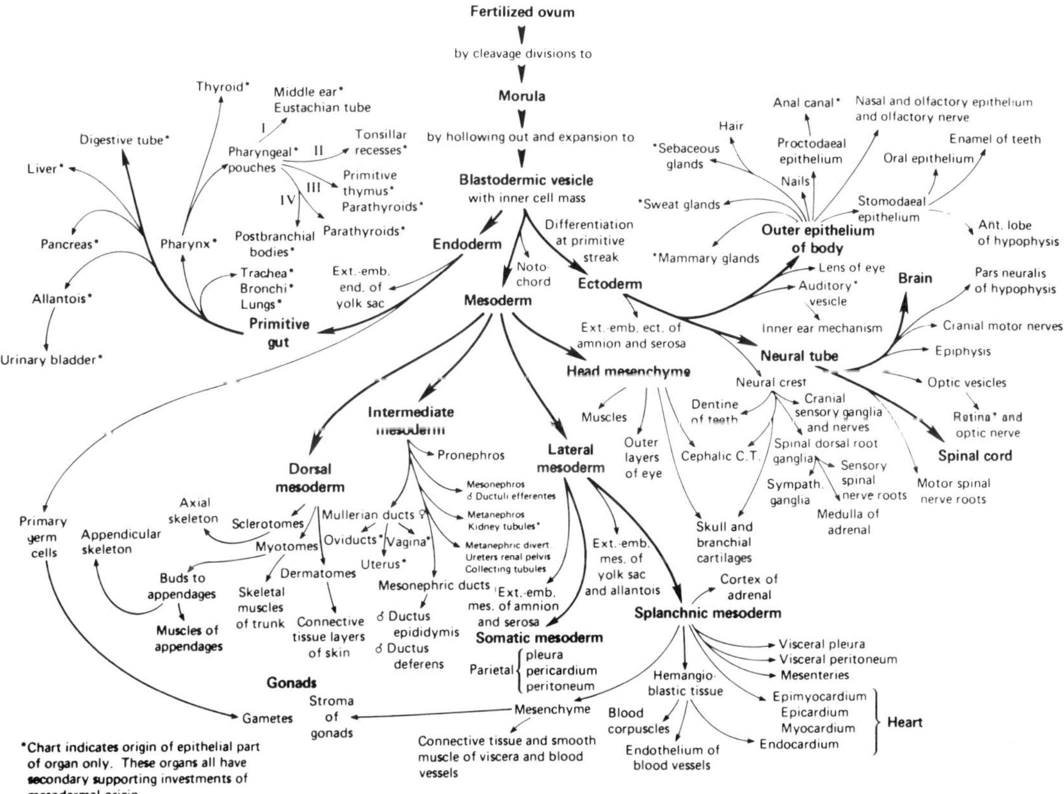

Figure 17.1 An outline of the progressive differentiation of cells to form the tissues of the body. (From Carlson (1985), reproduced with permission of publisher and author.)

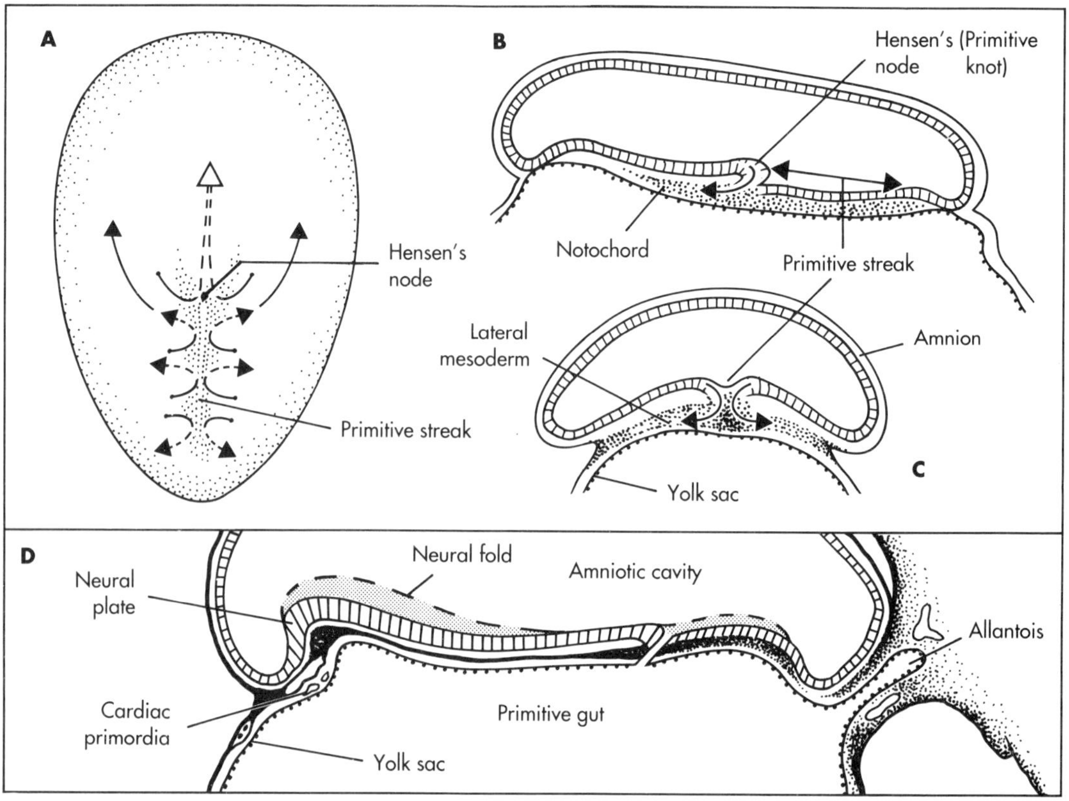

Figure 17.2 The embryonic disc at day 15, surface view (a) and longitudinal (b) and transverse (c) sections. From the ridges of the primitive streak cells are migrating through the groove cells to spread laterally and forward between the ectoderm and endoderm. Cells from the knot are also migrating, to form the notochord, which will extend forward between the epithelial layers above and below and the mesoderm on either side. The cavity of the primitive pit extends through the notochord and communicates with the york sac to form the neurenteric canal In (d) the notochord is fully developed and the ectoderm has formed the neural plate; the neural folds, indicted by the dotted line, lie outside the plane of the section, as does the lateral mesoderm whose two arms meet anteriorly and develop into the heart. The primitive node and the neurenteric canal are present, but the streak is regressing and submerging under the developing neural plate. (Redrawn from Carlson, 1985, with permission.)

fundamentals and their origin. In the former case, among the principles to be considered are:

- Cell migration
- Induction
- Position information
- Pattern formation
- Molecular genetics
- Morphogenesis

In the second case the question of intrinsic determinants at the molecular level, expressed in the self-assembly of at least some macromolecules, given that there is a mixture of the basic structural units, is paramount. A study of this activity is at the heart of molecular biology (Miller, 1984).

In the following account of the development of the musculoskeletal system, based on Moore (1988) and Patten (Carlson, 1985), there is no attempt to detail the operation of the foregoing mechanisms in controlling or determining successive stages. The interested reader is referred to the literature on developmental and cellular biology (e.g. Thorogood, 1983; Jacobson and Sater, 1988; Thorogood and Tickle, 1988; Alberts *et al.*, 1989).

The tissues of the musculoskeletal system arise from the intraembryonic mesoderm. To retrace the genealogy of the mesoderm is to arrive at the fertilized ovum. Going forward

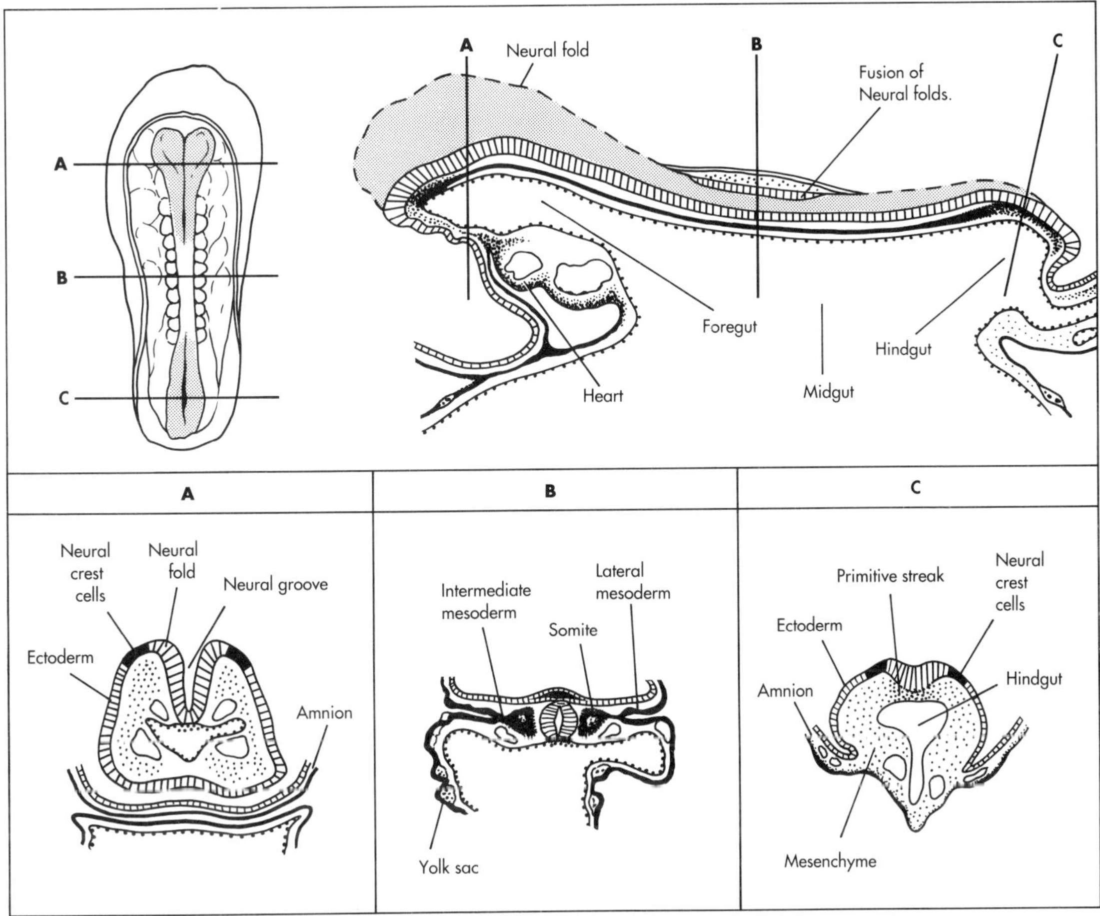

Figure 17.3 The embryonic disc at day 18–19 (7–8 somites): (a) surface view, (b) longitudinal and (c–e) transverse sections. The neural folds flank the neural groove at the cranial and caudal ends. In the mid-region the neural tube is complete and the somites (aggregations of mesodermal cells) have formed laterally at this level. The height of the neural folds are indicated by a dotted outline. At the cervical level the folds have fused, and the neural crest cells have detached and lie between the fused ectoderm and neural tube. The neurenteric canal has closed, the node has disappeared, and the streak has regressed to a cellular collection at the caudal end beneath the neural plate. The transverse sections show these changing relationships. Development of the mesoderm produces the somites, intermediate and lateral mesoderm. The last is in two layers; one becomes intimately associated with the ectoderm to form the somatopleure, the other with the endoderm, the splanchnopleure. This association is not stressed in Figure 17.1. (Redrawn from Carlson, 1985, with permission.)

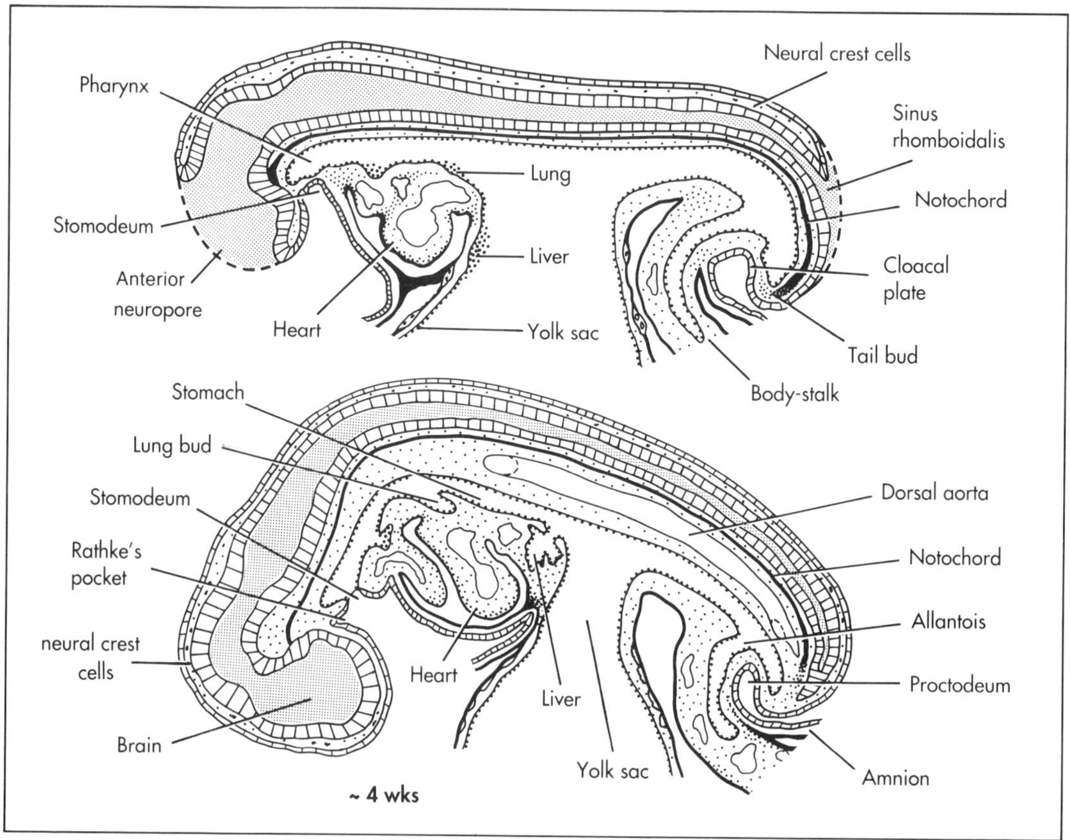

Figure 17.4 Longitudinal sections of the embryonic plate: (a) at 22 days (14 somites) and (b) at approx. 4 weeks (segmentation complete). As closure of the neural tube progresses neural crest cells are released. The streak regresses to become the tail bud and then disappears. Longitudinal (and lateral) folding (see Figure 17.8) contribute to the formation of the body cavity; attention is drawn to the stomodeum and the oropharyngeal membrane. The illustrations do not show the contemporaneous developments in the somites (see Figures 17.8–17.11). (Redrawn from Carlson, 1985, with permission.)

from this starting point, which itself is the end point of much biological activity at the cellular and molecular level, carries one through 15 days of human embryonic development before cells recognizable as mesodermal tissue are deployed. At the start of the 15th day the embryo is the bilayer disc at the conjunction of two sacs, the amnion and the secondary yolk sac. Near a margin of the disc, cells of the amniotic portion (epiblast) heap up in two parallel linear mounds with a groove between; the whole, identified as the primitive streak, expresses the orientation of the embryo. The streak is at the caudal edge of the disc, is short, terminates in the prominence of the primitive knot, and undergoes limited growth from its caudal end causing the whole to move cranially in the disc. These developments are accomplished towards the end of the 15th day.

Over the ensuing five days the developments of immediate concern to skeletal formation are the appearance of the mesoderm, and the formation of the notochord, of the primordia of the CNS, and of the neural crest. These developments are in part syn-

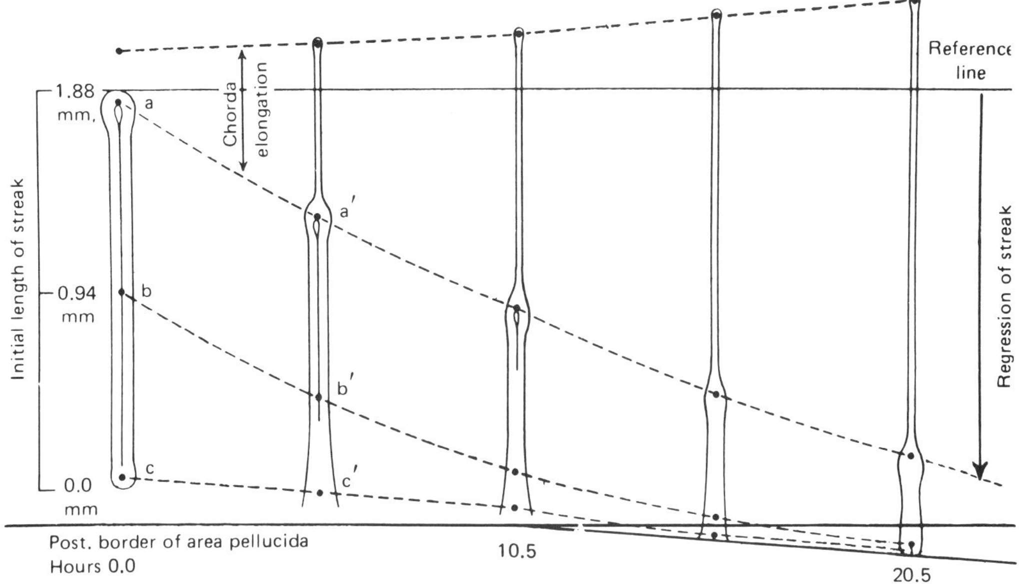

Figure 17.5 The regression of the primitive streak in the chick. It has virtually disappeared in 24 h. The complete developmental time for a chick is about 500 h. (Redrawn from Carlson, 1985, with permission.)

chronous and in part successive; to describe them briefly means describing them separately; but, their relationships are shown in the illustrations.

1. The mesoderm: cells migrate (Figure 17.2a, arrows) from the primitive streak, intruding as a third layer between the other two, extending forward, around the developments in the central axis.

2. The notochord is shown in Figures 17.2–17.4, 17.6 and 17.8–17.11. In the central axis, cells from the region of Hensen's node migrate into the plane between the bilayer to form the notochordal process, which, as it develops, acts as an inducer in developments of axial tissues. Under its influence, cells in the contiguous ectoderm develop into the neural plate. The extending notochordal process is canalized from a pit in the primitive knot. The pit in the knot is open to the amnionic cavity and further develop-

ment creates a communication between amnion and yolk sac, the neurenteric canal (Figure 17.2d). Growth of the notochord and of the neural plate and its gradual transformation to the neural canal is accompanied by closure of the neurenteric canal and the later atrophy of the knot and the primitive streak (Figure 17.5); failure of these to go to completion can result in sacrococcygeal teratoma and neurenteric cysts of the vertebral column, respectively.

3. The central nervous system: turning back to the neural plate, which is formed progressively, as the embryo lengthens, from ectoderm under the influence of the notochord: it soon acquires the paired, longitudinal neural folds which bound the neural groove (Figure 17.3). The folds rise up and then fuse to form the neural tube.

4. The neural crest (Figures 17.3 and 17.4): This is formed of cells at the

neuroectodermal junction, which come to lie at the crest of the neural folds, where they are continuous with the ectoderm. These three paired tissues are involved at the fusion which forms the neural tube: each pair establishes contact and separates from the other two. Thus, continuity of the ectoderm is established, the neural tube is formed, and the narrow band of neural crest tissue comes to lie between the other two.

The neural crest, an important tissue, is composed of migratory cells, which disperse widely and contribute to many tissues. Exact knowledge of this is still accumulating. There are some species variations; in mammals the following tissues can be listed (Figures 17.6 and 17.7):

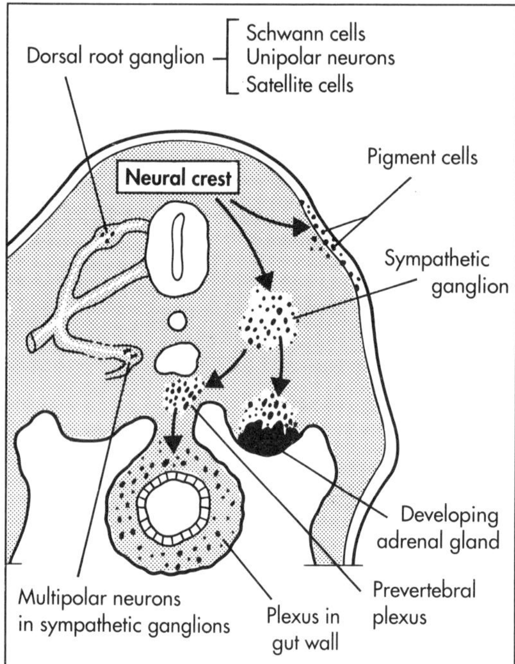

Figure 17.6 Schematic representation of neural crest cell migration and their destinations in the trunk. For the neural crest contribution to the skull see Figure 17.7. (Redrawn from Carlson, 1985, with permission.)

- Chondrocranium
- Jaws
- Teeth
- Ganglia
    spinal
    sympathetic
    enteric
- Chromaffin cells
- Melanophores
- Some APUD cells
- Schwann cells

The limit of the forward growth of the notochord and the neural plate is the site where the mouth will form (Figures 17.3, 17.4 and 17.9); at the stages discussed here this is known as the prochordal plate, but later is called the oropharyngeal membrane. The two extending sheets of mesoderm, one on either side of the neural plate, pass beyond and around this and meet (Figure 17.2); within the mesoderm of this conjunction is the cardiogenic area.

Even as the sheet of mesoderm is extending, developments within it are taking place (Figure 17.3b). Three regions are discernible: paraxial, intermediate and lateral. The first becomes a thick band parallel to the notochord which gradually segments transversely. Of the 42–44 somites finally formed (occipital, 4; cervical, 8; thoracic, 12; lumbar, 5; sacral, 5; coccygeal, 8–10), six to eight disappear; the remainder contribute to the axial skeleton (the base of the skull to the coccyx) and its soft tissues, and to the dermis. This is accomplished by divisions of the somites into three elements (Figure 17.8); each of these, following migration to them of neural crest cells, gives rise to various tissues:

1. The sclerotome – axial skeleton
2. The myotome – musculature
3. The dermal plate – dermal and subcutanous tissues

The intermediate layer of the mesoderm gives rise to the urogenital system through

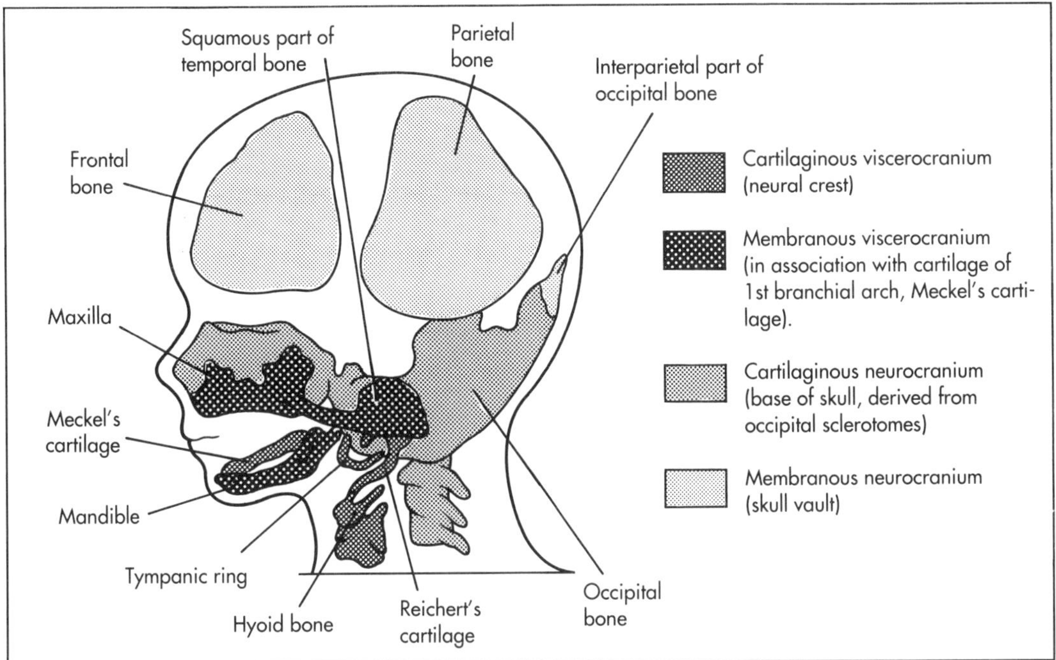

Figure 17.7 Diagram illustrating the origins and development of the major bones of the skull. (Redrawn from Carlson, 1985, with permission.)

its transformation into the nephrogenic cord which separates from the paraxial and lateral mesoderm and reaches a position in the posterior wall of the embryonic coelom (i.e. the peritoneal cavity) where it forms the nephrogenic ridge.

The lateral mesoderm is the thinnest portion. Within it, coalescing spaces form which result in a horseshoe canal extending from side to side around the cranial end. This is the intraembryonic coelom, which communicates laterally with the extraembryonic coelom (effectively the chorionic cavity). The dorsal wall of the intraembryonic coelom, a combination of mesoderm and ectoderm recognized as the somatopleure, will contribute to forming the body cavities, whereas the ventral wall, endoderm and mesoderm splanchnopleure, will form the connective tissue and smooth muscle of the viscera and vessels.

The foregoing events have been taking place in the embryonic disc, which has acquired a pear-shaped silhouette owing to more rapid growth of the cranial portion. The folding of the disc (Figures 17.4 and 17.6) at this stage, both in the longitudinal and the transverse axis establishes the corporate structure with the somatic and splanchnic mesoderm in their appropriate position to contribute to the development of the body.

Following the folding of the embryo the limbs develop as outgrowths of the somatic mesoderm and overlying ectoderm; the initial ectodermic cover has a controlling role in limb development and is identified as the ectodermal ridge. There is conflict of opinion about the role of migrant sclerotomal and myotomal cells as the source of bone and muscle in the limb bud, as opposed to differentiation of somatic mesoderm (Aoyama and Asamoto, 1988). In the limb the apical ectodermal ridge maintains a zone of undifferentiated mesenchyme at the tip, the progress zone; it is hypothesized that the pattern of development along the proximodistal axis depends on how long cells spend at the tip (Carrington and Fallon, 1988).

However it may be achieved, as the limb buds grow the rudiments of the bones, muscles and connective tissues appear and develop with time.

Cartilage and bone form within pre-existing mesenchyme (mesodermal connective tissue) by transformation of cells to the type which produces the appropriate interstitial matrix. With the exception of the craniofacial bones and the clavicle, cartilage models of the bones are formed, later to be ossified. Apart from those of the skull and face, there are some differences in detail between model formation in the axial and appendicular skeletons. In the latter, the mesenchyme of the limb bud is continuous and the models of individual bones occur as discrete foci of chondrification. The joint forms in the (interzonal) mesenchyme between them (Figure 17.11). This involves the formation peripherally of the capsule and ligaments (and centrally in the case of the knee); and the formation centrally of a cavity, lined by synovial cells which differentiate from the mesenchyme.

The difference in the detail of the models of the axial skeleton (comprising the skull, vertebral column, ribs and sternum, and pelvis) concern mainly the spine. Vertebrae develop from the segmented sclerotome of the paraxial mesoderm (see above). Cells migrate anteriorly to surround the notochord, posteriorly to envelop the neural tube, and into the body wall to form the ribs. Anteriorly, the paired segments fuse across the midline (Figures 17.8 and 17.9), enclosing the notochord. Additionally, each segment has a cranial and a caudal layer; the former of one segment fuses with the latter of the segment above to form a vertebral body, and the intervertebral disc appears at the boundary between the two layers of the segment. Although it is widely held that the notochord is responsible for the formation of the nucleus pulposus, not all the evidence supports this. As in other bones chondrification follows the establishment of the mesenchymal anlage (Figure 17.10).

The pattern of development of the skull and facial bones is depicted in Figure 17.7.

Joints are of three types. Synovial joints which have been described above, are the only ones with a defined interarticular space. In fibrous joints the two parts are joined by fibrous tissue; the joints of the cranium are typical, whereas the intervertebral joints are a modified form. In cartilaginous joints the connecting tissue is fibrocartilage (e.g. symphysis pubis) or hyaline cartilage (e.g. costochondral).

Myoblasts are responsible for the muscles.

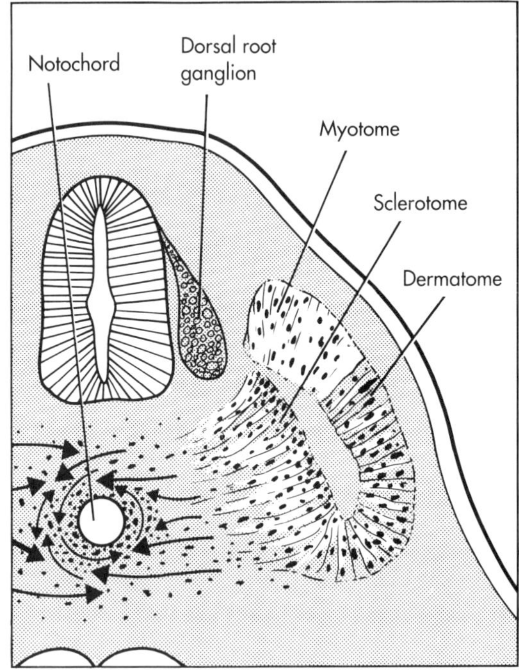

Figure 17.8 Schematic representation of the differentiation of the somite into myotome, dermatome and sclerotome. Cells from the last migrate to surround the notochord. Further developments here are depicted in Figure 17.9. (Redrawn fron Carlson, 1985, with permission.)

It seems more probable that their source is myotomal cells migrating at the time of limb bud formation. However that may be, they first form the main muscle mass (e.g. flexor) and later the individual entities. Myoblasts aggregate in syncytia in the form of myotubes within which muscle filaments are made and organized. Innervation is by penetration of axons from dorsal root ganglia, which establish both central and peripheral connections. The segmental innervation of the limb is probably achieved by a combination of guidance to the ingrowing axons (although the detail of how this is managed is far from clear) and the removal of those neurones that become wrongly connected (how this would be recognized and the removal accomplished is also unknown).

The vascular development throughout the body is said to be opportunistic. That is its control lies outside the presently known inductive/differentiative pathways, and the angioblasts appear to respond to local demand, a characteristic they retain in adults.

The following is a description of the external developments in the formation of the face, with a few details of the cellular and tissue developments (Wedden *et al.*, 1988). The time covered is roughly 4 to 10 weeks (Figures 17.12a, b and 17.13).

At the beginning of this period the prominent bulge of the head which will become the forehead and contribute the bridge and apex of the nose – the frontonasal process – overhangs the opening of the stomodaeum. Below the stomodaeum, as part of its floor, is the bulge of the pericardium. The space between these two prominences is bounded on either side by the first pair of branchial arches. The stomodaeum itself is cut off from the primitive gut by the oropharyngeal membrane which is at the point of disintegration. On the ventrolateral surface of the

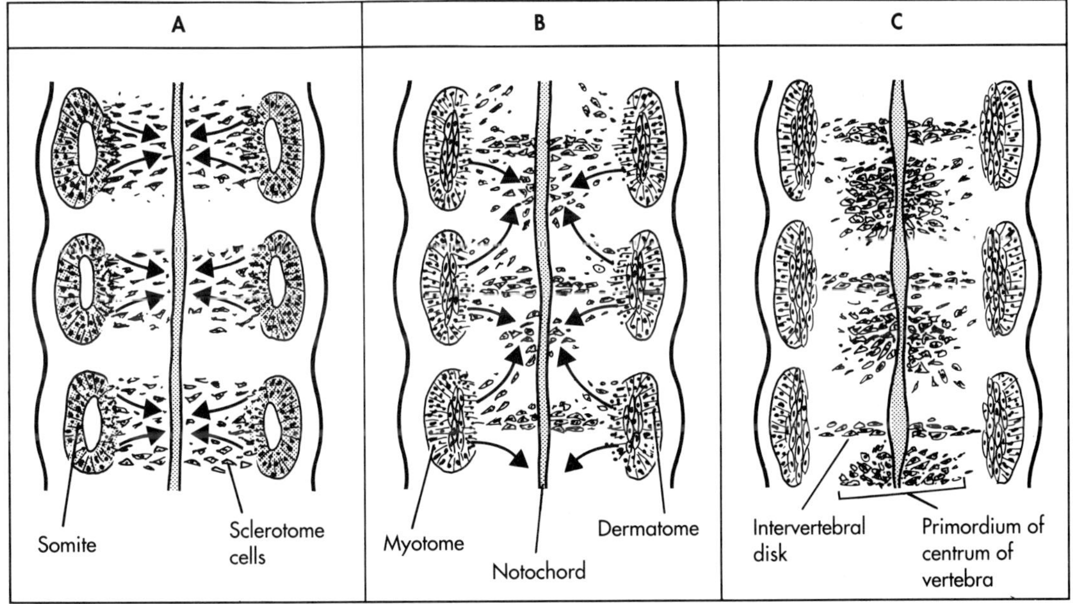

Figure 17.9 Coronal sections at the level of the notochord. In (a) the sclerotome cells have migrated to the mid-line. In (b) they are migrating from adjacent aggregations to meet in the intersegmental zone to form the primordia of the vertebral bodies. Cells remaining at the primary meeting place form the pre-intervertebral disc (c). (Redrawn from Carlson, 1985, with permission.)

head, on either side of the frontonasal process, there is formed at this early stage the nasal pit and the optic vesicle, both facing laterally. The eye apart, the anatomical entities that are here described are composed of mesenchyme (undifferentiated connective tissue derived from mesoderm) through most of the 4–10 week period.

The further developments required to produce a face are:

- to approximate the eyes to face forward
- to form a nose and establish its bridge
- to create the upper and lower jaws
- to create the palate, adapting the oronasal cavity for the simultaneous passage of air and food
- to form the oral opening (lips)

These can be described separately, and then put together in a composite picture.

1. **The eyes:** expansion of the skull may be

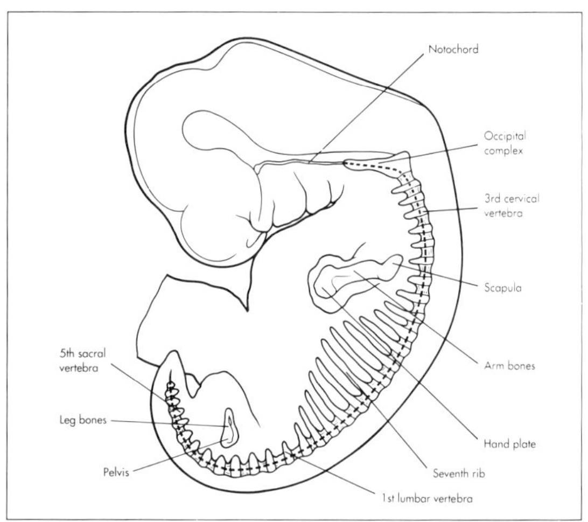

Figure 17.11 The precartilage skeletal primordia of a 9 mm (about 5.5 weeks) embryo. (Redrawn from Carlson, 1985, with permission.)

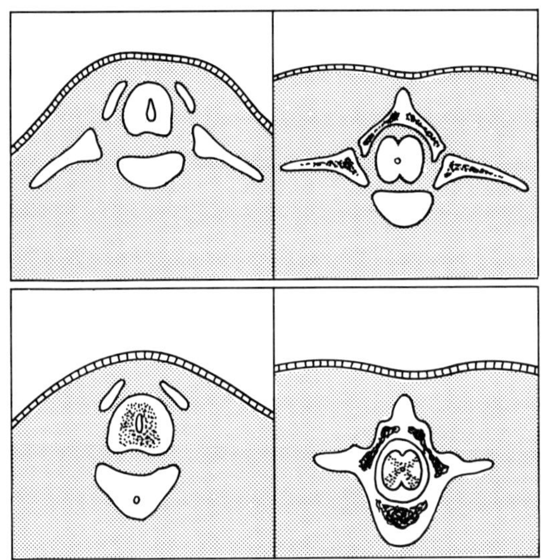

Figure 17.10 Successive stages in completing vertebrae. Cross sections of thoracic and lumbar regions. Cells from the centrum primordium migrate to form the other precartilaginous elements, including the ribs. Chondrification is followed by continuing growth and ossification. (Redrawn from Carlson, 1985, with permission.)

sufficient to bring the eyes to a position in front where they will face forward. But this must involve differential growth and modelling of tissues, both soft and bony, at various sites. In addition there is rotation of the external tissues around the eye: in early fetal life the long axis of the palpebral fissure slants downwards; gradually this changes to horizontal, and sometimes beyond.

2. **The nose:** the site of the nasal pits is first demarcated by an ectodermal thickening from whose periphery ridges arise in the form of a horse shoe with its arms pointing to the stomodaeum. The pits become cavities as the result of the growth of the ridges, and the gap between the tips becomes a groove which runs into the stomodaeum. The boundaries of the cavities and grooves are named the lateral and median nasal processes. The median processes are separated by a zone of tissue from which is derived, inter alia, the nasal septum that separates the nasal cavities as they are brought closer by growth and modelling. The floor of the now enlarged nasal

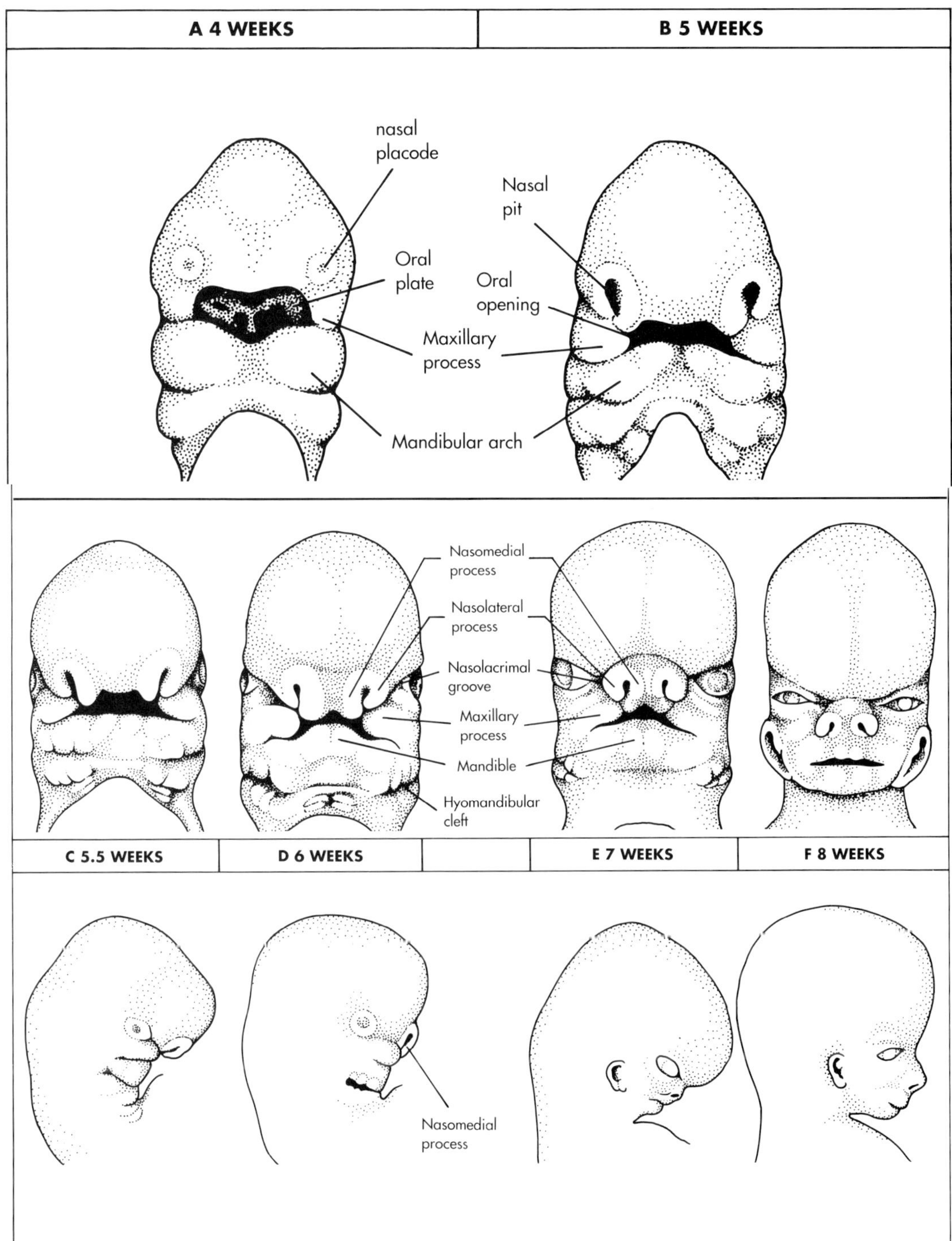

Figure 17.12 (a and b) Anteroposterior and lateral views, at several ages, of the developing face, indicating the basis of hypertelorism (wide spaced eyes), cleft lip, saddle nose and low set ears. (Redrawn from Carlson, 1985, with permission.)

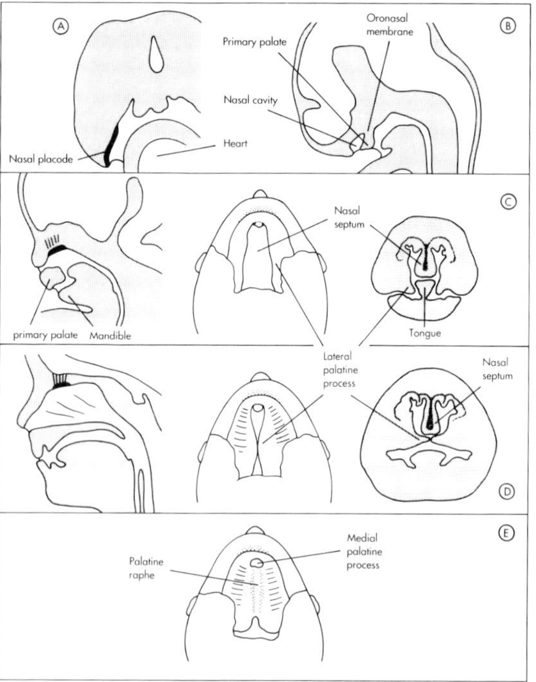

Figure 17.13 Schematic sagittal sections, at several ages, of human nasal and oropharyngeal regions to show their development together with views of the oral surface of the palate (based on developing pig) and coronal sections through it. Separation of the nasal and oral cavities is effected by the elevation of the lateral palatine processes and their fusion across the midline. (Redrawn from Carlson, 1985, with permission.)

cavities, derived from the median nasal process, overlies the front part of the primitive oral cavity (whose roof is principally the base of the skull); at their deep end the nasal cavities are closed by oronasal membranes. These rupture during the 7th week with the result that the nasal passage opens into the primitive mouth.

Externally the forepart of the nose is well formed by the 8th week, but there is only a deep depression between it and the forehead. After the 10th week there is an elevation of the tissue at this site to form the bridge and apex of the nose.

3. **The jaws:** early in the process of facial formation the first branchial arch, which borders the stomadaeum, divides horizontally to provide processes from which will be derived the maxilla and the mandible. The latter is the first to form, under the inductive influence of Meckel's cartilage. The mandibular processes grow forward (in concert with the other facial features, thereby deepening the oral cavity) to meet and fuse in the midline. At a somewhat later stage the maxillary processes follow. But the situation is more complicated by reason of the premaxilla, which is the lower portion of the median nasal process (developed in its turn from the frontonasal process). The premaxilla comes to lie between the advancing extremities of the maxillary process and fuses with them (7th week).

4. **The palate:** its formation is begun during the 8th week by outgrowths from the maxillary process laterally, and from the premaxilla anteriorly. At first they are vertically orientated masses with the tongue separating them. But during the 10th week they rotate to become horizontal, depressing the tongue and growing to meet and fuse in the midline. The nasal septum extends down, and posteriorly, meeting and fusing with the palate. The air passage now opens into the pharynx, making it possible to breathe and eat simultaneously.

5. **The lips:** these begin to form in the 7th week by the growth, from the free margin of the jaws, parallel with their external surface, of an ectodermal sheet (lamina). This separates the lips from the gums, and is completed when the central cells of the lamina degenerate. The cheeks are formed, and the opening of the mouth reduced, by fusion of the lips at the angles of the mouth. The process is complete at the 10/11th week.

There are many skeletal dysplasias in which features arising from some degree of failure of the foregoing processes are seen:

- Hypertelorism
- Down slanting palpebral fissures
- Saddle nose
- Degrees of cleft lip, maxilla, hard and soft palate
- Cleft mandible (very rare)
- Wide mouth
- Failure of dentition (not discussed above)

REFERENCES

Alberts, B., Bray, D., Lewis, L. *et al.* (1989) *Molecular Biology of the Cell*, 2nd edn, Garland Publishing, New York.

Aoyama, H. and Asamoto, K. (1988) Determination of somite cells: independence of differentiation and morphogenesis. *Development*, **104**, 15–28.

Carlson, B. (1985) *Patten's Foundations of Embryology*, 4th edn, McGraw-Hill, New York.

Carrington, J.L. and Fallon, J.F. (1988) Initial limb budding is independent of apical ectodermal ridge activity. *Development*, **104**, 361–7.

Jacobson, A.G. and Sater, A.K. (1988) Features of embryonic induction. *Development*, **104**, 341–59.

Miller, A. (1984) Self assembly. In *Developmental Control in Animals and Plants*, 2nd edn, (eds C.F. Sraman and P.P.F. Wareing), Blackwells, Edinburgh, pp. 373–95.

Moore, K.L. (1988) *The Developing Human*. WB Saunders, London.

Thorogood, P. (1983) Morphogenesis of cartilage. In *Cartilage*, Vol. 2, *Development, Differentiation and Growth* (ed. B.K. Hall), CRC Press, Boca Raton, FL.

Thorogood, P. and Tickle, C. (1988) Craniofacial development. *Development*, **103, supp**.

Wedden, S.E., Ralphs, J.R. and Tickle, C. (1988) Pattern formation in the facial primordia. In *Craniofacial Development*. (eds P. Thorogood, and C. Tickle) *Development*, **103, supp**. 31–40.

HISTOLOGICAL FEATURES OF CONNECTIVE TISSUES

Paul D. Byers

The bulk of the material that composes the supporting and connective tissues that result from the foregoing developmental processes is an extracellular matrix consisting of fibrous proteins and hydrated polysaccharide gels. These are made by the cells of the tissue, which usually occupy but a small proportion of the tissue mass (Fawcett, 1986).

The fibrous proteins are strong in tension but weak in compression. The hydrated polysaccharides are weak in tension but strong in compression; but in order to manifest this property they need to be contained, otherwise they disperse under load. Variation in proportions and organization of the fibrillar and gel components, provide a range of functional properties.

18.1 FIBROUS PROTEINS

The fibrous proteins are, in bulk, mainly a variety of collagens; but there are also elastin, fibronectin and osteonectin.

18.1.1 COLLAGENS

The basic structural unit is the alpha chain with about 1000 amino acid residues, of which glycine forms a third, and proline and lysine a distinctive feature because of their hydroxylation (Alberts *et al.*, 1989). Tropocollagen, the basic unit of collagen, consists of a helix formed of three polypeptide chains, 300 nm long and 1.5 nm in diameter. Twenty different polypeptides are known which form by varying proportions of eleven types of collagen, although theoretically 1000 different combinations are possible. Of these, three (types I,II,III) make up most of the body's collagen, and 90% of this is type I. All collagens represent 25% of the body's total protein (Miller and Gay, 1987).

The three main collagens are distributed as follows:

Type I: skin, tendon, bone, ligaments, cornea, internal organs.
Type II: cartilage, intervertebral disc, vitreous body.
Type III: skin, blood vessels, internal organs.

The sequence of events leading to the formation of collagen fibres in the matrix is depicted in Figure 18.1 (Alberts *et al.*, 1989). Pro-αchains are made in the cell (Leblond, 1989); they are kept separate by extension peptides, which are removed outside the cell allowing spontaneous formation of the molecule. The aggregation process continues under unknown control mechanisms, but the cell cytoskeleton, the cell membrane and components of the extracellular matrix are thought to play a part. Successive stages of polymerization produce ordered polymers, strengthened by covalent cross links. During assembly, molecules are staggered at 67 nm intervals, giving rise to the banding (Figure 18.2). Types I and II collagens form fibrils 10–300 nm in diameter and many μm long.

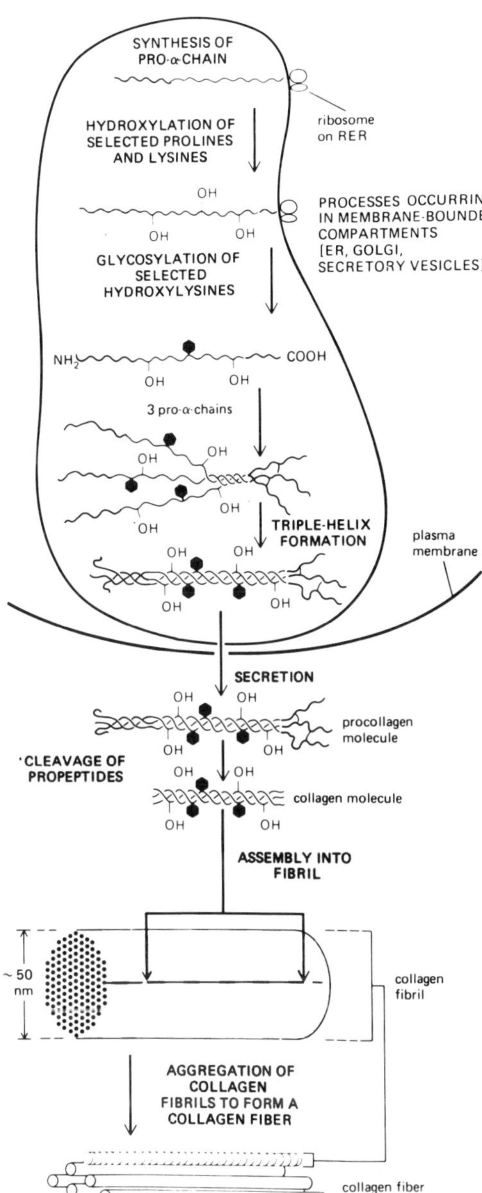

Figure 18.1 Intracellular and extracellular events in the formation of a collagen fibril. (Reproduced from Alberts *et al.* (1989) with permission.)

Type III fibrils are in the order of 50–55 nm in diameter, and constitute the argyrophil fibres that are recognized as reticulin. Collagen fibrils aggregate in their turn to form

fibres of a size that are recognizable by light microscopy: these are 0.5–20 μm in diameter in the case of types I and II; and 0.5–2 μm for type III.

Type IV collagen is a component of the basal lamina, together with fibronectin, protoeglycans and the glycoprotein laminin; there are thought to be other constituents as well. A feature of type IV collagen is long extension polypeptides which are not cleaved, which precludes the usual fibre formation. In addition to a structural role, basal lamina are a filtering mechanism and seem to induce cell differentiation, organize plasma membranes, affect cell metabolism and provide routes for cell migration. The laminae are secreted by the cells resting on it; these are mainly epithelial, but include muscle cells (the lamina has an important role at neuromuscular junctions).

18.1.2   ELASTIN

This is a large protein, 70 000 daltons, about which many details are uncertain. The molecules form filaments and sheets in a crosslinked random coil structure which permits stretching and recoil. Collagen fibres are

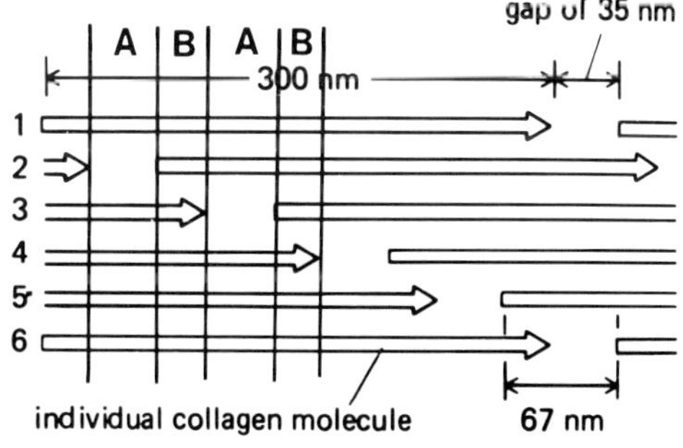

Figure 18.2 The staggered arrangement of the collagen molecules creates alternating regions in the fibrils where, when viewed transversely, intermolecular gaps are present or absent, creating the banded pattern. (Reproduced from Alberts *et al.* (1989), with permission.)

interwoven as a means of limiting extension. Microfibrils of a glycoprotein are attached to the surface of the fibres, whose function is thought to be the organization of the secreted elastic molecules.

18.1.3 FIBRONECTIN

This is a fibre-forming glycoprotein composed of two polypeptide chains of 220 000 daltons. It is produced by many types of connnective tissue and epithelial cell. Along its surface the molecule has many binding domains for macromolecules of cell surfaces and of extracellular matrix. Thus it contributes to cell/cell and cell/matrix adhesion. It is also present on platelets and is envisaged as contributing to their aggregation and adhesion in blood clot formation.

18.1.4 OSTEONECTIN

This is another glycoprotein with adhesive properties which binds strongly to collagen and hydoxyapatite.

18.2 HYDRATED POLYSACCHARIDE GELS
(HEINEGARD AND SOMMARIN, 1987; ALBERTS *ET AL.*, 1989; POOLE, 1989)

The 'functional units' of these gels are glycosaminoglycans (Figure 18.3). They are long chains of repeating disaccharide units, one of which is an amino sugar (*N*-acetylglucosamine or *N*-acetylgalactosamine) – hence the name glucosaminoglycan (GAG) and formerly labelled mucopolysaccharides. Four main groups are recognized by their chemical features:

- Hyaluronic acid
- Chondroitin sulphate, dermatan sulphate
- Heparan sulphate, heparin
- Keratan sulphate

These have differing, but overlapping, distribution in the connective tissues. Apart from hyaluronic acid they do not exist free in the tissues, but are aggregated by attachment to a protein core, to form a proteoglycan (PG), which can be thought of as an 'operational unit': upwards of 100 GAGs per protein molecule give a final molecular weight of millions of daltons (Figure 18.3). Since the length of the GAGs and of the core protein are variable, enormous heterogeneity is possible; but the extent to which it exists is not known. Before release from the cell GAGs are sulphated. Extracellularly, the high density of negative charges resulting from ionization of the sulphate radicals keeps the molecules extended and so occupying a very large volume relative to their mass. Moreover, the anions attract osmotically active cations; together they hold large amounts of water, creating a gel with a very high swelling pressure, resistant to compression, as in articular cartilage. An even larger structural unit can be created by the binding of core proteins at intervals along the length of hyaluronic acid. These are found particularly in cartilage (Figure 18.3). Maroudas (1979) discusses the physicochemical properties of articular cartilage.

In addition to its role in aggregating proteoglycans, hyaluronic acid is a major constituent of synovial fluid and vitreous humour. Its high viscosity makes it an excellent lubricant, and may also contribute to impeding movement of particulate matter, such as bacteria, through connective tissues.

The range of tissue types formed with these matrix components is readily categorized as: fibrous connective tissue, cartilage and bone.

Each of these categories has subdivisions within it. Those of the connective tissues have traditionally been based on the density of the fibrous element, namely loose, or dense which is subdivided into irregular and regular.

Loose tissues can be eclectically subclassified, with poorly defined boundaries, according to some prominent feature, e.g. areolar, reticular, adipose. Basically they are

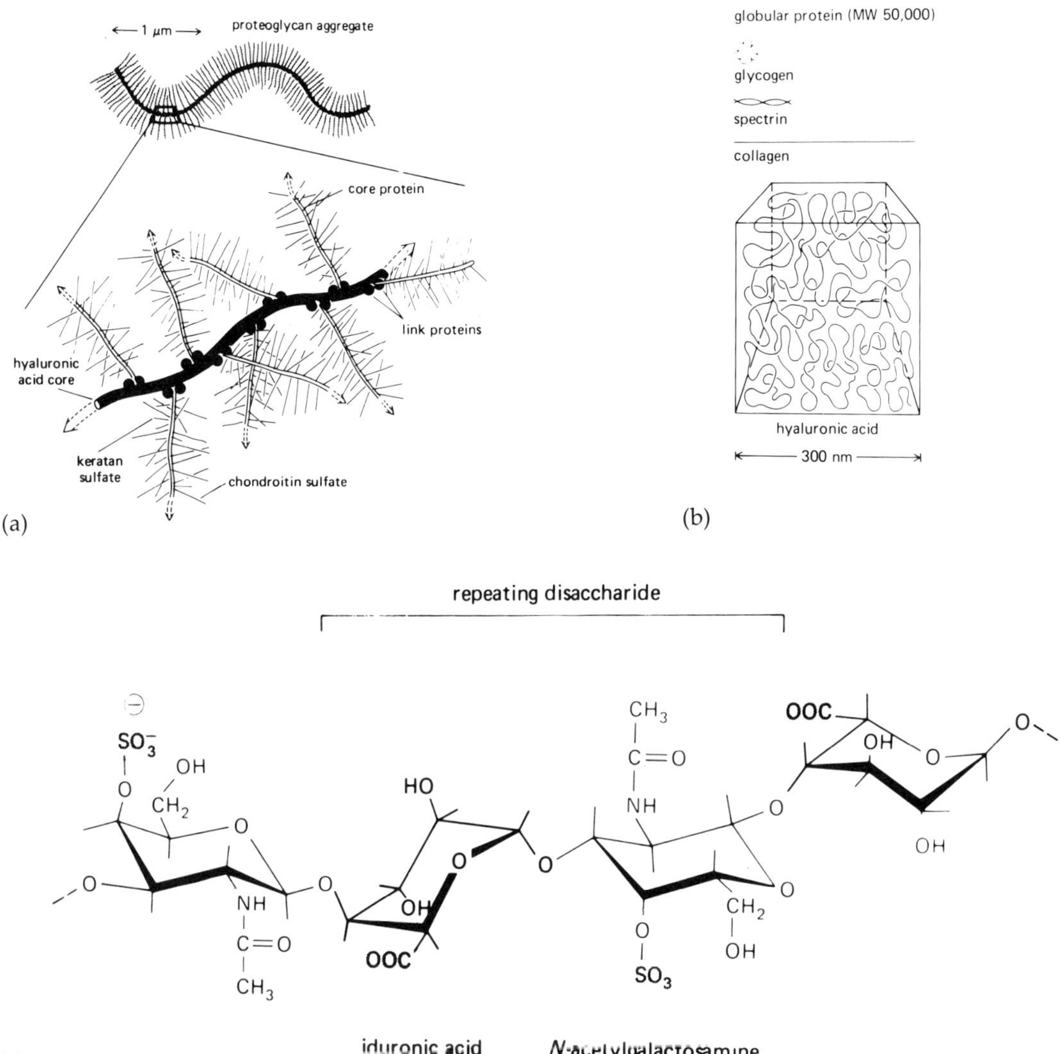

Figure 18.3 (a) Proteoglycan aggregate of cartilage. The glycosaminoglycans (GAGs) chondroitin and keratan sulphate are covalently attached to a protein core, forming a proteoglycan (PG) monomer. About 100 of these aggregate with an hyaluronic acid (HA) molecule, to which they are attached by link protein. (b) The relative volumes occupied by various molecules compared with hyaluronic acid. (c) Part of a GAG chain. These are in the range of 70–200 sugar residues in length. The high density of negative charges attracts an equal density of positive charges, which together create a high osmotic pressure: the retained water gives cartilage its stiffness and load-carrying capacity. (Reproduced from Alberts *et al.* (1989), with permission.)

an open three-dimensional network of collagen fibres, interlaced with some or none of elastic fibres. In the interstices are to be found:

1. The hydrated gels
2. Capillary networks,
3. Fixed and wandering cells
    (a) Fibroblasts, mesenchymal (undifferentiated) cells, lipocytes;
    (b) Mononuclear phagocytic cells (macrophages), lymphocytes, plasma cells, eosinophils, mast cells.

These tissues are widely distributed – subcutaneously, in the lamina propria and submucosa of gastrointestinal tract, mesentery and omentum, in planes and pockets of the musculoskeletal system and in support of parenchymatous organs. Throughout the body they are important in the distribution and availability of protective and reparative cells, and the physiology of interstitial fluid. The adipose tissues have a major role in energy metabolism with a daily turnover of 10% of fatty acids.

The dense collagenous tissues are of immediate concern to orthopaedics. As the name suggests, the amount of fibre is high and of gel low; but even so there is more fibre and less gel in those with a regular fibre arrangement.

18.3 OSTEOARTICULAR CONNECTIVE TISSUES

These tissues are classified as shown in Table 18.1.

Tendons and ligaments are the most uniformly arranged of these tissues, a design in keeping with their role to sustain strong forces in tension (Amiel *et al.*, 1984) (Figure 18.4). It is customary to consider them more or less identical in their structure. However, there are differences which warrant describing them separately.

18.3.1 TENDONS

Because repair of flexor tendons of the hand is so difficult they have been closely studied for their normal structure, which is generally applicable (Verdan, 1979). The final units of structure are the collagen fibres. These are variable in diameter, but fall into two groups, one with a mean of 60 nm and the other of 175 nm. They are intermingled to form fascicles, also of variable diameter which run the length of the structure. Each bundle is surrounded by a delicate fibrous sheath (endotenon), carrying the blood vessels, continuous externally with a thin layer of loose connective tissue enclosing the whole (ectotenon) and mingling with the adjacent soft connective tissues (paratenon). The external layers permit gliding motion. The vascular supply has three basic sources: the muscle of origin, the vessels running distally within the substance of the tendon; the site of attachment, the vessels running proximally within the tendon; the paratendinous tissue, the vessels running over the surface and penetrating the tendon to anastomose with the internal vessels. The vessels are small but numerous. The portions of tendons which pass over bony prominences or beneath retinacula are enclosed in a ten-

Table 18.1 Osteoarticular connective tissues

Fibre arrangement	Tissue
Regular	Tendon (and sheath)
	Ligament
Irregular	Joint capsule (and synovium)
	Fascia/aponeuroses
	Bursa
	Periosteum

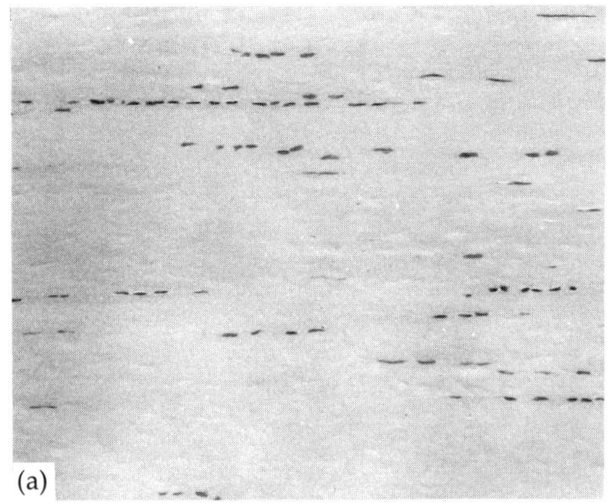

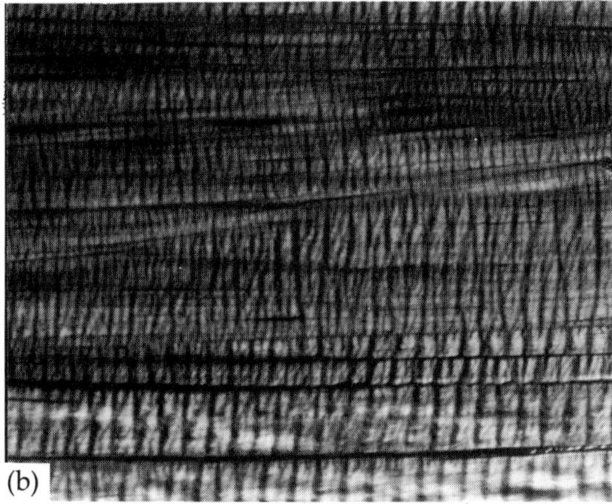

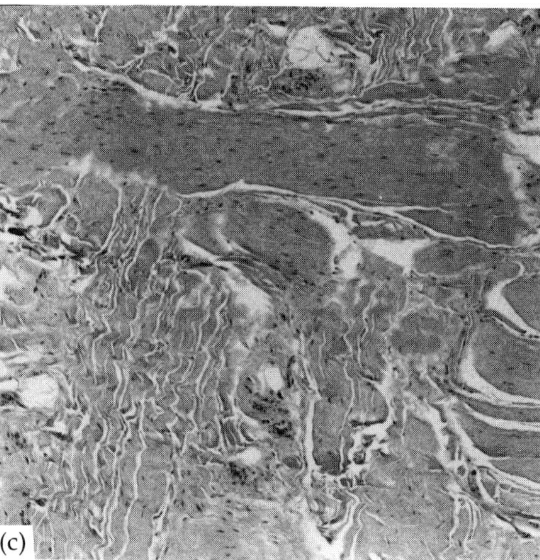

Figure 18.4 Dense collagenous tissues. (c) Joint capsule, constructed of bands of collagen fibres running in various directions. The wavy character of some bundles is an expression of the crimp.

Figure 18.4 Dense collagenous tissues. (a) Longitudinal section of tendon to show the sparse cellularity, and to emphasize the delicacy of the vasculature, which runs with the cells but is not visible at this power. (b) Longitudinal section of ligament. A thick section is light adjusted to show the crimp in the fibres, which is responsible for the banded appearance. A sparsely cellular tissue.

don sheath. This too is thin loose connective tissue arranged in a double layer, the inner attached to the tendon the outer to the contiguous tissues. The opposing surfaces are lined by a layer of synovial cells (section 8.1.1). The synovial space is traversed by blood vessels, fulfilling the function of those in the paratendinous tissue at other sites.

In longitudinal section the fibres are paral-

lel, tightly packed and slightly wavy, the crimp pattern which contributes to their functional capacity. Intensely birefringent, they present a distinctive picture. The cells are spindled in longitudinal section, round or oval transversely, and widely scattered, singly.

18.3.2 LIGAMENTS

Frank *et al.* (1985) identify, anatomically, cords and bands; sheets and capsular ligaments. The fibres in some are bundled; they suggest that potentially these are structural and functional features which might allow subclassification as details emerge from investigations. Histologically, ligaments are composed of parallel collagen fibres among which are scattered fibroblasts and rare blood vessels. Polarized light reveals a marked, regular wave arrangement of the fibres, the crimp, whose function is to act as a buffer when the structure is put under tension. Attachment to bone is via a transition in the tissue to fibrocartilage, mineralized fibrocartilage, and bone. In some preparations a mineralization front can be identified at the interface between the two zones of fibrocartilage.

In their comparative study of rabbit tendon and ligament Amiel *et al.* (1984) found that the cells of ligaments were more numerous and varied than in tendon, and the tissue DNA content was higher. Tendons had more collagen, but with a low proportion of type III, and lower GAG content compared with the ligaments. The two types of tissue also differed in their collagen cross linking. They concluded that the basis for these differences was still to be elucidated.

Irregular dense tissues have a broad spectrum of organization, which may not always be readily distinguished from the regular at one extreme and the loose at the other. In the middle ground they are composed of closely arranged collagen fibres, but without aggregation into the tight packaging of tendon bundles. The overall organization is into sheets, which is not readily apparent in histological sections, but is macroscopically. Many fibres cross over from one layer to another so that they are firmly laminated. The cells are as in tendon: spindled, single, and dispersed.

Although the density of proteoglycans is low in these tissues, nevertheless there is an intimate relationship between them and the collagen as evidenced by the spatial relationship of PG filaments to the cross banding of the collagen. But little is as yet known about this and many other aspects of connective tissues.

18.4 CARTILAGE AND BONE (JEE, 1988)

In the embryo, connective tissue matrix is a necessary prelude to the formation of cartilage and bone. Within limits this remains true in the child and adult, as exemplified by the formation of fracture callus. The bone of the skull, the facial skeleton and of the clavicle is formed in the embryo in connective tissue matrix. But the remainder of the skeleton is first established as a cartilage model which is converted into bone by the process of enchondral ossification.

18.4.1 CARTILAGE

Comprehensive details about cartilage can be found in Hall (1983) and Hall and Newman (1991). It exists in three forms: hyaline, elastic and fibrous. The last has the highest collagen content, and is strong in tension, but remains flexible and somewhat compressable. Elastic cartilage, with its large elastic fibre content provides flexible support. The bulk of skeletal cartilage is hyaline. In laboratory practice, it is most often seen in neoplasia, articular cartilage (Figure 18.5) and callus. The physis is also hyaline cartilage; although seldom encountered, knowledge of it is important. Basic details of hyaline cartilage are discussed here. Its attributes in particular situations will be discussed as they arise.

(a) The cartilage cells

Chondrocytes differentiate from spindled connective tissue cells. They round up, form a cluster and surround themselves with matrix. The cells form lacunae within the matrix, for whose production and maintenance they are responsible, both in further growth following cell division and functionally. The identification of chondrocytes histologically depends on the association with matrix: rounded cells in a hyaline metachromatic matrix. In conventional sections there is little about the cells *per se* that distinguishes them. In poorly differentiated neoplasms identification can be very difficult to resolve.

(b) Cartilage matrix

Articular cartilage matrix and its chondrocytes have been discussed by Meachim and Stockwell (1979), Stockwell and Meachim

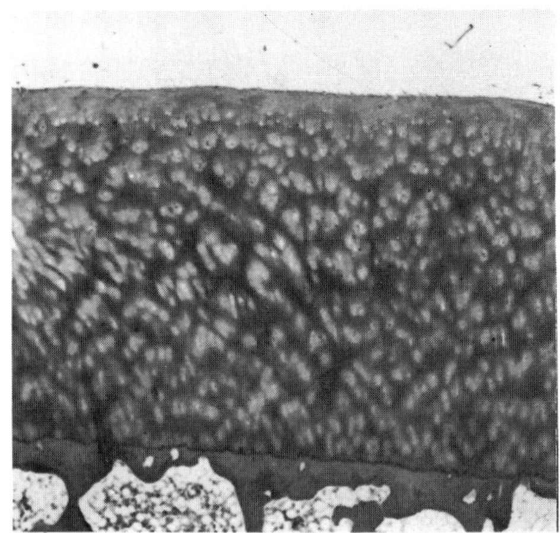

Figure 18.5 Normal adult articular cartilage. Decalcified, paraffin embedded, H&E stained. The bulk of articular cartilage is unmineralized, and is usually considered to have a superficial, middle and deep zones, but there are no precise landmarks. The cells of the superficial zone are flattened tangentially to the surface. In the deep zone the cells may show columnation. The distribution of glycosaminoglycans affects the staining properties, giving rise to a territorial (pericellular) and interterritorial pattern, which fades out towards the surface. The deepest layer of the cartilage is calcified; it is demarcated from the unmineralized cartilage by the haematoxophilic 'tide' line, which may be replicated. The calcified layer rests on a bone plate with which it interdigitates; there is a very thin, poorly staining zone between them, of unknown composition which is said not to be crossed by collagen fibres. There is great variability in the staining of normal articular cartilage; the example illustrated is strongly stained.

(1979) and in Hall (1983). The matrix is formed of a network of collagen fibres which entrap large complex molecules of protein polysaccharide. The latter have a very high osmotic pressure, owing to numerous ionizing terminal radicals, and imbibe and hold water which inflates the net. Details of the organization of the collagen net are unclear, although there is a great deal of information about the chemistry of collagen and the structure of collagen fibres. Fibres branch and anastomose; and they interweave; but it

is not known if and how they otherwise adhere to one another, although a number of hypotheses are extant. In adult articular cartilage the traditional model of collagen organization is the Benninghof arcade (Figure 18.6). More recent studies have shown aggregation of fibres to form parallel leaves held together by interconnecting fibres (Figure 18.7). At the surface the leaves fold over, and their collagen fibres meld with those of neighbouring leaves to form a mesh with a predominantly parallel structure, running at right angles to the plane of the leaves. If the surface is pierced with a pin over a wide area and then doused with Indian ink (Bullough and Goodfellow, 1968) and washed, the pinpricks will appear as oval splits whose long axes are parallel with the plane of the leaves – the 'split pattern' of articular cartilage (Jeffrey *et al.*, 1991).

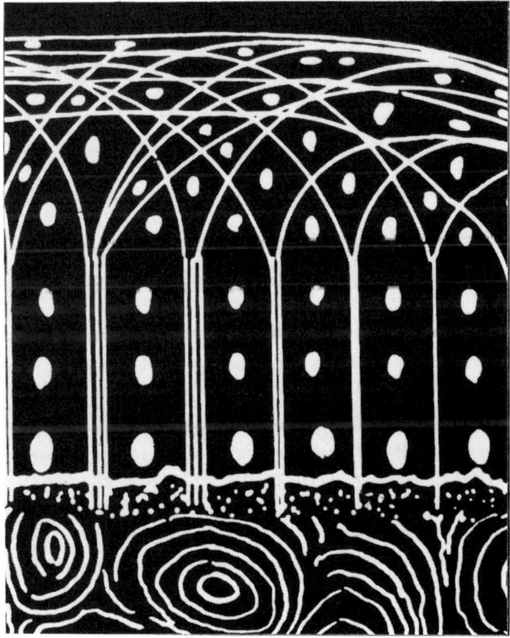

Figure 18.6 Benninghof arcade. The traditional hypothesis of articular cartilage collagen organization.

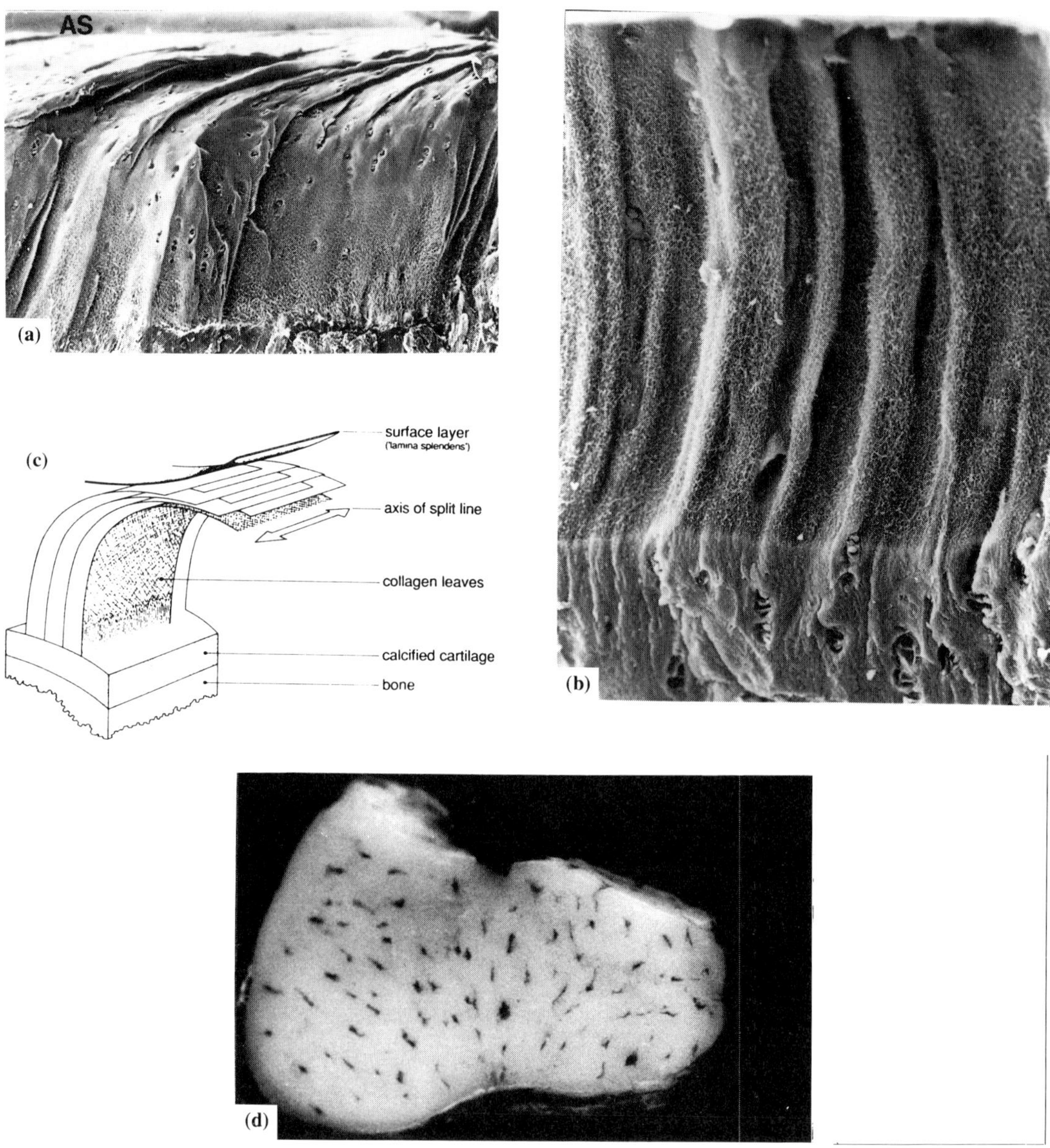

Figure 18.7 The leaf structure of articular cartilage. (a) Calf articular cartilage, freeze dried. Freeze fracture surface, at right angles to articular surface and oblique to the plane of the leaves. They arise as overlapping sheets from the calcified cartilage at the bottom and fold over and blend at the articular surface. (b) The fracture surface is at right angles to both the joint surface and to the plane of the leaves. The collagen structure of the leaves is denser than the intervening tissue; the latter serves to connect the leaves. (c) A diagram of the structure. At the surface the fibres of the leaves meld to form a collagenous cover with a predominantly unidirectional fibre orientation. This is covered by a thin amorphous layer of unknown composition, the lamina splendens. (d) Cuneiform of child. Split line pattern of articular cartilage. The surface is pierced by a pin, doused with Indian ink and then rinsed with water. The pin holes are slits running in the plane of the leaves. (Reproduced from Jeffrey *et al.* (1991) with permission of the author and publisher.)

18.4.2 BONE

(a) Bone matrix

The organic component of bone matrix is composed mainly of collagen fibres; but there is also an important glycosaminoglycan content (Table 18.2). These substances have been discussed above. There is extensive coverage of the matrix in Hall (1990–92). Bone is strong not only in tension, but also in compression and torsion as a result of the mineral component. The osteoblasts make the organic constituents, and are thought to act as agents for mineral deposition. Before mineral is added the matrix is referred to as osteoid, and after as bone. In immature osteoid (which, when it mineralizes is referred to as immature bone) the collagen fibres have a somewhat haphazard arrangement, weaving in and out relative to one another. The pattern is readily described as woven, and the term is used descriptively as synonymous with immature. To visualize this easily, a histological section can be examined in polarized light. Since collagen fibres are birefringent they appear as bright lines in the darker field of crossed polarizing lenses, and their arrangement can be assessed (Figure 18.8). The use of these lenses with the microscope is a simple, effective and essential method of examination of bone sections.

Woven osteoid can be laid onto any mineralized surface, e.g. cartilage, or be formed *de novo* in membrane bone formation (section 19.1). But the other type of collagen organiza-tion, lamellar, is only deposited on pre-existing bone surfaces, woven or lamellar. As bone matures, doing so in the modelling of growing bone, the collagen fibres are placed parallel to the surface on which they are formed, in layers with an alternating overall direction. The control mechanisms whereby this is achieved are not known. Viewed in polarized light they appear as light and dark parallel bands (Figure 18.9).

Because of the effect of the lifetime cellular activity of remodelling, as described in Chapter 19, the matrix is demarcated into units of structure, variously referred to as bone structural units or bone packets. The cells act on bone surfaces; osteoclasts resorb a small volume of bone; osteoblasts deposit osteoid in this. The new bone will be bounded by a thin haematoxyphilic line, called the reversal or cement line. On a trabecular surface in a histological section it will appear as a crescent (Figure 18.10); in osteonal bone it will be a ring. In each, the collagen layers will be light and dark bands parallel to the surface.

The recognition of woven and lamellar bone is important in osteoarticular pathology for classifying bone tissue. In general terms, woven bone (osteoid) matrix indicates rapid formation: this may be the result of immaturity, reactivity or neoplasia.

(b) Bone cells

These comprise the precursor cells (stem cells, preosteoclasts and preosteoblasts), the surface cells (osteoblasts, lining cells) and the

Table 18.2 Matrix constituents (Maroudas, 1979; Frost, 1986)

Substance	*% wet weight of*	
	Cartilage	*Bone*
Collagen	15–25	37
Proteoglycans	3–10	2
Water	65–80	12
Mineral	0	49

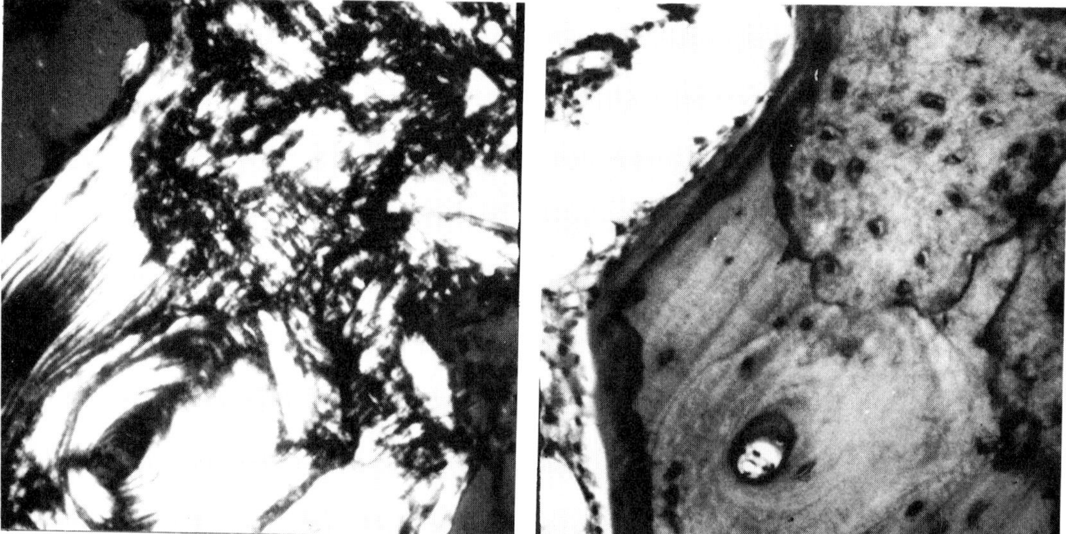

Figure 18.8 Woven and lamellar bone. The collagen pattern in polarized light of the histological section on the right. The distinction between woven and lamellar bone is clear.

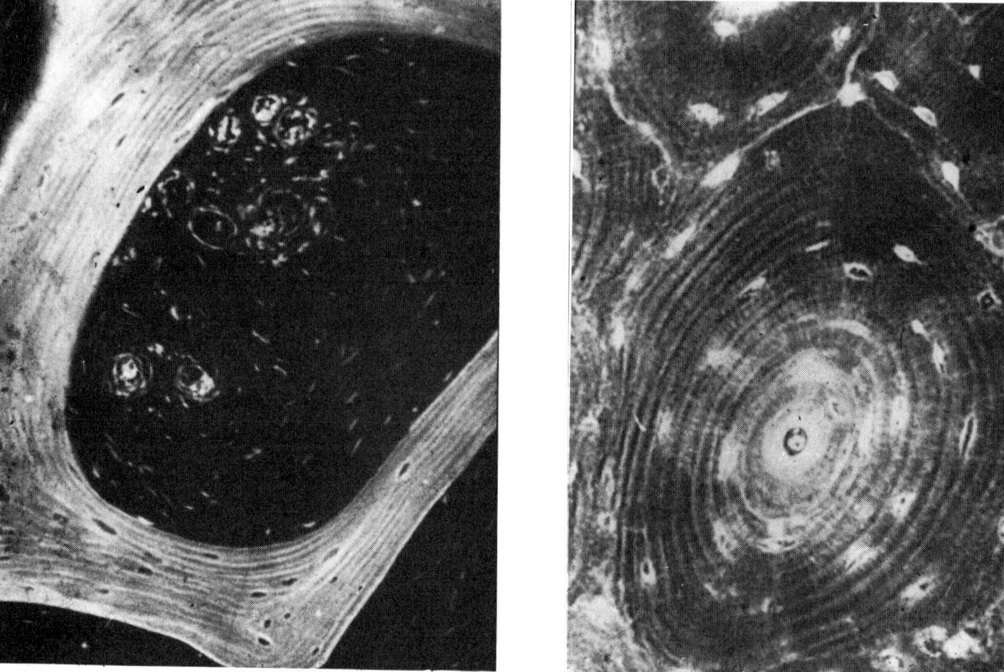

Figure 18.9 Lamellar organization of cancellous and cortical bone. In the latter each osteon is bounded by a cement (reversal) line, visible only at the top of the figure. In the trabeculum reversal lines will be found at sites where lamellar orientation changes, as at the bottom of the figure.

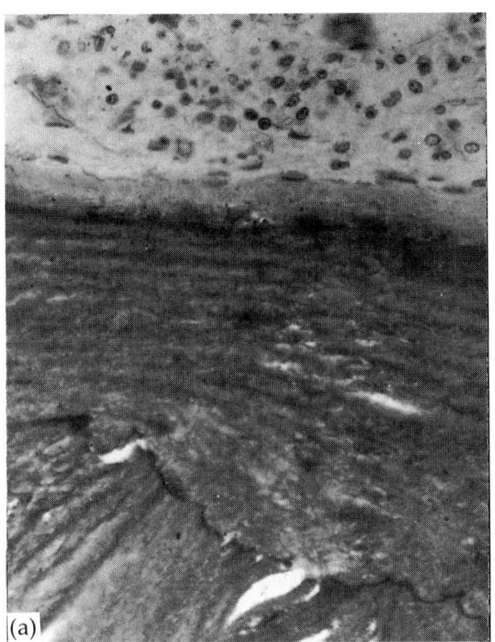

Figure 18.10 Undecalcified section of normal bone trabeculum. (a) Portions of a new and an old bone packet, or bone structural unit (BSU) are shown. At the top, marrow in contact with a pale, thin layer of osteoid on which are a few flattened osteoblasts. The successive layers are the calcification front (a thin, dark irregular band); lamellar bone (layers running parallel to trabecular surface); the reversal, or cement, line (dark, thin, slightly scalloped); lamellar bone, the lamellae almost at right angles to the preceding. The bone above the reversal line is a recently formed BSU which will soon be completely mineralized; the full length of the unit might be 5 or 10 times the portion depicted. Its terminations would be marked by the reversal line running up to the surface. The bone below the reversal line is the remnant of the old BSU.

internal cells (osteocytes).

It is now a reasonable proposition that the two classes of bone cell, resorptive and formative, are derived from different primary sources. The former, osteoclasts, develop from a marrow lineage that includes monocytic/phagocytic entities (Vaes, 1988; Burger and Nijweide, 1991). The latter stem from embryonic mesenchyme, responsible for skeletal tissue in the embryo, which in postembryonic life has given rise to osteoprogenitor stem cells in the marrow stroma, the periosteum and some connective tissues, notably muscle (Marks and Popoff, 1988). But many details remain unknown. There is uncertainty about the role of mononuclear cells in bone resorption (Holtrop, 1991). That they can resorb matrix under some circumstances is agreed, but whether they are of osteoclast lineage, or have the same operative mechanism for removing matrix, or play a significant role in bone metabolism are open questions. There is strong feeling that it is the multinucleated osteoclast with its clear zone and ruffled border that is the significant cell (Kahn and Partridge, 1991) (Figure 18.11).

(i)   Osteoclasts

In their active state, as described below, these are closely applied to the surface (Figure 18.11), but this attachment seldom survives routine preparatory treatment. The number of nuclei is variable, seldom above 10, but may on occasion appear to be one in the plane of the section. At the level of light microscopy there is nothing beyond the multinucleation that is distinctive about osteoclasts. They contain tartrate-resistant acid phosphatase which is an identifying marker, but requires special preparations for its demonstration. Nevertheless, in routine paraffin sections of good quality the presence of multinucleated, or even mononuclear cells in proximity to resorption bays (Howship's lacunae) in the surfaces of bone or calcified cartilage is firm presumptive evidence of identification. This shifts the problem to the identification of resorption bays, as distinct from artefact. With polarized light the abrupt interruption of the orderly course of lamellae is helpful; in artefacts there is disorder, such as folding or fragmentation. The fate of osteoclasts following completion

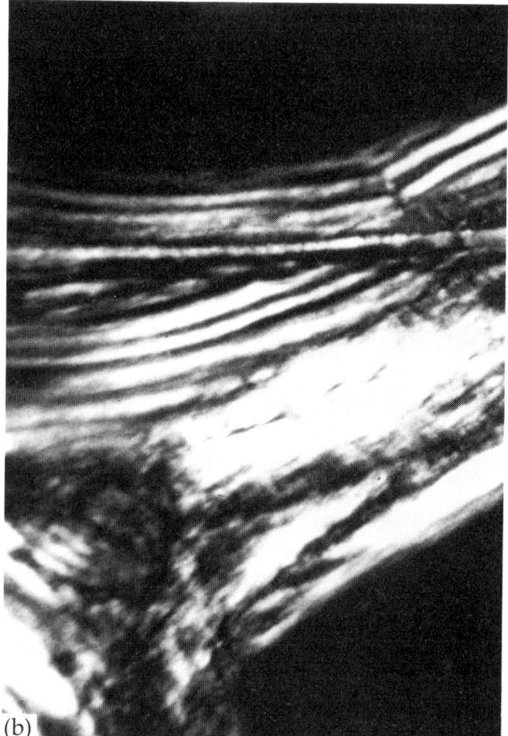

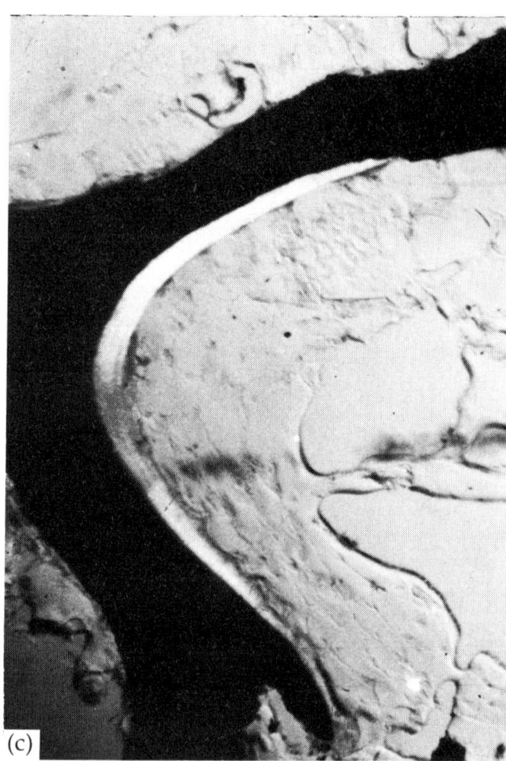

Figure 18.10 Undecalcified section of normal bone trabeculum. (b) Undecalcified trabeculum, H&E, in polarized light. The lamella of the most recent BSUs are at the surfaces, and remnants of older ones within. The collagen pattern would not be affected by decalcification. (c) Undecalcified trabeculum, von Kossa stain, polarized light. The plane of section is too close to that of the collagen lamellae for them to appear as alternating bright and dark lines.

of their task is not known. Osteoclasts are present in many bone tumours, both benign and malignant, and in some soft tissue lesions such as PVNS. It is assumed that a chemotactic factor draws them there (see below).

Current opinion (Vaes, 1988) is that osteoclasts derive from a multipotential haemopoietic stem cell with a capacity to develop along two lines to form tissue macrophages and osteoclasts. Several stages are postulated: stem cell; non-committed early progenitor, osteoclast progenitor, preosteoclast, multinucleated osteoclast. The non-committed progenitor can differentiate irreversibly along the route to either monocyte/macrophage or osteoclast. The former do not have the capacity to resorb bone even in their multinucleated form. The first two stages are believed to take place at sites of marrow formation, and then the (committed) osteoclast progenitors find their way via the bloodstream to the stromal tissue in and around bone, from where they can be called for further differentiation and directed to resorption sites.

The electron microscopic features of osteoclasts are, in addition to multiple nuclei, an abundance of mitochondria and lysosomes, free ribosomes and extensive Golgi complexes. The cytoplasm in contact with bone is a 'clear zone', a ring of contact which seals off

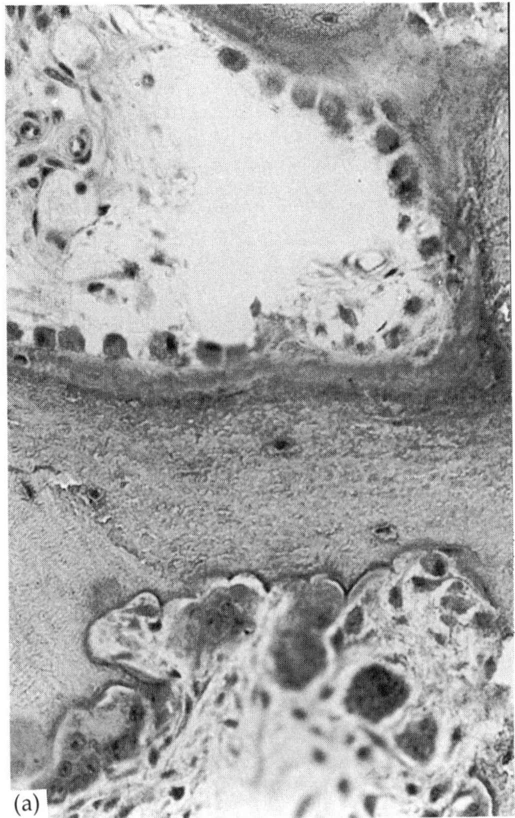 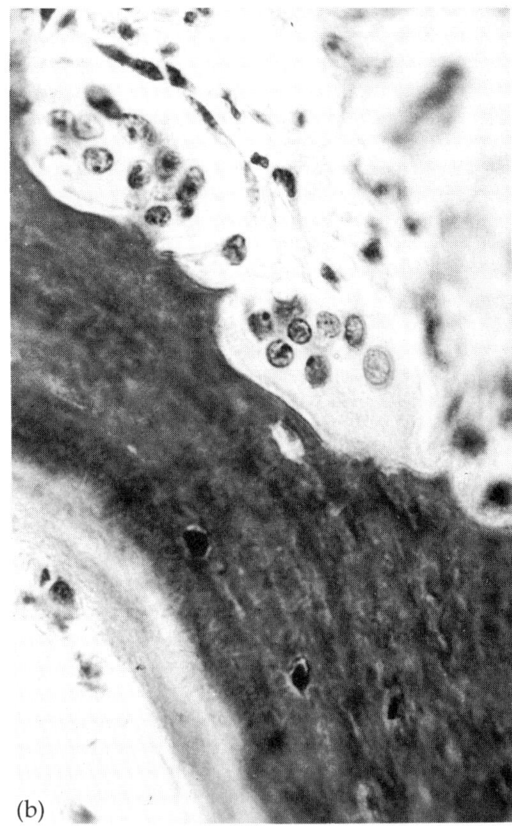

Figure 18.11 Bone cells. Undecalcified sections; (a) toluidine blue stain; (b) H&E. Osteoclasts, osteoblasts, and osteocytes are readily distinguished. A few mononuclear cells adjacent to the osteoclasts may be osteoblast precursors or recently differentiated osteoblasts.

a portion of the bone surface from the interstitial fluid. The plasma membrane within the sequestered zone is ruffled by an active system of pseudopodia which deliver the agents for resorption into the enclosed space. These agents are considered to be first, hydrogen ions secreted by an ATP-driven proton pump in the ruffled border, which dissolve the mineral; and second, acid hydrolases from lysosomes which remove the matrix. Osteoclasts move over the bone surface, eroding a succession of pits, as can be seen in SEM preparations of bone seeded with active osteoclasts, whose profile corresponds to Howship's lacunae in conventional sections.

Further clarification of the controls that determine osteoclast differentiation and switch on and off their resorptive activity is in progress. Current understanding is summarized in Figure 18.12, based on Hauschka (1990). However, the situation is not a simple one. There are numerous control substances which may be grouped into various classes, some into more than one. It appears that these may act in cascades as switches in many of the body's systems, and according to local conditions they may be instrumental in permitting or preventing, enhancing or retarding events.

Current ideas about the initiation of resorption derive from observations that, in

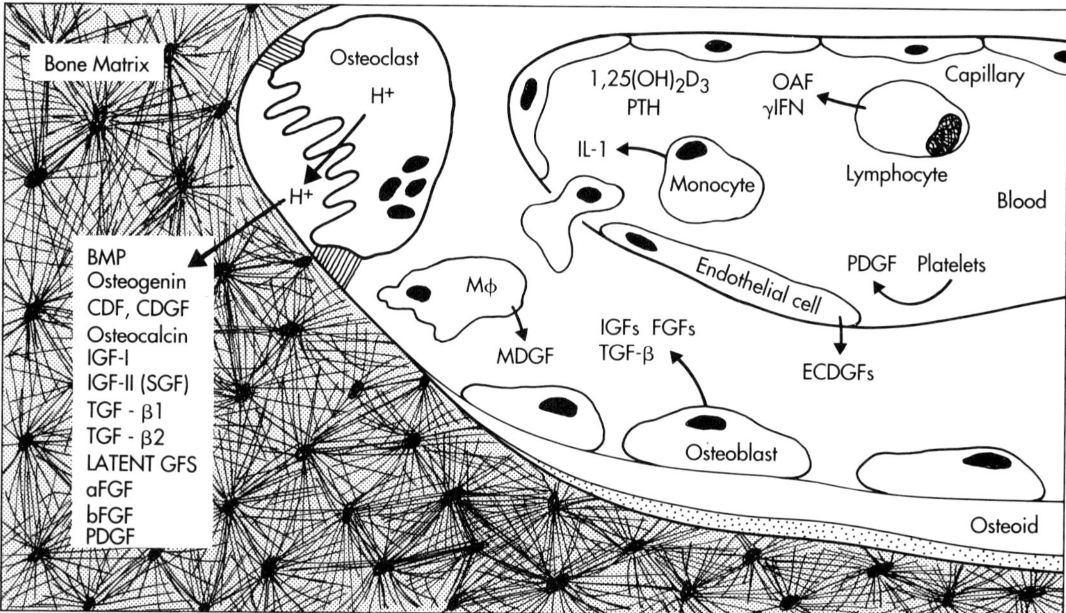

Figure 18.12 Schematic representation of bone cells of a BMU (Basic Multicellular Unit) and the sources of effector proteins that influence their actions and relationships. An osteoclast is shown attached to the bone by its clear zone, acidifying the enclosed space for action of resorbing enzymes, which will release matrix-bound growth factors, some of which will promote nearby osteoblast activity ('coupling' action). The many effector proteins in the neighbourhood will have a range of control over cellular responses. Modified from Hauschka (1990), reproduced with permission. Symbols: $1,25(OH)_2D_3$, vitamin D_3; PTH, parathyroid hormone; BMP, bone morphogenetic protein; GF, growth factor – PDGF, platelet derived; ECDGF, endothelial cell derived; TGF, transforming (several subtypes); FGF, fibroblast (acidic and basic types); MDGF, monocyte derived; CDGF, cell derived; IGF, insulin-like (types I and II) – IL-1, interleukin I; OAF, osteoclast activating factor; IFN, (gamma) interferon

experimental conditions, osteoblastic activity precedes that of osteoclasts. This suggests either that the osteoblasts stimulate osteoclasts, or that they clear the bone surface of a thin collagen cover by secreting collagenase. It is also postulated that peptides which stimulate osteoblastic activity are stored in bone matrix and are released by osteoclastic resorption thereby coupling resorption and formation in the remodelling process (Mundy, 1991a, b).

(ii)   *Osteoblasts, lining cells and osteocytes*

Specific cellular markers for osteogenic cells have not been identified (Tenenbaum, 1990). Thus the recognition of precursor cells in bone is by inference. Parfitt (1990) describes cells that are presumed to be preosteoblasts by reason of their location at sites of forming osteoid seams and deep resorption cavities which will soon be formation sites.

In established bone tissue, active osteoblasts are present as a monolayer on portions of the bone surfaces, an association by which they are recognized. Even when the marrow is very cellular, whether by reason of active haemopoiesis, inflammatory or neoplastic infiltration, active osteoblasts at a bone surface are recognizable by their close packed, cuboidal arrangement, which has been likened to a collar or necklace. Although they have an intensely basophilic cytoplasm, this does not survive acid fixatives and decalcifiers (Pritchard, 1972). Active cells will overlie osteoid seams (not visible in undecalcified sections), which they are forming. Forming surfaces are extensive in the child, but in adults they are less than 20%, and as little as about 5%. Elsewhere the cells are flat, sometimes being thinner than the resolving powers of the microscope, but up to 50 µm in diameter (Miller *et al.*, 1980) and are described as lining cells, more or less completely covering the surface. They communicate with the osteocytes via processes in the canaliculae. Collectively the quiescent surfaces of the adult amount to 80–95% of total surface.

The structure of the quiescent surface is discernible only by electron microscopy. On the bone surface is a thin dense mineralized layer of uncertain composition, the lamina limitans (Scherft, 1972). On this there is a 0.1–0.5 µm layer of connective tissue differently organized from osteoid, which can be confused with osteoid in the light microscope (Mathews, 1980). The bone lining cells rest on this. They are covered by a similar connective tissue layer when the adjacent marrow is fatty (Miller *et al.*, 1980), or, when the marrow is haemopoietic, by squamous cells of the marrow sac (Menton *et al.*, 1982).

It is currently postulated that lining cells are able to secrete collagenase, which removes the endosteal membrane, and that they themselves retract to expose calcified surface to the osteoclasts (possibly attracted by a chemical released from the bone).

In addition to their intimate association with bone, osteoblasts have the distinctive feature of containing alkaline phosphatase. It is difficult to take advantage of this in conventional histological preparations, but it is of great value in tumour diagnosis if films are made from the fresh tissue at the time of biopsy.

In addition to making bone matrix, they have a role in its mineralization.

The postulated line of development within bone of the osteoblast is from a stem cell, associated with the marrow stroma in bone, in two stages, the inducible osteoblast precursor cell and the differentiated osteoblast precursor cell. The latter is postulated to undergo some further divisions to terminal differentiation as an osteoblast. To account for the observation that bone formation can be induced in tissues with no connection to bone as well as in bone it is postulated that inducible osteoprogenitor cells are located in them. Thus decalcified bone matrix in muscle will give rise to cartilage which is ossified enchondrally to form an ossicle in which marrow is established. There is an abundance of experimental work concerned with these hypotheses (Tenenbaum, 1990).

Osteocytes are osteoblasts which have been incorporated in bone during its formation. They interconnect and communicate with the surface osteoblasts by means of cell processes which extend through the numerous canaliculi in the bone matrix (Figure 18.13). The processes of neighbouring cells communicate via gap junctions (Holtrop, 1990). Thus they constitute a network. The precise function of osteocytes is unknown, although there is every reason to believe that it is significant. There are two possible roles. One is related to communication; an obvious possibility is to 'report' on the internal state of the bone. The other is calcium metabolism. There are observations on which to postulate that bone extracellular fluid is different from systemic ECF, and that the lining cell/osteocyte complex maintains and regulates it.

It is no longer widely held that osteocytes are an agent in bone resorption as proposed by Belanger (1969). The osteocytes may be active in manipulating matrix within the limits of the lacunae, but even this is in dispute.

The life span of osteocytes follows one of two courses. They may be released in the course of remodelling; their ultimate fate here is not known, but is probably death. Or they may die *in situ*. The life span is calcu-

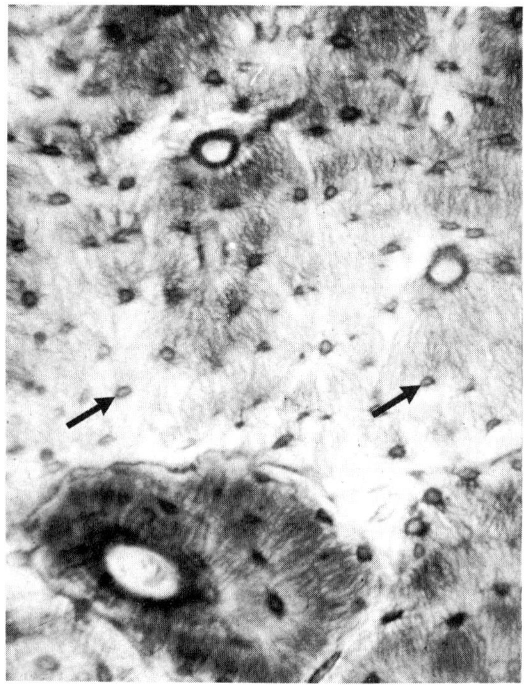

Figure 18.13 The canalicular system linking osteo-cytic lacunae (arrows), enabling osteocytic communication.

lated to be as long as 20 years. Death is signalled by pyknosis and dissolution, leaving empty lacunae. These and the canaliculi become densely calcified. The natural death of osteocytes is sporadic in distribution and is not considered an indicator of bone necrosis, although there may be obvious difficulties in making that distinction. As with most conundra arising from the study of histological sections, reference must be made to other sources of information about the case.

18.5 CONNECTIVE TISSUE MINERAL

Of all biologically formed minerals, about two-thirds are calcium with carbonates, phosphates, citrates, sulphates and oxalates (Williams and Frolik, 1991). Phosphates are most common in vertebrates, carbonates in invertebrates, and oxalates in plants. In primitive biological systems such as some bacteria and algae, mineralization occurs by bulk crystal formation within or outside the cell. In advanced systems an organic matrix serves as a framework. There are both common mechanisms and diverse regulatory systems throughout the biological kingdom.

Bone mineral, hydroxyapatite, plays a part in both the biomechanical and metabolic functions of bone within the bodily economy. Added to the organic matrix it gives rigidity. But it also provides a store of calcium, inorganic orthophosphate, sodium, magnesium, carbonate and other biologically necessary ions, and is a depository for unwanted ions such as lead, strontium, aluminium and others. At cellular and molecular levels there is an active interface between cells and minerals in which fluid circulation has a key role (Cooper *et al.*, 1966; Parfitt, 1979; Hughes *et al.*, 1986).

Calcium and phosphorus are able to combine with oxygen and hydrogen in a range of compounds, one class of which are the basic calcium phosphates. A species of this class is the apatites, all of which, at the dawn of time were bound up in igneous rocks (Posner, 1980, 1985). They were released by leaching into the earth's waters from where they were re-precipitated, via a biological cycle, in sedimentary rock, which in turn was subject to leaching (Figure 18.14).

The apatites are of wide interest and have been studied in a number of scientific fields. That formed by biological action, hydroxyapatite, is composed of very small crystals compared with those of igneous and hydrothermally altered rock. Consequently they have a high surface area per unit weight, which confers active surface chemistry. This and other details of their chemical structure are responsible for the biological actions listed above. They are not necessarily formed directly from the basic ingredients, but may result from transformation of amorphous calcium

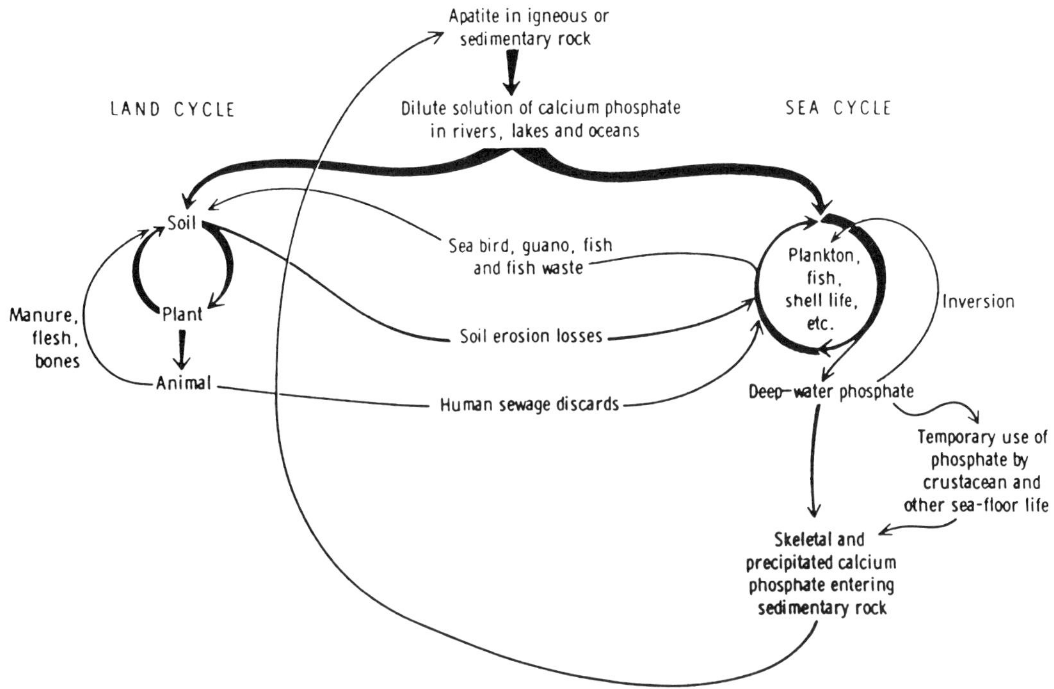

Figure 18.14 The calcium phosphate cycle in the earth's biosphere. (From Posner (1980), with permission.)

phosphate which is often formed from highly supersaturated solutions of calcium and phosphate.

The process of tissue mineralization is not finally established. There are at present two hypotheses. One gives primacy to the role of matrix vesicles in the deposition of hydroxyapatite crystals (Anderson, 1988). In the other it is factors in the matrix itself which are responsible (Glimcher, 1989). Each of these has been under investigation since the 1960s, contemporaneous with the burgeoning discoveries and understanding of the body's regulatory controls. It is not possible or necessary to present any of this in detail here. The object is to convey a sense of the dynamics of mineral metabolism in relation to bone and cartilage as active organs in the body economy over and above their locomotor function.

Most of the evidence in support of the vesicles is derived from observations of physeal cartilage (Anderson, 1969), with confirmatory observations from bone and teeth. The mineralization hypothesis based on them can explain some of the various forms of mineral deposition (Anderson, 1988). These are:

1. Normal
   (a) Cartilage ossification
   (b) Osteoid mineralization

2. Pathological extracellular
   (a) dystrophic (normal serum Ca^{2+} and PO_4^{3-}, tissue damage)

3. Pathological intracellular
   (a) dystrophic
   (b) metastatic (raised serum Ca^{2+} and PO_4^{3-}, normal tissues)

4. Calcium crystal deposition disorders (section 8.2.2)

Matrix vesicles are about 200 nm in diameter and are derived from the plasma membrane of cells. The membrane retains its phosphatases (alkaline phosphatase, ATP pyrophosphohydrolase, inorganic pyrophosphatase, Ca-ATPase, 5′ nucleotidase, p-nitrophenylphosphatase) which raise the level of PO_4^{3-} ; and the membrane lipids concentrate Ca^{2+}. This leads to phase 1 of the process – intravesicular crystal formation.

Extrusion of some or all of the crystal is followed by phase 2 – propagation of crystal growth. Hypothetically, the first phase is cell mediated and set in motion by alkaline phosphatase; the second is a physicochemical cascade in which matrix factors play an important part. These factors are collagen, carboxyglutamate proteins (GLA protein), phosphoproteins, glycoproteins (e.g. chondrocalcin) (Fisher and Termine, 1985), calcium–acidic phospholipid–phosphate complexes and proteolipids (Boyan *et al.*, 1989). Inhibitors play a role in the calcification process (Blumenthal, 1989); prominent among these in connective tissue matrices are the proteoglycans; others are Mg^{2+} pyrophosphate ion and ATP and ADP. Diphosphonates, synthetic compounds, also prevent

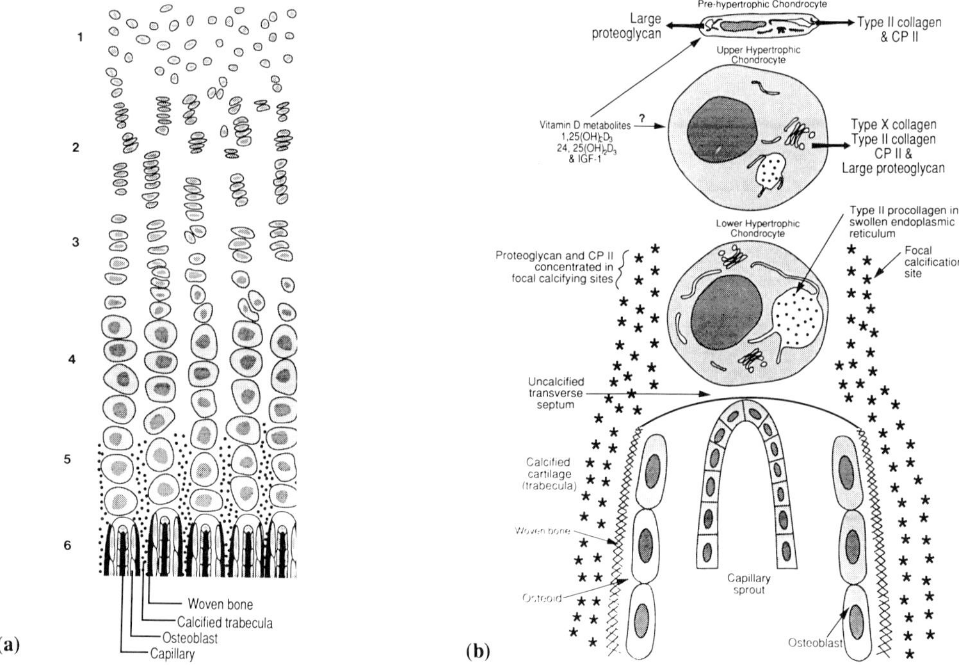

Figure 18.15 Schematic representation of an hypothesis for the mineralization of physeal cartilage. (a) The zones of the physis. 1, reserve; 2, proliferative, 3, maturation, 4, upper hypertrophic; 5, lower hypertrophic; 6, primary spongiosa. (b) The lower half of physis. Calcification starts in the lower hypertrophic zone at sites where large aggregating proteoglycans and the C-propeptide of type II collagen (CPII) are concentrated (see c). The last transverse septa of the hypertrophic zone, which marks the limit of the metaphysis is eroded by capillary sprouts. In the metaphysis osteoblasts deposited woven osteoid, which is mineralized to become bone. (Reproduced from Poole, 1991, with permission.)

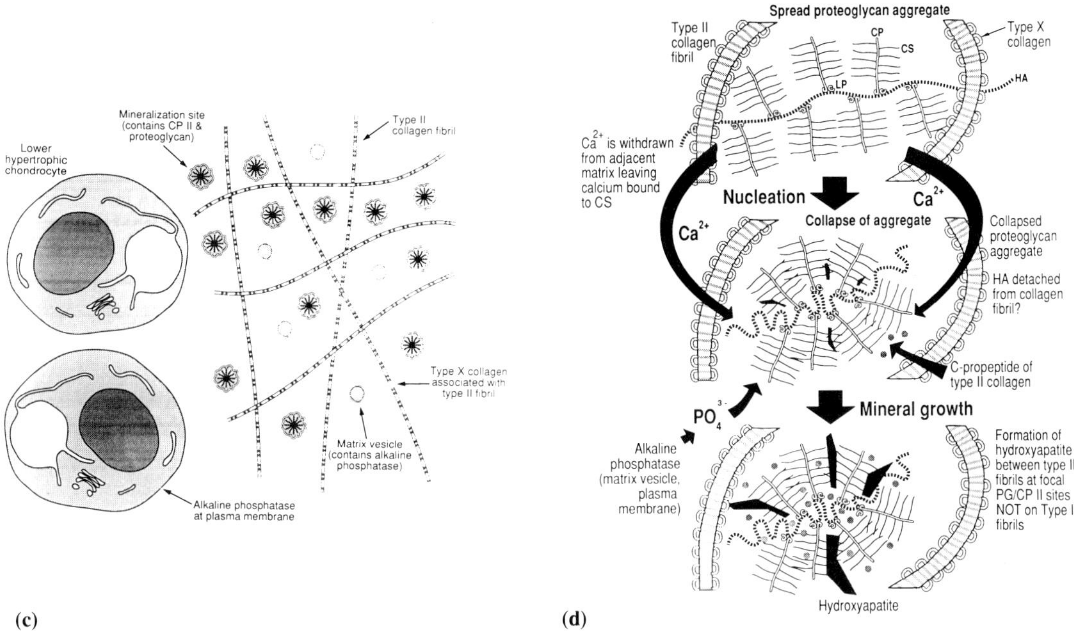

(c)   (d)

Figure 18.15 Schematic representation of an hypothesis for the mineralization of physeal cartilage. (c) The relationships of the participants in the calcification process: cells, collagens, proteoglycans and matrix vesicles. (d) The sites where large aggregating proteoglycans and the C-propeptide of type II collagen (CPII) are concentrated. The proteoglycans bind calcium to provide nucleation sites; crystal growth is enhanced by C-propeptide of type II collagen. Top drawing, the pre-mineralization state; middle, proteoglycan concentration and nucleation; bottom, crystal growth. (CP, core protein; CS, chondroitin sulphate; LP, link protein; HA, hyaluronic acid; PG, proteoglycan). (Reproduced from Poole (1991), with permission.)

apatite formation (Fleisch, 1989).

The protagonists of the matrix hypotheses have been largely concerned with bone (Glimcher, 1989). But others have studied the problem extensively in physeal cartilage (Matsui *et al.*, 1991; Alini *et al.*, 1992). None of these dispute the early action of vesicles in the process of calcification, but they regard them as but one of many initiating centres, and point to the fact that the vesicles are at a remove from the sites where the mineral deposition occurs. In osteoid the centres of initiation of importance in this hypothesis are in the collagen itself, giving rise to multiple minute foci, which may, or not, be synchronized (Glimcher, 1989). It is only in bone that collagen is physiologically involved in the mineralization process, even though type I collagen is the predominant form of collagen in many connective tissues; thus, it is unlikely that this is due to an intrinsic property of collagen but is enabled by a phosphoprotein. In physeal cartilage, foci of mineral deposition occur in the lower hypertrophic zone, beyond the location of maximum vesicle concentration in the proliferative zone, and are related to chemical alteration of proteoglycan molecules (Poole *et al.*, 1989; Poole, 1991) (Figure 18.15).

In all these hypotheses there are many unknowns. The control mechanisms are being slowly elucidated that make possible precipitation of calcium and phosphorus at some sites and not at others, with the formation of apatite crystals (Matsui *et al.*, 1991; Alini *et al.*, 1992).

18.6 MINERALIZATION AS SEEN IN HISTOLOGICAL SECTIONS

In practice, sites where mineral is being or has been deposited are difficult to recognize in decalcified sections. Sites in cartilage and in woven bone that have been mineralized frequently have a deeper staining in decalcified sections than non-calcified material. The same is true for woven bone. But in lamellar bone, it is unusual for osteoid and bone to be differentially stained in decalcified sections. To assess mineralization in bone requires undecalcified sections in which differential staining takes place with almost any stain.

Mineralization takes place at the interface between bone and osteoid. The narrow zone into which it is deposited is difficult to stain with complete reliability. The most satisfactory demonstration is by administering tetracycline, or similar fluorochrome, to the patient 48 hours before biopsy, and to view the section in polarized light (Figure 18.16). The seam of osteoid deposited in a resorption site begins to mineralize after an interval of some days, about 7–9, and then gradually proceeds more quickly than the rate of osteoid formation, until mineralization is complete after some 200 days. Patterns of mineralization are demonstrated in microradiographs, soft X-ray pictures of bone sec-

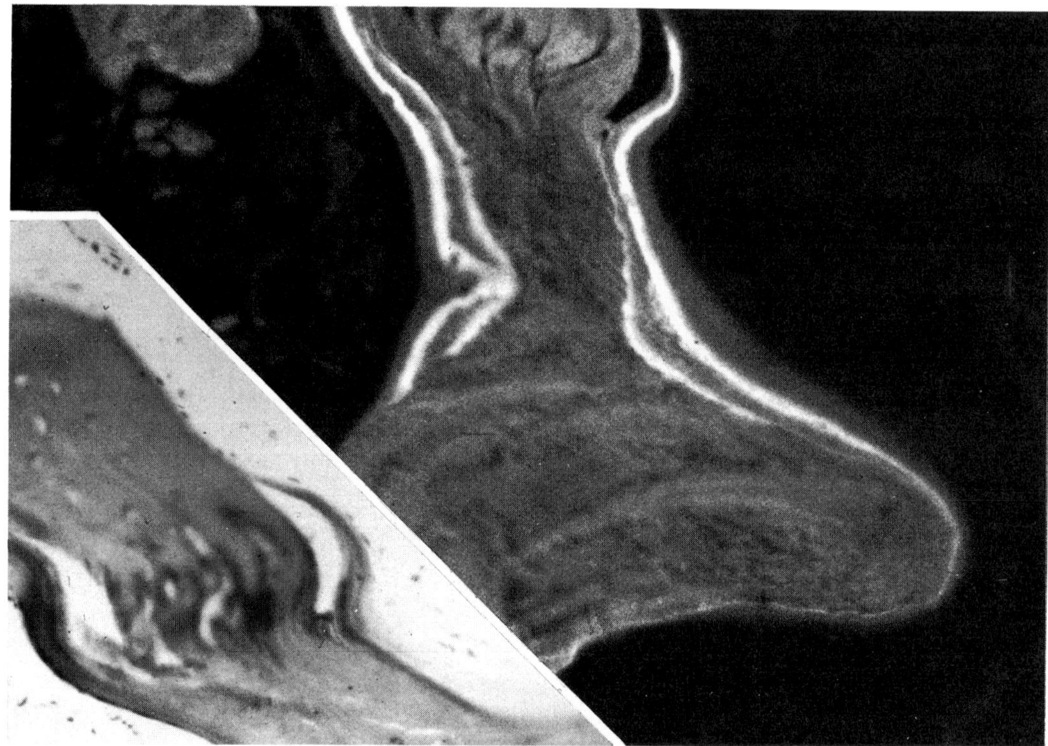

Figure 18.16 Tetracycline labelling of mineralization front. Fluorescence of double tetracycline label in a trabeculum. There is tissue over the second label which the inset (not a serial section) establishes as osteoid; the calcification front is visible in part.

tions in the range of 70–100 nm (Figures 18.17 and 18.18).

Pathological mineralization (Anderson, 1988) is frequently an intracellular process, particularly in the metastatic type. In that instance it is thought that some of the raised tissue fluid Ca^{2+} diffuses into the cytosol and the mitochondria take it up to maintain the low cytosol Ca^{2+} level. Over time this leads to $CaPO_4$ precipitation in the mitochondria and intracellular calcification. In dystrophic intracellular mineralization (Figure 18.19), cell damage destroys the plasma membrane Ca^{2+} pump, leading successively to raised cytosol and mitochondrial Ca^{2+} levels, and so to intramitochondrial $CaPO_4$ as before.

However, when dystrophic mineralization begins outside cells, it is postulated that membrane vesicles are derived from injured cells, although they have not been found in all examined cases, and are responsible for the onset of mineralization.

Evidence for a role of matrix vesicles is weakest in the calcium crystal deposition diseases, so called chondrocalcinosis or pseudogout, where the pathogenesis is largely unknown. The pathologist's most demanding encounter with these is likely to

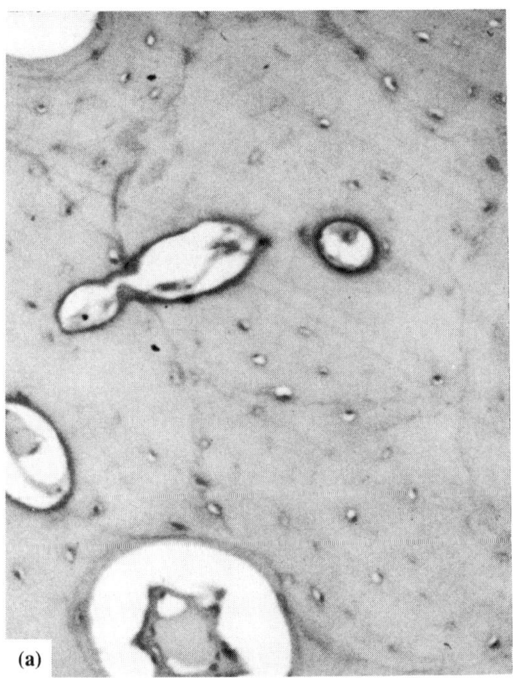

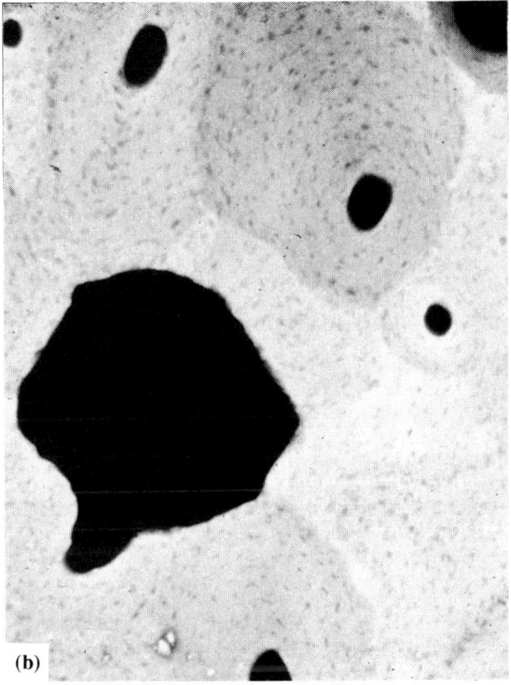

Figure 18.17 (a) A paraffin section of cortical bone showing one complete osteon and parts of several others. A Volkmann's canal is crossing the field (no related collagen lamellae). (b) Microradiograph of cross section of cortical bone. The osteonal canals are black; the mineralized bone shades of grey to white, according to density of mineral. The osteocyte lacunae are scattered grey flecks. Top right, a quadrant of osteon is seen with the least mineral density; this is a closing osteon. To its left is a recently completed osteon which has not yet achieved full mineralization. Other osteons, a paler shade of grey, are mature. The large cavity on the left is an osteonal canal in resorption phase; the surface is crenated by Howship lacunae; it is cutting into the territory of several adjacent osteons, creating an island of bone without a canal to which it is related: this is referred to as interstitial bone, which becomes the most densely mineralized tissue (palest grey).

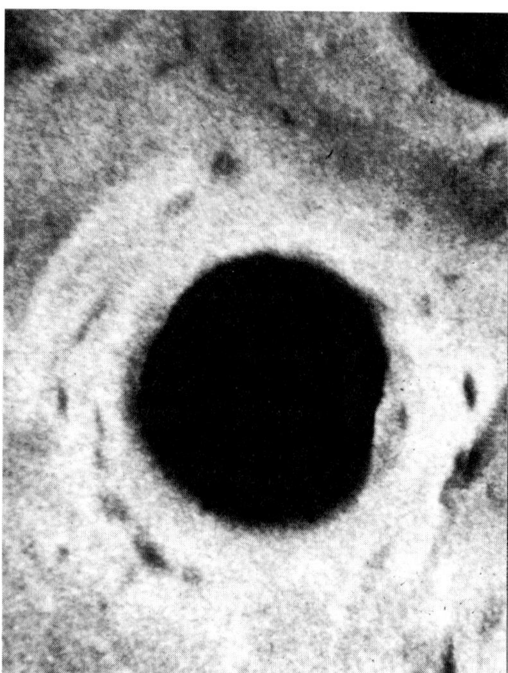

Figure 18.18 Microradiograph of bone in osteomalacia. The mineral density is very uneven, with the lowest density around osteocyte lacunae. This observation is indicative of an active role for osteocytes in the movement of mineral in mature bone.

be in the identification of crystals in synovial fluid (discussed in Chapter 8).

A number of crystals are to found in synovial fluid (McCarty, 1988):

- Monosodium urate monohydrate
- Calcium pyrophosphate dihydrate
- Basic calcium phosphate
     (carbonate apatite, octocalcium
     phosphate)
- Calcium oxalate mono/dihydrate
- Lipid
- Cholesterol
- Other particles and crystals
     Charcot–Leyden crystals
     Cryoglobulin crystals
     Amyloid fragments
     Aluminium phosphate crystals

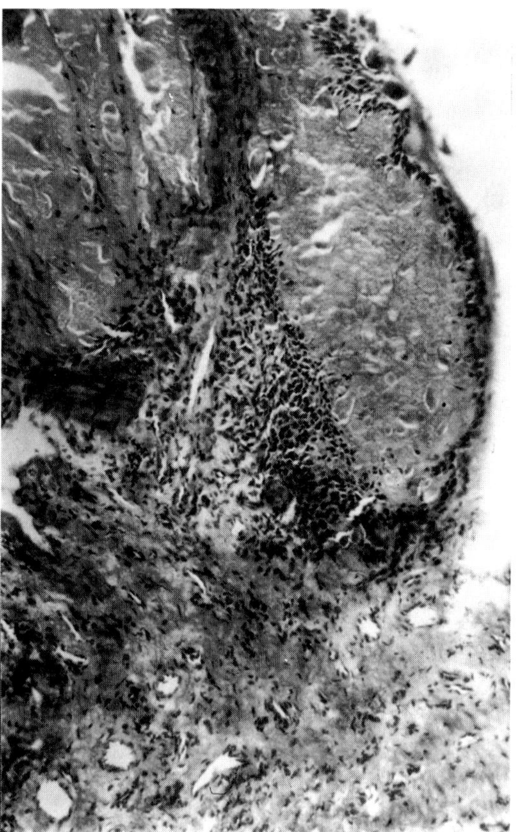

Figure 18.19 Female aged 32 years. Calcific deposit from shoulder. One large and two smaller foci of amorphous mineral surrounded by a zone of granulomatous reaction. Congested and poorly organized connective tissue below. Photograph courtesy of Professor S.Y. Ali.

     Metal fragments
     Cartilage fragments
     Particulate collagen

Of these only calcium pyrophosphate dihydrate (CPPD) and basic calcium phosphate are of concern here.

Westheimer (1987) discusses the dominant place of phosphates in biology, emphasizing their unique ability to confer on many compounds (DNA, RNA, energy-rich intermediate metabolites (ATP and others)) stability against hydrolysis and retention by lipid membranes. This plethora of phosphates leads to many intracellular synthetic reactions in which inorganic pyrophosphate is a by-product (Russell, 1976). Since this is not an energy source, nor an otherwise useful metabolic product it must be disposed of to prevent reversal of the reactions of which it is an end product. It is assumed that for this reason pyrophosphatases must be widespread and responsible for the low intra- and extracellular levels.

Inorganic pyrophosphate (PP_i) is a phosphate ester, a class of compound which is unable passively to cross lipid membranes. Since no transfer mechanism is known it is difficult to account for its extracellular presence. In the presence of CPPD crystal deposition, the synovial fluid level of PP_i is high and greater than that of the plasma. This infers intra-articular production, which has some experimental support from the finding that, *in vitro*, porcine cartilage produces PP_i (Rachow and Lawrence, 1988).

The mechanism of CPPD crystal deposition in tissues is not known, nor the determinants of which tissues are affected (mainly cartilage; to a lesser extent synovium), nor why of all the twelve reported calcium salts only two are formed *in vivo*. There are complexes formed with a number of other cations. This range of compounds reflects the range of inter- and intramolecular bonding configurations that inorganic pyrophosphate can form (Mandel and Mandel, 1988).

Basic calcium phosphate crystals are ultramicroscopic and consequently present problems in identification. They tend to form aggregations, but even these may be ultramicroscopic. At the level of imaging, macroscopic or light microscopic means it may not be particularly problematic to identify mineral deposition, but the complete identification of the composition of the deposits, which may often be a mixture of crystals, will be beyond the resources of routine diagnostic laboratories. These difficulties in identification have caused problems in classifying

and unravelling the pathogenesis of the associated disorders (Dieppe *et al.*, 1988; Reginato, 1991). For clinical purposes (Jensen, 1988), it may be adequate to distinguish between urate and pyrophosphate crystals, which can be done relatively easily by polarization (Figures 18.20 and 18.21).

18.7 THE REGULATION OF BONE AND CARTILAGE CELL ACTIVITY

Regulatory systems have been under independent investigation mainly in immunology, virology, haematology and cell biology (Nathan and Sporn, 1991) for some decades. Recently it has become evident, contrary to expectations, that the regulatory molecules are more or less common to all, but not before a confusing terminology was engendered. It is not the intention here to attempt a comprehensive review, but a brief summary of the most salient points of current theories of the operation of regulatory systems will be presented and some details about specific substances.

The regulators are classifiable as:

1. Endocrine (produced elsewhere, deliv-

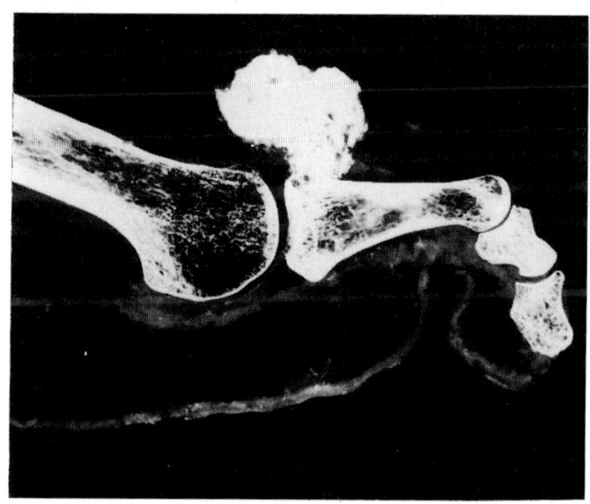

Figure 18.20 Mineral deposition in gouty tophus of long standing. The mineral is amorphous and will not affect the birefringence of the urate crystals.

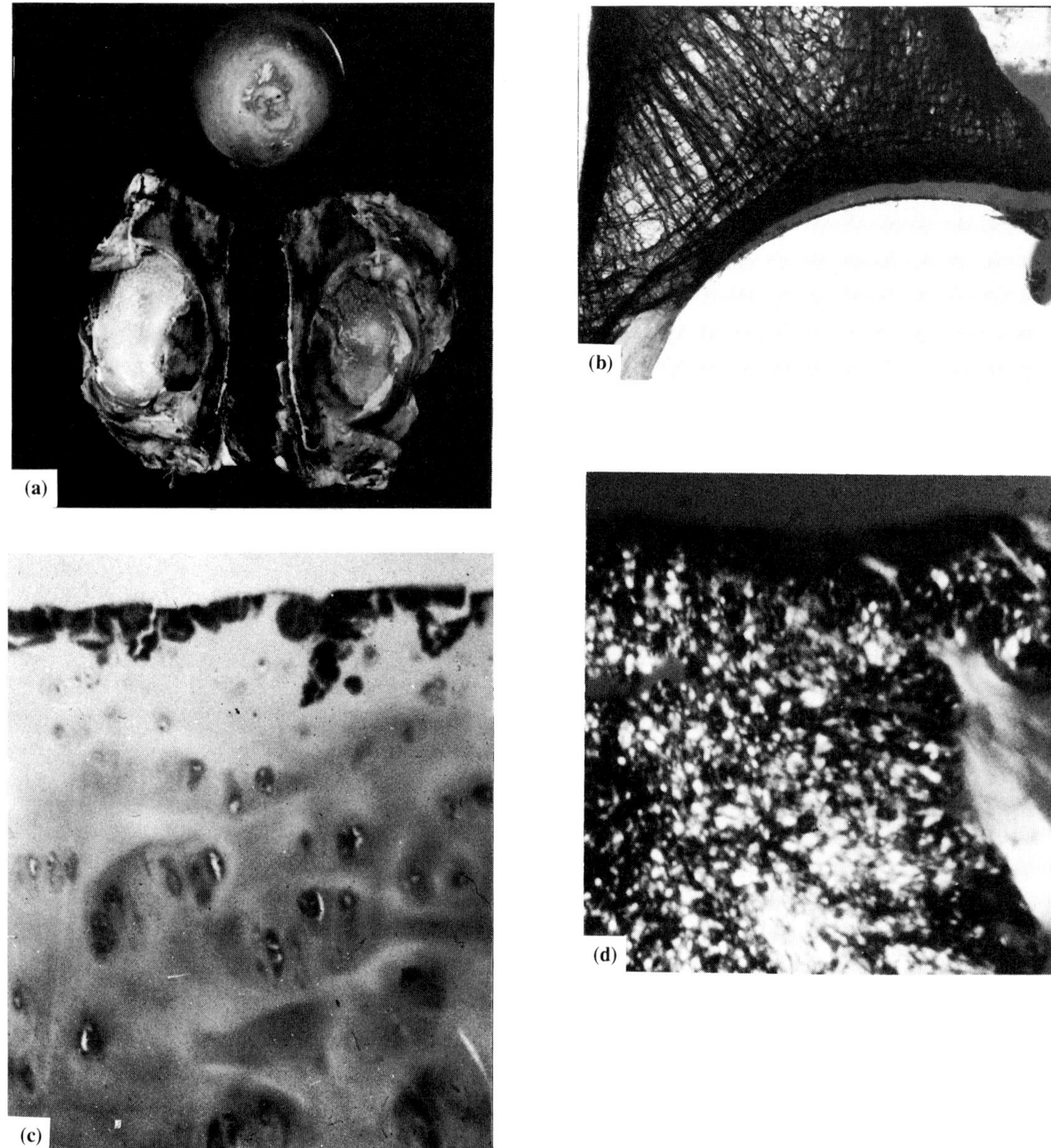

Figure 18.21 Calcium pyrophosphate deposition. Female aged 68 years. Incidental finding at autopsy. (a) Medial view of femoral head and lateral of bisected acetabulum. Several small chalky deposits around the fovea. Most of the surface of the acetabular cartilage is covered by deposit. (b) Fine detail radiograph of slab from acetabulum. The black line at the articular surface and the two foci in the labrum are crystal deposits. (c) Undecalcified section of articular cartilage with the retained mineral in surface deposits. (d) The crystals at high magnification in polarized light.

ered to all cells via the circulation);
2.   Paracrine (produced locally and active in the immediate neighbourhood);
3.   Autocrine/autocoid (intracellular);
4.   Neurotransmitter (synaptic, confined to the nervous system).

In this discussion it is important to recall that receptors are the means for introducing the message into the cell and starting the series of events to execute the command, and that they are themselves important in the regulatory system since their number, affinity, specificity and availability can also be controlled to provide a means of modulation (Brockes, 1990).

Knowledge of the paracrine/autocrine group has advanced as the result of research in the aforementioned disciplines. However, the outcome has often been confusing because of the contradictory actions of many regulators under different circumstances. It has been recognized that the operational environment is one determinant of cytokine effect. Nathan and Sporn (1991) have proposed a unifying concept. They use cytokine as the collective noun for polypeptide (protein) regulatory factors, which have been variously called interleukins, interferons, colony-stimulating factors and peptide growth factors. They define these as non-immunoglobulin, soluble (glyco)proteins produced by host cells, which, in minute amounts, act non-enzymatically to regulate host cell function (given the presence of receptor(s) on the target cell). They propose the central role of cytokines is the control of tissue (re)modelling, whether during embryological development, modelling/re-modelling of the developed body during growth and maturity, or in response to pathological events.

This proposal is inferred from seven types of interaction that have been observed between cytokines and matrix.

1.   Cells are induced to make cytokines by adherence to matrix.
2.   Cytokines induce cells to alter matrix.
3.   Cytokines affect cell adhesion receptors.
4.   Matrix presents cytokines to cells.
5.   Some adhesion receptors can act like cytokine receptors.
6.   Some cytokine receptors can promote cell–cell adhesion.
7.   Adhesion can control how cells respond to cytokines.

Control mechanisms are operated by cells for cells, organized as tissues, dependent on the infrastructure of the cells for such things as energy, protein production, intracellular transport and intercellular signalling, which means that any regulatory event is a cascade or a succession of cascades, within one or more types of cell or extracellularly. The intercellular signal molecules, the cytokines, may be rendered diffusible, cell bound or matrix bound, in a reactive state or latent and awaiting activation. Matrix, the product of cells, is complex in composition and rich in its store of molecules with a regulatory potential (Delmas *et al.*, 1984; Heinegard and Sommarin, 1987). The carbohydrate element of matrix macromolecules has the potential to store information rivalling that of the genome (Rademacher *et al.*, 1988). In addition, matrix under load produces electrical impulses with a potential role in signalling and communication. In the case of bone this has been recognized and exploited clinically (Luben, 1991).

Interest in the regulatory systems inherent to bone and cartilage was initiated by Urist and McLean's (1952) proposal that bone tissue contained a bone-inducing substance. This has been substantiated by the characterization of seven such proteins (section 18.7.2). Progress in the study of regulatory molecules has been greatly aided by recombinant DNA technology (Alberts *et al.*, 1989). In 1984 Delmas *et al.* separated from bovine bone 40 protein groups unrelated to collagen (non-collagenous proteins) constituted of 160 major entities; minor entities increased the total to above 200. At that time few had been characterized or their function postulated. The structure of several dozen is now known, and their role is becoming clearer. In cartilage the main non-collagenous proteins have long been recognized as proteoglycans. The unravelling of these complex molecules is leading to the recognition that their function is often more than inflating the collagen network, and is revealing other proteins (Heinegard and Sommarin, 1987). These non-collagenous matrix proteins, would probably meet Nathan and Sporn's definition of cytokine. A detailed account of factors controlling cartilage growth and differentiation is given by Seyedin and Rosen (1991).

Expansion of knowledge of regulators and how they act enables hypotheses about the operation of cellular activities. For bone, mechanisms have been suggested to account for the coupling of osteoclasts and osteoblasts (Chambers *et al.*, 1985; Mundy, 1991a, b), the control of remodelling and the healing of fractures. These are not fully established,

and they and many more aspects of bone physiology, normal and pathological, remain to be discovered. Similarly, for cartilage, there is a widening understanding of its molecular biology and the complexity of its regulation (Hall and Newman, 1991). Little by little, the details of the lower levels of Frost's Intermediary Organisation of the skeleton are being filled in.

The regulators usually considered in connection with bone (Williams and Frolik, 1991) and cartilage are shown in Table 18.3. The following thumbnail sketches are based on Williams and Frolik (1991), who give a substantial list of references. Hauschka (1990) discusses growth factor effects in bone with comprehensive references.

18.7.1 ENDOCRINE

(a) Parathyroid hormone (PTH)

PTH acts on bone, intestine and kidney. In the latter two it enhances calcium resorption.

Table 18.3 Bone and cartilage regulators

Endocrine	Parathyroid hormone
	Calcitonin
	Vitamin D
	Vitamin A
	Oestrogens
	Androgens
	Growth hormone
Paracrine/autocrine (synonyms: non-collagenous proteins; cytokines (Nathan and Sporn, 1991))	Proteoglycans
	Glycoproteins
	Phosphoproteins
	Gamma-carboxyglutamic acid proteins
	Proteolipids
	Growth factors (peptide growth factors)
	Transforming growth factor beta
	Bone morphogenetic proteins
	Insulin-like growth factor
	Epithelial growth factor
	Fibroblast growth factor
	Platelet-derived growth factor
	Cytokines

Receptors for PTH have been found on pre-osteoblasts, osteoblasts and chondrocytes, but not on osteoclasts. This supports the thesis that the action of the latter is dependent on osteoblast activity, either release of a signal or of collagenase which exposes mineralized tissue by removing a putative protective collagen layer. There is experimental evidence that PTH can lead to bone apposition, and that it modulates or is modulated by some growth factors.

(b)   Calcitonin

Calcitonin is produced by thyroid C cells, and acts on osteoclasts via a receptor to stop the resorption of bone. In addition, stimulating effects on bone and cartilage have been demonstrated experimentally, as well as interaction with other factors.

(c)   Vitamin D

The metabolism of vitamin D is principally in the kidney, but the major effect is on mineralization of bone and cartilage. The complex metabolic pathways, involving the osteoblast and interactions with other regulators, by which this is achieved are not entirely clear.

(d)   Vitamin A

In excess, retinoids decrease the formation of bone and cartilage matrix, whereas a deficiency tends to the opposite effect. They interact with other regulators, modulating vitamin D metabolism and influencing PTH production and activity, which may be their principal role in the development of bone.

(e)   Oestrogens

In women, and in female rats, reduced oestrogen leads to bone loss via turnover, which may be accelerated. This is now thought to be a direct effect on osteoblasts, and possibly on osteoclasts; the alternative is mediation through PTH and calcitonin.

(f)   Androgens

These contribute to the formation of bone and the maintenance of bone mass through a positive action via receptors on osteoblasts, and an indirect inhibition of osteoclasts, acting through PTH and calcitonin. There may be interaction with other growth factors.

(g)   Growth hormone

Much of the effect of this hormone on bone growth is via insulin-like growth factors. But there is also a direct effect on chondrocytes and osteoblasts where receptors can be found.

18.7.2   NON-COLLAGENOUS PROTEINS

(a)   Proteoglycans

The proteoglycans are a family of large and small members. In addition to inflating cartilage, some are proposed to have a role in matrix organization and mineralization (section 18.5).

(b)   Glyco- and phosphoproteins

This is not an easily separated group since some glycoproteins are also phosphorylated. In the former class are three proteins rich in sialic acid, hence bone sialoproteins BSP: BSP I, osteopontin (OPN); BSP II; bone acidic glycoprotein-75 (BAG-75). There is also a dentin SP. Attributed to these compounds is a role in the control of extracellular calcium, regulation of crystal growth and shape, and cell adhesion to bone surfaces. Phosphoproteins are believed to regulate (meaning to inhibit and/or promote, depending on circumstance) extracellular formation and mineralization. Specifically, osteonectin is a phosphorylated glycoprotein (Boskey, 1989; Butler, 1991; Wrana *et al.*, 1991).

(c) Gamma-carboxyglutamic acid proteins

Osteocalcin, found only in bone (hence bone GLA protein) is made by osteoblasts, and secreted into the matrix of osteoid after initiation of mineral. Secretion is under many controls, including vitamin D, TGF-β PTH. Serum levels reflect bone turnover. Their role appears to be the regulation of crystal growth and recruitment of osteoclasts. There is also a matrix GLA protein, found in bone, cartilage, lung, heart and kidney the function of which is not known (Hauschka and Wians, 1989; Balmain, 1991).

(d) Proteolipids

These are membrane proteins complexed with acidic phospholipids, especially phosphatidylserine. They cause hydroxyapatite deposition. Concentration in matrix vesicles is high, where they are thought to export protons and import calcium and phosphate (ionophore).

(e) Growth factors

Included under this heading are many peptides found in many tissues of many species, active in both development and growth, and in regulation in the mature animal. Structural and functional relationships, which often extend across species, exist. Moreover, all peptide 'growth factors' have multiple effects on cells, acting as multifunctional signalling molecules without intrinsic action (Sporn and Roberts, 1991). Transduction of the signal is by the receptor in the cell membrane, which switches on or off biochemical events (Luben, 1991).

(i) *Insulin-like growth factors (IGF I and II)*

These factors are produced by many types of cell, including those of bone (osteoblasts and chondrocytes). They act via receptors to promote proliferation, differentiation and matrix production of bone and cartilage. The action of growth hormone is closely integrated with the IGFs, although the mechanisms are not clear.

(ii) *Transforming growth factor β (Centrella et al., 1991)*

The name transforming growth factor comes from the effect of compounds, isolated from spontaneously formed colonies of neoplastic cells in soft agar, on normal cells, which otherwise do not colonize in soft agar. Two factors, named alpha and beta, were isolated: α is akin to epidermal growth factor, and is not found in bone; β is one of five closely related compounds which are produced in a large number of animals by many tissues. There are three human isoforms, the largest store being in bone matrix. A number of similar compounds have been described. All are collectively known as the TGF-β supergene family. Bone morphogenetic proteins are a subgroup. Knowledge about the actions of the TGFs in bone has been gained from osteoblast tissue culture systems. Results can be variable, dependent on dose and system. This is considered due at least in part to the influence of receptors, of which there at least four, and on the possibility of cross effects on and by other regulators (Boyd *et al.*, 1990). They increase DNA at low, but less effectively at high, concentrations; enhance synthesis of type I collagen and non-collagenous proteins; and reduce the activity of alkaline phosphatase. There is less information on the effect on osteoclasts; reports indicate stimulation by low concentrations and inhibition by high ones. The latter is associated with production of prostaglandins.

There is an hypothesis that the role of TGF-β is to induce bone formation in the BMU sequence of bone remodelling: osteoclasts release the regulator during resorption, which then stimulates osteoblasts to form bone at the site; it may also bring resorption to a close as the concentration of TGF-β at the site rises (Mundy, 1991a, b) (section 18.7.2).

(iii) Bone morphogenetic proteins (BMP)

A bone-inducing protein was first postulated in 1952 (Urist and McLean 1952, Urist *et al.*, 1967; Urist and Strates, 1971), since when seven related proteins (BMP1 – 7) with this property have been extracted from bone matrix and analysed (Wozney *et al.*, 1990). Their action is studied mainly in rats by subcutaneous implantation, where they induce infiltration, proliferation and differentiation of precursor cells into chondrocytes with subsequent formation and ossification of cartilage to form an ossicle containing bone cells and marrow. There is evidence to suggest that several growth factors may be involved. As mentioned above, the BMPs are part of the TGF-β supergene family.

(iv) Epithelial growth factor; Fibroblast growth factor; Platelet-derived growth factor; Cytokines (interleukins, colony-stimulating factors, tumour necrosis factor)

These compounds are thought to act on osteoblasts and, in some cases, osteoclasts by promoting proliferation and differentiation of precursors. Some are also believed to stimulate matrix production of osteoblasts and chondrocytes. It is also felt that they may have a direct or indirect part to play in mineralization (Williams and Frolik, 1991).

Finally, since regulation has to do with signalling and communication, there can be added **mechanosensory systems**. Bone responds to load by remodelling: Wolff's (1986) Law has been abundantly confirmed, as has the sensitivity, *in vitro*, of osteoblasts and chondrocytes to pressure; but the feedback mechanism whereby changes in load are registered, and resorption and formation are started, have not. Cowin *et al.* (1991) discuss possible mechanosensory systems in bone at the cellular and tissue level. The components are:

1. **The cell network**: osteocytes and their processes form an intraosseous network in communication with the surface cells, i.e. resting or active osteoblasts. Neighbouring cell processes communicate via gap junctions permitting passage of small molecules and ions. Postulated are stretch-sensitive ion channels in osteocytes; these are known to exist in fibroblasts and osteoblasts.

2. **Mineralized matrix**: stream-generated potentials are created when fluid, flowing through the spaces within the matrix, carries with it one class of ion whereas the other adheres to the matrix (Otter *et al.*, 1990). These spaces are the intercrystalline pores, and those lying between the plasma membranes of the cells and their processes, and the walls of the lacunae and of the canaliculae. These are continuous, but separated from the interstitial fluid of the marrow by the osteoblast layer.

Deformation of the matrix by load is postulated to have two effects: (a) distort the lacunae sufficiently to activate the pressure-sensitive ion channels; (b) to cause the movement of fluid through the system to generate streaming potentials which are also transduced to the osteocyte network. The transduced signals lead to the release of a second messenger which is carried to the surface osteoblasts, which set in motion the remodelling sequence.

A more detailed discussion is given in Cowin *et al.* (1991) together with references to supporting literature. They also quote the observation of Otter *et al.* (1990) that strain-related potentials have yet to be shown to affect or control remodelling.

REFERENCES

Alberts, B., Bray, D., Lewis, J. *et al.* (1989) *Molecular Biology of the Cell*, 2nd edn, Garland Publishing, New York, pp. 180–96.

Alini, M., Matsui, Y., Dodge, G.R. *et al.* (1992) The extracellular matrix in the growth plate before and during calcification: changes in composition and degradation of type II collagen. *Calcif. Tissue. Int.*, **50**, 327–35.

Amiel, D., Frank, C., Harwood, F. *et al.* (1984) Tendons and ligaments – a morphological and biochemical comparison. *J. Orthop. Res.*, **1**, 257–265.

Anderson, H.C. (1969) Vesicles associated with calcification in the matrix of epiphyseal cartilage. *J. Cell Biol.*, **41**, 59–2.

Anderson, H.C. (1988) Mechanisms of pathological calcification. *Rheum. Dis. Clin. North Am.*, **14**, 303–19.

Balmain, N. (1991) Calbindin-D9k. A vitamin D dependent binding protein in mineralised tissue. *Clin. Orthop.*, **265**, 265–76.

Belanger, L.F. (1969) Osteocytic osteolysis. *Calcif. Tissue. Res.*, **4**, 1–2.

Blumenthal, N.C. (1989) Mechanisms of inhibition of calcification. *Clin. Orthop.*, **247**, 279–89.

Boskey, A.L. (1989) Noncollagenous matrix proteins and their role in mineralisation. *Bone Miner.*, **6**, 111–23.

Boyan, B.D., Schwarz, Z., Swain, L.D. *et al.* (1989) Role of lipids in calcification of cartilage. *Anat. Rec.*, **224**, 211–19.

Boyd, F.T., Cheifetz, S., Andres, J. *et al.* (1990) Transforming growth factor Beta receptors and binding proteoglycans. *J. Cell Sci.*, Suppl. **13**, 131–8.

Brockes, J.P. (1990) Retinoic acid and limb regeneration. *J. Cell Sci.*, Suppl. **13**, 191–8.

Bullough, P. and Goodfellow, J. (1968) The significance of the fine structure of articular cartilage. *J. Bone Joint Surg.*, **73A**, 1418–28.

Burger, E.H. and Nijweide, P.J. (1991) Cellular origin and theories of osteoclast differentiation. In *Bone*, Vol. 2, *The osteoclast.* (Ed. B.K. Hall), CRC Press, Boca Raton, FL, pp. 31–59.

Butler, W.P. (1991) Sialoproteins of bone and dentin. *J. Biol. Buccale*, **19**, 83–9.

Centrella, M., McCarthy, T.L. and Canalis, E. (1991) Transforming growth factor-beta and remodelling of bone. *J. Bone Joint Surg.*, **73A**, 1418–28.

Chambers, T.J., Darby, A.J. and Fuller, K. (1985) Mammalian collagenase predisposes bone surfaces to osteoclastic resorption. *Calcif. Tissue. Res.*, **24**, 671–5.

Cooper, R.R., Milgram, J.W. and Robinson, R.A. (1966) Morphology of the osteon. *J. Bone Joint Surg.*, **48A**, 1239–71.

Cowin, S.C., Moss-Salentin, L. and Moss, M.L. (1991) Candidates for the mechanosensory system in bone. *J. Biomech. Eng.*, **113**, 191–7.

Delmas, P.D., Tracy, R.P., Riggs, B.L. *et al.* (1984) Identification of the noncollagenous proteins of bovine bone by two dimensional electrophoresis. *Calcif. Tissue Int.*, **36**, 308–16.

Dieppe, P., Campion, G. and Doherty, M. (1988) Mixed crystal deposition. *Rheum. Dis. Clin. North Am.*, **14**, 415–26.

Fawcett, D.W. (1986) Connective tissue proper. In *A Text Book of Histology*, 11th edn (eds L. Bloom and D.W. Fawcett) WB Saunders, London, Chapter 5, pp. 136–73.

Fisher, L.W. and Termine, J.D. (1985) Noncollagenous proteins influence the local mechanisms of calcification. *Clin. Orthop.*, **200**, 362–85.

Fleisch, H. (1989) Biphosphonates: a new class of drugs in diseases of bone and calcium metabolism. *Recent Results Cancer Res.*, **116**, 1–28.

Frank, C., Amiel, D., Woo, S.L-Y. *et al.* (1985) Normal ligament properties and ligament healing. *Clin. Orthop.*, **196**, 15–25.

Frost, H.M. (1960) Micropetrosis. *J. Bone Joint Surg.*, **42A**, 144–50.

Frost, H.M. (1986) *Intermediary Organisation of the Skeleton.* CRC Press, Boca Raton, FL.

Glimcher, M.J. (1989) Mechanism of calcification: role of collagen fibrils and collagen-phosphoprotein complexes in vitro and in vivo. *Anat. Rec.*, **224**, 139–53.

Hall, B.K. (ed.) (1983) *Cartilage.* Vol. 1, *Structure, function and biochemistry.* Vol. 2, *Development, differentiation and growth.* Vol. 3, *Biomedical aspects.* CRC Press, Boca Raton, Fl.

Hall, B.K. (ed.) (1990–2) *Bone.* Vol. 1 (1990) *The osteoblast and osteocyte.* Vol. 2 (1991) *The osteoclast.* Vol. 3 (1991) *Bone matrix and bone specific products.* Vol. 4 (1991) *Bone metabolism and mineralisation.* Vol. 5 (1992) *Fracture repair and regeneration.* CRC Press, Boca Raton, FL.

Hall, B.K. and Newman, S.A. (1991) *Cartilage: Molecular Aspects.* CRC Press, Boca Raton, FL.

Hauschka, P.V. (1990) Growth factors effects in bone. In *Bone*, Vol. 1. *The osteoblast and osteocyte.* (ed. B.K. Hall), The Telford Press, New Jersey, Vol. 1, Chapter 4, pp. 103–70.

Hauschka, P.V. and Wians, F.H. (1989) Osteocalcin–hydroxyapatite interaction in the extracellular organic matrix of bone. *Anat. Rec.*, **224**, 180–8.

Heinegard, D. and Sommarin, Y. (1987) Proteoglycans: an overview. *Methods Enzymol.*, **144**, 305–19.

Holtrop, M.E. (1990) Light and electron microscopic structure of bone forming cells, In *Bone* Vol 1: *The Osteoblast and the Osteocyte.* (ed. B.K. Hall), The Telford Press, New Jersey. Chapter 1, pp. 1–40.

Holtrop, M.E. (1991) Light and electron microscopic structure of osteoclasts. In *Bone*, Vol. 2. *The Osteoclast.* (ed. B.K. Hall), CRC Press, Boca Raton, FL. pp. 1–29.

Hughes, S.P.F., McCarthy, I.D. and Hooper, G. (1986) The vascular system in bone. *Clin. Orthop.*, **210**, 31–6.

Jee, W.S.S. (1988) The skeletal tissues. In *Cell and Tissue Biology: a Textbook of Histology*, 6th edn, (ed. L. Weiss), Elsevier, North Holland.

Jeffrey, A.K., Blunn, G.W., Archer, C.W. *et al.* (1991) Three dimensional collagen architecture in bovine articular cartilage. *J. Bone Joint Surg.*, **73B**, 795–801.

Jensen, P.S. (1988) Chondrocalcinosis and other calcifications. *Radiol. Clin. North Am.*, **26**, 1315–25.

Kahn, A.J. and Partridge, N.C. (1991) Bone resorption in vivo. In *Bone*, Vol. 2. *The osteoclast* (ed. B.K. Hall), CRC Press, Boca Raton, FL.

Leblond, C.P. (1989) Synthesis and secretion of collagen by cells of connective tissue, bone and dentin. *Anat. Rec.*, **224**, 123–38

Luben, R.A. (1991) Effects of low energy fields (pulsed and DC) on membrane signal transduction processes in biological systems. *Health Phys.*, **61**, 15–28.

Mandel, N. and Mandel, G. (1988) Calcium pyro phosphate crystal deposition in Model systems. *Rheum. Dis. Clin. North Am.*, **14**, 321–40.

Marks, S.C. and Popoff, S.N. (1988) Bone cell biology: the regulation of development, structure and function in the skeleton *Am. J. Anat.*, **183**, 1–44.

Maroudas, A. (1979) Physicochemical properties of articular cartilage. In *Adult Articular Cartilage*, 2nd edn, (ed. M.A.R. Freeman, Pitman Medical, Tunbridge Wells. pp. 215–90.

Mathews, J.L. (1980) Bone structure and ultrastructure. In *Fundamental and Clinical Bone Physiology* (ed. M.R. Urist), J.B. Lippincott, Philadelphia, pp. 4–44.

Matsui, Y., Alini, M., Webber, C. *et al.* (1991) Characterisation of aggregating proteoglycans from the proliferative, maturing, hypertrophic and calcifying zones of the cartilaginous physis. *J. Bone Joint Surg.*, **73A**, 1064–74.

McCarty, D.J. (1988) Crystal identification in human synovial fluids. *Rheum. Dis. Clin. North Am.*, **14**, 253–67.

Meachim, G. (1972) Light microscopy of Indian ink preparations of fibrillated cartilage. *Ann. Rheum. Dis.*, **31**, 457–64.

Meachim, G. and Stockwell, R.A. (1979) The matrix. In *Adult Articular Cartilage* (ed. M.A.R. Freeman), Pitman Medical, Tunbridge Wells. pp. 1–68.

Menton, D.N., Simmons, D.J., Orr, B.Y. *et al.* (1982) A cellular investment of bone marrow. *Anat. Rec.*, **203**, 157–64.

Miller, E.J. and Gay, S. (1987) The collagens: an overview and update. *Methods Enzymol.*, **144**, 3–41.

Miller, S.C., Bowman, B.M., Smith, J.A. *et al.* (1980) Characterisation of endosteal bone-lining cells from fatty marrow sites of adult beagles. *Anat. Rec.*, **198**, 163–73.

Mundy, G.R. (1991a) Inflammatory cell mediators and the destruction of bone. *J. Periodont. Res.*, **26**, 213–17.

Mundy, G.R. (1991b) The effects of TGF-Beta on bone. In *Clinical Applications of TGF-β*, Ciba Foundation Symposium 157 (eds G.R. Bock and J. Marsh), John Wiley, Chichester, pp. 137–51.

Nathan, C. and Sporn, M. (1991) Cytokines in context. *J. Cell Biol.*, **113**, 981–6.

Otter, M.W., Palmieri, V.R. and Cochran, G.V.B. (1990) Transcortical streaming potentials are generated by circulatory pressure gradients in living canine tibia. *J. Orthop. Res.*, **8**, 119–26.

Parfitt, A.M. (1979) Equilibrium and disequilibrium hypercalcaemia: new light on an old concept. *Metab. Bone Dis.*, **1**, 279–93.

Parfitt, A.M. (1990) Bone forming cells in clinical conditions. In *Bone* Vol 1, *The osteoblast and the osteocyte* (ed. B.K. Hall), Telford Press, New Jersey. Chapter 9, pp. 351–430.

Poole, A.R. (1981) Proteoglycans in health and disease: structure and function. *Biochem. J.*, **236**, 1–14.

Poole, A.R. (1991) The growth plate: cellular physiology, cartilage assembly and mineralisation. In *Cartilage: Molecular Aspects* (eds B.K. Hall and S. Newman), CRC Press, Boca Raton, FL. Chapter 6, pp. 179–211.

Poole, A.R., Matsui, Y., Hinek, A. *et al.* (1989) Cartilage macromolecules and the calcification of cartilage matrix. *Anat. Rec.*, **224**, 167–79.

Posner, A.S. (1980) Bone mineral. In *Scientific Foundations of Orthopaedics and Traumatology* (eds R. Owen, J. Goodfellow and P. Bullough), William Heinemann Medical Books, London, pp. 42–8.

Posner, A.S. (1985) The mineral of bone. *Clin. Orthop.*, **200**, 87–99.

Pritchard, J.J. (1972) The osteoblast. In *The Biochemistry and Physiology of Bone*. (ed. G.H. Bourne), Academic Press, London. pp. 21–43.

Rachow, J.W. and Lawrence, M.R. (1988) Inorganic pyrophosphate metabolism in arthritis. *Rheum. Dis. Clin. North Am.*, **14**, 289–302.

Rademacher, T.W., Parekh, R.B. and Dwek, R.A. (1988) Glycobiology. *Ann. Rev. Biochem.*, **57**, 785–838.

Reginato, A.J. (1991) Calcium pyrophosphate dihydrate, gout and other crystal deposition diseases. *Curr. Opin. Rheumatol.*, **3**, 676–83.

Russell, R.G. (1976) Metabolism of inorganic pyrophosphate (PP_i). *Arthritis Rheum.*, **19**, 465–78.

Scherft, J.P. (1972) The lamina limitans of the organic matrix of calcified cartilage and bone. *J. Ultrastruct. Res.*, **38**, 318–31.

Seyedin, S.M. and Rosen, D.M. (1991) Cartilage growth and differentiation factors. In *Cartilage: Molecular Aspects* (eds B.K. Hall and S.A. Newman), CRC Press, Boca Raton, FL, pp. 131–52.

Sporn, M.B. and Roberts, A.B. (1991) Introduction: what is TGF-β? In *Clinical Applications of TGF-β*. Ciba Foundation Symposium 157. (eds G.R. Bock and J. Marsh), John Wiley, Chichester, pp. 1–6.

Stockwell, R.A. and Meachim, G. (1979) The chondrocytes. In *Adult Articular Cartilage* (ed. M.A.R. Freeman), Pitman Medical, Tunbridge Wells. pp. 69–145.

Tenenbaum, H.C. (1990) Cellular origins and theories of differentiaion of bone forming cells. In *Bone* Vol 1, *The osteoblast and the osteocyte* (ed. B.K. Hall), The Telford Press, New Jersey. Chapter 2, pp. 41–70.

Urist, M.R. and McLean, F.C. (1952) Osteogenic potency and new bone formation by induction in transplants to the anterior chamber of the eye. *J. Bone Joint Surg.*, **34A**, 443–76.

Urist, M.R., Silverman, B.F., Buring, K. *et al.* (1967) The bone induction principle. *Clin. Orthop.*, **53**, 243–83.

Urist, M.R. and Strates, B.S. (1971) Bone morphogenetic protein. *J. Dental Res.*, **50**, 1392–406.

Vaes, G. (1988) Cellular biology and biochemical mechanism of bone resorption. A review of recent developments on the formation, activation, and mode of action of osteoclasts. *Clin. Orthop.*, **231**, 239–71.

Verdan, C. (1979) *Tendon Surgery of the Hand.* Churchill Livingstone, Edinburgh, Chapter 7, pp. 40–54.

Westheimer, F.H. (1987) Why nature chose phosphates. *Science*, **235**, 1173–8.

Williams, D.C. and Frolik, C.A. (1991) Physiological and pharmacological regulation of biological calcification. *Int. Rev. Cytol.*, **126**, 195–292.

Wolff, J. (1986) *The Laws of Bone Remodelling* (Translated by P. Maguet and R. Furlong), Springer-Verlag, Berlin.

Wozney, J.M., Rosen, V., Byrne, M. *et al.* (1990) Growth factors influencing bone development. *J. Cell Sci.* Suppl., **13**, 149–56.

Wrana, J.L., Kubota, T., Zhang, Q. *et al.* (1991) Regulation of transformation-sensitive secreted phosphoprotein (SPPI/osteopontin) expression by transforming growth factor-beta. Comparisons with SPARC (secreted acid cysteine-rich protein). *Biochem. J.*, **273**, 23–31.

Paul D. Byers and Colin G. Woods

19.1 INTRODUCTION

Bone tissue is fabricated throughout life as a normal physiological process. In the first instance it is in connection with increasing the size and achieving the shape of the skeleton: bone growth and skeletal modelling. In adulthood it is in connection with bone turnover, or skeletal remodelling. With exceptions, as noted later, the fabricated bone is added to pre-existing surfaces, a process of apposition, hence appositional formation. To be effective, both modelling and remodelling require a second component, namely, bone resorption. This too is a surface activity.

In the child, cartilage is responsible for growth in length of bones, leading to the term enchondral bone growth, comprising two processes: the growth of cartilage and its conversion into bone (ossification).

Before there can be cartilage or bone there must first be undifferentiated precursor cells. These usually occur in fibrovascular tissue: in the embryo this is the mesenchyme of mesodermal tissue; postnatally it is soft connective tissue and reparative/reactive granulation tissue. Within these, under the appropriate stimulation, cells may differentiate into fibro-, chondro- or osteoblasts and surround themselves with their respective matrices. This is growth by interstitial matrix formation. In the case of bone it is an alternative to appositional growth (formation), and

is often referred to as membrane (or intramembranous) bone formation, a term derived from the membranous character of the mesenchymal precursor tissue of the cranium (Figure 19.1).

In interstitial growth, cell number is increased either by division of already differentiated cells or by recruitment from undifferentiated cells in the surrounding mesenchyme (Jee, 1988). Increase in cell number will add something to the volume of the tissue, but the principal means of expanding the tissue (bone, cartilage, or fibrous (e.g. tendon)) is the secretion of more matrix by the cells. *A priori*, interstitial growth requires the existing collagen net, which is responsible for tensile strength, to be enlarged internally to accommodate the increase in proteoglycan molecules and their adsorbed water (Chapter 18). There are a few empirical observations on how this is done (Alini *et al.*, 1992). In cartilage genesis, precursor cells in mesenchyme differentiate and enclose themselves in matrix. Further growth is by division of the enclosed cells which add to the matrix, as can be observed in the physis. However, cells can also be recruited from the surrounding mesenchyme; the lateral enlargement of the physis is an example.

In the interstitial growth of bone, the initial formation is as for cartilage, but the unknown controls are such that trabeculae result and further growth is by differentiation of precursor cells adjacent to the trabe-

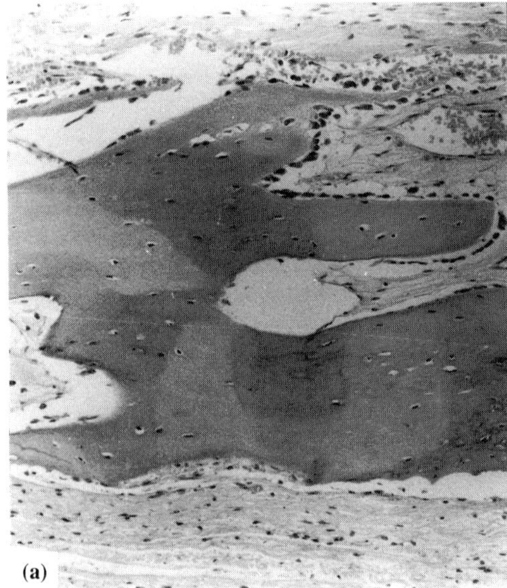

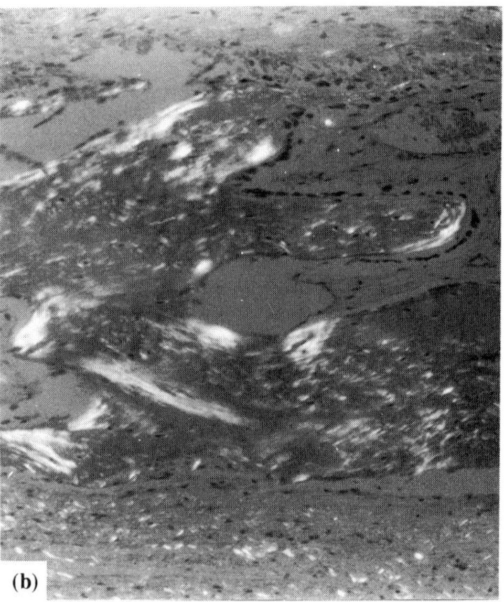

Figure 19.1 Photomicrograph of fetal skull showing woven bone forming 'in membrane'. At the top of the picture, a group of recently differentiated osteoblasts are initiating the formation of a bony trabeculum as an extension to the existing bone mass. Below this, a more substantial trabeculum is covered by osteoblasts, indicating that active formation is taking place. The bottom surface shows evidence of resorption indicated by the scalloped surface. (a) H&E; (b) polarized light.

cular surfaces which create matrix in continuity with that present. Division of the enclosed cells, now osteocytes, seems not to occur. In the periosteum the layer of precursor and differentiated osteoblastic cells (the cambium) are the source of the matrix-forming cells, and ostensibly of the fibrovascular tissue between the extending trabeculae, which could provide recruitable precursor cells. But the main source of growth is the cambium, the activity of whose cells carries the periosteum away from the bone surface.

The result of these growth activities, in the case of cartilage tissue, is a uniform mass; the embryonic model of most bones is formed in this way. In the case of bone tissue a collection of trabecular structures is produced within the fibrovascular tissue; this gives rise in the embryo to the membrane bones, namely: the frontal, parietal, occipital and temporal bones, part of the mandible, and the clavicle; postnatally the form is dictated by the local conditions (as in fracture callus). The collagen organization of this bone is woven. But it is subject to modelling and remodelling in the course of which it is converted into a lamellar structure and the adult architecture for the site.

Thus, for most of the skeleton, growth encompasses genesis of cartilage, chondral interstitial growth, and appositional bone fabrication and modelling. For some bones it entails intramembranous bone genesis, interstitial bone growth, and, later, appositional bone fabrication and modelling.

The shape of the growing bone is determined in part by the cartilage model, but the developing bone must be continually shaped throughout its growth to conform with regional needs and in response to the stresses and strains to which it is subjected. There are two mechanisms whereby this is achieved: modelling and remodelling (Frost, 1964, 1986).

Modelling acts mainly during growth. In this the bone cells act on extensive surfaces, removing (osteoclasts) and forming (osteoblasts) large volumes of bone. Co-ordination of this is by unknown mechanisms. The result is that in relatively a short time (measured in months, rather than years) the disposition and shape of substantial structures can be modified. As discussed in Chapter 16 these activities are called drifts – resorption, formation, or, collectively, formation drifts.

In remodelling, which is active throughout life, the activity of the cells is coupled, by mechanisms that are becoming understood, into a resorption/formation sequence acting over a small area of bone surface and affecting a small volume of bone. This unit of activity has been named the Basic Multicellular Unit (BMU), and resulting moiety of bone so formed the Bone Structural Unit.

On reflection it will be evident that, by varying the number of units, and rates (either as a unit, or of its constituent cells) and duration of their activity, the volume and disposition of bone can be modified. During growth this contributes to the increase of the skeleton and to its organization. In early adult life there is a steady state, after which there is a slow decline into old age, somewhat more marked in women after the menopause. Many facets of BMU activity can be quantified (Parfitt 1984 a,b), and form an integral part of bone morphometry.

Active resorption can be recognized from the presence of osteoclasts in the cavity. The completion of the resorptive phase is marked by a thin haematoxyphilic line, called the reversal or cement line. Its composition is uncertain, but it serves to identify the limits of a structural unit for purposes of quantitation. In trabeculae the completed unit will appear as a crescent, with the bone surface as one boundary, and the reversal line the other. In osteonal bone, the unit will be a ring, similarly bounded. Quantitative values can be obtained by mensuration. This is usually only done in trabecular bone, where the mean of its thickness at several points is used (the mean wall thickness).

During the formative phase the osteoid can be reliably identified in undecalcified sections. Active formation can be recognized by the presence of plump osteoblasts. Mineralization can be identified by the presence of a mineralization front at the interface between bone and osteoid. It is difficult to stain with complete reliability. The most satisfactory demonstration is by administering tetracycline, or similar fluorochrome (Melsen and Mosekilde, 1978). The seam of osteoid deposited in a resorption site begins to mineralize after an interval of some days, about 7–9, and then gradually proceeds more quickly than the rate of osteoid formation, until mineralization is complete after some 200 days. The administration of two labels with a time interval between allows a deter-

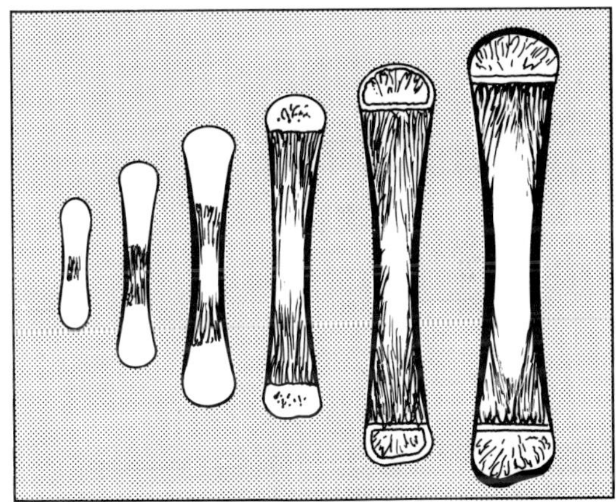

Figure 19.2 The progress of the conversion of the cartilage tissue into bone tissue in the cartilage model of a long bone. When growth ceases, all the physeal cartilage is converted into bone. In the epiphysis, it can be assumed that the portion of the cartilage devoted to growth becomes the subchondral bone plate. Nevertheless, adult articular cartilage retains a calcified zone adjacent to the bone plate and is capable of ossifying, and of growing and ossifying as in osteophytes.

mination of the rate of mineralization, and, by inference, the rate of formation.

Enchondral ossification is the process of converting the cartilage model into bone. It begins in the diaphysis (Figure 19.2) with differentiation of the perichondrium to a periosteum, which surrounds the mid-region with a collar of bone formed interstitially, and is responsible for the further growth in the diameter of the diaphysis. Vascular penetration of the model then takes place at this level, enabling the conversion of cartilage into bone. The details of this are given below. The conversion takes place more rapidly than growth in length of the cartilage model until, in the case of a long bone, for example, the ossification front reaches the level of the metaphyseal/epiphyseal junction. These two regions are then separated by a band of growing, ossifying cartilage, properly called the physis, but commonly referred to as the epiphyseal growth plate.

The conversion of perichondrium into periosteum parallels the advance of bone, until only the physis is left with perichondrial tissue. After an interval, which varies for different bones, the epiphysis is vascularized and its ossification begins. This extends in all directions at a rate exceeding

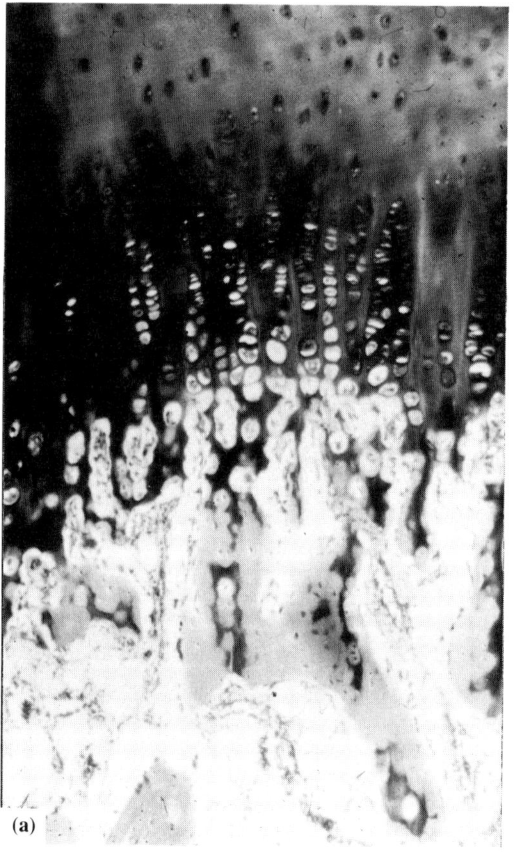
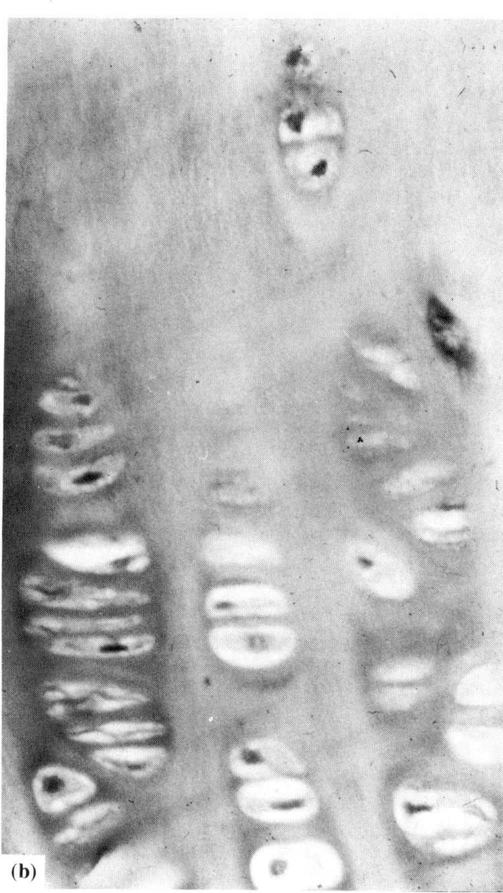

Figure 19.3 Photomicrographs of the physis. (a) A low power view of the physis. Compare with Figure 18.15a. (b) The upper hypertrophic zone.

growth until the cartilage of the epiphysis is reduced to a hemispherical rim. As the ossification of the epiphysis approaches the boundary of the physeal cartilage its activity slows and stops, leaving an osseous layer on this surface of the physeal cartilage.

The conversion of cartilage into bone is by a sequence of developments in the cartilage and linked functions of endothelial and bone cells. The principles apply to any circumstance where cartilage is being converted into bone tissue. However, there are signifi-cant variations in detail between physes and epiphyses, and probably other cartilages as well.

19.2 THE PHYSIS: ITS ORGANIZATION FOR GROWTH, MINERALIZATION AND OSSIFICATION

19.2.1 PHYSEAL GROWTH

Within the physis there are layers of interdependent activity. Five zones are recognized (Figure 19.3). First, a reserve zone of small

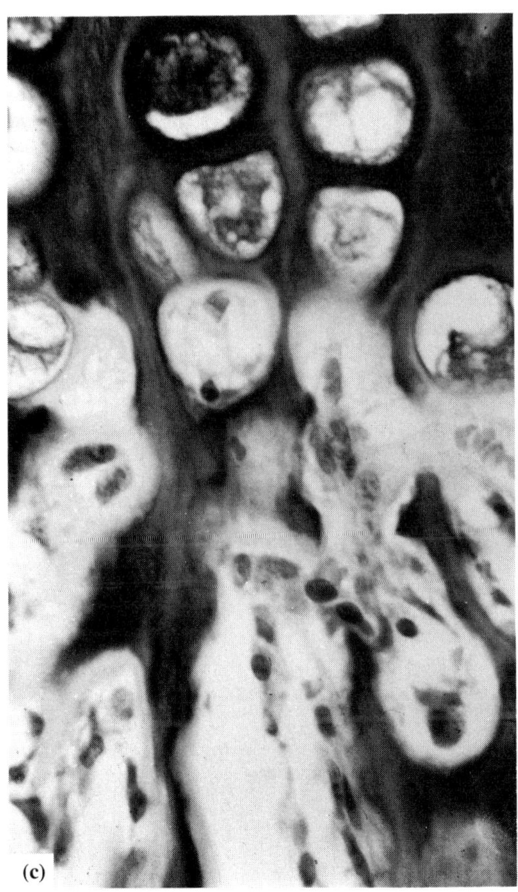

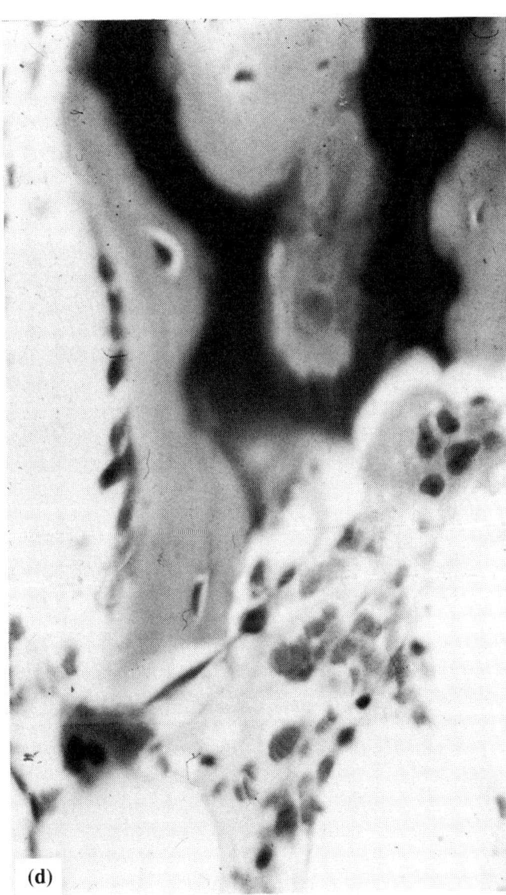

Figure 19.3 Photomicrographs of the physis. (c) The lower hypertrophic zone and primary spongiosa. Vascular penetration of the cell columns has disrupted the unmineralized transverse intercellular septae. (d) The secondary spongiosa. The calcified intercolumnar tissue has been clothed with osteoid by osteoblasts and is undergoing remodelling.

rounded cells. At its junction with zone two, the proliferative, dividing cells produce a daughter cell and a reserve cell; the latter continues to divide and to produce daughters (Kember, 1960). These cells are flattened and the organization is such that the daughters are in effect added to a mounting column of cells. This multiplication of cells is necessarily accommodated by some addition to the matrix. This also takes place in the third zone (maturation), where the cells mature by rounding up and enlarging slightly. But the major increase in substance takes place in the next zone (4, upper hypertrophic) marked by an abrupt cellular hypertrophy, each increasing five to tenfold (Buckwalter *et al.*, 1986). There must therefore be a commensurate production of matrix. The net effect is to move all cells except the last of the hypertrophic zone yet further from the centre of the bone, The cells proximal to this (5, lower hypertrophic, or mineralizing) mineralize the surrounding matrix, which is thus stabilized and fixed in position relative to the centre, i.e. no growth in length takes place here.

19.2.2 PHYSEAL MINERALIZATION

Calcification occurs in the lower hypertrophic zone with the appearance of mineral deposits in the matrix close to the cells, and extends throughout the intercolumnar matrix; it rarely appears in septal matrix. Some details of the current hypotheses of mineralization (Poole, 1991), which is not a fully understood process, can be found in Chapter 18.

19.2.3 PHYSEAL OSSIFICATION (FIGURE 19.3D)

Bone fabrication at this site is appositional, i.e. bone tissue is added to existing surfaces; this is analogous to the building of a brick wall. This necessitates that osteoblasts gain access to surfaces. In order to make available

the surface of the now-mineralized cartilage matrix it is necessary to open up the cell column. One can change the metaphor and think of the cell column as a tube, or tunnel, penetrating the matrix, segmented by the septae between cells. Proliferating endothelial cells, forming a vessel with a blind end, penetrate the column. A function of these cells is resorption of unmineralized matrix, whereby they open up the tube and expose the mineralized tubular surface, which the endothelial cells are incapable of resorbing. Osteoblasts enter the tube and lay down (appose) osteoid of woven collagen structure on its surface. This zone is the primary spongiosa. The first stage of ossification has begun.

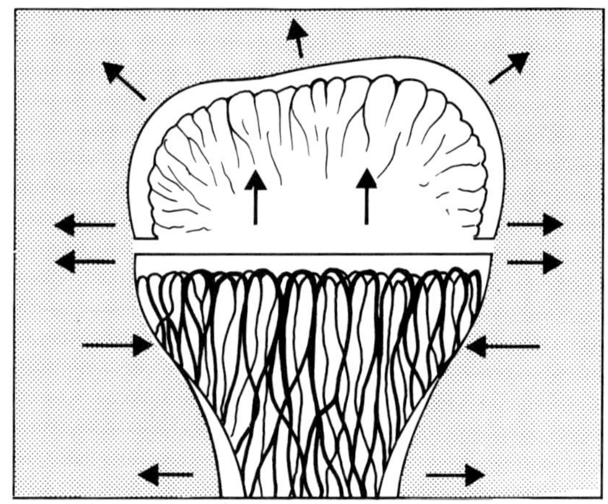

Figure 19.4 The modelling of the metaphysis during long bone growth. The arrows indicate the movement in space of the growing tissues. The epiphysis grows commensurately with the physis. Physeal growth (upwards here) adds to the metaphyseal bone, which must be reduced to the width of the diaphysis by periosteal resorption. The diameter of the diaphysis increases in harmony with the increasing physeal diameter by periosteal apposition (see Figures 19.5 and 19.6).

19.3 METAPHYSEAL GROWTH

After mineralization of the osteoid, this hybrid tissue (calcified cartilage core encased by immature bone) is subject to the first manifestation of the migratory, focal, coupled interplay between osteoclasts and osteoblasts that will continue throughout the rest of the life of the bone in the process known as remodelling, but sometimes called turnover.

The physis increases in diameter over time by recruiting cells from the perichondrium. The diaphysis, smaller in diameter, keeps pace with this through periosteal apposition, while its internal diameter is adjusted by osteoclastic resorption of the internal surface (endosteum). Lying betwen physis and diaphysis is the metaphysis, with a funnel shape. Thus, today's wide metaphysis with its cancellous architecture is next year's narrow tubular diaphysis. To achieve the transition from a broad metaphysis of uniform trabecular architecture to a narrower thick-walled tube requires (Figure 19.4):

1. Progressive removal of trabecula internally to create the cavity; this is accomplished by BMU remodelling as described above;
2. Progressive periosteal reduction in the external diameter to that of the diaphysis, accomplished by osteoclasts working on the whole extent of the periosteal

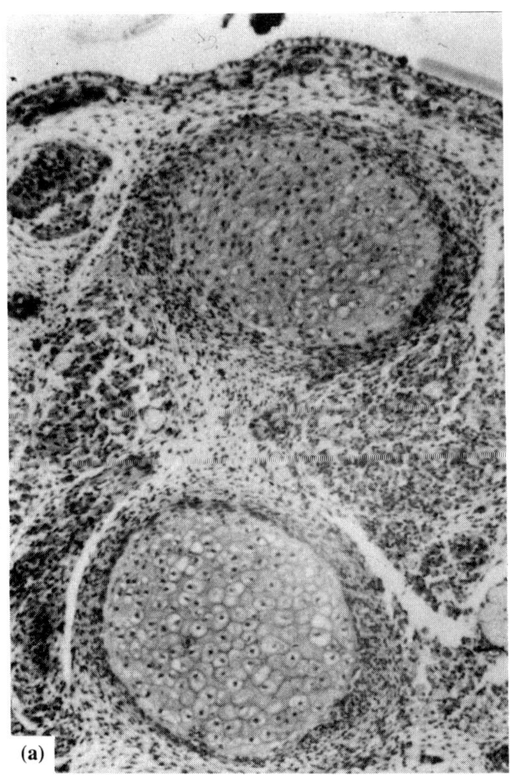

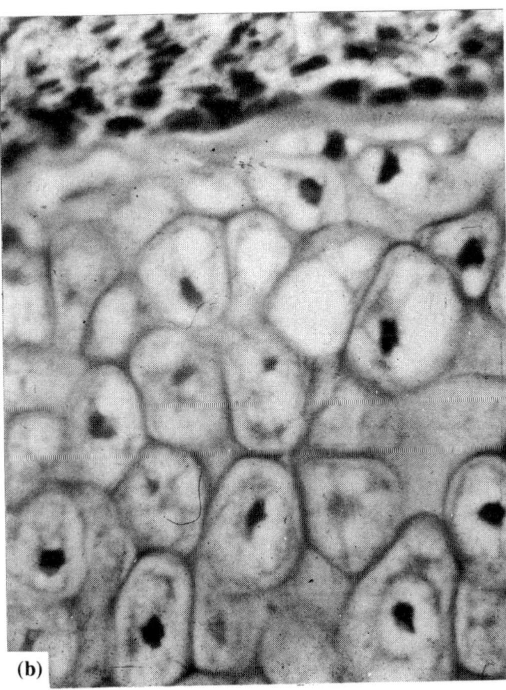

Figure 19.5 (a) Transverse section of the forearm of a fetus. Both bones are wholly cartilaginous. In one the cells are beginning to hypertrophy preparatory to vascular invasion. (b) In a high power view of a segment of this a narrow layer of osteoid encloses the shaft. Periosteal osteoblasts are prominent (the cambium) and are overlain by the fibrous periosteum.

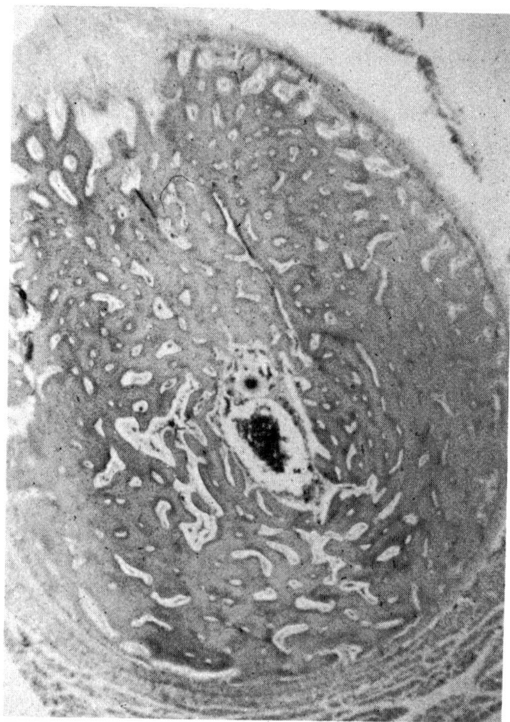

Figure 19.6 Mid-shaft of femur at about 1 year. There is a small marrow cavity and thick cortex. The many irregular channels are primary osteons and Volkmann canals. The periosteum is a pale band of tissue enclosing the bone. It is relatively inactive in the lower half of the illustration. In the upper half the dark line between the fibrous periosteum and the bone is the cambium layer, which is actively producing the network of bone and primary osteons. Deeper in the substance it is possible to discern many secondary osteons: round holes surrounded by a ring of bone, accentuated by variations in staining of matrix.

surface (or envelope) of the metaphysis. This is an example of a resorption drift.
3. Progressive endosteal osteoblastic activity to build a thickening cortex to meld with that of the diaphysis. Formation of this order is a formation drift.

19.4   DIAPHYSEAL GROWTH (FIGURES 19.5–19.7)

At the same time there must be provision for the diaphysis to expand pro rata with the overall growth. Not long after the appearance of the ossification centre, there is only bone to be found in the diaphysis, increasing in external diameter by the periosteum (this is in effect a formation drift). In due course a marrow cavity is created and enlarged by osteoclastic activity on the endosteal surface (and here a resorption drift). In this way the diaphysis continues to enlarge and achieve its adult size.

The internal osteonal architecture of the diaphyseal cortex is achieved by BMU remodelling. As the diameter of the bone increases, periosteal blood vessels are incorporated within canals, the primary osteons. Eventually, the surfaces of these are the seat of remodelling. The osteoclasts work along the surface as a cutting cone, enlarging the diameter of the canal; behind them come the osteoblasts laying osteoid lamellae circumferential to the axis of the canal, closing the diameter of the canal. Successive waves of BMU activity gradually create the secondary osteonal structures, each bounded by a reversal line.

19.5   THE GROWTH OF THE EPIPHYSIS

This takes place in its cartilage cover. This tissue has a dual function. Its outer aspect serves articulation; its inner aspect is for growth. Mankin (1964), using ^{3}H-thymidine labelling in rabbits, demonstrated in immature animals two annuli of mitotic activity, concluding that the inner was for epiphyseal growth. Mankin (1964), using [^{3}H]thymidine that here was a clear indication that the two functions of the terminal cartilage were anatomically distinct, and the tissue is a bi-layer (Figure 19.8).

It is widely held that ossification here is the same as in the physis, i.e. columnation of cells, mineralization of intervening matrix, vascular penetration of the cell column, bone deposition on the exposed surfaces, and, finally, remodelling of the mixed tissue to pure bone. The epiphyseal

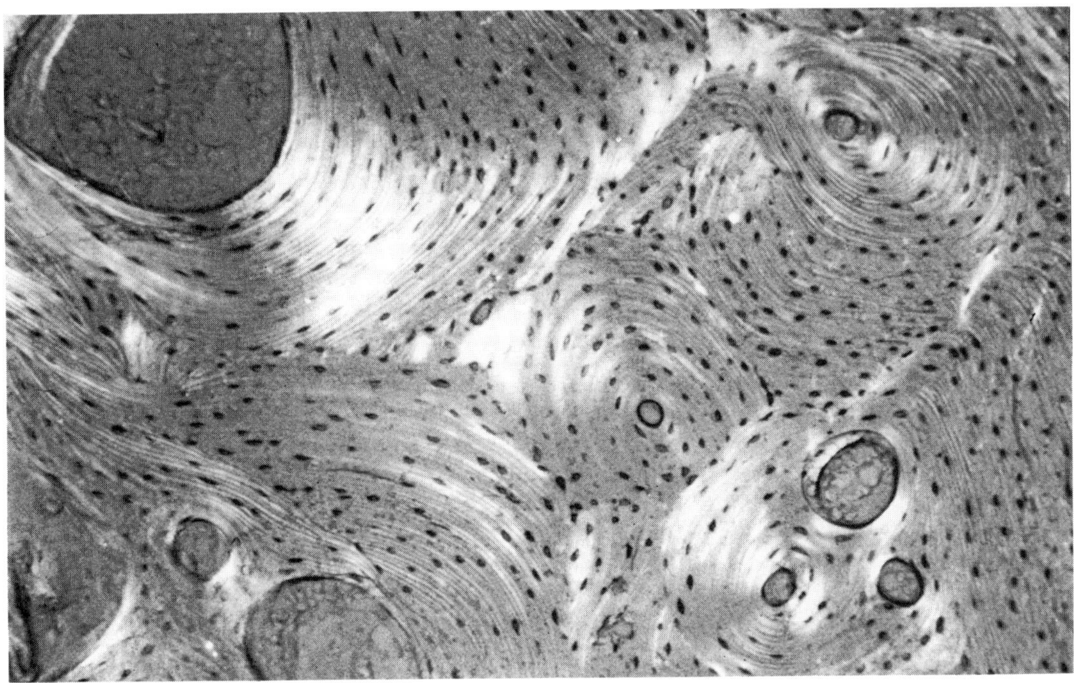

Figure 19.7 Adult cortex, midshaft of femur, in polarized light. Circumferential lamellae enclose the osteonal canals. There are several generations of osteon. The older ones have been partially eroded to provide space for new osteons. Some remnants of old osteons have lost their canal; these are referred to as interstitial tissue.

growth cartilage does have columns of cells; presumably this is an efficient way to pack proliferating cells for purposes of growth. By comparison with the physis the columns are irregular. Moreover, the mineralization extends between cells, so that in macerated specimens instead of tubes extending through a zone of calcification as in the physis (Figure 19.9) there is a continuous layer of mineral with only occasional holes through it (Figure 19.10) (Brown *et al.*, 1993). The surface of these preparations is irregular because the mineral is deposited from below upward and around the cells which exist in a cup-shaped hollow until the mineral closes over them (Figure 19.10). This layer of mineralized tissue is remodelled into bone. Bone multicellular units (BMUs) are activated:

osteoclasts resorb bays into the calcified tissue, which are then lined by osteoid and mineralized through osteoblastic activity (Figure 19.11). The tissue between BMUs stands out from the receding surface, cores of calcified cartilage encased in bone, similar to those of the physis. These will in turn be remodelled, eventually to produce the trabecular structure of the epiphysis. Thus, the basis for the difference from the physis lies in the pattern of mineralization: in the physis mineral deposition is polar, occurring only at the sides of the cell columns and leaving the septa free; in epiphyseal growth cartilage there is continuous deposition of mineral; i.e. the inter cell septa are also mineralized so that there is no non-mineralized tissue susceptible to endothelial cell resorption and the advance of

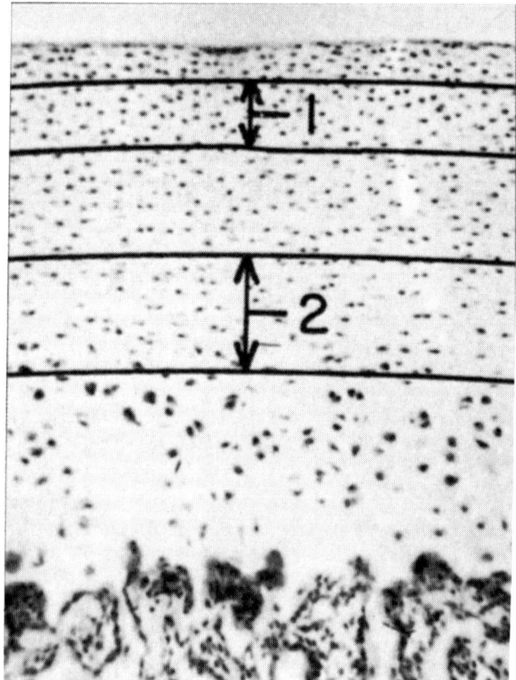

Figure 19.8 Articular cartilage of an immature, actively growing rabbit. Tritiated thymidine revealed two zones of mitotic activity: 1, serving the growth of the articular layer and 2, serving the growth of the epiphysis. (From Mankin (1964), with permission.)

ossification must be by osteoclastic resorption. It is logical to postulate that the termination of a child's growth must be marked by the ossification of the growth layer, with the formation of a continuous subchondral bone plate beneath the articular layer. However, in contrast to the physis where all cartilage is consumed, the articular cartilage remains. In the adult this can progressively mineralize and subsquently be ossified. Moreover, the cartilage can grow, as manifested by osteophytes arising in articular cartilage (Figure 19.12). The ossification process is as in epiphyseal growth cartilage (Figure 19.13).

19.6   THE BONE MULTICELLULAR UNIT/AND THE RESULTING BONE STRUCTURAL UNIT

Remodelling is the result of osteoclasts and osteoblasts, coupled and restricted in the sense that osteoclasts, moving over a surface, resorb a small amount of bone, and osteoblasts follow behind filling in the cavity. In the child, remodelling substitutes one tissue for another during the conversion of the primary spongiosa into its secondary state, forms the shape of trabecular bone, and converts primary osteons into their secondary structure. In the adult it replaces new for old tissue, in both cancellous and cortical bone, presumably in the repair of microdamage, but possibly with other purposes as well. At all ages, the net result of BMU activity, the removal and replacement of bone, is a determinant of bone volume (Figure 19.14). In the child, as a whole, the balance is positive and contributes to growth. But regionally, local balances can be varied, thereby contributing to modelling. Remodelling persists into adult life, with some dynamic modifications. Treated as a whole, the bone balance of adults continues to be positive for a few years, stabilizes at about 20–30 years of age, and then declines steadily with age, somewhat more precipitately in postmenopausal women (Meunier and Courpron, 1973; Vedi *et al.*, 1982).

However, on a regional basis the findings are not uniform. This led Frost to recognize the importance of different classes of bone surface: (a) periosteal; (b) osteonal (or Haversian); (c) endosteal (or corticoendosteal) and (d) trabecular.

He used 'envelope' to convey the sense that each is functionally discrete, a concept and terminology generally recognized. The changes in the envelopes with age, as the result of differences between resorption and formation by the BMUs, are as follows:

1.   Periosteal: continually enlarges.

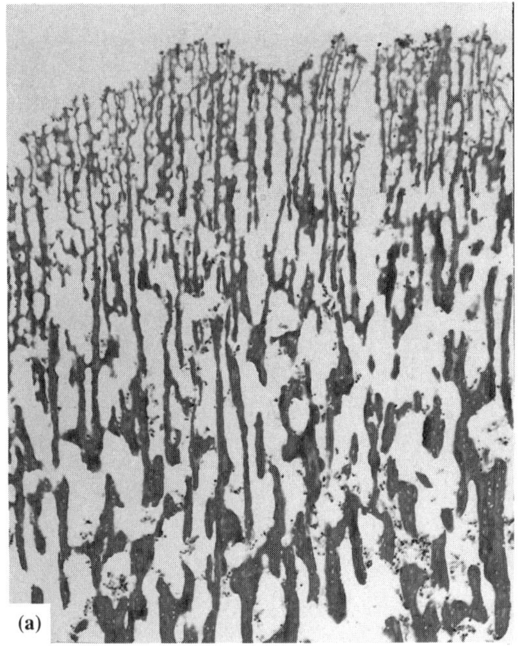

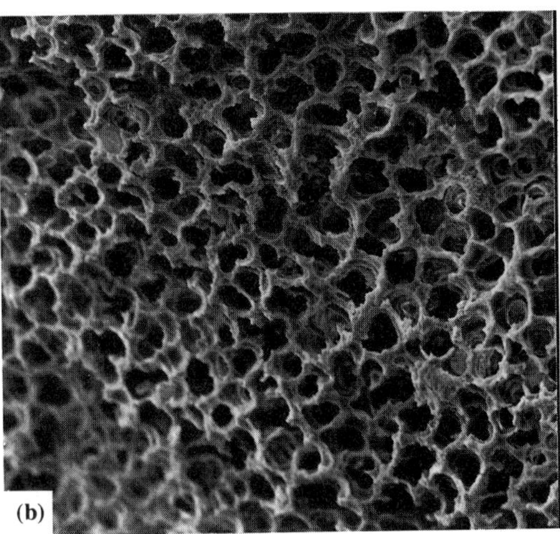

Figure 19.9 Macerated physis of growing rabbit. (a) A histological section emphasizing the 'organ pipe' structure that results from restriction of mineralization to intercolumnar matrix (b) SEM of the epiphyseal surface of the specimen showing the uniform pattern of holes penetrating to the marrow space. (Reproduced from Brown *et al.*, 1993, with permission.)

2. Osteonal: enlarges only slightly, mainly in the outer two-thirds of the cortex.
3. Endosteal: continually enlarges.
4. Trabecular: trabeculae continually thin, and eventually reduce in number.

The BMUs have been studied intensively by histomorphometrists, resulting in a wealth of empirical and hypothetical detail, some of which will contribute to the following discussion. The sequence of events in the cycle of a BMU is activation → resorption → formation. The number of active BMUs is variable, a function of the activation rate. The performance of the cells is variable both in terms of rate and time, so that the area covered and the volume of tissue removed and replaced can vary. There are normal values for these parameters from various centres, and some knowledge of how they vary in relation to age and disease, particu-larly osteoporosis (Foldes *et al.*, 1991). Two outcomes have been observed: the gradual thinning of trabeculae; and the disappearance of portions of trabeculae when resorption cavities extend through them (Parfitt, 1983; Compston *et al.*, 1989; Mellish *et al.*, 1989) (Chapter 10). Some values for cortical and trabecular bone are given in Table 19.1 (Jee, 1988).

19.7 BLOOD SUPPLY OF BONE

A final comment can be made about the blood supply to bone, since it is of relevance to appreciating the changes that occur in bone following fracture without or with nailing, and to the pathogenesis of osteomyelitis (Figure 19.15).

The nature of the circulation in bone has led Rhinelander (1980) to classify it under

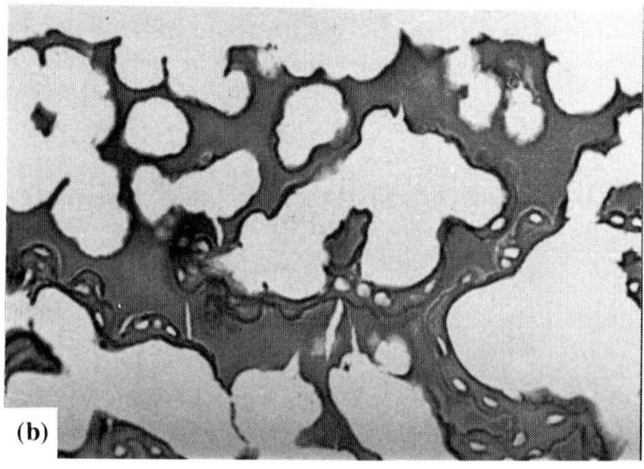

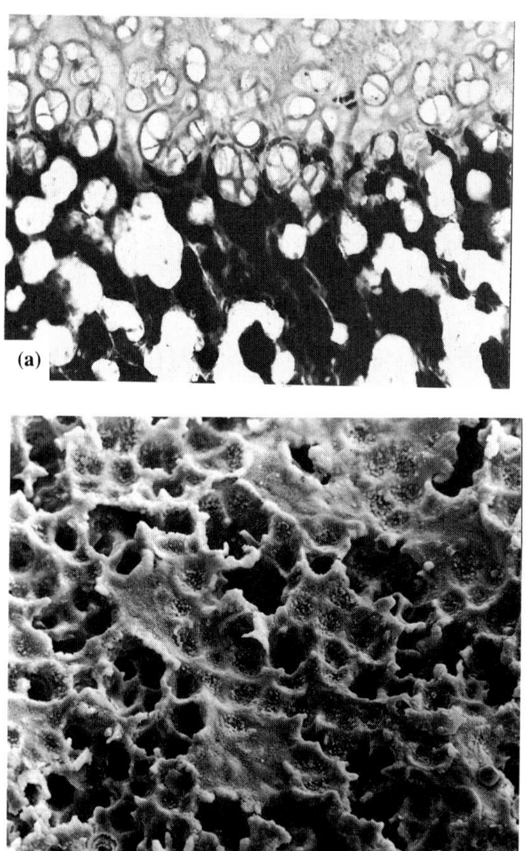

Figure 19.10 Undecalcified preparations of epiphysis of growing rabbit. (a) von Kossa stain. Mineral has been deposited around individual and clusters of cells in the calcified zone. Remodelling is forming the spongiosa, opening one channel to the cartilage. (b) Macerated preparation. The pattern reflects the appearances in (a). A channel opens to the surface and the mixed tissue structure of the spongiosa is evident. (c) SEM of the articular surface of the macerated specimen. The surface is formed of cupped depressions. Shallow ones occur in irregular sheets of the mineralized tissue; deeper ones break up the surface, in many the basal layer is evident, but a few others extend through to the marrow space. (Reproduced from Brown *et al.*, 1993, with permission.)

three headings: (a) afferent system; (b) efferent system; (c) intermediate system of compact bone.

The afferent system has three components which arise from: (a) the principal nutrient artery; (b) multiple periosteal arterioles and (c) multiple metaphyseal arteries

The nutrient artery passes through the cortex without branching, and within the medullary cavity divides into ascending and descending branches. These give off branches to the marrow and the endosteal surface, dividing successively through the metaphysis in the approach to the epiphysis.

The marrow branches feed a system of sinusoids from which the blood enters a central vein and is returned to the heart.

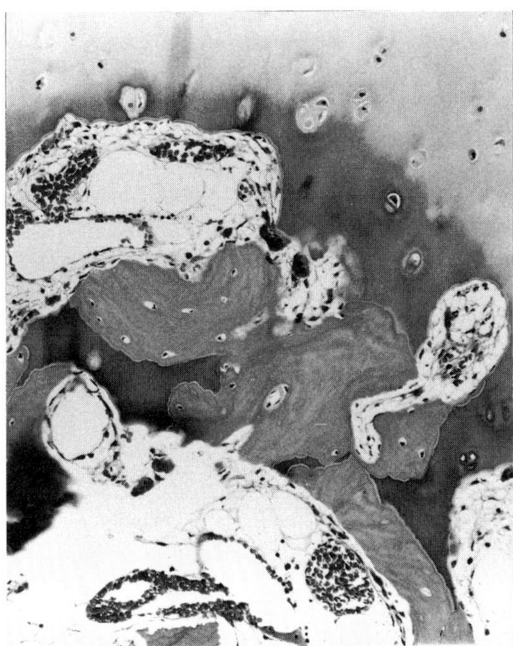

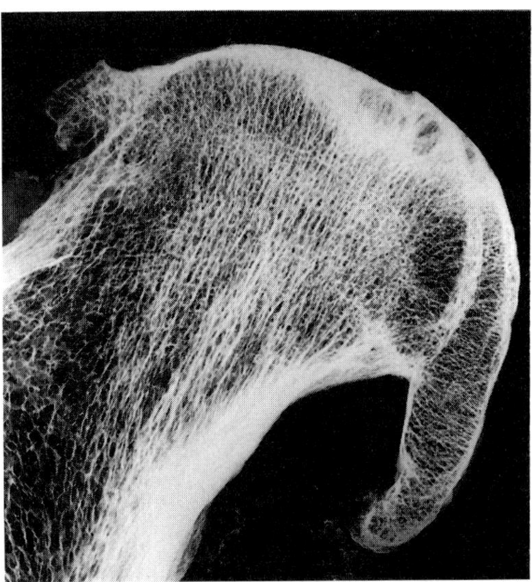

Figure 19.11 Photomicrograph of normal navicular from the foot of a girl aged 7 years to demonstrate normal epiphyseal endochondral ossification (compare with Figure 19.3, physeal growth and ossification). The articular surface is at the top. The calcified zone of the cartilage is a dark band; much of it is being resorbed. Two struts of mixed osseous and cartilage tissue connect it to a supporting arc, also of mixed structure. On the right three resorption bays extend into the calcified zone; two have bone formed on parts of the surface. The mixed supporting arc is in the process of remodelling. As the cartilage grows, the calcification front advances, even as it is converted into bone by remodelling.

Figure 19.12 Slab radiograph of a femoral head resected in the treatment of osteoarthritis. The inferior osteophyte arises from the whole of the subfoveal articular cartilage, whose growth has covered the original subchondral plate with cancellous bone. The articular surface provided by the osteophyte has been involved in the arthritic process.

19.7.1   THE METAPHYSEAL ARTERIES

In addition to the vessels reaching the metaphysis from the nutrient artery there are also vessels entering on all sides through the metaphyseal cortex. These two sources anastamose. There is an important difference between the adult and the child owing to the presence of the physis in the latter.

In the child, on the metaphyseal side of the physis most arterioles turn back to enter large venous channels, which are thought to have an important role to play in the pathogenesis of osteomyelitis (Chapter 7). However, until the formation of the epiphyseal ossification centre some blood vessels extend from the medulla into the cartilaginous epiphysis. But when the ossification centre forms and the bone plate backing it up on the epiphyseal side is established these transphyseal vessels are greatly reduced, with

From the endosteal branches vessels enter the cortex, traversing it via Volkmann canals and feeding the osteonal system en route. Both types of vessel finally anastamose with the periosteal system. The periosteal arterioles reach it via the intermuscular septae. They ramify through the periosteum, providing a local supply to just the outer third of the cortex.

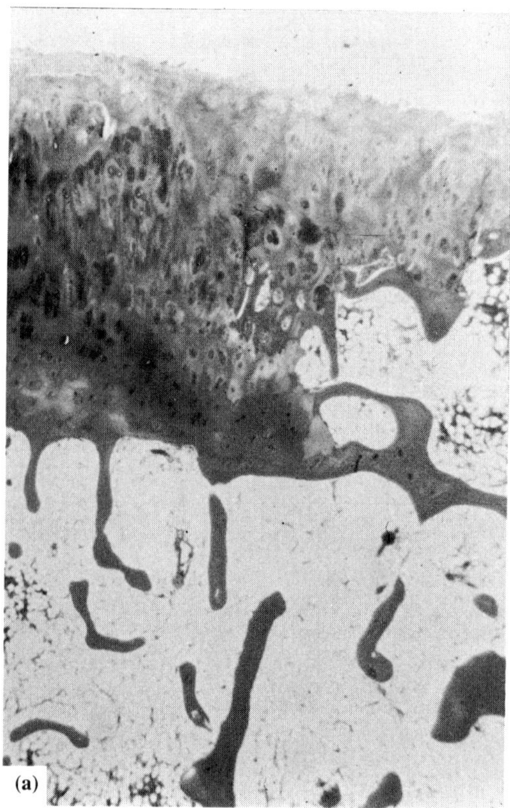
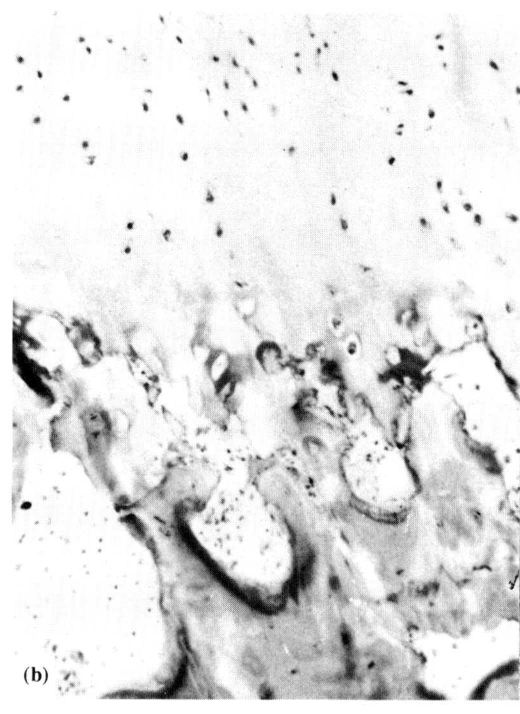

Figure 19.13 Ossification of articular cartilage forming an osteophyte. (a) The ossification process is advancing from the right into the body of the articular cartilage. The cartilage overlying the encroaching bone is growing and undergoing ossification to add to the substance of the osteophyte. (b) Articular cartilage above forming bone below. The pattern of ossification is similar to that in Figure 19.11.

only occasional vessels crossing this barrier. When growth is completed and the bone plate remodelled, there is again a freer vascular entry into the epiphysis from the metaphysis (Trueta, 1957, 1959; Ogden, 1979; Alderson *et al.*, 1986).

19.7.2 THE EPIPHYSEAL CIRCULATION

In the child, epiphyseal ossification begins when it is penetrated by vessels from a surrounding vascular complex. These form multiple branches which supply the ossifying surfaces, and continue to supply bone plate formed to back the physis. There are vessels which cross the physis but their

number varies with age (Trueta, 1957). When the physeal ossification is completed the epi- and metaphyseal systems anastomose. The pattern of vascular supply in the metaphyseal/epiphyseal region is thought to influence the pathogenesis of osteomyelitis (Trueta, 1959; Ogden, 1979; Alderson *et al.*, 1986).

The circulation through this system is now considered to be centripetal (Williams *et al.*, 1989): blood enters via the medullary artery, passes through the cortex and the Haversian system, and is collected by the periosteal vessels. Some observations have indicated that the flow may also be in the other direction (Sevitt, 1981), at least in as far as provid-

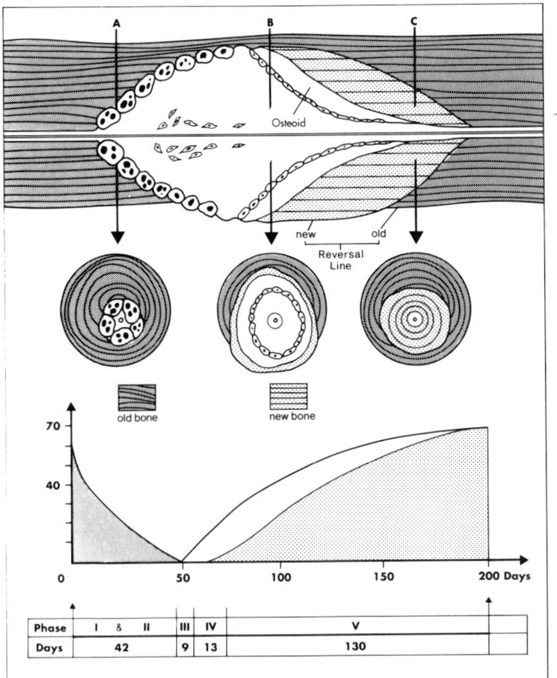

Phase	I & II	III	IV	V
Days	42	9	13	130

Figure 19.14 A diagrammatic representation of the Basic Multicellular Unit (BMU). The illustrations may be seen as longitudinal and transverse sections of a BMU working on an osteonal canal surface; but, hemisected by obscuring the upper half, they also serve to illustrate a BMU on a trabecular surface. The cells clustered around the vessel are precursor cells. A is at the front end of the cutting cone which has enlarged the cavity to the size at B, the reversal zone where the reversal (cement) line is formed. Osteoblasts are in position but have yet to form osteoid. At C the cavity is being closed by osteoblast activity. At D osteoid formation and mineralization are complete and the osteoblasts are in the form of lining cells. After Parfitt (1976). Below is a depiction of the total remodelling period: duration of phases and depth/thickness measures as determined by Eriksen *et al.* (1984). The phases are I, osteoclast resorption; II, mononuclear cell resorption (see osteoclasts in Chapter 18); III, reversal phase; IV, mineralization lag time; V, mineralization.

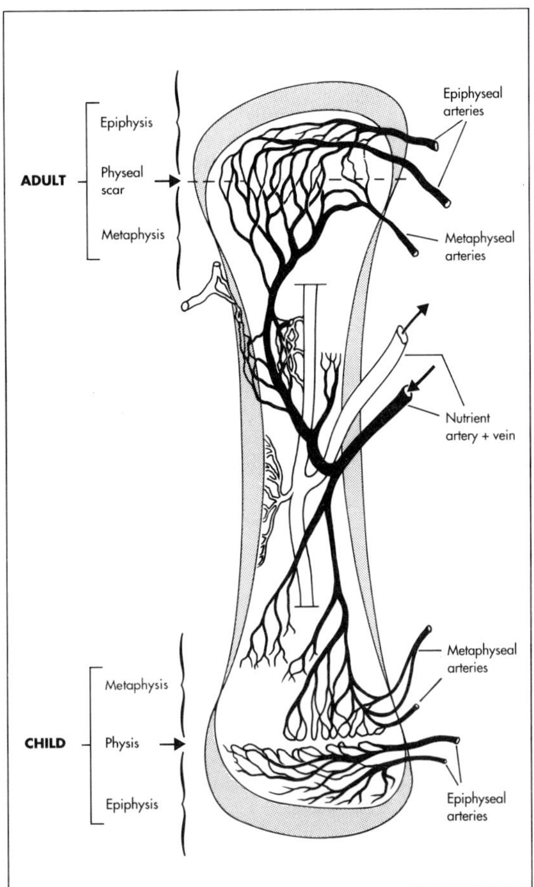

Figure 19.15 Schematic representation of the vascular supply to bone. Blood enters via the nutrient artery, the periosteal arteries, the metaphyseal and epiphyseal arteries. The nutrient artery gives off branches to the endosteum, which traverse the cortex, supply the osteonal system, anastomose with periosteal branches and drain into the periosteal veins. The periosteal arteries support the outer third of the cortex (Sevitt, 1981). The nutrient artery divides progressively into the metaphysis: in the child it supplies the physis in conjunction with arteries entering at the metaphyseal level. The epiphysis has its own supply during growth, but amalgamates with the metaphyseal when the physis disappears. There is epiphyseal and metaphyseal drainage, in addition to that into the central sinus. The nutrient artery also supplies the blood for the marrow sinusoids, which is returned via the central sinus.

Table 19.1 Some values for cortical and trabecular bone (Jee, 1988)

	Cortical	*Trabecular*
Fractional volume (mm^3/mm^3)	0.95	20
Surface/bone volume (mm^2/mm^3)	2.5	20
Total bone volume (mm^3)	1.4×10^6	0.35×10^6
Total internal surface (mm^2)	3.5×10^6	7.00×10^6
BSUs (number/mm^3 bone volume)	21×10^6	14×10^6
(length, mm)	2.5	1.0
(wall thickness, mm)	0.075	0.040
BMU resorption period (days)	24	21
formation period (days)	124	91
total birth rate (per hour)	180	720
Bone turnover rate (%/year)	3	26

ing a supply to the outer third of the cortex. Since the system is difficult to visualize, and the flow to bone can be variable under both physiological and pathological conditions it is possible that in such a highly anastomosed system the direction of circulation varies.

The effect of interrupting the system by fracture alone, or with medullary nailing is discussed in Chapter 6.

The blood supply to the femoral head is of importance because of the prevalence of avascular necrosis following fracture of the femoral neck. Wertheimer and Fernandes Lopes (1971) give a bibliography of many studies of this subject in their report of an injection study of 81 cadaveric specimens using radio-opaque medium. They found considerable variability in the arterial pattern. Three sources were found:

1. Two to six large calibre arteries entering superiorly, in all specimens;
2. Two to three small calibre arteries inferiorly in all specimens;
3. Arteries of the ligamentum teres in 28 specimens.

These combine in various ways to form anastomotic arches within the head (Figure 6.8), namely; in 55 the superior and inferior; in 12 the superior and ligamental and in 14 all three sources. Within the head the anastomoses form a variety of loops or circles from which subsidiary branches arise to ramify to all parts of the head.

To investigate the reliability of the radiographs of the ligamentum teres, serial histological sections were made of 11 specimens with injected vessels and of 11 in which none were seen. In the former group the vessel diameter ranged from 200 to 511 μm; whereas the other group had arteries less than 200 μm in diameter.

The effect of interrupting the blood supply to the femoral head is discussed in Chapter 6.

Mention must be made of the vascular anatomy of the vertebral column because of the effect it has been proposed to have on the unusually high proportion of cases of adult osteomyelitis due to coliform organisms. This is attributed to the spinal venous drainage which Batson (1957) had shown to be intimately linked to that of the urinary bladder and genitalia, which could allow organisms to reach the vertebrae by retrograde flow. It is postulated (but not universally accepted) that the conditions under which this is prone to occur are cystitis or manipulative procedures of pelvic organs in the presence of infections. The alternative explanation being that these same procedures induce a conventional haematogenous spread (Wiley and Trueta, 1959).

REFERENCES

Alderson, M., Speers, D., Emslie, K. *et al.* (1986) Acute haematogenous osteomyelitis and septic arthritis. *J. Bone Joint Surg.*, **68B**, 268–74.

Alini, M., Matsui, Y., Dodge, G.R. *et al.* (1992) The extracellular matrix in the growth plate before and during calcification: changes in the composition and degradation of type II collagen. *Calcif. Tissue Int.*, **50**, 327–35.

Batson, O.V. (1957) The vertebral vein system. *Am. J. Roentgenol.*, **78**, 195–212.

Brown, R., Blunn, G.W., Salisbury, J.R. *et al.* (1993) Two patterns of calcification in primary and secondary growth cartilage. *Clin. Orthop.*, **294**, 318–324.

Buckwalter, J.A., Mower, D., Ungar, J. *et al.* (1986) Morphometric analysis of chondrocyte hypertrophy. *J. Bone Joint Surg.*, **68A**, 243–55.

Compston, J.E., Mellish, R.W., Croucher, P. *et al.* (1989) Structural mechanisms of trabecular bone loss in man. *Bone Miner.*, **6**, 339–50.

Eriksen, E.F., Gundersen, H.J.G., Melsen, F. *et al.* (1984) Reconstruction of the formative site in iliac trabecular bone in 20 normal individuals employing a kinetic model for matrix and mineral apposition. *Metab. Bone Dis.*, **5**, 243–52.

Foldes, J., Parfitt, A.M., Shih, M.S. *et al.* (1991) Structural and geometric changes in iliac bone: relationship to normal ageing and osteoporosis. *J. Bone Miner. Res.*, **6**, 759–66.

Frost, H.M. (1964) Dynamics of bone remodelling. In *Bone Dynamics* (ed. H.M. Frost), Little, Brown, Boston, pp. 315–33.

Frost, H.M. (1986) *Intermediary Organisation of the Skeleton.* CRC Press, Boca Raton, FL, pp. 133–46.

Jee, W.S.S. (1988) The skeletal tissues. In *Cell and Tissue Biology: A Textbook of Histology*, 6th edn (ed. L.Weiss), Elsevier, North-Holland, Amsterdam, pp. 211–55.

Kember, N.F. (1960) Cell division in endochondral ossification: a study of proliferation in rat bones by the method of tritiated thymidine autoradiography. *J. Bone Joint Surg.*, **42B**, 824–39.

Mankin, H.J. (1962) Localisation of tritiated thymidine in articular cartilage of rabbits, I. Growth in immature cartilage. *J. Bone Joint Surg.*, **44A**, 682–8.

Mankin, H.J. (1964) Mitosis in articular cartilage of immature rabbits. A histological, stathmokinetic (colchicinic) and autoradiographic study. *Clin. Orthop.*, **34**, 170–85.

Mellish, R.W., Garrahan, N.J. and Compston, J.E. (1989) Age-related changes in trabecular width and spacing in human iliac crest biopsies. *Bone Miner.*, **6**. 351–8.

Melsen, F. and Mosekilde, L. (1978) Tetracycline double labelling of the iliac trabecular bone in 41 normal adults. *Calcif. Tissue Res.*, **26**, 99–102.

Meunier, P. and Courpron, P. (1973) Iliac trabecular bone volume in 236 controls – representativeness of iliac samples. *Proceedings of the first workshop on Bone Morphometry*, University of Ottawa Press, pp. 100–5.

Ogden, J.A. (1979) Paediatric osteomyelitis and septic arthritis: the pathology of neonatal disease. *Yale J.Biol. Med.*, **52**, 423–48.

Parfitt, A.M. (1983) The stereologic basis of bone histomorphometry. Theory of quantitative. microscopy and construction of the third dimension. In *Bone Histomorphometry. Techniques and Interpretations* (ed. R. Recker), CRC Press, Boca Raton, pp. 53–87.

Parfitt, A.M. (1984a) The cellular basis of bone remodelling: the quantum concept re-examined in light of recent advances in cell biology. *Calcif. Tissue Int.*, **36**, S37–S45.

Parfitt, A.M. (1984b) Age related structural changes in trabecular and cortical bone: cellular mechanisms and biomechanical consequences. *Calcif. Tissue Int.*, **36**, suppl. 1, S123–8.

Poole, A.R. (1991) The growth plate: cellular physiology, cartilage assembly and mineralisation. In *Cartilage: Molecular Aspects* (eds B.K. Hall and S.A. Newman), CRC Press, Boca Raton, FL, pp. 179–211.

Rhinelander, F.W. (1980) The blood supply of the limb bones. In *The Scientific Foundations of Orthopaedics and Traumatology* (eds R. Owen, J. Goodfellow and P. Bullough), William Heinemann, London, pp. 126–51.

Sevitt, S. (1981) *Bone Repair and Fracture Healing in Man*, Churchill Livingstone, London, pp. 21–3.

Trueta, J. (1957) The normal vascular anatomy of the human femoral head during growth. *J. Bone Joint Surg.*, **39B**, 358–94.

Trueta, J. (1959) Three types of acute haematogenous osteomyelitis. *J. Bone Joint Surg.*, **41B**, 671.

Vedi, S., Compston, J.E., Webb, A. *et al.* (1982) Histomorphometric analysis of bone biopsies from the iliac crest of normal British subjects. *Metab. Bone Dis. Rel. Res.*, **4**, 232–6.

Wertheimer, L.G. and Fernandes Lopes, S.D.L.

(1971) Arterial supply of the femoral head. *J. Bone Joint Surg.*, **53A**, 545–56.

Wiley, A.M. and Trueta, J. (1959) The vascular anatomy of the spine and its relationship to pyogenic vertebral osteomyelitis. *J. Bone Joint Surg.*, **41B**, 796–809.

Williams, P.L., Warwick, R., Dyson, M. *et al.* (1989) *Gray's Anatomy*, 37th edn, Churchill Livingstone, Edinburgh, pp. 299–300.

REACTIONS OF BONE 20

Paul D. Byers and Colin G. Woods

It is possible to analyse the reactions of bone by means of practical and theoretical considerations. However, in the real world of diagnostic pathology it is only their practical visualization that counts. That can be done at the macroscopic or microscopic level. Microscopical visualization is by sampling, and although it gives abundant information at the tissue and cellular levels, it tells little or nothing of the extent and distribution. Such information can be gained by inspecting the site in amputation or postmortem material. In biopsy diagnosis the source of macroscopic information is imaging. Thus, as is emphasized in Chapter 4, the two disciplines are complementary. The most useful imaging modality for the pathologist is the radiograph. Its limitation in orthopaedic pathology is that only calcified tissues are shown in detail. The following discussion assumes recognition of the place and importance of radiographs in skeletal pathology. Chapter 4 gives descriptions of imaging.

The reactions of bone are in effect the response of cells in bone to stimuli, the response and, usually, the stimulus being beyond the range of normal.

The stimuli to which bone reacts are either systemic (generalized) or local (Table 20.1).

The distribution of the responses is a prime observation, reflecting the disease process which gives rise to them. In broad terms the distribution may be generalized, which includes regional; or local, which may be unifocal or multifocal. Setting these against the disease processes shows the pattern in Table 20.2. A line of division, which is far from absolute, runs through this table and separates the focal processes from the regional and generalized: traumatic, inflammatory, circulatory and neoplastic from congenital/developmental and metabolic.

In the most general of terms it can be said that the focal group is characterized by the imposition of a 'noxious' agent at one or more sites. The reaction to this is in the nature of a modelling response: large, geographically distinct surfaces devoted to resorption or formation, 'drifts' in Frost's lexicon (see Chapter 16 for definition of

Table 20.1 Stimuli which cause bone reactions

	Stimulus	*Response*
Generalized	Hormonal	Physiological/
	Nutritional	Pathological
	Exogenous substances	
Localized	Mechanical forces	Physiological/
		Pathological
	Agents of other	Inflammatory/
	disease processes	Circulatory/
		Neoplastic

Table 20.2

Distribution	Congenital/ developmental	Metabolic bone dis.	Traumatic	Inflammatory	Circulatory	Neoplastic
Unifocal		+	+++	+++	+++	+++
Multifocal						
One bone			+	+	+	
Two plus bones	+	+	+	+	+	++
Regional	+++	+++	+	+	+	
General	+++	+++				+

'drift'). When resorption and formation surfaces are back to back, as on either surface of the cortex or threaded over a plane running through cancellous bone, large volumes of bone are moved. An example of the second case is resorption of cancellous bone in the face of an expanding neoplasm with, slightly further away, an osteoblastic drift forming a sclerotic zone. Thus, drift activity will alter the volume of the bone, leading to degrees of porosis or sclerosis. This response may, or may not, be associated with bone genesis.

Of the regional and generalized groups, the congenital/developmental, being affections of growth, are in broad terms, a derangement of the modelling of growth. The manifestations of the metabolic disorders are brought about mainly by modifications of remodelling. It is necessary to recognize that the response of bone to the generalized stimuli is the tissue manifestation of the disease process.

Nevertheless, those generalized stimuli are sometimes manifest as focal lesions which can draw attention away from the general manifestations if they are present, necessitating their inclusion in a discussion of focal reactions. In the latter, the tissue of the disease process, the lesional tissue, is different from the reactive response of the bone to its presence. The nature of the response reflects to a degree some of the characteristics of the lesion. But since many lesions have similar characteristics, the degree of specificity is most

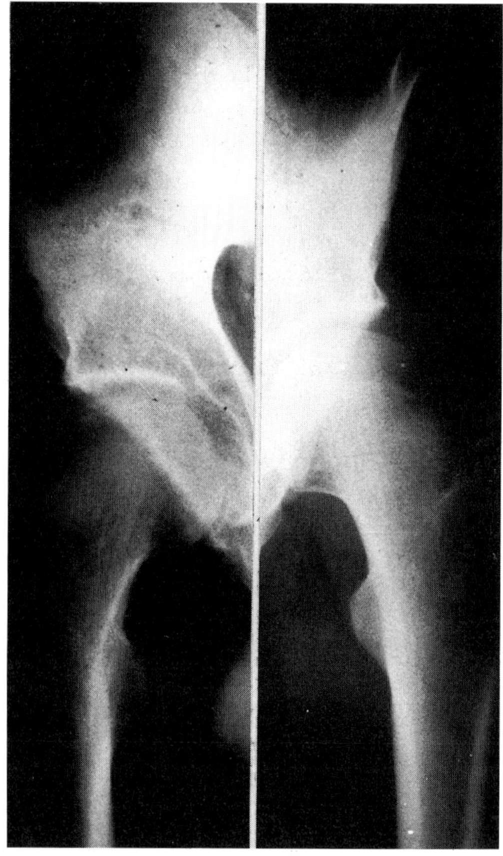

Figure 20.1 Post-traumatic osteoporosis, or the regional acceleratory phenomenon. Male aged 37 years with sports injury to right leg. Pronounced osteoporosis of the right hemi-pelvis and femur. The extent of the bone loss can be judged by comparing the two sides.

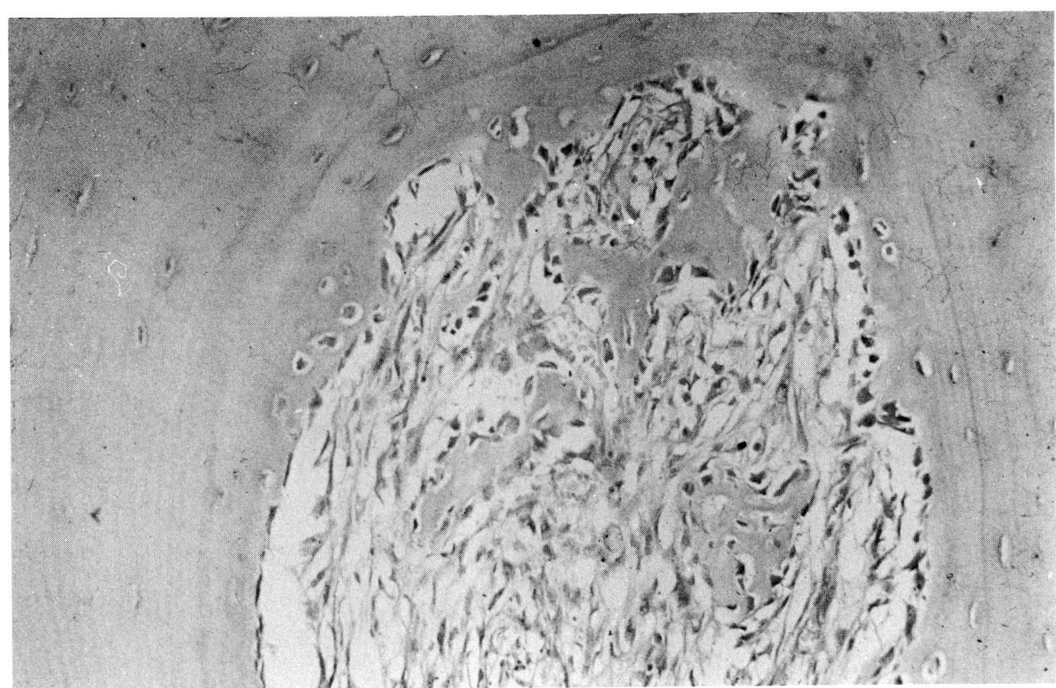

Figure 20.2 Marrow reaction. The marrow is replaced by fibrous tissue in which bone trabeculae, with a surface layer of normal osteoblasts, have formed. In addition there has been deposition of woven bone on the pre-existing lamellar bone surface (the immaturity of the bone, suggested by its tissue pattern and texture and the disposition of the osteocytes, is confirmed by polarized light). The old and new bone are demarcated by a smooth cement line: the inference is that there was no preceding resorption, and the sequence was activation/formation. Such cement lines are spoken of as arrest lines, implying that formation stopped and then resumed after an interval (see Figure 20.6 for another example). (Compare this illustration with Figure 20.3.)

useful in establishing broad categories at the macroscopic level, which in biopsy pathology means imaging. The topic 'reactions of bone' is a discussion of the bone response to focal lesions.

The agents of the reaction are cells (discussed in Chapter 18), namely:

- Osteoclasts and osteoblasts acting on surfaces:
      trabecular: in bone
      endosteal: in bone
      osteonal: in bone
      periosteal: on bone
- Fibroblasts, endothelial cells and bone cell precursors acting

      in marrow: in bone
      in periosteum: on bone
      extraosseous: in soft tissue

Working separately or together the cells can reduce or produce bone of mature or immature quality, produce and reduce collagenous tissue, create granulation tissue which can develop into fibrous tissue, and in which both cartilage and immature bone can be formed, i.e. membrane formation, and the latter from the former by enchondral ossification.

Table 20.2 emphasizes an important aspect of the distribution of reactions, and, *a priori*, the lesions giving rise to them: they may be

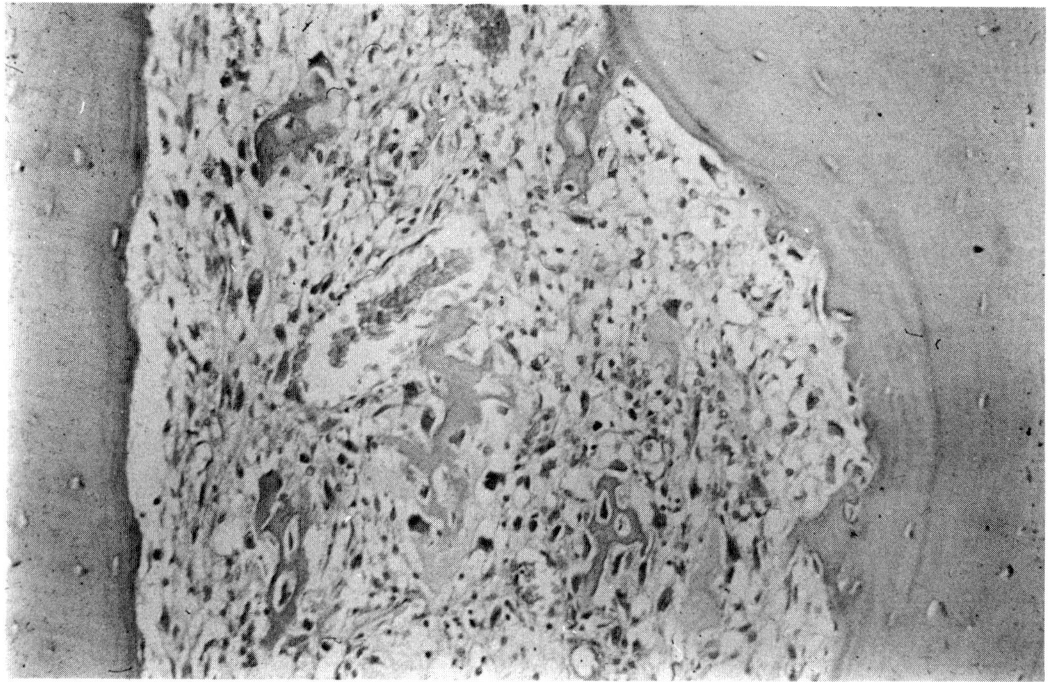

Figure 20.3 A field comparable with Figure 20.2 in which the marrow is fibrotic and infiltrated by osteosarcoma cells (scattered, pleomorphic, hyperchromatic). They are implicated in the formation of the bone spicules by their intimate association and the absence of normal osteoblasts. On the left reactive bone overlies an arrest line. But on its surface tumour cells are depositing bone; demarcating arrest lines are evident lower left.

in bone, on bone (anatomical), or in soft tissues. Additionally, only particular locations within bone may be involved, namely: epiphyseal, metaphyseal, diaphyseal; central or eccentric; medullary or cortical.

Information about macroscopic location alone serves to narrow the range of possibilities to be considered histologically, and in some cases, because additional features are unique, can with certainty offer the definitive diagnosis. Nevertheless, it is not unusual for there to be an element of ambiguity in the radiographic appearance of the morbid anatomy at the specific diagnostic level owing to the limited mechanisms for altering bone patterns.

An important reaction of bone which occurs in association with many focal lesions is a regional acceleratory phenomenon, conveniently abbreviated to RAP (Figure 20.1). This term is from Frost's lexicon (Frost, 1983). Cuthbertson (1976) in discussing the response to injury in general terms mentions features with which some of Frost's points about the RAP are in accord. The reaction to which it applies had been recognized, mainly as post-traumatic osteoporosis, with an implication that it was a consequence of disuse. But Kolar *et al.* (1965) had recognized a general metabolic shift in mineralized tissues following injury (Frost, 1985). Frost has studied it in some detail in clinical circumstances and provided a working hypothesis concerning its pathogenesis and function. Others have also undertaken investigations with results

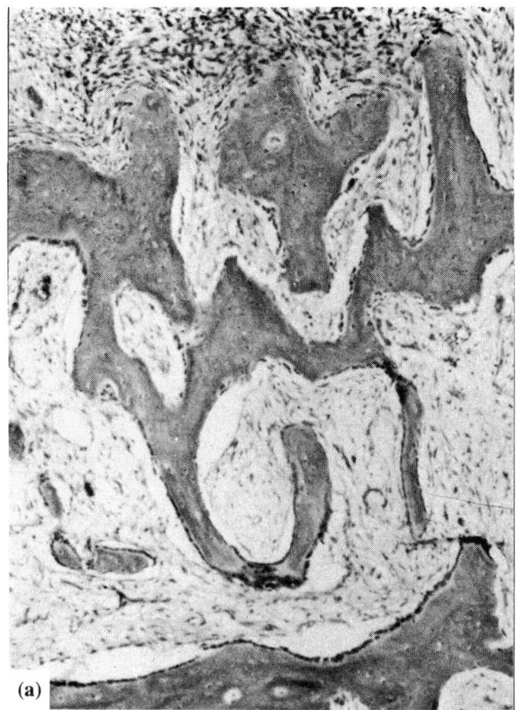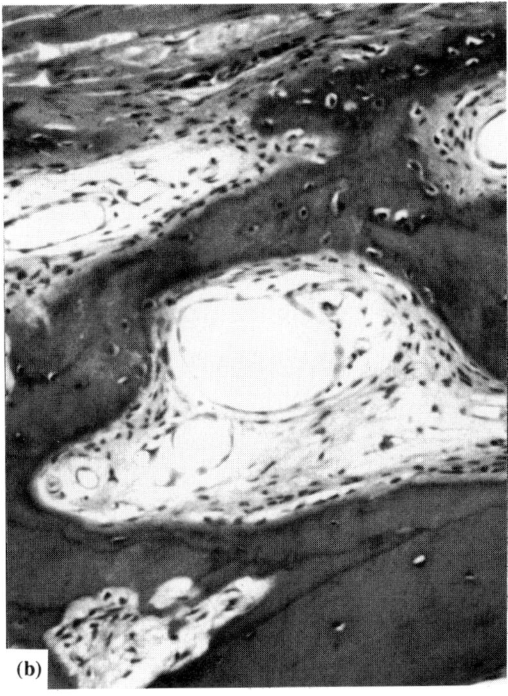

Figure 20.4 Reactive bone tissue. (a) Reactive tissue surrounding an abscess cavity in sclerosing osteomyelitis of the clavicle. Abscess at the top; endocortex at the bottom; fibrovascular tissue between with abundant reactive bone. At most bone surfaces bone cells are active: osteoblasts are obvious, but it is mainly the ragged surface that indicates resorption. Blood vessels are not strikingly prominent. (b) Periosteal reaction. Immature bone forming beneath the periosteum. The texture of the woven bone is different from the lamellar bone at the bottom.

which substantiate some aspects; nevertheless, much remains to be done (Verschooten *et al.*, 1989; Mueller *et al.*, 1991; Yasuoka and Oka, 1991).

In summary, any regional noxious stimulus (trauma, infection, non-infectious inflammation, infarction, some neoplasia) of sufficient magnitude to bone, joint or soft tissue, and acute peripheral denervation or central paralysis, as well as acute disuse can cause RAP.

The nature of the reaction is that in the region of the injury most active vital processes are accelerated: perfusion; growth of skin, bone, cartilage, hair; BMU turnover of woven and lamellar bone; turnover of connective tissues; and enhancement of healing and metabolism of regional cell populations (but see Mueller *et al.*, 1991; for a systemic effect). The manifestations are local warmth, increased uptake of bone-seeking isotopes (e.g. technetium), decreased bone density due to increased remodelling space (the proportion of bone undergoing turnover: as BMU activation increases more bone has been resorbed, and more surface is covered by osteoid), which is often manifest as minute focal osteolytic foci – so-called rain-drop osteoporosis. This enhanced activity is detectible histologically as vascular dilatation and increased cellular activity at bone surfaces (Mueller *et al.*, 1991).

The duration of RAP is in the range of months to several years.

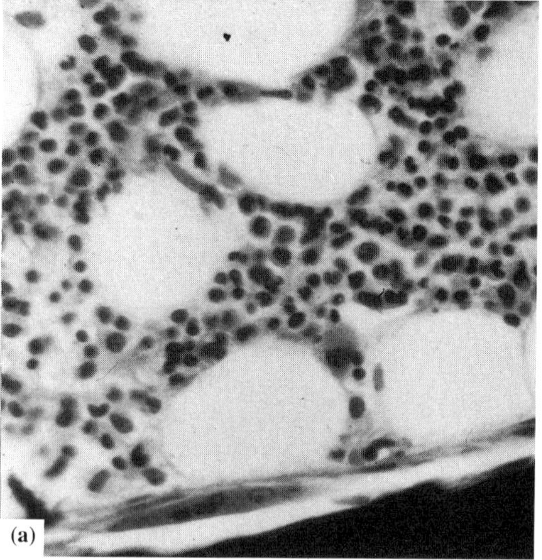

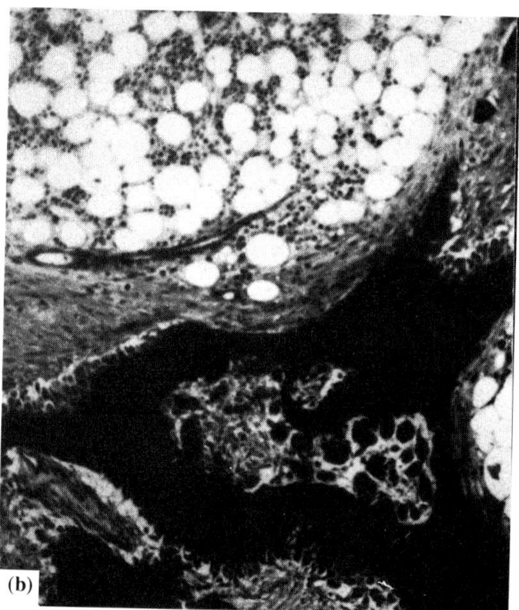

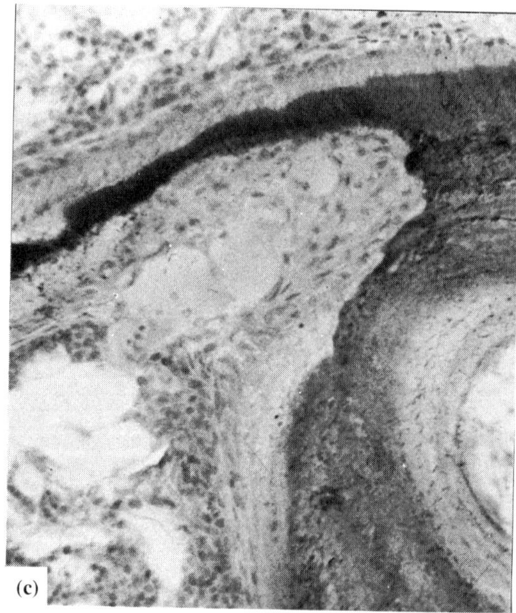

Figure 20.5 Fibrous replacement of bone. (a) Minimal fibrous deposition on a resorption surface of bone. (b) Advanced fibrous replacement of large resorption cavities in hyperparathyroidism. (c) Osteomalacia with secondary hyperpathyroidism. All the bone surfaces are active; the osteoid is abundant and some seams abnormally thick. A deep resorption bay is filled by fibrous tissue which merges with the osteoid. The marrow is normal in all three figures.

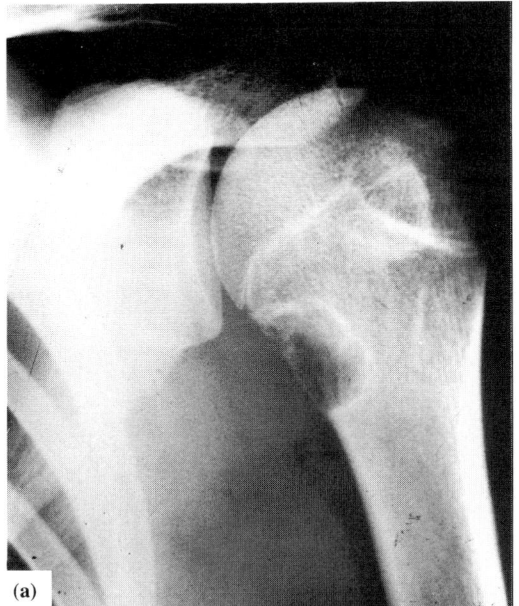
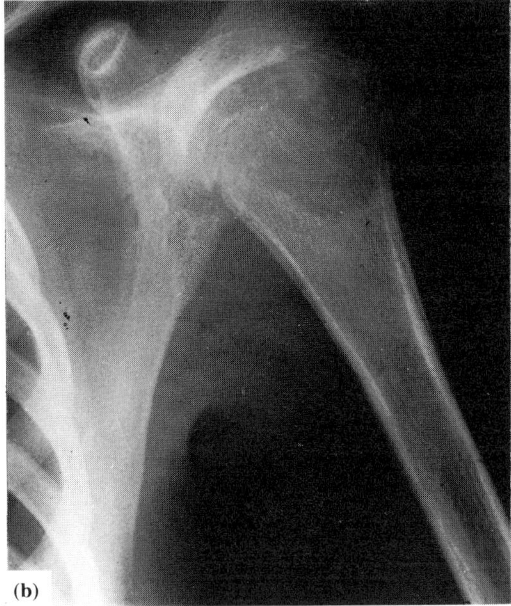

Figures 20.6 At the lesion's edge. (a) Osteolytic lesion in the neck of humerus. The edge of the lesion is defined by a well-developed sclerotic margin. The cortex has disappeared except for a pencil line of periosteal mineral. There is no soft tissue swelling, and thus no stimulus for a Codman triangle. (b) A large osteolytic lesion involving epiphysis and metaphysis, showing spotty mineralization in the lesion. There is a well-defined edge with a diffuse blush of reaction in cancellous bone; periosteal reaction extends well down the shaft. A benign relationship, but the size, limited cancellous reaction and the extent of the periosteal reaction indicate more active growth.

Frost believes that the RAP has a role in promoting healing, a view based on the observation that some non-unions occur in patients who do not develop the phenomenon.

Focal lesions do things, or cause things to be done, to a bone through control mechanisms. What these things are reflects in some measure the character of the lesion. In diagnostic pathology the simplest way to see the bone's reaction is in radiographs, which can give a global view. All the reactions have a cellular basis and can be analysed histologically. But, since it is usual to avoid reactive tissue in taking a biopsy, except where it is in contact with the lesion and may hold information about its behaviour, and even then the sample will be restricted, little information will be forthcoming from biopsy sections that can compare with the global view of the radio-graph. It behoves the pathologist therefore to be able to interpret the radiographs in histological terms. Much of the basic histological information has been given in preceding chapters and can be deployed here in a discussion largely concerned with radiographic appearances.

In a discussion of focal reactions of bone the term 'bone' is used as a referrent to both the organ and the tissue. As organ, bone contains the marrow, whose tissue reactions contribute to the microscopic and macroscopic appearances. Equally, so do the bone tissue responses. The summation of those responses gives the morbid anatomical architecture.

From the many choices of framework in which to discuss focal reactions of bone, the following anatomical framework has been adopted here:

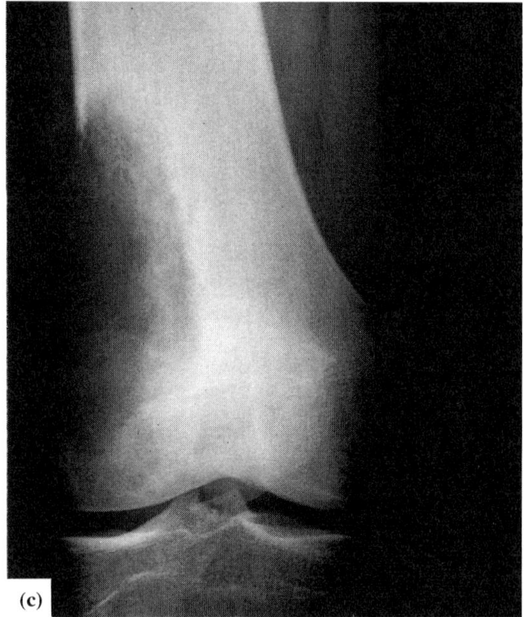

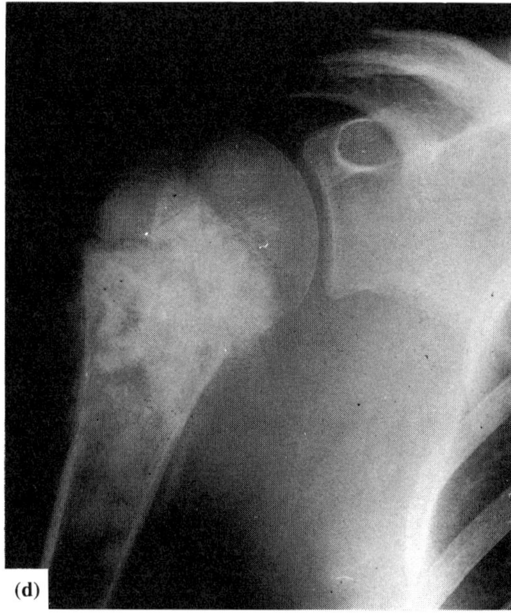

Figures 20.6 At the lesion's edge. (c) It is possible to discern a boundary here, but it has much irregularity; the lower edge is obscure. The loss of cortex with a soft tissue swelling (which may still be within the periosteum), the beginning of a Codman triangle at the upper pole, and the large size all indicate malignant tumour, but the invasiveness is restricted. (d) Metaphyseal lesion of humerus. It is not possible to know from this one film whether the fluffy mineralized tissue is in or on the bone; however experience has shown that this is the pattern of intraosseous osteosarcoma, so the experienced have no hesitation over inferring the site. A film at right angles to the plane of this would be confirmatory, and establish the widespread infiltration of the marrow, and extension into the epiphysis. There are clouds of mineralization, but no edge or definable border. The periosteum is reacting, especially on the medial side; the interruption of the reaction here indicates a soft tissue mass.

1. In bone
   (a) marrow reactions
   (b) reactions leading to loss of bone
   (c) reactions leading to increase of bone
2. On bone
   (a) reactions leading to loss of bone
   (b) reactions leading to increase of bone
3. In soft tissue
   (a) reactions leading to formation of bone

20.1 FOCAL REACTIONS WITHIN BONE

20.1.1 BONE MARROW REACTIONS (FIGURES 20.2–20.4)

These reactions include marrow fibrosis; vascular dilatation; fibrovascular proliferation (granulation tissue); bone genesis (as opposed to the bone fabrication of apposition, either as in BMU or drift activity) which is truly a reaction of marrow giving rise to increases in bone; membranous bone; and cartilaginous bone.

Fibrosis of marrow is a non-specific reaction. It is to be distinguished from fibrous replacement of bone, where the tissue deposited in Howship's lacunae is fibrous rather than osteoidal. In the early stages of hyperparathyroidism this may be seen without any accompanying marrow fibrosis.

Vascular dilatation is also a common response in bone, a component of the general

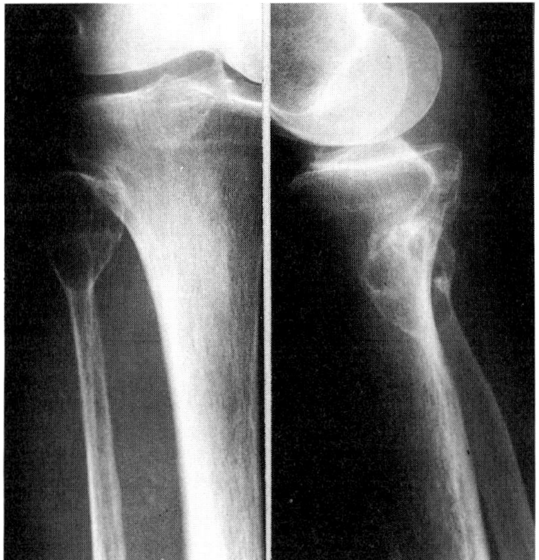

Figure 20.7 Expanding lesion of the head of the fibula. This lesion has been growing at an overall uniform rate, resulting in a smooth endocortex, as compared with the 'erosive' appearance in the preceding illustration. This and the clear demarcation from the fibula favour a benign lesion.

response to injury (RAP), and of many other conditions.

Fibrovascular tissue proliferation can occur in association with a variety of lesions. The prominent vessels lined with endothelium can be mistaken for vascular hamartoma or neoplasia.

There comes a stage when new bone may appear in the fibrovascular tissue through membrane formation. This occurs soonest and to the greatest degree in callus, where it is the expected development, and to a much lesser extent in the presence of other lesions. The resultant bone can develop and mature by remodelling, become stable, or resolve if circumstances lead to resolution of the lesion.

20.1.2 REACTIONS LEADING TO LOSS OF BONE (FIGURES 20.5–20.7)

Focal loss of bone is nearly always due to an expanding or infiltrating (synonyms: invasive, permeating) lesion. Acute regional osteoporosis can mimic this, as can the porotic phase of Paget's disease. Such lesions are neoplastic, dysplastic and other tumour-like conditions, or inflammatory. Non-invasive lesions have what some call a pushing front, resulting in a large hole in the bone through inciting a resorption drift. If there is an accompanying formation drift, the site will be surrounded by a zone of increased density. Lodwick (1964, 1966) applies the term geographic to the resulting radiographic appearance. It is apparent that the margin is going to reflect the pattern of growth of the lesion: uniform, unequal, lobulated, satellitic, invasive, slow, rapid. As one progresses along this catalogue of behaviour, the mind's eye can picture the pattern altering through a progressively disorderly arrangement to arrive at a stage with no major focus and an irregular, almost osteoporotic loss of bone from rapid infiltration of osteomyelitis or a round cell neoplasm. Descriptive terminology is hard put to match this kaleidoscope, and many are the terms employed. But the essence is simple: the more ragged the pattern, the more aggressive the lesion in terms of its invasive potential. The radiologist's job is to recall from his or her experience conditions that have given rise to the pattern under review. The pathologist must ensure that his interpretation of the tissue is a condition that can give rise to it.

Some tissues and cells, including some neoplasms, permeate the marrow without giving rise to any resorptive activity. Invasion does not necessarily imply rapid growth, as many slowly growing chondrosarcomas of adults demonstrate. Nor does it necessarily imply neoplasia: inflammation is equally invasive, and often indistinguishable in radiographs.

One of the consequences of marrow invasion by any type of tissue may be the creation of sequestra that result from compromising the blood supply to the bone. In time the sequestra appear relatively more

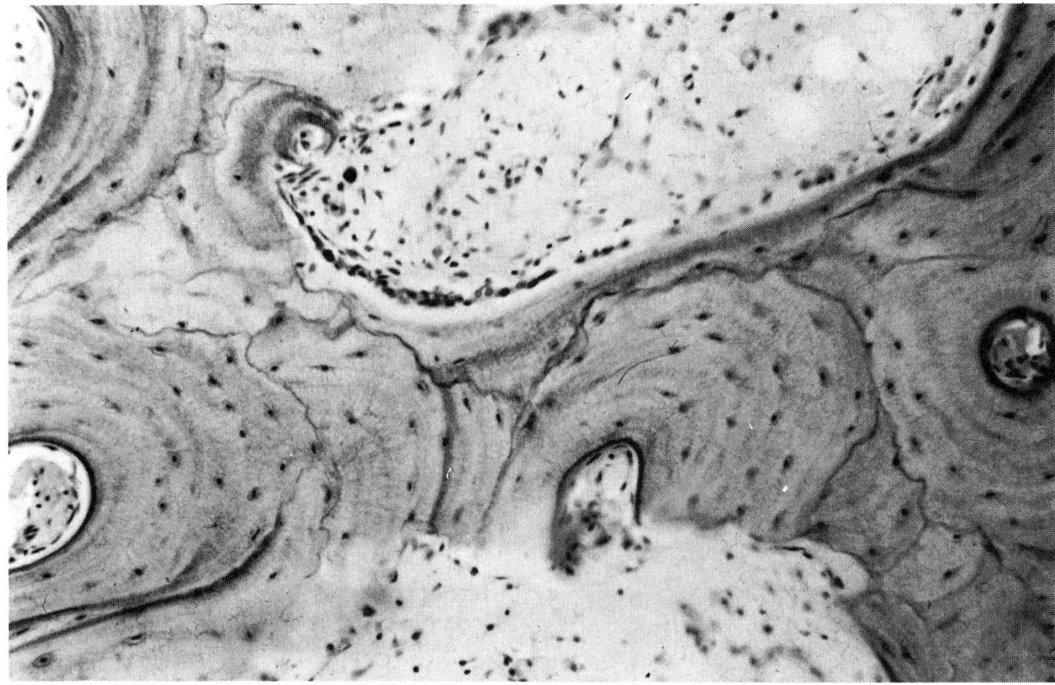

Figure 20.8 Increased bone density. Trabecular bone has been grossly altered by remodelling, and its volume increased. Much remodelling has produced many small packets (BSUs) of bone with a mosaic pattern. Corticalization of the bone has occurred in the sense that osteons have been formed.

dense than the viable bone; this is caused by progressive osteoporosis of the latter rather than an increase in the mineral content of the former.

Erosion implies resorption of bone cortex from its surface by osteoclasts in response to a contiguous lesion; in the context of lesions within bone that would be the endosteal surface. In general, the implication is relatively rapid osteoclastic activity with little compensatory osteoblastic activity. This contrasts with expansion, where there is accompanying periosteal apposition, as seen in slowly growing intraosseous tumours, e.g. benign tumours, some low-grade chondrosarcomas in adult long bone. The thickness of the cortex will be determined by the relative amounts removed and added (Figure 20.7).

20.1.3　REACTIONS LEADING TO INCREASES IN BONE (FIGURES 20.8–20.13)

Increased density and osteosclerosis are qualitative terms that describe sectors on a continuous scale of increasing bone volume. Since there are no quantitative values, there are no points of demarcation and it is a matter of choice as to which is used. Generally, sclerosis is used to describe the more striking increases. The increases come about through several mechanisms.

1. Remodelling during which formation exceeds resorption in BMUs, and there may be increased activation frequency. The bone formed may be lamellar or woven. The reversal line pattern begins to assume a mosaic pattern (Figure 20.8).

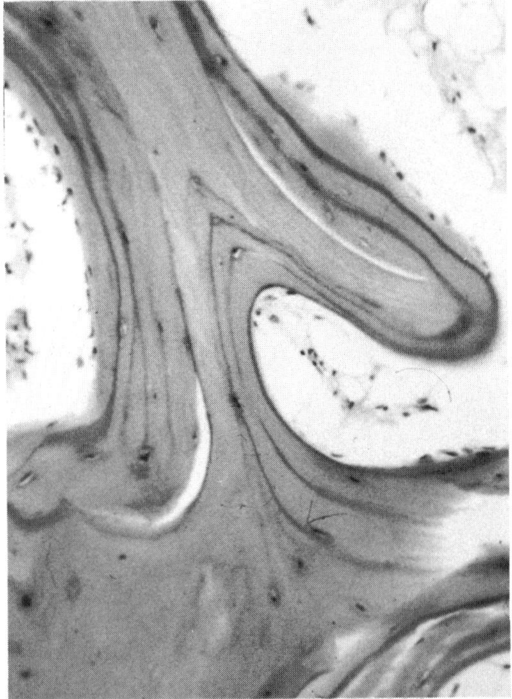

Figure 20.9 Increased bone density as the result of the successive activation of linear apposition. The original trabeculum is recognizable at the centre of a number of layers of lamellar bone demarcated by arrest cement lines (see legend Figure 20.2). The bone, although poorly cellular (as in older people) is viable, a conclusion supported by the viable marrow. This is a non-specific response. In avascular necrosis, successive episodes of necrosis can be recognized from necrosis of the original and reactive layers.

2. Lamellar apposition to surfaces without preceding resorption, sometimes in successive waves, demarcated from the pre-reactive bone, and from each other, by long sweeping cement lines, which are also called arrest lines (meaning that no resorption has taken place between successive waves of apposition).
3. The genesis of bone in the marrow (Figure 10.2.3).

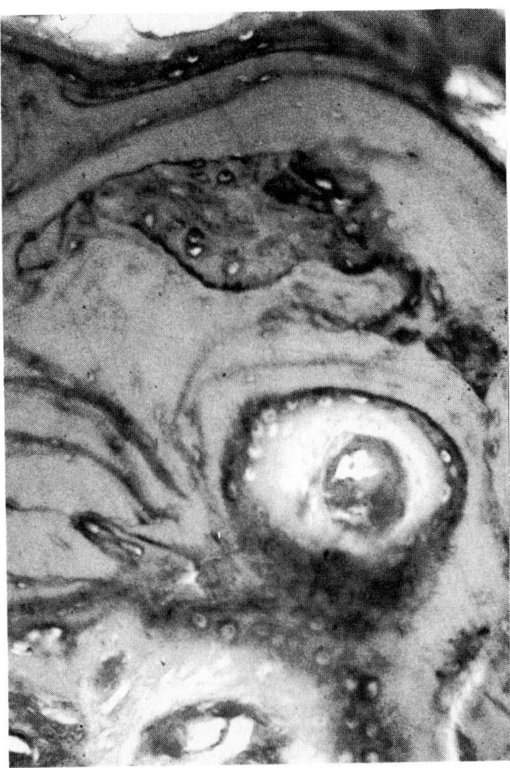

Figure 20.10 A more complex reaction in cancellous bone in osteoarthritis of the femoral head. In addition to linear apposition of lamellar bone, there are pockets of woven bone and of calcified chondroid material. The result is very dense bone to which the term osteosclerosis would apply.

20.2 FOCAL REACTIONS ON THE BONE SURFACE

20.2.1 REACTIONS LEADING TO LOSS OF BONE (FIGURE 20.14)

Erosion is the resorption of bone cortex from its surface by osteoclasts in response to a contiguous lesion. It is a hallmark of inflammatory lesions of the synovium, as in rheumatoid arthritis or tuberculosis, resulting in excavation of bone at the site of attachment of the synovium on both sides of the joint cavity. The resorption may extend beyond the immediate vicinity of the inflammation and reduce the subchon-

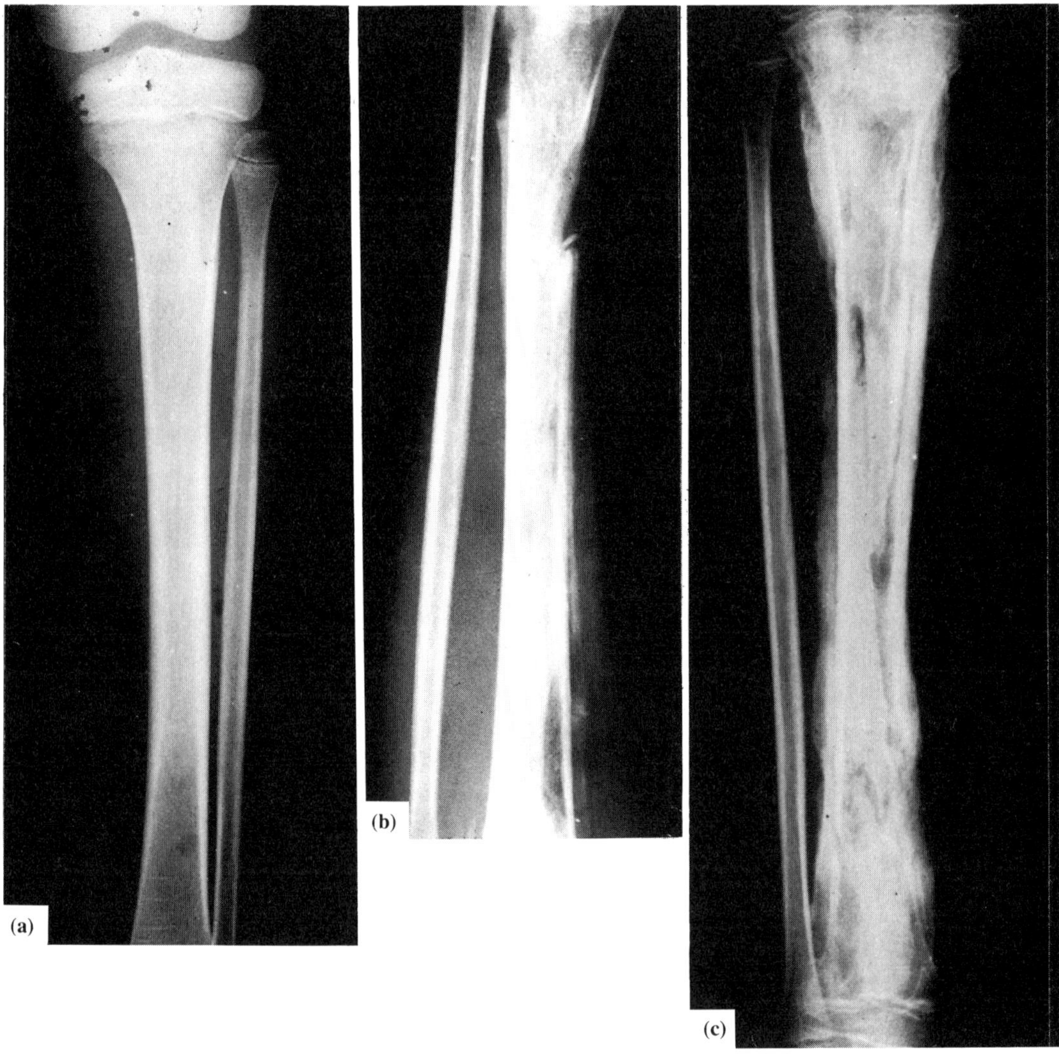

Figure 20.11 Osteomyelitis of the tibia, pre-antibiotic era. (a) Initial radiograph after a few days of acute pain, tenderness and fever. There is virtually nothing to be seen beyond a suggestion of a periosteal reaction on the lateral side of the proximal metaphysis even though much of the marrow must have been involved by the inflammation. (b) After 6 weeks, and an attempt to drain the shaft, a periosteal reaction is developing. (c) After three months the necrotic shaft, a sequestrum, is encased in periosteal bone, the involucrum. After several more months and a massive sequestrectomy the patient was on the way to recovery.

dral bone as well as removing the subchondral plate (Chapter 7). Neoplastic penetration of the joint can also cause erosion, but this affects only one bone.

In hyperparathyroidism, focal subperiosteal erosion is common, and may be one of the early skeletal signs. However, this is not at the site of synovial attachment so there is no confusion with the erosion associated with synovial inflammation.

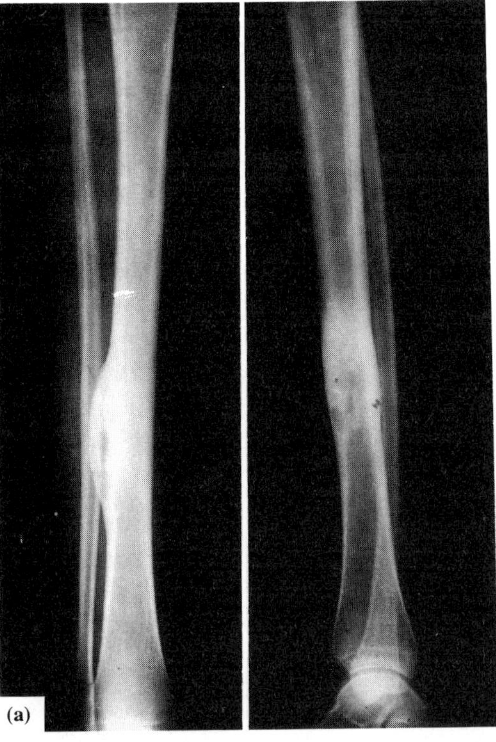

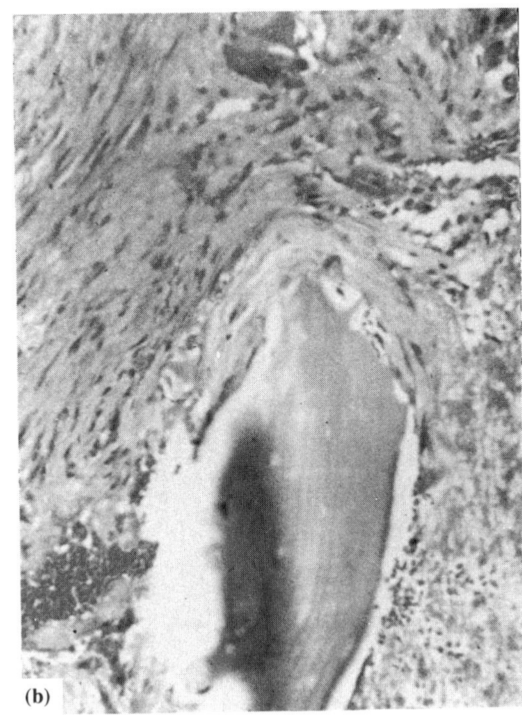

Figure 20.12 Periosteal bone abscess in a young man. (a) A small lucent lesion on the cortex enclosed by a marked local periosteal reaction. (b) Removal of the lesion reveals a small sterile abscess, with a fibrous wall, containing a sequestrum and a little inspissated pus.

Resorption of the outer end of the clavicle is an exception since it is within the structure of the acromioclavicular joint. In hyperparathyroidism, focal pronounced resorption and fibrous replacement of bone may produce a spindle cell reactive lesion with many osteoclasts, which is usually multifocal, but may be solitary. The latter can be confused macroscopically and histologically with giant cell tumour and aneurysmal bone cyst (Murray *et al.*, 1990), a difficulty resolved biochemically.

20.2.2 REACTIONS LEADING TO INCREASES IN BONE ON THE EXTERNAL SURFACE (FIGURE 20.15)

(a) Periosteal remodelling

The age-related enlargement of bone has been excluded from this discussion (see Chapter 10), but in Paget's disease of bone, characterized by high turnover on all envelopes at affected sites, the net result of BMU activity is positive and enlarges the bone (see section 10.5.7).

(b) Periosteal apposition

In this case lamellar bone is added where the invoked activity is slow – the expansion of the cortex around a slowly growing cartilage tumour was cited above.

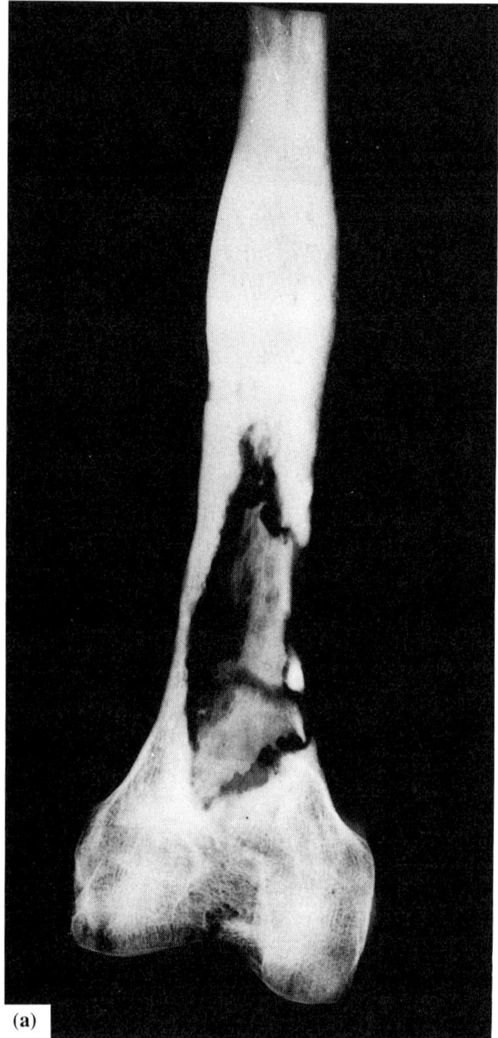

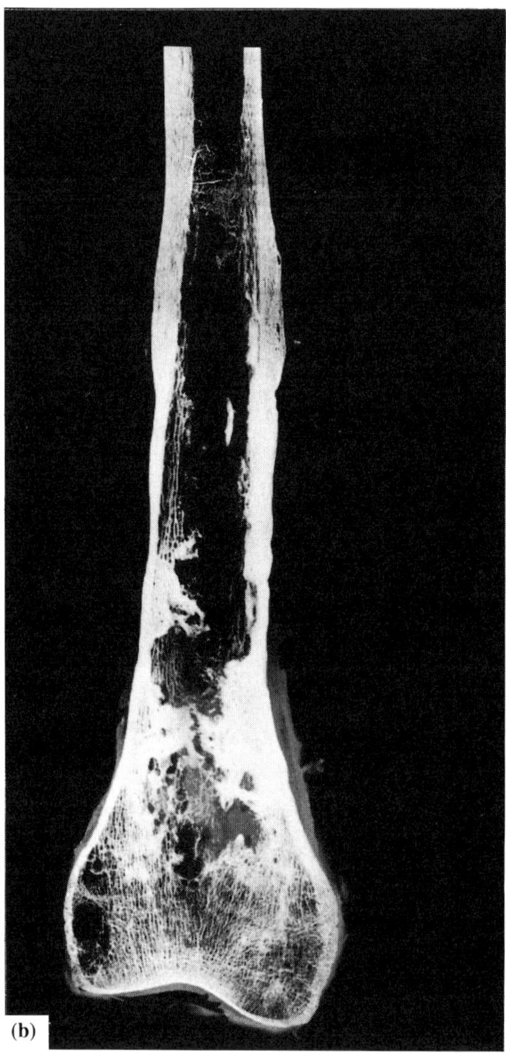

Figure 20.13 (a) and (b) Chronic osteomyelitis following war injury to the femur. Persistence of the lesion led to amputation. Two slab radiographs from the specimen. The morbid anatomy has been influenced by surgical sequestrectomy and debridement over the years. For present purposes the points to note are the reactive changes. There is a large diaphyseal cavity bounded above by delicate reactive trabeculae. The endocortical surface is irregularly eroded, the diameter of the diaphysis is increased by uneven periosteal apposition: these are features of any expanding lesion of moderate aggression. There is a smaller metaphyseal cavity, irregular in shape, with ill-defined margins in part, surrounded by sclerotic bone which extends irregularly into the epiphysis where the inflammmation has permeated the marrow. There are several small and large sequestra of cortical and/or cancellous bone throughout.

(c) Periosteal bone genesis

A periosteal reaction, provoked by more active lesions within the bone (giving rise to the radiographic patterns described above in section 20.1.2), gives rise to the formation of woven bone by the periosteum. The

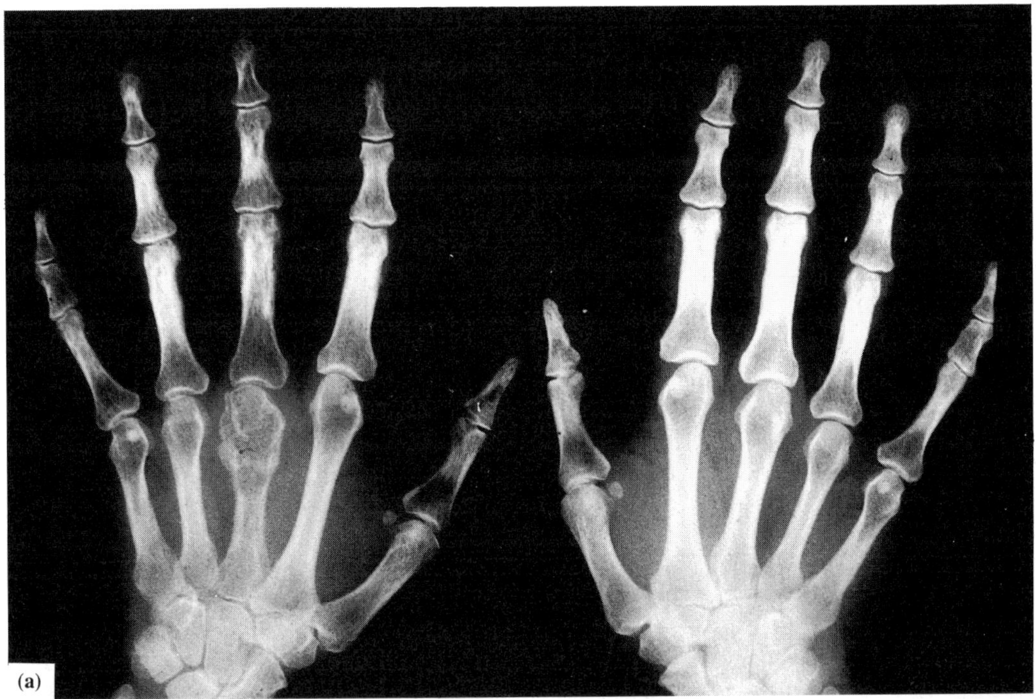

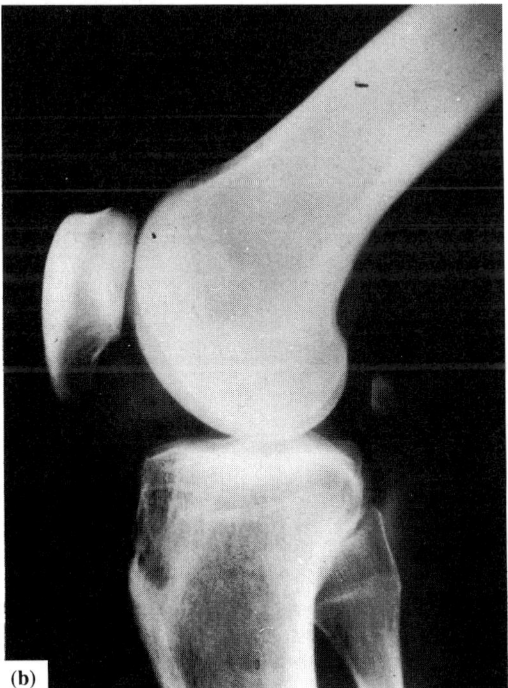

Figure 20.14 Periosteal erosions. (a) Female aged 58 years, swelling in hand. The benign expanding lesion of the head of the third left metacarpal comes immediately to notice; then the osteoporosis of this ray as compared with its neighbours, the osteoporosis of this hand as compared with its fellow: all consistent with a benign neoplasm. Further careful observation shows subperiosteal erosions of proximal phalanges of rays 2–5 in the left hand and 2 and 3 on the right; the middle phalanx of right ray 3 is similarly affected. The prime diagnosis is now hyperparathyroidism, confirmed biochemically. (b) Male aged 32 years. Boggy swelling of knee. The soft tissue swelling is just evident in the illustration. There is erosion of the lower pole of the patella and of the anterior surface of the tibia. Erosion on both sides of a joint are indicative of synovial inflammation; in this case pigmented villonodular synovitis.

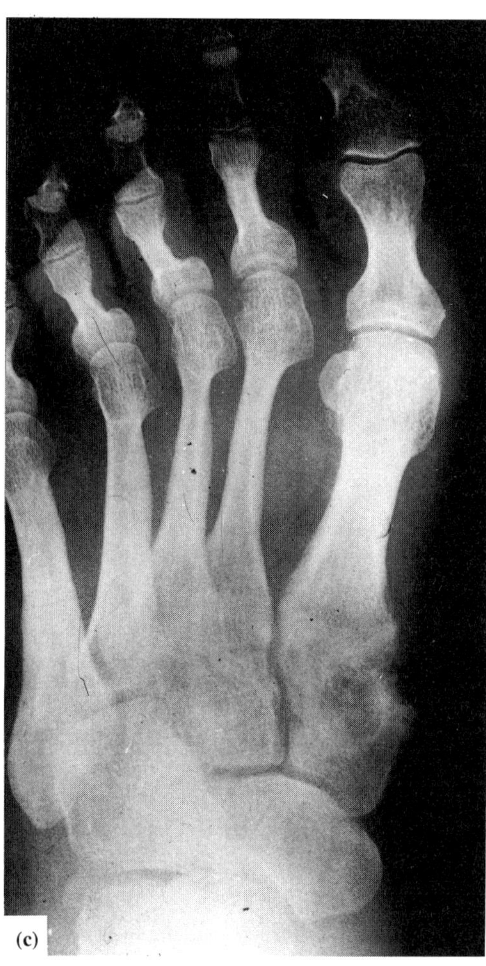

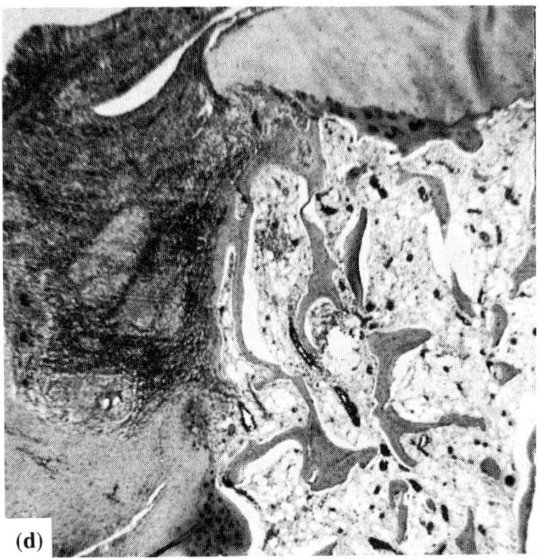

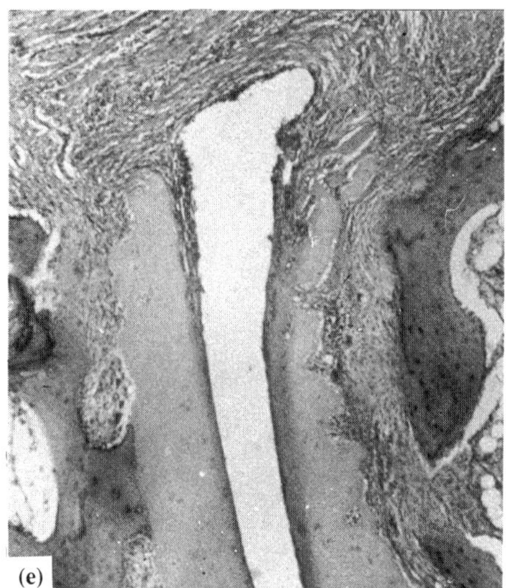

Figure 20.14 Periosteal erosions. (c) Marginal bone erosion on both sides of the first tarsometatarsal in a tuberculous infection. (d) Histological section from the resected 1st cuneiform: granulomatous inflammation in the synovium, erosion of cortex and subchondral bone plate; pannus extending onto cartilage surface; inflamed villus. Note, top right, resorption of subchondral plate in association with minimal non-specific fibrovascular tissue in the marrow. (e) Chronic psoriatic arthropathy (histologically similar to rheumatoid arthritis). Marginal erosion of bone and articular cartilage, of subchondral plate, and articular surface on both sides of the joint by a now quiescent inflammation.

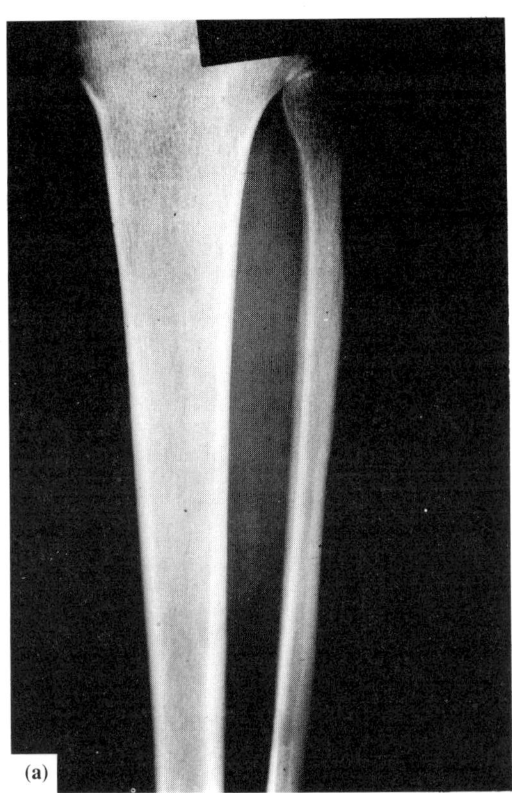

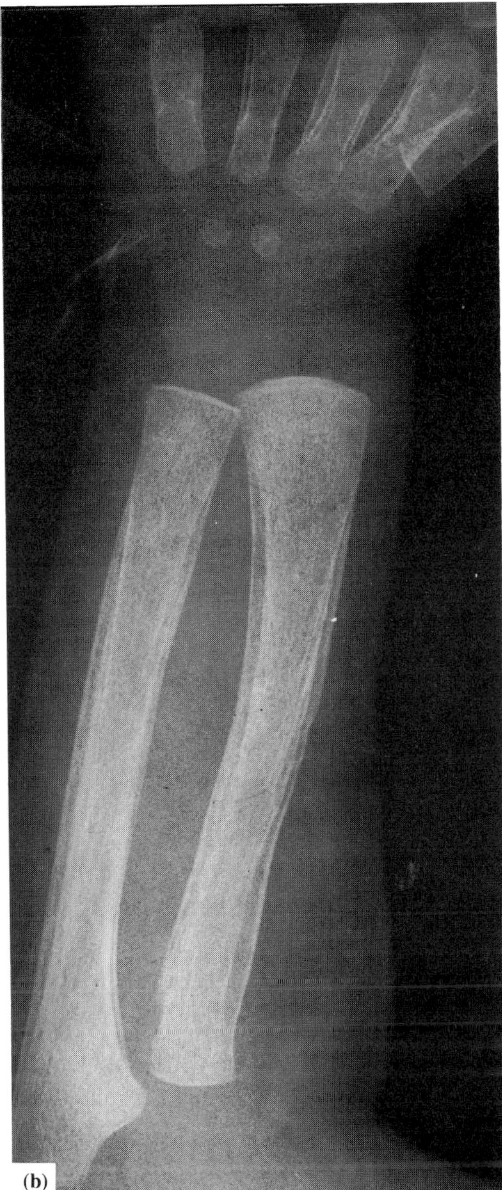

Figure 20.15 Periosteal (formative) reactions. (a) Slight periosteal reaction of the upper fibular diaphysis. Attributed to stress. (b) Diffuse reaction involving the short and long tubular bones of the forearm in congenital syphilis.

architecture of this is trabecular. The trabeculae may be arranged parallel to the surface, may be arranged parallel to the surface, perpendicular to it, or irregularly, giving a laminar ('onion skin'), spicular ('sunray' or 'hair on end') or diffuse appearance in radiographs. These patterns are not readily discernible in histological sections unless the sample is large and well-orientated. The first two patterns tend to be associated with particular causes, but these are not perfect associations and lack a high degree of specificity. Some infiltrating neoplasms extend through the Volkman and osteonal canals to lie beneath the periosteum, which is then lifted from the surface by tumour growth; reactive bone appears where the periosteum attaches to the surface, forming Codman's triangle.

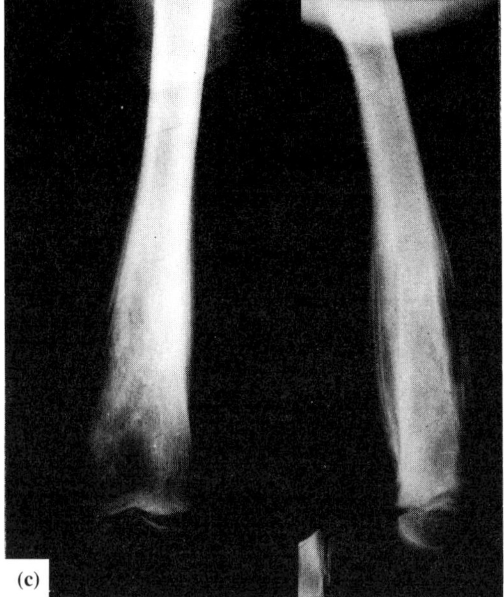

Figure 20.15 Periosteal (formative) reactions. (c) Ewing's tumour of the distal femur with a laminated periosteal reaction. (d) Osteosarcoma of distal femur with sun-ray reactive spiculation. The extraosseous tissue is a mixture of neoplasm and vertically orientated bone spicules formed from the periosteum.

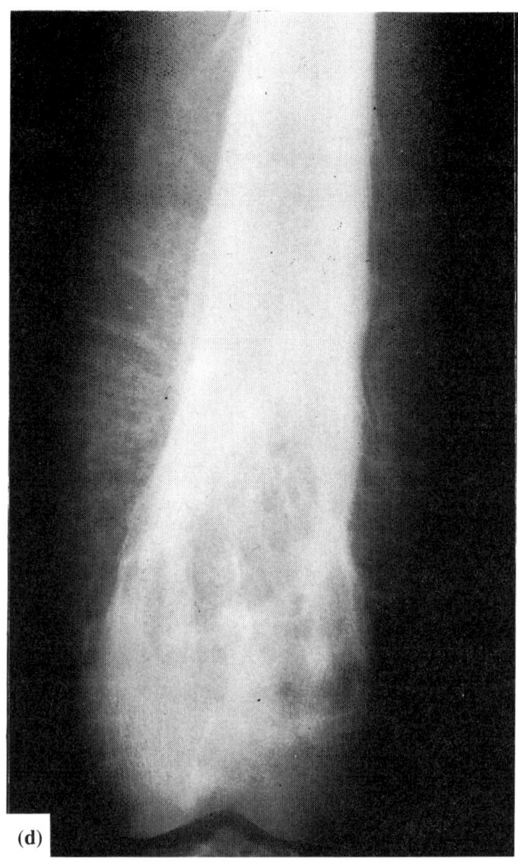

(d) Fibrovascular proliferation and bone genesis

In effect this is callus, usually provoked by traumatic disruption of the periosteum, in which membrane bone formation occurs, often accompanied by cartilagenous bone formation.

20.3 FOCAL REACTIONS IN SOFT TISSUE HETEROTOPIC BONE FORMATION

There being no pre-existing bone in soft tissue there are no reactions related to the modelling or remodelling. However, the bone forming reactions are subject to remodelling, and thus may mature (Figure 20.16), remodel and be resorbed.

Bone reactions involving soft tissues may retain a base on bone, although external to the periosteum, as exemplified by many lesions of myositis ossificans, and belong in the category 'on bone'. Such lesions must be distinguished from avulsions, which invoke callus. The solitary lesion must also be differentiated from parosteal (and periosteal) osteosarcoma. This is not easy, or even possible in the early stages before the parosteal neoplasm has developed unequivocal features of malignancy. In practical terms the matter is resolved by behaviour. If the lesion does not resolve or mature in the course of a few weeks, and has occurred without good and sufficient cause, then it must be regarded as low grade osteosarcoma (section 13.4.4)

Pseudomalignant osseous tumour of soft tissue, usually classed as myositis ossificans,

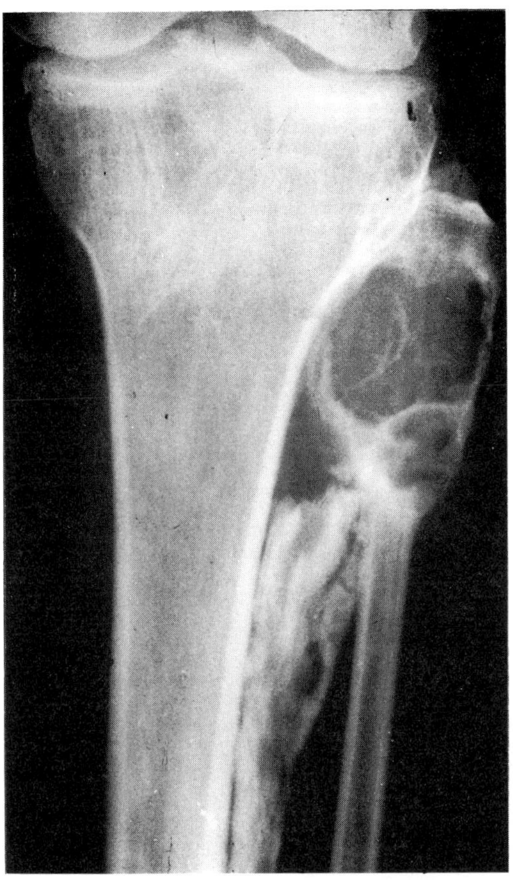

Figure 20.16 Soft tissue mineralization. Female aged 34 years. Pain in the knee due to pathological fracture of chondromyxoid fibroma of proximal fibula. Five years earlier an injury was sustained to the leg resulting in ossification of the interosseous ligament.

occurs in soft tissue at a remove from bone (Figure 6.13). Although uncommon it is a well-recognized lesion, and is discussed in connection with myositis ossificans in Chapter 6.

Material in soft tissue from giant cell tumour, as a result of spillage at operation, will induce the formation around it of reactive bone. This is but one example of bone induction by transposed tissue (see section 18.7.2 for further discussion).

REFERENCES

Cuthbertson, D.P. (1976) Surgical metabolism: historical and evolutionary aspects. In *Metabolism and the Response to Injury* (eds A.W. Wilkinson and D. Cuthbertson), Pitman Medical, Kent, pp. 1–34.

Frost, H.M. (1983) The regional acceleratory phenomenon. *Henry Ford Hosp. Med. J.*, **31**, 3–9.

Frost, H.M. (1985) The pathomechanics of osteoporosis. *Clin. Orthop.*, **200**, 198–225.

Kolar, J., Babicky, A. and Vrabec, R. (1965) *The Physical Agents and Bone*. Czech Academy of Science, Prague.

Lodwick, G.S. (1964) Reactive response to local injury in bone. *Radiol. Clin. North Am.*, **2**, 209–19.

Lodwick, G.S. (1966) Solitary malignant tumours of bone. The application of predictor variables and diagnosis. *Semin. Roentgenol.*, **1**, 293–313.

Mueller, M., Schilling, T., Minne, H. *et al.* (1991) A systemic acceleratory phenomenon (SAP) accompanies the regional acceleratory phenomenon (RAP) during heaing of a bone defect in the rat. *J. Bone Miner. Res.*, **6**, 401–10.

Murray, R.O., Jacobson, H. and Stoker, D.J. (1960) *The Radiology of Skeletal Disorders*. Churchill Livingstone, Edinburgh, pp. 431–8.

Verschooten, F., Roels, J., Lampo, P. *et al.* (1989) Radiographic measurement from the lateromedial projection of the equine foot with navicular disease. *Res. Vet. Science*, **46**, 15–21.

Yasuoka, T. and Oka, N. (1991) Histomorphometric study of trabecular bone remodelling during condylar process fracture healing in the growing period: experimental study. *J. Oral Maxillofac. Surg.*, **49**, 981–8.

Jonathan R. Salisbury and Colin G. Woods

21.1 BONE SAWS

Bone saws used for the sawing of gross specimens vary from small hand-held 'junior' hacksaws to large band saws designed for the butchery trade. Small electric-driven band saws are suitable for small specimens (Figure 21.1a) and produce flatter cut surfaces than hand-held saws. Large band saws are required for limbs, etc. (Figure 21.1b). These machines are dangerous and must be treated with respect. It is essential that they are properly installed, maintained and used in accordance with both the manufacturer's instructions and Health and Safety regulations. A plastic apron and surgical gloves are required. Safety goggles are necessary to protect the eyes from bone dust and splinters. Fingers must be kept well away from the blade. Large band saws have a steel guiderail to hold the specimen as it passes the blade. Wooden 'push sticks' are an alternative. A large, highly visible, emergency cut-off button should be within easy reach. Ideally, a second person should be present at the time of use. The saw-blade must be adequately cleaned and sterilized after use; this may involve partial dismantling for large saws.

21.2 SPECIMEN AND SLAB RADIOLOGY

Radiographs of tissue slabs, or of whole smaller specimens, provide a permanent record of macroscopic detail. As a consequence of the national breast screening programme in the United Kingdom, many

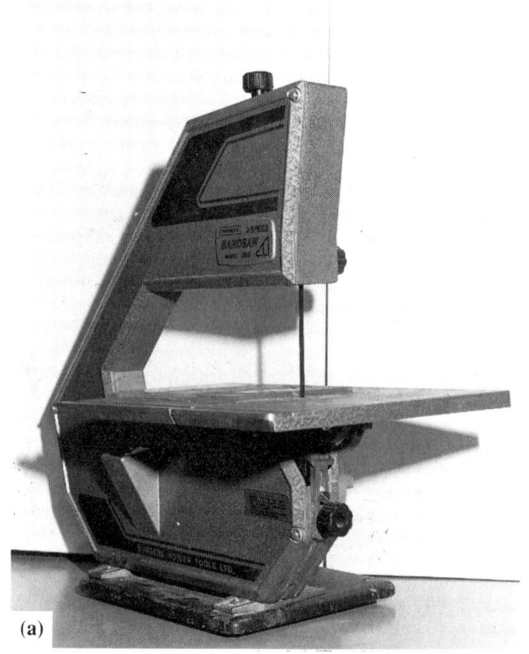

Figure 21.1 Band saws suitable for large and small specimens. (a) A home workshop band saw with an 8 cm jaw adequate for handling small bone specimens in the cut-up room.

pathology laboratories have been provided with small X-ray machines (e.g. Faxitron or Microfocus Imaging) for the detection of calcifications that have been demonstrated mammographically and then surgically excised. These machines produce excellent radiographs of all but the largest bone specimens. If the pathology laboratory does not have its own X-ray facilities, and for very large specimens, the co-operation of col-

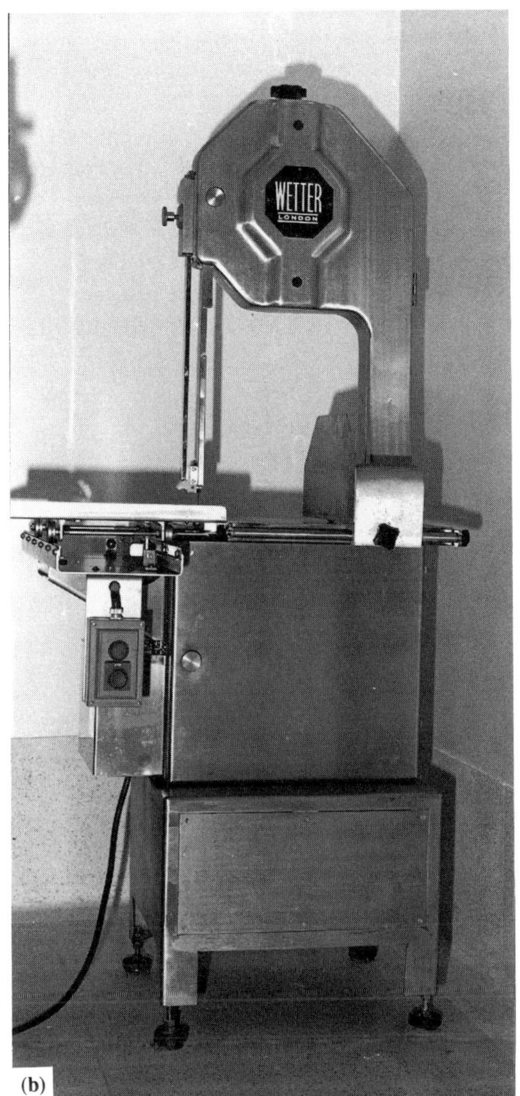

Figure 21.1 Band saws suitable for large and small specimens. (b) A commercial meat saw. The jaw size is sufficient to accommodate an amputated leg.

leagues in the local radiology department must be sought.

The outlines of the tissue blocks taken for histology can be marked on specimen sketches or, even better, on the radiographs themselves (Figure 21.2). Such a record allows the histological observations to be related to successively higher levels of anatomical organization. In any case, the observations can be related to higher levels of organization through the radiological and clinical information.

Radiography of bone samples is used as a record of the size of a trephine biopsy, for the purpose of selecting an area for examination (for example a femoral head which may be involved by Paget's disease), and as a check on decalcification (see below).

Fine-detail radiographic examination can be useful for small specimens as it will reveal the location of any mineralized tissues. Patterns of mineralization can also be distinguished within broad categories, e.g. reactive bone, pre-existing bone, osteoid osteoma (see Figure 13.3).

21.3 FIXATION

Fixation in 'buffered' formalin is satisfactory for all general purposes including the identification of tetracycline label. However, 100% ethanol is essential for the preservation of gout crystals which are water-soluble.

The choice of fixative for a sample of bone to be examined for evidence of metabolic bone disease has been much debated. Unless some of the specimen is to be examined in an electron microscope, 10% formalin which has been brought to a pH of 7.0 or more is perfectly satisfactory for most purposes. A 70% solution of ethanol is preferred by some when there is tetracycline labelling but is not mandatory. There are occasions when an urgent report is required on a biopsy and a decalcified section is adequate for the purpose: in this circumstance 5% trichloroacetic acid can be used as a combined fixative and decalcifying agent to reduce processing time. Fixation in formalin or 70% ethanol at 4°C followed by methacrylate embedding is required for histochemical staining for phosphatases.

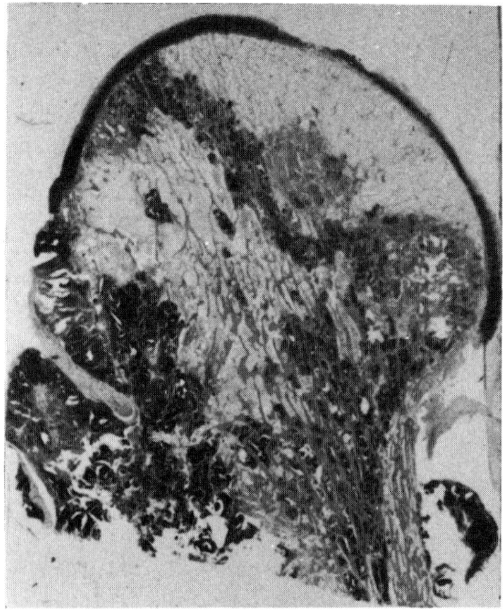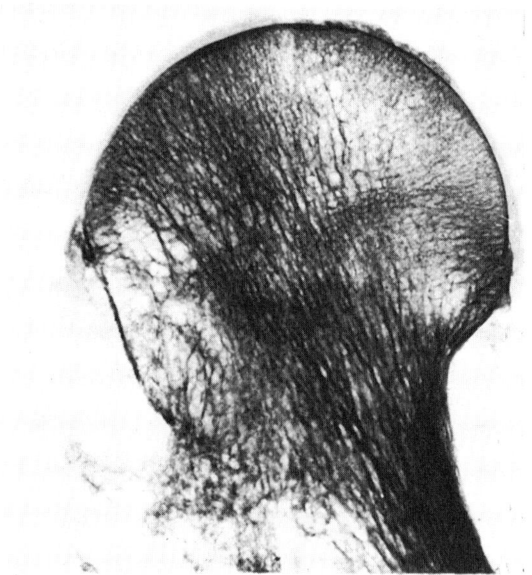

Figure 21.2 Photograph of a stained whole mount preparation and radiograph of a slab of the femoral head and neck in a case of chondrosarcoma. A comparison shows that there has been extensive permeation of marrow with little or no bone destruction. The position of the histology blocks marked on the radiograph would facilitate interpretation.

21.4 SECTION PREPARATION

Sections of bone for light microscopy may be prepared with or without the retention of the mineral content. Choice of method is influenced principally by the information required but may also depend on the availability of equipment and to some degree the urgency for a report.

What follows is a short review of the methods of section preparation which may be used, together with the stains which can be applied.

21.4.1 UNDECALCIFIED SECTIONS

Sections can be cut with a microtome if the bone is adequately supported by the embedding material and the cutting instrument is sufficiently robust. Paraffin wax alone will not support the brittle structure of thin slices of bone but if the tissue is first impregnated with nitrocellulose before embedding in paraffin it is possible to obtain 8–10 µm sections of cancellous bone, a process described as 'double embedding'. Tissue embedded in plastic is better supported and this is now the most commonly used medium for the preparation of undecalcified sections. There is a choice of materials suitable for the purpose including mixtures of butyl and methyl methacrylate and resins such as Spurr, 'Beetle' and 'London'. All require special storage and careful handling because of their irritant, toxic or explosive properties; only properly trained persons should be involved in their storage and handling. The appropriate Hazard Data Sheets and the Control of Substances Hazardous to Health (COSHH) Regulations (1988) should be consulted and followed.

When cutting hard tissue, microtome knives tend to vibrate and shatter the section. Microtome knives must therefore be inherently robust and firmly clamped on either side of and close to the cutting area with the 'cutting angle' as small as possible to obviate this problem. If those conditions can be fulfilled, it is easily possible to cut sections of cancellous bone 1 cm square. Compact bone such as is found in ribs, vertebrae and ilium can also be sectioned if plastic embedded. Motor-driven microtomes are now commonly used to cut sections of bone. The Jung 'K' microtome was the only machine available for several years but smaller instruments that will cut thinner sections and have knives which are more easily sharpened are now on the market. The smaller machines can also be used for cutting other tissues which are resin embedded. Undecalcified sections are essential for the proper evaluation of osteoid. Plastic-embedded sections are superior to those which are double embedded for the staining and identification of cement lines, aluminium deposits and tetracycline labels. If the embedding medium is retained in the section, staining schedules may have to be varied from those given in standard texts of histological methods (section 21.5).

The following schedule for processing bone samples into London Resin (LR) white resin is convenient for general purposes.

1. Fix in 70% alcohol for 1 day
2. Absolute alcohol for 3 days (change each day)
3. Chloroform overnight on the third day
4. Absolute alcohol for 1 day
5. Absolute alcohol: LR white resin 50:50 for 2 days
6. LR white resin for 2 or 3 days, preferably under vacuum
7. Polymerize in fresh resin at 60°C in water bath for about 24 hours (less for small volumes of resin)

An alternative research technique for the measurement of the extent of *in vivo* tetracycline labelling has been described (Gardner *et al.*, 1990; Gardner and Oates, 1993). Briefly, images of wet bone slices, sawn from iliac crest bone with a diamond knife, are captured by a confocal scanning optical microscope and presented to an IBAS image analyser. The image quality is so high that fully automated morphometry can be used to determine trabecular bone volume (TBV). The technique is fast so that TBV can be calculated within 1 hour of biopsy.

21.4.2 GROUND SECTIONS

In this histological sections are prepared by sawing thin slices from a block of bone and grinding them, either by hand or machine, to appropriate thinness between glass plates previously roughened, 'sharpened', by carborundum dust. Cancellous bone may be embedded in a hard plastic such as methyl methacrylate after being sawn; other plastics and resins do not give enough strength to the sections which then break during handling, but this is optional for cortical bone or whole transverse sections of rib (Frost, 1958). Transverse sections of tubular bones with a substantial cortex are best for this technique. Despite the crude image evoked by sawing and grinding, it is a practical method, albeit one that requires great skill to produce sections less than 25–50 μm thick without shattering the specimen. It produces sections of superb quality that are flat and defect-free; at 15–25 μm they are in many ways ideal for bone histology. The only stains which can be used are trichrome stains, which will discriminate bone from osteoid, but are virtually useless for assessment of the marrow space. It is the only method for producing the 70–100 μm sections for microradiography. This technique was used in a few research departments, but has been superseded by thin plastic embedded microtome sections and is of mainly historical interest.

21.4.3 DECALCIFIED SECTIONS

Decalcification is usually effected by chemical action; electrolytic methods are less convenient. The chemicals used may be inorganic acids, organic acids or chelating agents used at pH 7.0. Acidic solutions have the disadvantage that prolonged immersion of tissue destroys the haematoxyphilic constituents (nuclei and cement lines). It is therefore essential that tissue should be removed from these decalcifying solutions as soon as decalcification is complete. For this reason a radiographic check of decalcification is superior to chemical checks which confirm the removal of calcium one day after it is complete. Provided that radiographic checking is available the inorganic acids (nitric or hydrochloric at 5% concentration) have the advantage of speed of action. The use of trichloroacetic acid as a combined fixative/decalcification agent is described above; other organic acids (citric and formic at 10% concentration) are cheaper (because chemical titration is used to determine endpoint rather than radiography). Immunocytochemical reactions which may be of value are not inhibited by acidic decalcification. Chelating agents (10% di-sodium ethylenediaminetetra-acetic acid neutralized with sodium hydroxide solution) have a very slow action but produce good histology.

Block staining with silver nitrate followed by decalcification was introduced by Tripp and McKay (1972) as a method to combine the advantages of the von Kossa technique with the convenience of decalcified tissue processing. It has the disadvantages of being slow and of not always staining the mineralized tissue in the centre of trabeculae. It is of value when the facilities for processing mineralized bone are not available.

21.5 SECTION STAINING

Various methods of staining decalcified histological sections are described in textbooks of histological techniques (Bancroft and Stevens, 1990) which should be consulted for routine methods.

An economical modern method of producing undecalcified sections is to embed in methylmethacrylate resin and cut on a motorized rotary microtome using a tungsten knife. Sections (10 µm) are stained free floating and then picked up on glass slides. A modified von Kossa technique for calcium (von Kossa, 1901) is used to demonstrate the calcified bone with a modified Van Gieson's (1889) method as a counterstain to demonstrate osteoid. Morphometric analysis can be done with these von Kossa–Van Gieson sections and it is usual to sample the biopsy at four levels (leaving some tissue as reserve). Sections (8 µm) are stained with a modified haematoxylin and eosin for cellular assessment and by a modified Goldner's (1938) technique. Unstained sections (15 µm) are cut to observe tetracycline fluorescence (the thicker sections give brighter lines).

The following staining techniques have been modified for resin-embedded sections.

(a) Modified H & E for bone samples in LR white resin

1. Sections cut and stained free-floating from distilled water
2. Erlich's haematoxylin, 1 h
3. Distilled water, 10 min
4. Differentiate in 1% acid alcohol, four dips
5. Blue in tap water, 15 min
6. 5% eosin, 1 h
7. Rinse in tap water
8. Distilled water
9. Mount on clean glass slides, remove excess water by blotting and clip together with waxed paper and slides, and leave to dry on hot plate at 15°C for 1 or 2 days
10. Dip in xylene and mount in DPX

(b) Modified von Kossa's technique for bone samples in LR white resin

1. 1% silver nitrate solution freshly made under lamp for 1 h

2. Wash in three changes distilled water
3. Hypochlorite for 1.5 min diluted to 2.5%
4. Wash well in three changes distilled water, 5 min each
5. Running tap water in baskets with clip for 1 h
6. Van Gieson (equal parts 1% acid fuchsin and saturated aqueous picric acid) for 2 h
7. Rinse quickly in distilled water and mount on slides
8. Remove excess water and clip and dry as for H & E
9. Dip in xylene and mount in DPX

(c) Modified Goldner's technique for bone samples in LR white resin

1. Sections in solution of 45 ml 80% alcohol and 5 ml 25% ammonia for 1 h
2. Distilled water, 15 min
3. Weigert's haematoxylin, 1 h
4. Distilled water, 10 min
5. Fresh distilled water, further 5 min
6. Ponceau/fuchsin/azophloxine solution for 20 min (1. Ponceau de Xylidine soln 5 ml + 2. azophloxine soln 1 ml + 3. 0.2% acetic acid up to 50 ml)
7. Rinse 1% acetic acid, 15 s
8. PMA/Orange G solution for 1 h
9. Rinse 1% acetic acid, 15 s
10. Stain in light green for 5 min
11. Rinse in three changes 1% acetic acid
12. Rinse in distilled water, mount and clip together as for H & E, dry at 15°C for 1 or 2 days
13. Dip in xylene and mount in DPX

(i) Solutions for Goldner's technique

1. Ponceau de Xylidine solution

Ponceau de Xylidine	3.75 g
Acid fuchsin	1.25 g
Acetic acid	5 ml

Mix and add to 500 ml distilled water

2. Azophloxine solution

Azophloxine	2.5 g
Acetic acid	3 ml

Mix and add to 500 ml distilled water

3. Light green

Light green	1.0 g
Acetic acid	1.0 ml

Mix and add to 500 ml distilled water

4. PMA/Orange G

Molybdophosphoric acid	3 g
Orange G	2 g

Mix and add to 500 ml distilled water, add thymol crystal, dissolve

21.6 POLARIZED LIGHT AND BLUE LIGHT FLUORESCENCE

Frequent reference has been made throughout this book to the value of polarized light microscopy in the study of connective tissues. Most modern microscopes can be easily fitted with polarizing and analysing filters, and quartz interference plates for the identification of crystals. Manufacturers' handbooks provide details.

Blue light fluorescence takes advantage of the short wavelength of the ultraviolet light that is part of the emission of halide light sources. This excites the tetracycline to fluoresce. A BG 12 blue filter is placed on the substage diaphragm and Blau-abs blocking filters are placed into the eyepieces. The intensity of the blue light fluorescence is less than that of ordinary fluorescence viewed in a fluorescence microscope; nevertheless it is a cheap and perfectly satisfactory alternative for visualizing tetracycline labels.

21.7 IMMUNOHISTOCHEMISTRY

Almost all applications of immunohistochemistry to bone pathology for diagnostic purposes are concerned with the differential diagnosis of tumours, and most antigens that can be demonstrated in routine histopathological practice can also be demonstrated in decalcified sections. Immunohistochemical information on individual bone tumours is provided with the entries in Chapters 13–15. The following is a summary account of those areas of bone tumour pathology where immunohistochemistry has proved most useful. These are secondary tumours, myeloma and malignant lymphoma, tumours of cartilage and their mimics, the small round cell tumours of childhood and Langerhans' cell histiocytosis.

It is not possible to remove cross-linked acrylic resins from sections. Immunohistochemical staining can usually be done if the blocks are trimmed of any excess resin and then placed in water for about one week before cutting (water penetrates most resins at a rate of about 1 mm every 2 days). Sections are then cut from the block and immunostained with no further treatment.

21.7.1 SECONDARY TUMOURS

Metastatic deposits in bones are an unfortunately common problem and are much commoner than primary bone tumours. The large majority are never biopsied because their nature is clear from the clinical history. A solitary metastasis, a metastasis in an unusual site or a metastasis causing symptoms before the primary tumour announces itself are all biopsied on occasion. The important task is to recognize that the tumour is a secondary deposit and not a primary bone tumour. Immunohistochemistry can be of help here as the large majority of secondary deposits are from carcinomas. The commonest carcinomas giving rise to bone secondaries are those of bronchus, breast, prostate, kidney and thyroid. Clearly, demonstrating the presence of cytokeratins or epithelial membrane antigen will be invaluable (exclusion of chordoma or adamantinoma is not usually a practical problem in these cases). The finding of a tissue-specific product, e.g. thyroglobulin or prostate-specific antigen can accurately identify the primary site and focus clinical investigation with obvious savings to the patient.

Occasionally, a secondary deposit turns out to be a bony metastasis from a malignant melanoma. Like the primary tumours (Nakajima *et al.*, 1982a,b), these are positive for S-100 protein and, more specifically, for cytoplasmic melanoma antigens such as those recognized by HMB45. Secondary deposits in bone from primary sarcomas elsewhere are very rare in adults but do occasionally occur (Bramwell *et al.*, 1982).

21.7.2 MYELOMA

Although strictly of bone marrow origin, this, the commonest primary bone tumour (Dahlin, and Unni, 1986), is a tumour of malignant plasma cells – mature antibody-producing B lymphocytes. As such, plasma cells are normally readily identifiable by their morphological features. The role of immunohistochemistry is to confirm that the plasma cell proliferation is monoclonal, and hence malignant, and this is usually done by demonstrating restricted expression of immunoglobulins. As malignant clones, myeloma cells from an individual tumour usually produce a single type of light chain, either kappa or lambda, and often a single type of heavy chain as well. Showing whether a plasma cell proliferation is monotypic or polytypic in its light chain expression is therefore an important procedure. Some plasmacytic malignancies react positively with EMA antibodies such as HMFG-2 and negatively with LCA (Salter *et al.*, 1985), which can be confusing if forgotten.

21.7.3 MALIGNANT LYMPHOMA AND BONE

The non-Hodgkin's lymphomas can present as primary bone tumours (Dahlin and Unni, 1986) but secondary involvement of bone is much commoner. Identification of a tumour as a non-Hodgkin's lymphoma can be confirmed by staining for LCA (Kurtin and

Pinkus, 1985). Primary malignant lymphomas of bone can be of either B or T cell lineage and B and T cell markers are used to make this distinction.

Hodgkin's disease will also involve bone, up to 29% of cases at presentation, or as the disease progresses. Strict histopathological criteria have been laid down for the identification of Hodgkin's disease in the bone marrow (Lukes, 1971) and membrane surface marker studies may be necessary to distinguish true Reed–Sternberg cells from mimics. Involvement of bone by Hodgkin's disease is always a sign of widespread disease and is commonest with the nodular sclerosis and mixed cellularity subtypes (which are the common subtypes). About 50% of cases of the rarer lymphocyte-depleted subtype have marrow involvement at presentation.

21.7.4 CARTILAGE TUMOURS AND THEIR MIMICS

S-100 protein is present in normal chondrocytes (Stefansson *et al.*, 1982) and in tumours showing cartilaginous differentiation such as chondrosarcomas (Salisbury and Isaacson, 1985). The assessment of cartilaginous tumours, vis-à-vis their malignant potential, can be very difficult (Chapter 13) but immunohistochemistry is of no help here. The importance of immunohistochemistry is in excluding some of the tumours that may enter the differential diagnosis of chondrosarcoma in the axial skeleton. Chordomas are rare bone tumours, believed to be derived from notochord rests (Willis, 1962; Salisbury and Isaacson, 1985), that occur most often in the spheno-occipital area and the sacral vertebrae. In histological appearance they can resemble chondrosarcomas, especially the more myxoid variants. Chordomas however, like human notochord, contain cytokeratins (Miettinen *et al.*, 1983) and so are positive with antibodies such as CAM 5.2,

and with EMA-like antibodies such as HMFG-2 (Salisbury and Isaacson, 1985). Chondrosarcomas do not stain with these 'epithelial' markers but are positive for lysozyme, as is normal cartilage, whereas chordomas are negative (Salisbury and Isaacson, 1984). The other tumour that can enter the differential diagnosis of chondrosarcoma in the sacral region is the myxoid papillary variant of ependymoma. Ependymomas, however, are positive with GFAP (Miettinen *et al.*, 1983). As chondrosarcomas, chordomas and ependymomas are all positive with S-100 protein (Nakamura *et al.*, 1983), this cannot be used as a discriminant.

21.7.5 SMALL ROUND CELL TUMOURS OF CHILDHOOD

The problem here is that the cells that make up a number of the malignant tumours that occur in children and adolescents can look very similar by conventional histological stains. Malignant non-Hodgkin's lymphomas and leukaemias, Ewing's sarcoma and variants, Askin's tumour/peripheral neuroepithelioma, primitive neuroectodermal tumour of bone and metastatic neuroblastoma are the bone tumours that fall into the category of small round cell tumours of childhood (the category also contains the soft tissue sarcoma designated embryonal rhabdomyosarcoma). Obviously information obtained from the clinical history (e.g. age), radiographs and investigations (e.g. blood count, VMA levels) may be vital in reaching the correct diagnosis. To arrive at the histopathological diagnosis of 'small round cell tumour' is fairly straightforward but the further separation of the group usually requires immunohistochemistry. The very large majority of non-Hodgkin's lymphomas, but not all, will stain with LCA. The other small round cell bone tumours of childhood (Ewing's sarcoma and variants, Askin tumour/peripheral neuroepithelioma, primitive neuroectodermal tumour and neuroblastoma) all show some degree of 'neural' differentiation – as some of their names suggest. That degree ranges from immunohistochemical positivity with a few 'neural' markers in the case of Ewing's sarcoma, which appears composed of undifferentiated mesenchymal cells by light and electron microscopy, to the obvious neurites seen in neuroblastoma. Immunohistochemistry is clearly important in confirming that a small round cell tumour belongs to this group but the exact placement of any one tumour within the group usually depends on a combination of morphological and histochemical features (Triche and Cavazzana, 1989). It is usual to perform staining for neurone-specific enolase, S-100 protein and neurofilaments. Initial studies using PAP techniques suggested that it might be possible to assign a tumour within the group on the basis of positivity or negativity with either neurone-specific enolase or Leu7 but use of the more sensitive ABC or streptavidin techniques has shown these markers to be fairly ubiquitous within all categories of the group. Embryonal rhabdomyosarcoma not infrequently metastasizes to the bone marrow.

21.7.6 LANGERHANS' CELL HISTIOCYTOSIS

The proliferating cells in the group of diseases that make up the spectrum of Langerhans' cell histiocytosis or histiocytosis X, namely eosinophilic granuloma, Hans–Schuller–Christian disease and Letterer–Siwe disease, have been extensively studied by immunohistochemical methods. Positive staining for S-100 protein (Nakajima *et al.*, 1982b) and CD1 (T6) (Fithian *et al.*, 1981) have been incorporated into the disease definition (Writing Group of the Histiocyte Society, 1987) and LCA (Flotte *et al.*, 1984), CD4 (T4) (Wood *et al.*, 1983) and HLA-Dr are also usually expressed (Rowden, 1980). All can be useful in establishing the diagnosis in difficult cases.

REFERENCES

Bancroft, J.D. and Stevens, A. (1990) *Theory and Practice of Histological Techniques*, 3rd edn, Churchill Livingstone, Edinburgh.

Bramwell, V.H.C., Littley, M.B., Chang, J. *et al.* (1982) Bone marrow involvement in adult soft tissue sarcomas. *Eur. J. Cancer Clin. Oncol.*, **18**, 1099–106.

Control of Substances Hazardous to Health Regulations (COSHH) (1988) HMSO, London.

Dahlin, D.C. and Unni, K.K. (1986) *Bone Tumors*, 4th edn, Charles C. Thomas, Springfield, IL.

Fithian, E., Kung, P., Goldstein, G. *et al.* (1981) Reactivity of Langerhans cells with hybridoma antibody. *Proc. Natl. Acad. Sci. USA*, **78**, 2541–4.

Flotte, T.J., Murphy, G.E. and Bhan, A.K. (1984) Demonstration of T200 on human Langerhans cell surface membranes. *J. Invest. Dermatol.*, **82**, 535–7.

Frost, H.M. (1958) Preparation of thin undecalcified bone sections by rapid manual methods. *Stain Technol.*, **33**, 273–7.

Gardner, D.L. and Oates, K. (1993) Impact of confocal scanning optical microscopy on pathological practice. *Br. J. Hosp. Med.*, **49**, 160–73.

Gardner, D.L. Elliot, D. and Simpson, R. (1990) Rapid bone morphometry with blocks, not sections. Application of confocal scanning microscopy to the diagnosis of metabolic bone disease. Abstract. *J. Pathol.*, **160**, 166.

Goldner, J. (1938) Modification of the Masson trichrome technique for routine laboratory purposes. *Am. J. Pathol.*, **14**, 237–43.

Kurtin, P.J. and Pinkus, G.S. (1985) Leucocyte common antigen. A diagnostic discriminant between hematopoietic and nonhematopoietic neoplasms in paraffin sections using monoclonal antibodies. Correlation with immunologic studies and ultrastructural localization. *Hum. Pathol.*, **16**, 353–65.

Lukes, R.J. (1971) Criteria for involvement of lymph node, bone marrow, spleen and liver in Hodgkin's disease. *Cancer Res.*, **31**, 1755–67.

Miettinen, M., Lehto, V.-P., Dahl, D. *et al.* (1983) Differential diagnosis of chordoma, chondroid and ependymal tumours as aided by anti-intermediate filament antibodies. *Am. J. Pathol.*, **112**, 160–9.

Nakajima, T., Watanabe, S., Sato, Y. *et al.* (1982a) Immunohistochemical demonstration of S100 protein in malignant melanoma and pigmented nevus, and its diagnostic applications. *Cancer*, **50**, 912–18.

Nakajima, T., Watanabe, S., Sato, Y. *et al.* (1982b) S-100 protein in Langerhans cells, interdigitating cells and histiocytosis X cells. *Gann*, **73**, 429–32.

Nakamura, Y., Becker, L.E. and Marks, A. (1983) S-100 protein in human chordoma and human and rabbit notochord. *Arch. Pathol. Lab. Med.*, **107**, 118–20.

Rowden, G. (1980) Expression of Ia antigens on Langerhans cells in mice, guinea pigs and man. *J. Invest. Dermatol.*, **75**, 22–30.

Salisbury, J.R. and Isaacson, P.G. (1984) Application of immunohistochemistry and histochemistry to the differential diagnosis of chordomas. *J. Pathol.*, **143**, 330A.

Salisbury, J.R. and Isaacson, P.G. (1985) Demonstration of cytokeratins and an epithelial membrane antigen in chordomas and human fetal notochord. *Am. J. Surg. Pathol.*, **9**, 791–7.

Salter, D.M., Krajewski, A.S., Miller, E.P. *et al.* (1985) Expression of leucocyte common antigen and epithelial membrane antigen in plasmacytic malignancies. *J. Clin. Pathol.*, **38**, 843–4.

Stefannson, K., Wollman, R.L., Moore, B.W. *et al.* (1982) S-100 protein in normal chondrocytes. *Nature*, **295**, 63–4.

Triche, T. and Cavazzana, A. (1989) Round cell tumors of bone. In *Bone Tumors* (ed. KK. Unni), Churchill Livingstone, New York, pp. 199–223.

Tripp, E.J. and McKay, E.H. (1972) Silver staining of bone prior to decalcification for quantitative determination of osteoid in sections. *Stain Technol.*, **47**, 129–36.

Van Gieson, J. (1889) Laboratory notes of technical methods for the nervous system. *N. Y. Med. J.*, **50**, 57–60.

von Kossa, J. (1901) *Beitr. Anat. Pathol.*, **29**, 163.

Willis, R.A. (1962) *The Borderland of Embryology and Pathology*. Butterworths, London.

Wood, G.S., Warner, N.L. and Warnke, R.A. (1983) Anti Leu 3/T4 antibodies react with cells of the monocyte/macrophage and Langerhans lineage. *J. Immunol.*, **131**, 212–16.

Writing Group of the Histiocyte Society. (1987) Histiocytic syndromes in children. *Lancet*, **i**, 208–9.

INDEX

(Data for each tumour or tumour-like lesion is presented under the headings of: clinical features, skeletal distribution, prognosis, treatment, radiology, pathology, morbid anatomy, histopathology, differential diagnosis)